Vitamin D in Chronic Kidney Disease

Pablo A. Ureña Torres • Mario Cozzolino
Marc G. Vervloet

Editors

Vitamin D in Chronic Kidney Disease

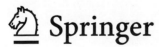 Springer

Editors

Pablo A. Ureña Torres
Ramsay-Générale de Santé
Clinique du Landy
Saint Ouen
France

Marc G. Vervloet
VU University Medical Center
Amsterdam
The Netherlands

Mario Cozzolino
San Paolo Hospital
DiSS University of Milan
Milan
Italy

ISBN 978-3-319-32505-7   ISBN 978-3-319-32507-1   (eBook)
DOI 10.1007/978-3-319-32507-1

Library of Congress Control Number: 2016952637

Printed on acid-free paper

This Springer imprint is published by Springer Nature
The registered company is Springer International Publishing AG Switzerland

Foreword

Chronic kidney disease (CKD) is a global public health problem, affecting up to 10 % of the world's population and increasing in prevalence and adverse outcomes. The progressive loss of kidney function is invariably complicated by disorders of bone and mineral metabolism and cardiovascular disease, resulting in premature death. The disturbances in mineral metabolism begin early in the course of progressive CKD with a reduced capacity to fully excrete a phosphate load and to convert vitamin D into the biological active 1,25-dihydroxy-vitamin-D, resulting in a compensatory secondary hyperparathyroidism, elevated levels of FGF23, and disturbed klotho levels in addition to hyperphosphatemia, vitamin D deficiency, bone disease, and extraskeletal calcifications. During the past decade there has been a substantial focus on the pathophysiology and the interrelations between and the understanding of the fundamental mechanisms, which are involved in the regulation of the many hormones and factors employed in the disturbances in CKD-mineral and bone disorder (CKD-MBD). The new knowledge comes both from clinical and experimental studies, and the need for confirmatory randomized clinical trials is often stressed.

A distinguished group of contributors under the editorship of Dr. Pablo Ureña Torres have produced an extremely concise synopsis on some of the major areas of importance in the field of vitamin D. Thus, this textbook updates in a relevant and clear way all aspects of vitamin D in CKD with special focus on metabolism, measurements of the different analogs and metabolites, assessment of vitamin D status, physiological and pathophysiological actions, non-classical pleiotropic beneficial and or deleterious effects, and on the endemic insufficiency or deficiency in CKD. A section is dedicated to the effects of vitamin D deficiency and treatment in kidney transplantation. Finally, the last part reviews the therapeutical aspects of vitamin D supplementation and the use of vitamin D analogs in CKD. The purpose of this textbook is to provide a state-of-the-art overview of both basic and clinical aspects of vitamin D in CKD-MBD. The chapters are written in a very clear-cut and updated way to enlighten the novice and to extend the knowledge of clinicians and clinical investigators of the recent progress in the many exiting aspects of vitamin D in CKD.

Klaus Olgaard, MD
Nephrological Department P 2132
University of Copenhagen
Rigshospitalet, 9 Blegdamsvej
DK 2100 Copenhagen, Denmark

Introduction

In the actual and revolutionary "numerical" era we are living, the writing of a classical textbook on vitamin D might appear relegated to a second- or third-line priority, probably even lower for geek peoples. In addition, since the exploding and exponentially increasing number of vitamin D publications appearing every week, it is highly probable that many of the data presented in this book will be already obsolete at the moment of its release. Nevertheless, the growing interest manifested by the general public and health caregivers for all aspects of vitamin D, including metabolism, measurement and assessment of vitamin D status, physiological actions, unexpected pleiotropic beneficial/deleterious effects, and the endemic insufficiency/deficiency status observed in patients with chronic kidney disease (CKD), as well as the lack of high-quality and evidence-based guidelines, motivate us to embark in this exciting adventure.

This textbook is divided into five major sections: the first one considers the metabolism of vitamin D in normal and pathological situations, the assessment of vitamin D status based on actual methods of measuring vitamin D molecules as well as its binding protein, and the epidemiology of vitamin D deficiency in CKD worldwide. The second section discusses the classical biological and biochemical effects of vitamin D on mineral and bone metabolism in case of CKD. The third section reviews the non-classical and potential pleiotropic effects of vitamin D in CKD. The fourth section is dedicated to the metabolism of vitamin D and the effects of vitamin D treatment in CKD beneficing of a kidney graft. Finally, the fifth section reviews the therapeutical aspects of vitamin D supplementation and the use of vitamin D analogs in CKD. In the next pages, I will summarize, in a non-exhaustively manner, the most relevant issues developed here by internationally renowned experts on vitamin D.

Generalities, Measurement, and Epidemiology

We believed that we knew everything about vitamin D physiology, however, in the first chapter Drs. Zierold and DeLuca reminded us that there are still many unanswered questions. Vitamin D is a pro-hormone synthesized in the skin from the precursor 7-dehydrocholesterol by the action of sunlight. Low amounts of vitamin D are present in food, fortified dairy, and fish oils. Vitamin D undergoes two-step bio-activation process required to produce its active form. It is converted in 25-hydroxyvi-tamin D in the liver by 25-hydroxylation, followed by the conversion to $1,25(OH)_2D$ by the 1α-hydroxylase in kidney under very tightly regulated physiological condi-tions. $1,25(OH)_2D$ is responsible for maintaining adequate serum calcium and phos-phate levels, which are essential for a healthy mineral and bone metabolism. In addition, $1,25(OH)_2D$ plays an important role in many biological non-calcemic func-tions throughout the body. $1,25(OH)_2D$ must bind to the vitamin D receptor to carry out its functions. The highly active and lipid-soluble $1,25(OH)_2D$ is inactivated by the 24-hydroxylase, which is the enzyme responsible for the major catabolic pathway that ultimately results in the water-soluble calcitroic acid for excretion in the urine. Regulation of key players in vitamin D metabolism is reciprocal and very tight. The activating enzyme 1α-hydroxylase and the catabolic enzyme 24-hydroxylase are reciprocally regulated by PTH, $1,25(OH)_2D$, and fibroblast growth factor 23 (FGF23).

Chronic kidney disease (CKD) leads to an altered vitamin D metabolism, mainly a decreased production and circulating levels of $1,25(OH)_2D$. Several mechanisms contribute to this phenomenon, including decreased renal mass, decreased delivery of DBP-bound 25-hydroxyvitamin D to the 1α-hydroxylase enzyme, inhibition of 1α-hydroxylase activity by FGF23 and uremic toxins, reduced renal tubular megalin expression, reduced intestinal absorption of vitamin D, and finally increased $1,25(OH)_2D$ degradation by FGF23-stimulated 24-hydroxylase activity. These alterations are asso-ciated with abnormalities of calcium and phosphate metabolism, an increased risk of cardiovascular calcifications, and significant high morbidity and mortality rates.

Vitamin D deficiency and insufficiency is a global health problem and Dr. Metzger and Stengel elegantly reviewed this issue in case of CKD. They emphasized the fact that there is not a clear-cut definition of vitamin D status in CKD patients. Currently, it is defined as a circulating 25(OH)D level below 20 ng/ml (50 nmol/L), which has been recognized as a major risk factor for bone and mineral disorders and has been related to increased risk of non-skeletal health outcomes including mortality, diabe-tes, and cardiovascular disease. A greater prevalence of deficiency is expected in patients with CKD because they are older and more likely to have dark skin, obesity, and associated comorbidities such as diabetes and hypertension. In clinical-based studies, the mean circulating 25(OH)D levels ranged from 18 to 29 ng/ml for patients with non-end-stage renal disease, and from 12 to 32 ng/ml for those on dialysis. Large population-based clinical studies, however, are inconsistent regard-ing the association between kidney function and vitamin D level. While some stud-ies reported significant positive, and independent association between glomerular filtration rate and circulating 25(OH)D values, others showed low levels only in advanced CKD stages. Other studies show no or even an inverse association, with paradoxically higher serum levels of 25(OH)D in individuals with moderate CKD than in those without CKD. Whether the observed relations are direct and causal, or indirect because of confounders, is not established. Only few studies examined the relations between proteinuria or albuminuria and circulating 25(OH)D levels and generally reported significant negative associations.

Dr. Adriana Dusso extensively treats the complex genomic and non-genomic actions of vitamin D, and their modification by CKD. She pointed out that the most characterized calcitriol/VDR genomic actions include the suppression of PTH synthesis, the stimulation of the phosphaturic hormone FGF23, the longevity gene klotho, the calcium channel TRPV6 in enterocytes, the rate-limiting step in intestinal calcium absorption, the parathyroid calcium sensing receptor, and the receptor of the canonical Wnt pathway LRP5 in bone, all essential effectors for normal skeletal development and mineralization. The "non-genomic" actions of vitamin D occur within minutes of exposure to calcitriol. Some of these not yet well-characterized rapid actions involve the cytosolic VDR, although other potential vitamin D receptors have been identified. These rapid actions regulate intracellular calcium fluxes, the degree of protein phosphorylation, stability and/or processing of microRNAs, acetylation and subcellular localization, which, by affecting protein function, greatly modify classical and non-classical direct and indirect genomic signals.

CKD is a state in which there is resistance to the action of many hormones including $1,25(OH)_2D_3$. As vitamin D requires binding to the VDR to exert its physiological role, the resistance to the action of vitamin D, which has never been clearly defined, may partially be explained by a disturbed VDR function. Here, Dr. Bover et al. made a comprehensible and in-depth review of VDR in CKD. They stressed out that the uremic ultrafiltrate contains chemical compounds that significantly reduced the VDR interaction with DNA binding and with the VDRE. When normal VDR were incubated with uremic ultrafiltrate, they lose 50 % of their maximal binding capacity to the VDRE. Beyond altered receptor interaction with target genes, decreased MRN expression and VDR concentration in target organs, such as in the parathyroid glands, the osteoblasts, and the intestine, might also explain the diminished biological action of vitamin D in CKD. Various mechanisms have been proposed to explain the decrease of VDR in CKD: First, $1,25(OH)_2D_3$ is known to upregulate its own receptor; consequently, the low circulating calcitriol levels leads to VDR downregulation. Second, SHPT may decrease VDR concentration of in CKD, as suggested by the fact that PTH downregulates the VDR and VDR messenger RNA and also blocks $1,25(OH)_2D_3$-induced upregulation of rat intestinal and renal VDR. Third, uremic ultrafiltrate in normal animals suppresses VDR synthesis, possibly at translational sites, and consequently accumulation of uremic toxins in CKD may reduce VDR concentration. They finally revised the development of new VDR activators that would induce unique conformational changes in the VDR that allow them being more specific and selective, and probably with improved biological profile for therapeutic application.

Undoubtedly, measuring 25(OH)D is actually one of the most relevant, frequent, and debated dosage in daily clinical practice. Indeed, this is the most employed measurement to assess global vitamin D status. In this book, Dr. Cavalier et al. describe the potential clinical and biological indications and methods available to measure vitamin D molecules including cholecalciferol, 25(OH)D, and 1,25 and 24,25 vitamin D in CKD as well in the general population. They also critically revised the measurement and utility assessing circulating vitamin D binding protein

(VDBP) concentration and the new concept of "free" or "bioavailable" vitamin D. Indeed, the low circulating levels of total 25(OH)D frequently observed in Black Americans do not probably indicate a true vitamin D deficiency. According to a particular VDBP gene polymorphism, these subjects also show reduced circulating VDBP and a lower affinity VDBP for 25(OH)D, which renders 25(OH)D more bioavailable, suggesting that the measurement of the free form might be more appropriate than total 25(OH)D to detect vitamin D sufficiency.

The transition with the precedent chapter is perfectly done by Dr. Gutierrez who described the racial differences in vitamin D metabolism in CKD. Compared to white individuals, black individuals have lower circulating concentrations of 25-hydroxyvitamin D (25(OH)D), leading to the widespread assumption that blacks are at higher risk of vitamin D deficiency. Since low 25(OH)D is associated with adverse cardiovascular and kidney outcomes, this has supported the notion that low circulating 25(OH)D concentrations partly underlie racial disparities in health outcomes, including faster progression of CKD in blacks versus whites. However, the finding that black peoples maintain better indices of musculoskeletal health than whites throughout their life span despite having lower circulating 25(OH)D concentrations suggests that the relation between vitamin D deficiency and racial health disparities may not be so straightforward. This has been further underscored by epidemiologic studies showing major racial heterogeneity in the association of 25(OH)D with cardiovascular outcomes. When coupled with emerging data showing genetically determined differences in the bioavailability of vitamin D by race, these data suggest that there are important differences in vitamin D metabolism by race, which need to inform and perhaps revise our current understanding of the role of vitamin D in racial disparities in CKD outcomes.

Classical Mineral and Bone Effects

The second section considers the classical biological and biochemical effects of vitamin D on mineral and bone metabolism in case of CKD. It started by the excellent review made by Dr. Rodriguez et al. that tried untangling the tight link between vitamin D and parathyroid gland function. The presence of both VDR and CaR in parathyroid chief cells enables the parathyroid gland to respond to vitamin D and calcium, two of the main inhibitors of the parathyroid function. Vitamin D also upregulates its own receptor as well as the CaR, which makes parathyroid gland more sensitive to the suppressive action of calcium. Vitamin D upregulates vitamin D receptor only if calcium is normal or high. Conversely, the VDR is downregulated in case of hypocalcemia and upregulated by activation of the CaR. Thus, the inhibition of parathyroid function by vitamin D is impaired in the presence of hypocalcemia. In CKD, the prolonged stimulation of parathyroid glands promotes parathyroid hyperplasia and a severe secondary hyperparathyroidism develops, which may become resistant to medical treatment – such is the case of nodular and monoclonal parathyroid hyperplasia. Hyperplasia is accompanied by a decrease in the expression of parathyroid receptors, including FGFR-1 and klotho. Although the exact mechanisms whereby parathyroid hyperplasia is developed are not completely understood, several factors such as hypocalcemia, phosphorus retention, and deficiency in vitamin D have been directly associated to an increase in cell proliferation.

PTH regulates mineral and bone metabolism as well as vitamin D synthesis through its specific type I receptor (PTH1R). Dr. Urena et al. concisely treated this chapter and detailed that in the kidney, PTH inhibits proximal tubular reabsorption of phosphate, stimulates the synthesis of $1,25(OH)_2D_3$, and enhances calcium reabsorption in the thick ascending limb of Henle's loop. In the skeleton, the physiological action of PTH is more complex. PTH has a paradoxical anabolic/catabolic effect and combines the simultaneous modulation of resorption and formation of bone tissue, and ultimately of bone remodeling rate. This paradoxical anabolic/catabolic effect relies on its mode of administration. Intermittent or pulsatile PTH has a bone anabolic effect, while chronic administration or excessive production of PTH, as in case of primary and secondary hyperparathyroidism, is detrimental for the skeleton due to stimulation of bone resorption. The PTHR1 is an 84-kDa glycosylated protein that belongs to the seven transmembrane domains G protein-coupled receptors family. It activates two intracellular signaling pathways, protein kinase A and phospholipase C, through the stimulation of Gs and Gq proteins. The differential use of one or another of these two signaling pathways depends on the connection of PTH1R with the sodium-dependent hydrogen exchanger regulatory factor-1 (NHERF-1). In early CKD, PTH1R is downregulated in bone and kidney, which may favor the development of SHPT. Such a downregulation may be exacerbated by vitamin D since daily and intermittent administration of active vitamin D inhibits PTH1R expression and function in bone cells, which may partially explain the skeletal resistance to the hypercalcemic action of PTH in CKD.

Drs. Komaba and Lanske revisited the anti-aging klotho as well as the modifications of the axis FGF23/klotho in CKD. They emphasized that by acting as a cofactor for FGFR in FGF23 signaling, klotho is a key player in the pathogenesis of disturbances of phosphate and vitamin D metabolism in CKD. Both the transmembrane and soluble forms of klotho are deficient in patients with CKD and ESRD and such klotho deficiency is likely to contribute to the pathogenesis of SHPT, vascular calcification, left ventricular hypertrophy, and worsening of kidney injury. Moreover, as previously described in this textbook, vitamin D is a potent inducer of the klotho gene, and that the loss of renal klotho fully reproduces the *accelerated aging and the short life span* of global klotho absence in mice and men. Interestingly, they reported that klotho is also present in bone cells and that FGF23 in osteocytes increased the expression of *Egr-1* and *Egr-2*, downstream targets of FGF23 signaling. This observation suggests that bone is another target organ for FGF23 with klotho acting as a co-receptor. This might help resolving the question whether FGF23 had a direct effect on the skeleton and explaining some peculiar features of MBD in CKD.

To further investigate the FGF23/klotho axis, Dr. Prié reviewed in extent FGF23 physiology and pathophysiology in CKD. It denotes that FGF23, by contrast with many other FGF, belongs to the small hormone-like FGF subfamily with FGF15/19 and FGF21. FGF23 is secreted by osteocytes and osteoblast in response to high phosphate or calcitriol levels. FGF23 inhibits the expression of renal sodium phosphate transporters, which augments phosphate excretion in urine. Its physiological action requires the expression at the cell surface of a FGFR and the co-receptor αklotho. FGF23 concentration increases at the early steps of renal insufficiency to maintain plasma phosphate concentration within normal range. This participates to the genesis of secondary hyperparathyroidism. High concentrations of FGF23 induce cardiac hypertrophy in the absence of klotho. The decrease in circulating calcitriol concentration induced by FGF23 may contribute to its deleterious cardiac effects in CKD.

Sclerostin and vitamin D in CKD is a passionate topic emotionlessly treated by Drs. Apetrii and Covic. Sclerostin is a 22 kDa glycoprotein product of the SOST gene. Inactivating mutations of this gene lead to two rare genetic diseases characterized by high bone mass, including sclerosteosis and Van Buchem disease. This finding led to the conclusion that sclerostin must be a natural brake for bone formation, preventing the body from making too much bone. When mechanical forces are applied to the bone, the osteocytes stop secreting sclerostin and bone formation is initiated on the bone surface. Circulating sclerostin concentrations clearly increase in CKD; however, whether this is due to reduced renal clearance, increased skeletal production, or both is still a subject of debate, as well as if sclerostin could be another useful biomarker in the prediction of CKD-MBD. Experimental and clinical studies suggest that high circulating sclerostin levels are associated with the presence of cardiovascular calcifications, and vitamin D might modulate bone homeostasis and sclerostin production.

Then, Dr. Martine Cohen-Solal et al. illustrate the complexity of bone abnormalities observed during CKD-MBD, which relies on the presence of several confounding factors that include mineral metabolism, bone structure, and regulation of bone remodeling. All these factors contribute to the bone fragility and the promotion of skeletal fractures, which when occurring greatly impair the quality of life of CKD subjects. The failure of 25(OH)D 1α-hydroxylation in patients with CKD is responsible for low circulating 1,25(OH)2D levels that increases PTH, increases bone resorption, and contributes to bone loss and skeletal fractures. Low circulating vitamin D concentrations are constantly and independently associated with reduced bone mineral density at almost all skeletal sites, increased subperiosteal bone resorption, and the risk of skeletal fractures. Administration of calcitriol derivatives reduces PTH, but insufficient data are available on the impact on bone mineral density and fractures. In contrast, calcidiol only partially reduces PTH in end-stage renal disease, but contribute to ameliorate bone mineralization and subsequently the bone capacity and pain.

This section ends up with a wonderful chapter written by Drs. Bachetta and Salusky on the relation between vitamin D status and longitudinal bone growth in children with CKD. Indeed growth retardation is a common complication of childhood CKD, resulting from a combination of abnormalities in the growth hormone axis, vitamin D deficiency, SHPT, hypogonadism, inadequate nutrition, cachexia, and drug toxicity. As in adult CKD patients, vitamin D metabolism is completely modified by CKD, and children with CKD are particularly prone to 25(OH)D deficiency, while beneficial effects of vitamin D on immunity, anemia, and cardiovascular outcomes have been described in pediatric CKD. Native vitamin supplementation and active vitamin D analogs are currently the mainstay of therapy for children with CKD-MBD, decreasing serum PTH levels while increasing FGF23. However, oversuppression of PTH in dialyzed children using vitamin D analogs may lead to adynamic bone disease, growth failure, cardiovascular calcifications, and growth plate inhibition.

Non-classical Effects of Vitamin D

The third section of this textbook reviews the non-classical and potential pleiotropic effects of vitamin D in CKD. It starts probably with one of the most important issues, which is CKD progression, wonderfully written by Dr. Marc DeBroe. Besides regulating mineral and bone metabolism, vitamin D possesses many other pleiotropic effects on vascular function, blood pressure, proteinuria, insulin resistance, lipid metabolism, inflammation, and immunity which all may play a role in the progression of CKD. Angiotensin-converting enzyme inhibitors (ACEi) for renin-angiotensin-aldosterone system (RAAS) blockade are routinely used to slow CKD progression. Natural vitamin D and active vitamin D analogs may further reduce proteinuria in CKD patients in addition to these current treatment regimens. The effects of vitamin D on renal fibrosis and slowing down/preventing progressive renal damage have been investigated thoroughly in vitro, in vivo, and in humans, but currently limited to a promising item. The increase in serum creatinine levels observed during several studies is not attributable to a decreased GFR but on the increased creatinine generation, an anabolic effect of vitamin D. The inverse correlation of blood pressure and serum vitamin D levels as well as promising data from small intervention studies of vitamin D supplementation provides a rationale for the design of well-performed RCT addressing efficacy and safety of vitamin D in hypertension/cardiovascular diseases. Unfortunately, up to now three RCTs have not been able to support this hypothesis.

Another recognized pleiotropic effect of vitamin D is to regulate the pancreatic endocrine function as evocated by Dr. Gonzalez Parra et al. in this chapter. It stimulates pancreatic beta cells proliferation and insulin secretion. And several studies suggest that vitamin D status may have a significant role in glucose homeostasis in general, and on the pathophysiology and progression of metabolic syndrome and type-2 diabetes in particular. Low circulating vitamin D levels are associated with a reduced insulin secretion, which might be an important factor for the susceptibility of developing diabetes. Therefore, supplementing with native vitamin D has been proposed as a therapeutic agent in the prevention and treatment of type-1 and type-2 diabetes. In diabetic patients at various CKD stages, circulating 25(OH)D levels are negatively correlated with glycosylated hemoglobin values. Unfortunately, the level of scientific evidence supporting an eventual 25(OH)D therapy for preventing or

treating diabetes mellitus in CKD patients is low. Several studies of nutritional
vitamin D supplementation in patients with CKD and type-2 diabetes are actually
ongoing, although their results are not yet available.

Vitamin D deficiency is a well-known factor associated with reduced muscle
mass, strength, physical performance, and of increased risk of falls. Drs. Chauveau
and Aparicio analyzed all the information on vitamin and muscle physiology gath-
ered so far in CKD patients. They proposed that muscle wasting, weakness, and
structural changes, fundamentally as atrophy of type II muscle fibers, but also insulin resistance is common finding in CKD patients. Among the different mechanisms
liable to contribute to such muscle wasting, vitamin D deficiency, which is present
in 50–80 % of incident dialysis patients, appears to be an important one. In these
circumstances, vitamin D supplementation appears to be a reasonable, simple, and
potentially adequate therapy. However, only few observational studies have been
performed, and there are not enough data to draw definitive conclusions about the
effects of natural vitamin D supplementation on muscle disorders and their mechanical and metabolic properties.

Whether vitamin D deficiency or insufficiency favors infection in CKD is also a
matter of intense debate. Here Dr. Viard examines the mechanisms by which the
vitamin D status may influence the immune response in CKD subjects. Infections
are the third cause of death in CKD patients and this is because uremia, the dialysis
condition, and the high frequency of vitamin D deficiency lead to an impaired
immune system at several levels: decreased innate and adaptive immunity, and
increased inflammation. Moreover, low circulating vitamin D levels in CKD may
also contribute to the decreased innate immunity and increased inflammation or
immune cell activation by modulating the microbiome and intestinal permeability.
Monocytes/macrophages express both toll-like receptors (TLRs), recognizing
ligands originating from pathogens. They have also CYP27B1 (1α-hydroxylase)
that can locally transform 25(OH)D in calcitriol and activate the VDR. This makes
an intracrine system that plays an important role in the production of bactericidal
peptides, such as cathelicidin, with largely proven activity against *Mycobacterium
tuberculosis* and β-defensin 4A. There are convincing data from epidemiological
studies and meta-analyses demonstrating the association between vitamin D deficiency with inflammation, all-cause mortality, cardiovascular mortality, and infection. However, interventional RCTs are still needed to validate the causality
relationship and determine whether vitamin D supplementation can reduce infections in CKD patients.

Infection goes always in parallel with inflammation. Dr. Donate-Correa from
Dr. Gonzalez-Navarro's team reminds us that CKD and the dialysis condition are
especially characterized by a chronic state of micro-inflammation or an overt
inflammation, which represent an important factor contributing to the rapid progression of CKD and the high cardiovascular morbidity and mortality observed in these
patients. Inflammation is associated with vitamin D deficiency in CKD, and several
mechanisms have been proposed including the regulation, synthesis, and production
of several cytokines (TNF-α, interferons (IFNs), interleukins (IL-1, IL-2, IL-6,
IL-8, IL-10, and IL-12)), transcription factor NF-kB, fibrogenesis, leptin, adiponec-

tin, RAAS, immune response, and monocyte/macrophage growth and differentiation. Vitamin D also inhibits the activation of TNF-α converting enzyme (TACE), also called ADAM17, which plays an important role in the generation of renal fibrosis, glomerulosclerosis, and proteinuria. They discuss some of preclinical and clinical data suggesting the existence of modulatory effects on the immune system and the decrease of inflammatory biomarkers after treatment with VDRAs. However, there is a lack of RCTs on the immunomodulatory effects of vitamin D in CKD.

Cardiovascular complications, including sudden death, are the leading cause of mortality in CKD patients. Dr. Pilz relates here the consequences of vitamin D deficiency on heart structure and function in CKD. The VDR is expressed in the heart and the vessels, and experimental studies have documented various molecular effects of vitamin D that may protect against heart diseases. There are numerous epidemiological studies showing an association between low vitamin D levels and adverse cardiovascular outcomes in CKD patients. However, the few RCTs performed in CKD subjects showed that vitamin D treatment has no effect on myocardial hypertrophy. Whether vitamin D treatment can significantly reduce cardiovascular events in CKD patients is still unclear. One example of this complexity is illustrated by the results of the PRIMO study where paricalcitol treatment did not reduce left ventricular mass index in dialysis patient. Further large RCTs are urgently needed to better characterize the cardiovascular effects of vitamin D treatment in CKD. Fortunately, several studies, on active as well as on natural vitamin D supplementation, are ongoing in CKD patients and will hopefully help to clarify the role of vitamin D treatment for heart structure and function soon.

Many of the abovementioned cardiovascular complications are closely related to endothelial dysfunction, which represents the initial arterial lesion that eventually leads to atherosclerosis and arteriosclerosis. Dr. Covic has also connected endothelial dysfunction in CKD to vitamin D deficiency in CKD as explained in this chapter. Vitamin D has direct effects on the endothelium: endothelial cells are capable of activating 25(OH)D to $1,25(OH)_2D_3$, which acts locally to regulate vascular tone, prevent vascular inflammation and oxidative stress, and promote cell repair and survival. Low circulating vitamin D levels also favor the development and/or perpetuation of metabolic abnormalities including hyperglycemia, dyslipidemia, SHPT, chronic inflammation, and RAAS activation, conditions that trigger endothelial dysfunction. Finally, CKD-associated perturbations of the vitamin D-FGF23-klotho axis additionally promote endothelial dysfunction. Unfortunately, we are still waiting for RCT demonstrating that vitamin D supplementation or treatment improves endothelial function in CKD.

Obviously, the next step, after the description that in CKD vitamin D deficiency was associated with disturbed immune system, chronic inflammation, endothelial dysfunction, and structural and functional changes of cardiac and vascular structures, was the development of cardiovascular calcifications. Dr. Hénaut et al. from Massy's research team recall that preclinical and clinical studies have shown that both abnormally low and extremely high circulating vitamin D levels have local and systemic effects promoting cardiovascular calcification in CKD.

And one of the most devastating complication of CKD and cardiovascular complications is the calciphylaxis or calcific uremic arteriolopathy (CUA). As reviewed by Dr. Brandenbourg, CUA is characterized by the stepwise development of superficial painful sensations and cutaneous lesions similar to livedo reticularis, skin necrosis, and ulceration. Its etiology is incompletely understood, but disturbed vitamin D as well as mineral and bone and mineral metabolism are frequently involved. Previous or concomitant treatment with vitamin K antagonists for oral anticoagulation therapy is considered as a major triggering and risk factor. Unfortunately, evidence-based therapeutic options are absent, since controlled treatment trials have not been conducted yet.

Anemia is a common finding in CKD with more than 80 % of dialysis patients requiring a treatment by erythropoiesis-stimulating agents (ESAs) such as exogenous human recombinant erythropoietin, iron or inhibitors of propyl hydroxylase activity, or hypoxic-inducible factor stabilizers. Drs. Breda and Vervloet describe putative links between vitamin D and erythropoiesis in this chapter. They reported several studies demonstrating an association between abnormal vitamin D status and low hemoglobin levels and resistance to ESA, suggesting a cross talk between the vitamin D system and erythropoiesis. The administration of either inactive or active vitamin D has been associated with an improvement of anemia and reduction in EPO hyporesponsiveness.

Finally, Dr. Cunningham closes this section by revising the scientific evidence that we have regarding whether disturbed vitamin D metabolism, and if the correction of it, results in any improvement of patient survival in CKD. It is striking seeing that virtually all of the available data at hand at the moment fall some way short of being able to establish clear-cut cause and effect in regard to mortality in CKD. Nevertheless we still lack convincing data from randomized intervention controlled trials demonstrating that any formulation of vitamin D results in improved patient level outcomes, although many are actually in progress. In spite of this, he concludes that for the nephrologist it was clear to keep using active vitamin D compounds in appropriate pharmacological doses, often supra-physiological, for established indications based on the classical actions of vitamin D on the parathyroids, bone and mineral metabolism, and that they also should keep giving generous supplementation of native vitamin D to all CKD patients with the aim of supporting widespread extrarenal generation of calcitriol and facilitating the putative pleotropic effects of vitamin D that could mitigate some of the cardiovascular and other attrition faced by these patients.

Kidney Transplantation

Renal transplantation is undoubtedly the best treatment of end-stage CKD. The fourth section of this textbook is dedicated to the metabolism of vitamin D and the effects of vitamin D treatment in CKD patients beneficing of a kidney graft. The kidney graft partially restores renal function and corrects metabolic and many hormonal disturbances observed in CKD. As a consequence, circulating $1,25(OH)_2D_3$ levels rapidly restore after successful renal transplantation. However, serum $1,25(OH)_2D_3$ concentrations remain relatively low in the early posttransplant period despite the persistent SHPT and hypophosphatemia. Both, vitamin D deficiency and insufficiency remain very common among renal transplant recipients. Hypovitaminosis D may contribute to persistent hyperparathyroidism and post-transplant bone and vascular disease. Limited epidemiological evidence also suggest that hypovitaminosis D may foster malignancies and infections in renal transplant recipients. Disappointingly, intervention studies with vitamin D supplementations or active vitamin D analogs are scanty and inconclusive. Hard endpoint interventional RCT are lacking at all.

Vitamin D is susceptible to improve renal graft survival and protect against chronic graft rejection because of its nephroprotective and immunomodulatory properties. As above mentioned and recalled here by Dr. Courbebaisse, vitamin D attenuate CD4+ and CD8+ T-cell proliferation and their cytotoxic activity; decrease plasma cell differentiation, B-cell proliferation, IgG secretion, and differentiation; and stimulate maturation of dendritic cells, all of these mechanisms may protect against acute kidney graft rejection. Observational studies and small interventional trials in renal transplant recipients support the potential protective role of active vitamin D against acute rejection. Regarding chronic rejection, in addition to potentially inducing tolerogenic dentric cells, VDR agonists could also inhibit the production of chemokines, responsible for leukocytes infiltration in vessels allograft, and may downregulate TGF-β pathway, which has a profibrotic activity. Other reno-protective effects of vitamin D, such as inhibition RAAS and of NF-kB activation, may participate in the prevention of chronic allograft rejection. The results of three ongoing randomized controlled trials are testing native vitamin D supplementation in renal transplantation and determining whether vitamin D reduces or not the risk of acute and chronic allograft rejection.

Therapeutical Aspects of Vitamin D Supplementation and the Use of Vitamin D Analogs in CKD

The fifth section of this textbook reviews therapeutical aspects of vitamin D supplementation and the use of vitamin D analogs in CKD. Dr. Souberbielle recalls that the main source of vitamin D resides on the total amount synthesized in the skin, and that the amount of nutritional vitamin D is limited. Some foods contain significant amounts of vitamin D such as fatty fish liver oil such as cod liver and fatty fish. White fish, offal (liver, kidney), egg yolk, and to a lesser extent meat (muscle) also contain significant amounts of vitamin D3, while dairy products (non fortified) contain very small amounts of vitamin D3 with the exception of butter that can provide significant amounts of vitamin D3. Mushrooms are the only non-animal-based foods containing vitamin D2. Some animal foods, including meat, offal, egg yolk, contain 25(OH)D, which can be better and more quickly absorbed than native vitamin D and significantly contributes to the optimal vitamin D status. Food fortification may be the best way to eradicate severe vitamin D deficiency (i.e., 25(OH)D <12 ng/mL) in the general population. However, in CKD patients and because of the putative higher target values, an individualized pharmacological supplementation should probably be preferred.

Then, Dr. Basile et al. provide an updated review of the sources and pharmacological characteristics of natural vitamin D compounds, their most important clinical uses, and results obtained in CKD patients. They stated that native vitamin D supplementation usually corrects vitamin-deficiency-related mineral and bone disorders; however, the scientific evidence demonstrating its beneficial effect on non-classical target organs in the general population as well as in CKD are still inconsistent and await confirmation by large RCTs. Additionally, CKD besides its altered mineral and bone metabolism is associated with low circulating 25(OH)D (calcidiol) and $1,25(OH)_2D_3$ (calcitriol) levels as well as vitamin D resistance in most of target tissues. They stressed out that the major health care organizations worldwide have been unable to define a unique and consensual desirable circulating 25(OH)D concentration for the CKD population.

The next chapter by Dr. Negri et al. outlines the available evidence on the controversy about which vitamin D is better for CKD patients. As CKD patients cannot completely convert 25(OH)D to its more active form, $1,25(OH)_2D_3$ because of their reduced renal 1α-hydroxylase activity, nephrologists have traditionally treated patients with CKD with active vitamin D (calcitriol) or related analogs. Multiple observational studies in patients with CKD have shown that they not only have low circulating levels of $1,25(OH)_2D_3$ but also 25(OH)D. The fact that in CKD there is also extrarenal conversion of 25(OH)D to $1,25(OH)_2D_3$ in multiple tissues leading to paracrine and autocrine vitamin D actions has led to the speculation that CKD patients must also be supplemented with nutritional vitamin D. However, numerous questions remain unanswered. For example, do we need to measure circulating 25(OH)D levels in all CKD patients, or can we replete knowing which of them most are vitamin D deficient? Can we combine nutritional and active vitamin D or does this is harmful in CKD patients increasing the risk of hypercalcemia, hyperphosphatemia, and soft tissues and cardiovascular calcification? Does vitamin D has to be replaced in renal transplant patients and does this affect graft function?

Drs. Floreani and Cozzolino wrestle with the intricate question: Which vitamin D receptor activators (VDRAs) are prescribed to CKD subjects? They stated that the rationale behind the prescription of vitamin D sterols in CKD is rapidly increasing due to the coexistence of growing expectancies close to unsatisfactory evidences, such as the lack of RCTs proving the superiority of any vitamin D sterol against placebo on patient-centered outcomes, the scanty clinical data on head-to-head comparisons between the multiple vitamin D sterols currently available, the absence of RCTs confirming the crescent expectations on nutritional vitamin D pleiotropic effects even in CKD patients, and the promising effects of VDRAs against proteinuria and myocardial hypertrophy in diabetic CKD cohorts. They reviewed the results of several known RCTs including VITAL, OPERA, PRIMO, ACHIEVE, and IMPACT.

Finally, Dr. Mazzaferro et al. recapitulate the interactions between vitamin D and calcimimetics in particular in CKD, beginning with briefly describing the characteristics of the parathyroid CaSR and the properties of new compounds capable to stimulate it, the calcimimetics. Cinacalcet, the first calcimimetic available for clinical uses, is currently successfully employed to reduce serum PTH levels in dialysis patients. At variance with vitamin D, calcimimetics, while decreasing PTH, also decrease serum levels of calcium and phosphate. The effect on serum calcium often requires the concomitant prescription of vitamin D. Importantly, vitamin D administration increases the CaSR expression on parathyroid cells and, reciprocally, calcimimetics increase VDR expression. This interaction allows presuming potential clinical advantages to control uremic SHPT. Further, since both VDR and CaSR are expressed also in tissues not involved with mineral metabolism, other still unpredicted clinical effects could be possible.

I hope that after reading all, or some chapters of your interest, you have refreshed your knowledge and discovered the new latest developments in the vitamin D field and its relation with CKD. It was my principal objective marrying advances in basic scientific research and trying to bring them to clinical management, so you could translate and apply them in your daily patient care. I also hope that it will do as much to excite the readers about the right future studies to be undertaken in order to decipher the putative, delightful, and pleiotropic effects of vitamin D in CKD.

Saint Ouen, France   Pablo A. Ureña Torres

Contents

Part I   Generalities, Measurement and Epidemiology

1   **Vitamin D Metabolism in Normal and Chronic Kidney
Disease States**.   3
Claudia Zierold, Kevin J. Martin, and Hector F. DeLuca

2   **Epidemiology of Vitamin D Deficiency in Chronic
Kidney Disease**   19
Marie Metzger and Bénédicte Stengel

3   **Molecular Biology of Vitamin D: Genomic and Nongenomic
Actions of Vitamin D in Chronic Kidney Disease**   51
Adriana S. Dusso

4   **Vitamin D Receptor and Interaction with DNA:
From Physiology to Chronic Kidney Disease**   75
Jordi Bover, César Emilio Ruiz, Stefan Pilz, Iara Dasilva,
Montserrat M. Díaz, and Elena Guillén

5   **Measurement of Circulating 1,25-Dihydroxyvitamin D
and Vitamin D–Binding Protein in Chronic Kidney Diseases**   117
Etienne Cavalier and Pierre Delanaye

Part II   Classical Mineral and Bone Effects

6   **Vitamin D and Racial Differences in Chronic Kidney Disease**.   131
Orlando M. Gutiérrez

7   **Vitamin D and Parathyroid Hormone Regulation
in Chronic Kidney Disease**   147
María E. Rodríguez-Ortiz, Mariano Rodríguez,
and Yolanda Almadén Peña

8   The Parathyroid Type I Receptor and Vitamin D
     in Chronic Kidney Disease.................................... 163
     Pablo A. Ureña Torres, Jordi Bover, Pieter Evenepoel,
     Vincent Brandenburg, Audrey Rousseaud, and Franck Oury

9   Vitamin D and Klotho in Chronic Kidney Disease 179
     Hirotaka Komaba and Beate Lanske

10   Vitamin D and FGF23 in Chronic Kidney Disease 195
     Dominique Prié

11   Wnt/Sclerostin and the Relation with Vitamin D
     in Chronic Kidney Disease................................... 207
     Mugurel Apetrii and Adrian Covic

12   Vitamin D and Bone in Chronic Kidney Disease................. 217
     Martine Cohen-Solal and Pablo A. Ureña Torres

13   Vitamin D in Children with Chronic Kidney Disease:
     A Focus on Longitudinal Bone Growth 229
     Justine Bacchetta and Isidro B. Salusky

Part III   Non-classical Effects of Vitamin D

14   Vitamin D and Progression of Renal Failure 249
     Marc De Broe

15   Vitamin D and Diabetes in Chronic Kidney Disease.............. 267
     Emilio González Parra, Maria Luisa González-Casaus,
     and Ricardo Villa-Bellosta

16   Vitamin D and Muscle in Chronic Kidney Disease 285
     Philippe Chauveau and Michel Aparicio

17   Vitamin D Deficiency and Infection in Chronic Kidney Disease 295
     Jean-Paul Viard

18   Vitamin D and Inflammation in Chronic Kidney Disease 305
     Javier Donate-Correa, Ernesto Martín-Núñez,
     and Juan F. Navarro-González

19   Vitamin D and Heart Structure and Function in Chronic
     Kidney Disease 321
     Stefan Pilz, Vincent Brandenburg, and Pablo A. Ureña Torres

20   Vitamin D and Endothelial Function in Chronic
     Kidney Disease 343
     Mugurel Apetrii and Adrian Covic

**21   Vitamin D and Cardiovascular Calcification in Chronic
      Kidney Disease** 361
      Lucie Hénaut, Aurélien Mary, Said Kamel,
      and Ziad A. Massy

22   Calciphylaxis and Vitamin D 379
      Vincent M. Brandenburg and Pablo A. Ureña Torres

23   Vitamin D and Anemia in Chronic Kidney Disease 391
      Fenna van Breda and Marc G. Vervloet

24   Vitamin D and Mortality Risk in Chronic Kidney Disease 405
      John Cunningham

Part IV   Kidney Transplantation

25   Vitamin D in Kidney Transplantation 423
      Pieter Evenepoel

**26   Vitamin D in Acute and Chronic Rejection
      of Transplanted Kidney** 443
      Marie Courbebaisse

27   Nutrition and Dietary Vitamin D in Chronic Kidney Disease 453
      Jean-Claude Souberbielle

28   Natural Vitamin D in Chronic Kidney Disease 465
      Carlo Basile, Vincent Brandenburg, and Pablo A. Ureña Torres

**29   Which Vitamin D in Chronic Kidney Disease: Nutritional
      or Active Vitamin D? Or Both?** 493
      Armando Luis Negri, Elisa del Valle,
      and Francisco Rodolfo Spivacow

30   Use of New Vitamin D Analogs in Chronic Kidney Disease 515
      Riccardo Floreani and Mario Cozzolino

**31   Interaction Between Vitamin D and Calcimimetics
      in Chronic Kidney Disease** 537
      Sandro Mazzaferro, Lida Tartaglione, Silverio Rotondi,
      and Marzia Pasquali

Index 563

Contributors

Michel Aparicio, MD Service de Néphrologie Transplantation Dialyse, Centre Hospitalier, Universitaire de Bordeaux, Bordeaux, France

Mugurel Apetrii, MD, PhD Nephrology Unit, Dr CI Parhon University Hospital, Iasi, Romania

Justine Bacchetta, MD, PhD Centre de Référence des Maladies Rénales Rares, Service de Néphrologie Rhumatologie Dermatologie Pédiatriques, Hôpital Femme Mère Enfant, Bron, France

Carlo Basile, MD Division of Nephrology, Miulli General Hospital, Acquaviva delle Fonti, Italy

Jordi Bover, MD, PhD Department of Nephrology, Fundació Puigvert, IIB Sant Pau, REDinREN, Barcelona, Spain

Vincent M. Brandenburg Department of Cardiology and Center for Rare Diseases (ZSEA), RWTH University Hospital Aachen, Aachen, Germany

Etienne Cavalier, PhD Department of Clinical Chemistry, University of Liège, Liège, Belgium

Philippe Chauveau, MD Centre Hospitalier Universitaire de Bordeaux, Bordeaux, France

Martine Cohen-Solal, MD, PhD Rheumatology Department, Hospital Lariboisiere, Inserm U1132 and University Paris-Diderot, Paris, France

Marie Courbebaisse, MD, PhD Functional Renal Explorations Service, Department of Physiology, Georges Pompidou European Hospital, Paris, France

Adrian Covic, MD, PhD, FRCP (London), FERA Nephrology and Internal Medicine, University "Grigore T. Popa", Iasi, Romania

Mario Cozzolino, MD, PhD, FERA Renal Division, Department of Health Sciences, San Paolo Hospital, University of Milan, Milan, Italy

John Cunningham, MD Centre for Nephrology, CL Medical School, Royal Free Campus, London, UK

Iara Dasilva, MD Department of Nephrology, Fundaciò Puigvert, IIB Sant Pau, REDinREN, Barcelona, Spain

Marc De Broe, MD, PhD University Antwerpen, Antwerp, Belgium

Elisa del Valle, MD IDIM Instituto de Investigaciones Metabólicas, Universidad del Salvador, Buenos Aires, Argentina

Pierre Delanaye Department of Nephrology, Dialysis and Transplantation, University of Liege, Liege, Belgium

Hector F. DeLuca, BA, MS, PhD Department of Biochemistry, University of Wisconsin-Madison, Madison, WI, USA

Montserrat M. Díaz-Encarnacíon, MD, PhD Department of Nephrology, Fundaciò Puigvert, IIB Sant Pau, REDinREN, Barcelona, Spain

Javier Donate-Correa, PhD Research Unit, University Hospital Nuestra Señora de Candelaria, Santa Cruz de Tenerife, Spain

Adriana S. Dusso, PhD Bone and Mineral Research Unit, Instituto Reina Sofía de Investigación Nefrológica (IRSN), Hospital Universitario Central de Asturias, Asturias, Spain

Pieter Evenepoel, MD Department of Medicine, Division of Nephrology, Dialysis and Renal Transplantation, University Hospital Leuven, Leuven, Belgium

Riccardo Floreani, MD Renal and Dialysis Unit, San Paulo Hospital, Milan, Italy

Maria Luisa González-Casaus, MD Laboratory of Nephrology and Mineral Metabolism, Biochemistry/biopathology, Hospital Central de la Defensa Gomez Ulla, Madrid, Spain

Elena Guillén, MD Department of Nephrology, Fundaciò Puigvert, IIB Sant Pau, REDinREN, Barcelona, Spain

Orlando M. Gutiérrez, MD, MMSc Division of Nephrology, Department of Medicine, School of Medicine, Department of Epidemiology, School of Public Health, University of Alabama at Birmingham, Birmingham, AL, USA

Lucie Hénaut, PhD Laboratory of Renal and Vascular Pathophysiology, Fundación Jiménez Díaz, Madrid, Spain

Said Kamel, PharmD, PhD INSERM Unit 1088 and Department of Biochemistry, University Hospital, University of Picardie Jules Vernes and CHU d'amiens, Centre Universitaire de Recherche en Santé (CURS), Amiens, Picardie, France

Hirotaka Komaba, MD, PhD Division of Nephrology, Endocrinology and Metabolism, Tokai University School of Medicine, Shimo-Kasuya, Isehara, Japan

Beate Lanske, PhD Department of Oral Medicine, Infection & Immunity, Harvard School of Dental Medicine, Boston, MA, USA

Kevin J. Martin, MB, BCh, FASN Division of Nephrology, Department of Internal Medicine, Saint Louis University, Saint Louis, MO, USA

Ernesto Martín-Núñez Research Unit, University Hospital Nuestra Señora de Candelaria, Santa Cruz de Tenerife, Spain

Aurélien Mary, PharmD, PhD INSERM Unit 1088, University of Picardie Jules Vernes, Amiens, France

Ziad A. Massy, MD, PhD, FERA Division of Nephrology, Ambroise Paré University Hospital, Boulogne, France

Sandro Mazzaferro Department of Cardiovascular, Respiratory Nephrologic Anesthetic and Geriatric Sciences, Sapienza University, Nephrology and Dialysis Unit, Policlinico Umberto I, Rome, Italy

Marie Metzger, MD Inserm UMR 1018, Centre de Recherches en Epidémiologie et Santé des Populations (CESP), Villejuif, France

Juan F. Navarro-González, MD, PhD, FASN Research Unit and Nephrology Service, University Hospital Nuestra Señora de Candelaria, Santa Cruz de Tenerife, Spain

Armando Luis Negri, MD, FACP Instituto de Investigaciones Metabólicas, Buenos Aires, Argentina

Klaus Ølgaard, MD Nephrological Department, University of Copenhagen, Copenhagen, Denmark

Franck Oury, MD Institut National de la Santé et de la Recherche Médicale (INSERM) U115, Institut Necker Enfants Malades (INEM), Université Paris Descartes, Paris, France

Emilio González Parra, MD Servicio de Nefrología, Universidad Autónoma, Fundación Jiménez Díaz, Madrid, Spain

Marzia Pasquali, MD, PhD Department of Cardiovascular, Respiratory, Nephrologic and Geriatric Sciences, Sapienza University of Rome, Rome, Italy

Yolanda Almadén Peña, PhD Lipid and Atherosclerosis Unit, Instituto Maimónides de Investigación Biomédica de Córdoba (IMIBIC), Reina Sofia University Hospital/University of Cordoba, Córdoba, Spain

CIBER Fisiopatologia Obesidad y Nutricion (CIBEROBN), Instituto de Salud Carlos III, University of Cordoba, Córdoba, Spain

Stefan Pilz, MD, PhD Department of Endocrinology and Metabolism, Medical University of Graz, Graz, Styria, Austria

Dominique Prié, MD INSERM U845, Centre de Recherche Croissance et Signalisation, Université Paris Descartes, Hôpital Necker Enfants Malades, Paris, France

Mariano Rodríguez, PhD Service of Nephrology, University Hospital Reina Sofía, University of Córdoba, Instituto Maimónides de Investigación Biomédica de Córdoba (IMIBIC), Córdoba, Spain

María E. Rodríguez-Ortiz, PhD IIS-Fundación Jiménez-Díaz, Madrid, Spain

Silverio Rotondi, MD Department of Cardiovascular, Respiratory, Nephrologic and Geriatric Sciences, Sapienza University of Rome, Rome, Italy

Audrey Rousseaud Institut National de la Santé et de la Recherche Médicale (INSERM) U115, Institut Necker Enfants Malades (INEM), Université Paris Descartes, Paris, France

César Emilio Ruiz, MD Department of Nephrology, Fundaciò Puigvert, IIB Sant Pau, REDinREN, Barcelona, Spain

Isidro B. Salusky, MD David Geffen School of Medicine at UCLA, Division of Pediatric Nephrology, University of California Los Angeles, Los Angeles, CA, USA

Jean-Claude Souberbielle, MD Laboratoire d'explorations fonctionnelles, Hôpital Necker-Enfants maladies, Paris, France

Francisco Rodolfo Spivacow, MD IDIM Instituto de Investigaciones Metabólicas, Universidad del Salvador, Buenos Aires, Argentina

Bénédicte Stengel, MD, PhD Center for Research in Epidemiology and Population Health (CESP), Renal and Cardiovascular Epidemiology Team, University Paris-Saclay, Paris, France

Lida Tartaglione, MD Department of Cardiovascular, Respiratory, Nephrologic and Geriatric Sciences, Sapienza University of Rome, Rome, Italy

Pablo A. Ureña Torres, MD, PhD Ramsay-Générale de Santé, Service de Néphrologie et Dialyse, Clinique du Landy, Saint Ouen, France

Department of Renal Physiology, Necker Hospital, University of Paris V, René Descartes, Paris, France

Fenna van Breda, MD Department of Nephrology and Institute for Cardiovascular Research, VU University Medical Center, Amsterdam, The Netherlands

Marc G. Vervloet, MD, PhD, FERA Department of Nephrology, VU University Medical Center, Amsterdam, The Netherlands

Jean-Paul Viard, MD UF de Thérapeutique en Immuno-infectiologie Hôtel-Dieu, Paris, France

Ricardo Villa-Bellosta, PhD Department of Nephrology, IIS-Fundación Jiménez Díaz, Madrid, Spain

Claudia Zierold, PhD DiaSorin, Stillwater, MN, USA

Part I
Generalities, Measurement and Epidemiology

Chapter 1
Vitamin D Metabolism in Normal and Chronic Kidney Disease States

Claudia Zierold, Kevin J. Martin, and Hector F. DeLuca

Abstract Vitamin D is a prohormone synthesized in the skin from the precursor molecule 7-dehydrocholesterol by the action of sunlight. It is found in low amounts in food, with fortified dairy and fish oils being the most abundant source. Vitamin D undergoes an important 2-step bio-activation process required to produce the active metabolite 1,25-dihydroxyvitamin D (1,25(OH)$_2$D). The bio-activation process comprises the synthesis of 25-hydroxyvitamin D in the liver by 25-hydroxylation, followed by the conversion to 1,25(OH)$_2$D by the 1α-hydroxylase in kidney under very tightly regulated physiological conditions. 1,25(OH)$_2$D is responsible for maintaining adequate levels of calcium and phosphorus in the blood. Calcium is essential for muscles and nervous system functions, and through the actions of 1,25(OH)$_2$D on intestine, kidney, and bone, the body prevents imbalances of both calcium and phosphate via an intricate system. In addition, 1,25(OH)$_2$D plays an important role in many biological non-calcemic functions throughout the body. 1,25(OH)$_2$D must bind to the vitamin D receptor to carry out its functions. The highly active and lipid soluble 1,25(OH)$_2$D is inactivated by the 24-hydroxylase, which is the enzyme responsible for the major catabolic pathway that ultimately results in the water soluble calcitroic acid for excretion in the urine. Regulation of key players in vitamin D metabolism is reciprocal and very tight. The activating

C. Zierold, PhD (✉)
DiaSorin, 1951 Northwestern Ave, Stillwater, MN 55082, USA
e-mail: claudia.zierold@diasorin.com

K.J. Martin, MB, BCh, FASN
Department of Internal Medicine, Saint Louis University,
3635 Vista Ave, Saint Louis, MO 63110, USA
e-mail: martinkj@slu.edu

H.F. DeLuca, BA, MS, PhD
Department of Biochemistry, University of Wisconsin-Madison,
433 Babcock Drive, Madison, WI 53706-1544, USA
e-mail: deluca@biochem.wisc.edu

© Springer International Publishing Switzerland 2016
P.A. Ureña Torres et al. (eds.), *Vitamin D in Chronic Kidney Disease*,
DOI 10.1007/978-3-319-32507-1_1

enzyme 1α-hydroxylase, and the catabolic enzyme 24-hydroxylase are reciprocally regulated by PTH, 1,25(OH)$_2$D, and FGF23. Chronic kidney disease is associated with abnormalities of phosphorus homeostasis and altered vitamin D metabolism, and if left untreated, result in significant morbidity and mortality.

Keywords Vitamin D • VDR • Cholecalciferol • Ergocalciferol • Calcium • Phosphate • FGF23 • Intestine • Kidney • Bone • CKD

1.1 Vitamin D

Vitamin D is a general term covering vitamin D$_2$ and D$_3$. Vitamin D$_3$ is also known as cholecalciferol. It is produced in skin upon exposure to sunshine. Although it was discovered and classified as a vitamin, the fact that it can be produced in skin and thus not required in the diet makes it different from other vitamins. Vitamin D should more properly be considered a prohormone, and not a vitamin. It is found in low amounts in food, with fortified dairy and fish oils being the most abundant source. The most important role of vitamin D is to regulate the homeostasis of two key players in bone mineralization, calcium and phosphorus, but it also plays an important role in many biological functions throughout the body. Vitamin D is synthesized from the precursor molecule 7-dehydrocholesterol found in skin by the action of sunlight via a non-enzymatic reaction to the intermediary pre-vitamin D molecule, which in turn slowly isomerizes to vitamin D (Fig. 1.1). For the conversion to occur, a UV light of a specific wavelength (280–315 nm) is required to irradiate the skin. In nature, the sun is able to provide this radiation depending on season and latitude. In northern populations, the winter sun lays too low for light at 280–315 nm to penetrate the skin with enough intensity, resulting in increased incidence of vitamin D deficiency in the populations of those regions. The high incidence of deficiency in northern countries is remarkable, and emphasizes the importance of the sunlight in the synthesis of vitamin D. Furthermore, people with darker skin synthesize vitamin D less efficiently due to the large amount of the pigment,

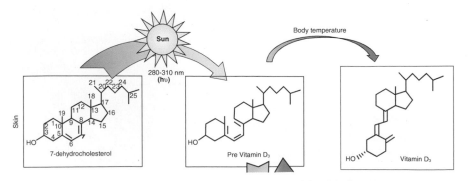

Fig. 1.1 Synthesis of vitamin D$_3$ (cholecalciferol) from 7-dehydrocholesterol in the skin

melanin, which effectively absorbs UV light. Factors that decrease exposure of the 280–310 nm sunlight have had significant impact on vitamin D status. Such factors include pollution, increased indoor lifestyle, sunscreen usage, and ethnic clothing all of which have contributed to the increased occurrence of vitamin D deficiency worldwide. Vitamin D is obtained from the diet or supplements in the form of cholecalciferol (Vitamin D_3, animal origin) or ergocalciferol (Vitamin D_2, plant/fungal origin). The difference between vitamin D_2 and vitamin D_3 lies in the structure of their side chains. The side chain of vitamin D_2 contains a double bond between carbons 22 and 23, and a methyl group on carbon 24 (Fig. 1.2) [1–7]. Vitamin D is absorbed through the proximal segments of the small intestine by incorporation into bile salt micellar solutions [8].

Vitamin D and its metabolites are hydrophobic molecules. Eighty-eight percent of the vitamin D metabolites in circulation are bound to the vitamin D–binding protein (DBP), while the rest loosely associate with albumin, and less than 0.05 % of 25-hydroxyvitamin D (25(OH)D) is found in free form (<0.5 % for 1,25-dihydroxyvitamin D or 1,25(OH)$_2$D). The DBP, also known as G$_c$-globulin, has been characterized as a multifunctional protein, but its major roles are to bind vitamin D metabolites, and to capture extracellular monomeric actin that is released following cellular trauma. Interestingly, only 2 % of the DBP in circulation is occupied by vitamin D metabolites, a very low fraction when compared to other steroid carrier proteins such as thyroxine binding globulin, cortisol binding globulin, and sex hormone binding globulin whose binding sites are approximately 50 % occupied by their specific ligands. Though all vitamin D metabolites bind to DBP, their affinities vary, with 25(OH)D having the highest affinity (5×10^8 M^{-1}) while vitamin D, and 1,25(OH)$_2$D bind with affinities at about one order of magnitude less [9].

The DBP is a highly polymorphic protein that has been used in population genetic studies, yet no humans have been identified with null mutations, leading to speculations that one or more of its functions are vital. Phenotypic alterations due to DBP polymorphisms have also been studied in relation to their affinity to vitamin D

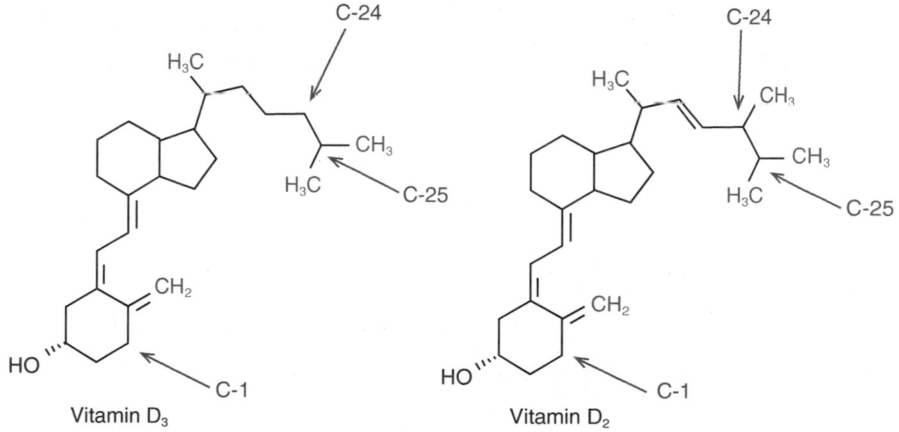

Fig. 1.2 Structure of vitamin D_3 and vitamin D_2 with carbon 1, 24, and 25 highlighted as the most important sites in the metabolism of vitamin D

metabolites and circulating DBP concentration with corresponding effect on various diseases, but conclusive evidence is not available. DBP knockout mice, however, show no impairment of the basic vitamin D functions [9–11].

1.2   25-Hydroxyvitamin D

25(OH)D is produced when vitamin D enters the circulation bound to DBP and is carried to the liver. There it gets hydroxylated at carbon 25, an important step in a 2-step bio-activation process required to produce the active hormone (Figs. 1.1 and 1.3). This important conversion to 25(OH)D was discovered in the late 1960s when radiolabeled vitamin D with high specific activity was first synthesized and administered to vitamin D-deficient animals. Conversion to more polar radiolabeled compounds was observed. The major one was identified as 25(OH)D$_3$, and is the major circulating form of vitamin D in the body. Animals with complete hepatectomy produce little 25(OH)D$_3$, providing evidence that the major, if not exclusive, site of production is the liver. It is now well established that 25-hydroxylation occurs primarily in liver microsomes and mitochondria by 25-hydroxylase

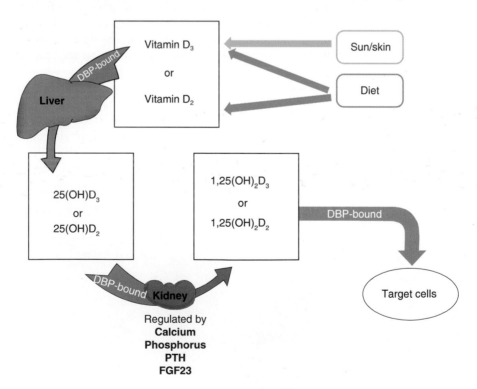

Fig. 1.3 Two-step bioactivation process of vitamin D to 25-hydroxyvitamin D in liver (unregulated) and 1,25-dihydroxyvitamin D in kidney (tightly regulated)

enzymes. The 25-hydroxylation step is minimally regulated, resulting in a relationship of vitamin D dose to circulating levels of 25(OH)D. As more vitamin D is synthesized in the skin or ingested, the levels of circulating 25(OH)D rise; thus, the measurement of serum or plasma 25(OH)D has been adopted as an indicator of an individual's vitamin D status [4, 6, 7].

25-Hydroxylation is executed primarily in liver microsomes with CYP2R1, a cytochrome P450 mixed function monooxygenase, being the major contributor to 25-hydroxylation of vitamin D. In addition, less specific liver 25-hydroxylases, which also hydroxylate other sterols, catalyze the same reaction when large doses of vitamin D are administered. A number of enzymes belonging to the cytochrome P450 family have been considered candidates for this enzymatic transformation, and include CYP27A1, CYP2C11, CYP2D25, CYP34A, and CYP2J2/3. The CYP27A1, a sterol 27-hydroxylase, has broad substrate specificity and is able to 25-hydroxylate vitamin D. The generation of the CYP2R1-null mice has provided evidence that this liver 25-hydroxylase enzyme is responsible for a large part of the conversion of vitamin D to 25(OH)D, but not all. Mice with ablation of both CYP2R1 and CYP27A1 did not have significantly different circulating levels of 25(OH)D than the CYP2R1 mice alone, indicating that other enzymes contribute to this step. Very few patients with CYP2R1 mutations have been identified, yet those with mutations have symptoms of vitamin D deficiency. The scarcity of symptomatic cases may be due to the fact that alternate 25-hydroxylation pathways exist, and that mutations go unnoticed in most cases. It is interesting that the symptomatic cases (vitamin D deficiency symptoms) have been in darker skinned patients of Nigerian or Arabic decent, perhaps because lower levels of vitamin D are generated in these subjects to begin with, and concomitant impaired first-step activation increases susceptibility to the mutation [12].

1.3   1,25-Dihydroxyvitamin D

1,25(OH)$_2$D is the active metabolite or hormonal form of vitamin D. Synthesis of radiolabeled vitamin D, made possible the discovery of vitamin D conversion to 25(OH)D. In later studies the synthesis and administration of radiolabeled 25(OH)D$_3$ resulted in the observation that 25(OH)D$_3$ was converted to a more polar metabolite that accumulated in the nucleus of cells in target tissue. Isolation of the metabolite from 1,600 chicken intestines led to the identification by a combination of mass spectrometry and specific chemical reactions of the active metabolite of vitamin D, 1,25(OH)$_2$D$_3$. 1,25(OH)$_2$D$_3$ is a steroid hormone that is highly active in calcium transport and bone mineralization. Synthesis of 1,25(OH)$_2$D$_3$ occurs primarily in kidney (Fig. 1.3), where 25(OH)D is hydroxylated on carbon-1 by the 1α-hydroxylase (CYP27B1) enzyme. The 1α-hydroxylase enzyme displays properties similar to adrenal cytochrome P450 enzymes, including a requirement for magnesium ions, molecular oxygen and a source of reduced pyridine nucleotides. 1α-hydroxylase also requires the cofactors ferredoxin and ferredoxin reductase to set up an electron transport chain. The need for magnesium for the optimal function of 1α-hydroxylase has important dietary implications, as deficiency of magnesium may cause this activation step to be less efficient. The 1α-hydroxylase is localized to the mitochondria of proximal tubular cells, and is a critical component of the vitamin D system. Circulating levels of the active hormone are produced by the kidney, as was shown in anephric animals that do not produce circulating 1,25(OH)₂D. The function of 1,25(OH)₂D is reflected in calcium absorption, and in bone calcium mobilization. Nephrectomized rats given 1,25(OH)₂D are able to absorb calcium from the intestine, and, because their circulating levels of PTH are high, mobilize calcium from bone; they cannot function if provided with 25(OH)D instead. On the other hand, animals with intact kidneys can function with normal amounts of 25(OH)D [1–7].

1,25(OH)₂D is responsible for maintaining adequate levels of calcium and phosphate in the blood. Calcium is essential for muscles and nervous system functions. The body is equipped with an intricate system to prevent imbalances, through the actions of 1,25(OH)₂D on intestine, kidney, and bone (the classical target organs) to prevent hypocalcemic tetany (Fig. 1.4a). In addition, 1,25(OH)₂D is important for mineralization of the skeleton. 1,25(OH)₂D maintains mineral homeostasis by enhancing the efficiency of calcium and phosphorus absorption from dietary sources in the small intestine. 1,25(OH)₂D is the only substance that can stimulate transport of calcium from the lumen of the intestine through the enterocyte to the blood against an electrochemical gradient. Phosphorus transport occurs via unrelated mechanisms, but it is also an active transport mechanism which is calcium-dependent. In the event that the dietary calcium supply is not sufficient, 1,25(OH)₂D can increase the mobilization of calcium from bone into the circulation, but this only occurs in conjunction with parathyroid hormone (PTH) at sufficiently high levels. Furthermore, 1,25(OH)₂D, also in conjunction with PTH, acts on the kidney to reduce the excretion of calcium in urine by increasing reabsorption of the last 1 % of the filtered calcium load from the distal tubule in the kidneys. This amount is significant considering 7 g of calcium are filtered in humans each day. To maintain neutral phosphate balance, the kidney responds to hormonal stimuli, such as fibroblast growth factor 23 (FGF23) and PTH, to excrete phosphate into the urine, thus counterbalancing the phosphate absorbed in intestine and mobilized from bone (Fig. 1.4a,b) [2, 5–7, 13,14].

Synthesis and catabolism of 1,25(OH)₂D are highly regulated. Under conditions of low serum calcium, a calcium-sensing receptor in the parathyroid gland stimulates the synthesis and release of PTH, an 84-amino acid peptide. PTH acts on membrane receptors of proximal tubule kidney cells resulting in increased 1α-hydroxylase activity, while also decreasing activity of the catabolic enzyme 24-hydroxylase. 1,25(OH)₂D acts on intestine, bone, and kidney to increase circulating calcium. When circulating calcium levels return to normal, PTH production and secretion is suppressed by signaling from the calcium sensing receptor and by direct inhibition of PTH gene transcription by 1,25(OH)₂D. 1α-hydroxylase activity is then diminished by 1,25(OH)₂D and a lack of PTH. An increased breakdown of 1,25(OH)₂D results from the 1,25(OH)₂D stimulation of the 24-hydroxylase [2, 5–7].

Regulation of phosphorus homeostasis is less precise than that of calcium homeostasis. The discovery of FGF23, which is produced by osteocytes/osteoblasts, has led to better understanding of phosphate regulation and a better understanding of the disorders of bone and mineral metabolism in chronic kidney disease (CKD). The

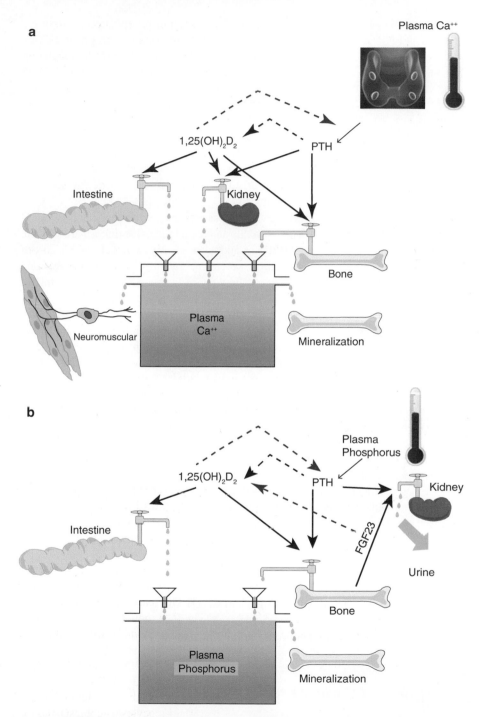

Fig. 1.4 Regulation of 1,25-(OH)₂D, PTH, and FGF23 for maintenance of calcium (**a**) and phosphorus (**b**) homeostasis

main function of FGF23 is to decrease the level of sodium-phosphate cotransporters (NTP2a and NPT2c) that results in increased renal excretion of phosphate. FGF23 also suppresses $1,25(OH)_2D$ by down-regulating the 1α-hydroxylase and up-regulating the 24-hydroxylase. Administration of $1,25(OH)_2D$ increases production of FGF23 independent of serum phosphorus levels. FGF23 acts through FGF-receptors and requires a cofactor, the membrane-bound form of klotho, which are both expressed in target tissues. The importance of FGF23 in phosphorus homeostasis and vitamin D metabolism is evidenced by genetic mouse models, where excess FGF23 causes hypophosphatemia, aberrant vitamin D metabolism, impaired growth, and rickets/osteomalacia. Inversely, ablation of FGF23 results in hyperphosphatemia, excess $1,25(OH)_2D$ and soft tissue calcification. Loss of function by genetic mutations of klotho results in phenotypes resembling FGF23 deficiency [13–15].

Inactivation of the 1α-hydroxylase enzyme causes the genetic disorder Vitamin D Dependent Rickets Type I. Patients with this autosomal recessive disease are not able to make the active metabolite $1,25(OH)_2D$, and subsequently cannot efficiently absorb calcium. They develop hypocalcemia, secondary hyperparathyroidism, retarded growth, and severe rickets despite adequate vitamin D intake, and exposure to UV light. Administration of physiological doses of $1,25(OH)_2D_3$ completely corrects the symptoms. Gene sequence analysis has confirmed that Vitamin D Dependent Rickets Type I is caused by mutations in the 1α-hydroxylase gene. In the absence of functional 1α-hydroxylase activity rickets that is identical to vitamin D deficiency results. The generation of mutant mice lacking the 1α-hydroxylase enzyme (CYP27B1-null) has produced mice with a phenotype that is very similar to that observed in human Vitamin D Dependent Rickets Type I. Rescue of the phenotype was clearly shown by treating mutant animals with $1,25(OH)_2D$. In addition, a high-calcium lactose-containing diet was able to normalize blood biochemistry and correct hypocalcemia, secondary hyperparathyroidism, and bone abnormalities, emphasizing the primary importance of $1,25(OH)_2D$ in calcium absorption to normalize serum calcium [1, 4].

Extra-renal production of $1,25(OH)_2D$ and autocrine and paracrine actions have been proposed. Anephric rats are unable to synthesize $1,25(OH)_2D_3$, and human patients with bilateral nephrectomy or chronic renal failure have low or undetectable levels of serum $1,25(OH)_2D_3$. There exist, however, certain disease states, such as sarcoidosis and immune-proliferative disease, where serum $1,25(OH)_2D$ rises to high levels in spite of hypercalcemia, due to extra-renal production by macrophages and lymphoid cells. Additionally, during pregnancy, extra-renal production of $1,25(OH)_2D$ occurs in the placenta. In these altered or diseased states, extra-renal production is regulated differently, and results in increased circulating $1,25(OH)_2D$ levels with corresponding marked physiological effects. The role of $1,25(OH)_2D$ synthesis at other sites besides kidney, immune cells, and placenta in normal conditions remains to be determined [1–3].

1.4   Effects of Chronic Kidney Disease

The closely related abnormalities of phosphorus homeostasis and altered vitamin D metabolism that occur in chronic kidney disease (CKD) are characterized by progressive secondary hyperparathyroidism, bone disease, and extra-skeletal

Table 1.1 Factors leading to decreased circulating 1,25(OH)$_2$D levels in chronic kidney disease

Factors	Effects
Decreased synthesis of vitamin D in the skin	↓ Circulating 25(OH)D
Decreased circulating 25(OH)D	↓ Substrate for 1α-hydroxylase
Increased FGF23	↓ 1α-hydroxylase and ↑24-hydroxylase
Decreased GFR/renal mass	↓ Delivery of 25(OH)D to 1α-hydroxylase
Decreased renal tissue	↓ 1,25(OH)$_2$D production
Decreased renal megalin	↓ Reabsorption of DBP-bound 25(OH)D into proximal tubules for 1α-hydroxylation
Accumulation of uremic toxins	↓ Production and action of 1,25(OH)$_2$D

calcifications, including vascular calcification. This often occurs early in the course of CKD and if left untreated, results in significant morbidity and mortality. The levels of 1,25(OH)$_2$D progressively decrease as kidney disease progresses and glomerular filtration rate (GFR) declines. This facilitates the development of secondary hyperparathyroidism by both hypocalcemia and the lack of suppression of the pre-proparathyroid hormone gene by the absence of 1,25(OH)$_2$D. Retention of phosphate also contributes to hyperparathyroidism, and is associated with increases in FGF23. FGF23 acts together with PTH to increase phosphate excretion in an effort to maintain phosphorus homeostasis, but this is limited by the loss of renal mass [16, 17].

Several mechanisms contribute to the decreased production of 1,25(OH)$_2$D in the course of CKD as shown in Table 1.1. It was initially thought that decreased renal mass limits the amount of 1α-hydroxylase available to synthesize 1,25(OH)$_2$D. The reduction in GFR, however, may also limit the delivery of 25-hydroxyvitamin D to the 1α-hydroxylase enzyme, thereby, limiting the ability of the kidney to produce 1,25(OH)$_2$D. This occurs because circulating 25(OH)D is bound to the DBP and is filtered at the glomerulus and absorbed into the proximal tubule by a receptor-mediated mechanism involving megalin. This mediates the endocytosis of 25(OH)D bound to its carrier protein, DBP, and thus, regulates the delivery of 25(OH)D to the site of the 1α-hydroxylase in the mitochondria. This becomes problematic in CKD because low levels of circulating 25(OH)D are common in patients with CKD, particularly in those with proteinuria, when 25(OH)D, bound to DBP is excreted in the urine. CKD has also been associated with reductions the expression of megalin in the kidney, which can further aggravate this process. The intestinal absorption of dietary and supplemental vitamin D could also be reduced in CKD subjects as suggested by the results of experimental studies in uremic animals [18]. An additional factor, and potentially the major one, that contributes to decreased levels of 1,25(OH)$_2$D in CKD is the progressive increase in the levels of FGF23 that occur early in the course of CKD. FGF23 directly suppresses the activity and expression of 1α-hydroxylase, and therefore, this is an important factor that contributes to the decreased ability of the failing kidney to maintain 1,25(OH)$_2$D production. In addition, FGF23 is also known to increase the expression of 24-hydroxylase, which is the enzyme responsible for the degradation of 1,25(OH)$_2$D. Finally, the accumulation of "uremic toxins" may limit the production and actions of 1,25(OH)$_2$D in CKD [16, 17].

1.5   The Vitamin D Receptor

$1,25(OH)_2D$ must bind to the vitamin D receptor (VDR) to carry out its functions. The VDR is a nuclear receptor that belongs to the nuclear steroid receptor family. It binds $1,25(OH)_2D$, with very high affinity ($K_D = 10^{-10}$ to 10^{-11} M), consistent with the low levels of the hormone found in circulation (10^{-10}–10^{-11} M). The affinity of 25(OH)D and other metabolites for the VDR is two orders of magnitude lower, and 25(OH)D will only bind to the VDR when present at high enough levels to compensate for its lower affinity. Vitamin D-dependent rickets Type I patients, having no $1,25(OH)_2D$, were able to be treated when given large doses of 25(OH)D, demonstrating the ability of 25(OH)D to act as an analog to $1,25(OH)_2D$. In healthy subjects, 25(OH)D becomes toxic once concentrations are so high that it begins to bind the VDR eliciting physiological actions in an unregulated manner. Thus in the presence of toxic 25(OH)D levels, calcium and phosphorus levels in serum are greatly elevated, resulting in calcification of soft tissues [4–6].

The VDR is a nuclear receptor, and has an overall structure characteristic of other steroid receptors in the superfamily, such as the glucocorticoid receptor and the estrogen receptor. These receptors possess a ligand binding domain, a DNA binding domain, activation domains, and a hinge area. The VDR binds to regulatory regions of target genes with its partner the retinoic X receptor (RXR), another member of the steroid receptor superfamily, to regulate gene transcription. The specific binding sites are known as vitamin D response elements (VDRE). They are two direct repeats of six specific nucleotides, separated by three non-specified nucleotides. Once bound to the VDRE, the VDR forms transcriptional complexes that increase or decrease target gene transcription [1, 4–6, 19].

The VDR is expressed at low levels in several target tissues, but specific physiologic conditions can alter VDR levels, adding a regulation step in addition to regulation of the metabolites. The strongest regulation is observed during development, when VDR is absent at birth, but begins to be expressed 16–18 days after. Other examples include upregulation of the VDR by $1,25(OH)_2D$ itself in many tissues, as well as downregulation of VDR in parathyroid glands by hypocalcemia to relieve some of the $1,25(OH)_2D$-suppressive effects on PTH [5].

The most crucial evidence that the VDR is essential for function are Vitamin D Dependent Rickets Type II patients who possess a dysfunctional VDR. They are resistant to $1,25(OH)_2D$, have high circulating levels of this hormone, yet they have hypocalcemia, severely impaired bone formation, alopecia, and infertility. VDR-null mice show typical features of vitamin D deficiency. However, the hypocalcemia in these mutant mice can be normalized by feeding a diet high in calcium and lactose (rescue diet), to aid passive calcium absorption, resulting in the normalization of the bone phenotype, indicating again that one of the important roles for $1,25(OH)_2D$ and its receptor is to increase calcium absorption to maintain calcium homeostasis and allow for proper bone mineralization [1, 4].

Detecting VDR in tissues beyond intestine, kidney and bone, led to the realization that $1,25(OH)_2D$ has a broader spectrum of actions that are not related to the classical functions of mineral homeostasis. The VDR has since been found in the pancreas, pituitary cells, skin, ovarian cells, aortic endothelial cells, placenta, activated T-cells, and a number of cancer cells. Because of these findings, there are suggestions that vitamin D deficiency is associated with diabetes, infectious and autoimmune diseases, hypertension, cancer, and complications during pregnancy [1, 3, 5].

1.6 24,25-Dihydroxyvitamin D and 1,24,25-Trihydroxyvitamin D

The 24-oxidation pathway is the major catabolic pathway for $1,25(OH)_2D$ metabolism: the highly active and lipid soluble $1,25(OH)_2D$ is inactivated and over multiple steps transformed into the water soluble calcitroic acid for excretion in the urine (Fig. 1.5). Inactivation of $1,25(OH)_2D$ serves to control physiological levels of $1,25(OH)_2D$ and guard against the toxic effect of excessive levels. 24-hydroxylation is the first step in this oxidation pathway, and 24-hydroxylase is generally

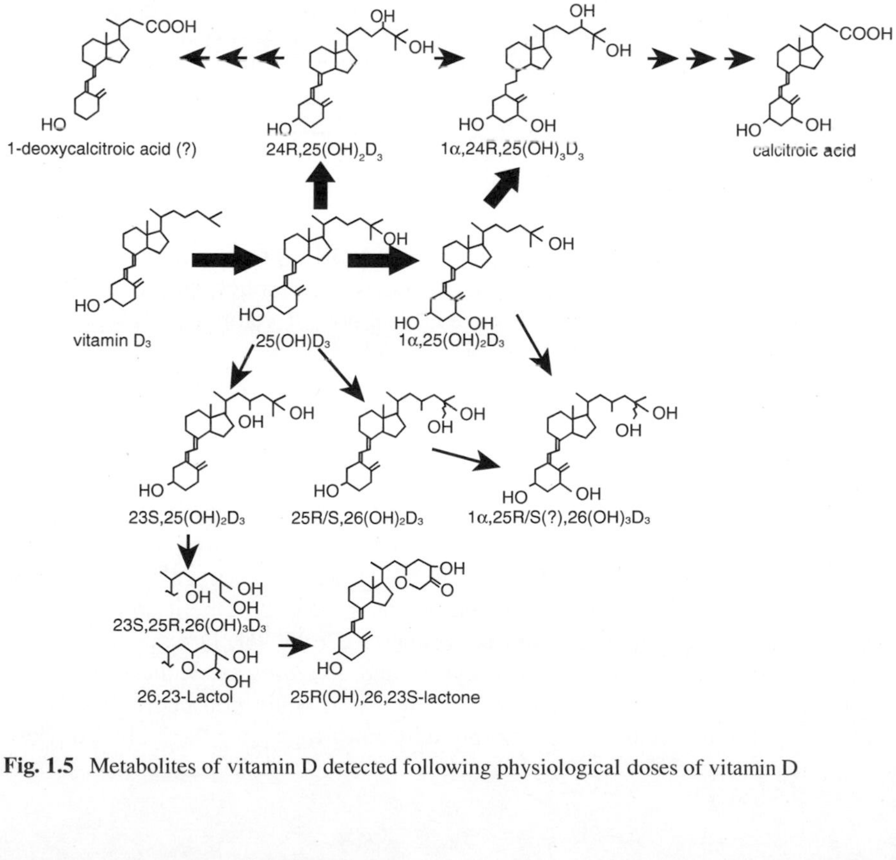

Fig. 1.5 Metabolites of vitamin D detected following physiological doses of vitamin D

present in the inner membrane of the mitochondria of target cells. This enzyme, also known as CYP24A1, is a cytochrome P-450 mixed function monooxygenase that requires nicotinamide adenine dinucleotide phosphate oxidase (NADPH), ferrodoxin, and ferrodoxin reductase to introduce molecular oxygen on the carbon 24 of $1,25(OH)_2D$ or $25(OH)D$. Both metabolites are substrates for the 24-hydroxylase, but the affinity is tenfold higher for $1,25(OH)_2D$ than $25(OH)D$, yet the $25(OH)D$ circulates at 1,000-fold higher concentrations (ng/mL versus pg/mL). Recently, human patients with infantile idiopathic hypercalcemia were identified with mutations in the CYP24A1 gene, and found to have accumulation of serum $1,25(OH)_2D$, further supporting the role of 24-hydroxylase in the clearance of vitamin D metabolites [1, 2, 6].

A biological role for 24-hydroxylated vitamin D metabolites remains controversial. While inactivation of the active $1,25(OH)_2D$ makes physiological sense, the role of inactivation of the not-yet-active $25(OH)D$ has been questioned. However, that 24-hydroxylation of $25(OH)D$ decreases the available substrate for 1α-hydroxylation does afford a viable regulatory step. Animals fed a diet with $24,24$-difluoro-25-OH-D_3 as their sole source of vitamin D for two generations had normal growth, reproduction and skeletal mineralization. The difluoro compound cannot be 24-hydroxylated, but behaves as $1,25(OH)_2D$ when 1α-hydroxylated, and the metabolism of vitamin D is not unbalanced, yet $24,25(OH)_2D$ is absent. Furthermore, 24-Hydroxylase-null mice were generated and show 50 % perinatal lethality. Interestingly the mice that survived past weaning were able to catabolize $1,25(OH)_2D$ by an alternate pathway, and showed normal levels of circulating calcium and phosphate. These surviving homozygous 24-hydroxylase-null mice can be bred, and have offspring with abnormal bone development, which can however be rescued when CYP24/VDR double null mutants are generated. This can be explained by the fact that 24-hydroxylase-null dams have elevated levels of $1,25(OH)_2D$ during gestation which cause the bone abnormalities in the developing offspring when VDR is present. In the absence of VDR, $1,25(OH)_2D$ cannot carry out its function even though circulating at elevated levels, and the offspring now have normal bone development in spite of the absence of $24,25(OH)_2D$. In light of this, $24,25(OH)_2D$ does not appear to be necessary for normal bone development during development, and is likely the product of the first catabolic step for $25(OH)D$, with no known function. This confirms the early conclusions reached using the $24,24$-difluoro-25-OH-D as a sole source of vitamin D [7, 20].

Regulation of key players in vitamin D metabolism is reciprocal and very tight. The activating enzyme 1α-hydroxylase, and the catabolic enzyme 24-hydroxylase are reciprocally regulated by PTH, $1,25(OH)_2D$, and FGF23. PTH up-regulates 1α-hydroxylase when calcium is needed, while at the same time it downregulates the 24-hydroxylase. When calcium is normalized, $1,25(OH)_2D$ regulates its own breakdown by activating the 24-hydroxylase, and decreases its synthesis by downregulating the 1α-hydroxylase. FGF23 is increased when phosphorus levels are elevated, and shuts down further absorption by down-regulating the 1α-hydroxylase and up-regulating the 24-hydroxylase [2].

1.7 Other Metabolites

Over 33 metabolites of vitamin D have been isolated and identified, and most are formed only when high doses of vitamin D are administered. The metabolites that have been isolated under physiological conditions are shown in Fig. 1.5. In addition to the above mentioned pathways, other important metabolic pathways of vitamin D that occur at physiologic concentrations are the 23-hydroxylation of 25(OH)D with subsequent 26-oxidation, and cyclization to form a lactone, and the 26-hydroxylation of 25(OH)D. Animals maintained on 25(OH)D fluorinated at positions 23, 26, and 27 to prevent hydroxylation at these carbons, were shown to have normal growth, reproduction, and bone mineralization thus suggesting that the 23- and 26-hydroxylated metabolites do not have important functions in calcium and phosphorus homeostasis, and that these compounds are likely metabolites of another catabolic pathway that leads to excretion [4, 6].

1.8 C3-Epimer of 25(OH)D

The C3-epimer of 25(OH)D is an isomer of 25(OH)D, having the hydroxyl group on carbon 3 in the β orientation instead of α. It has been measured in some infant blood samples, and it can be found at levels similar to or greater than 25(OH)D. Since its initial detection in pediatric samples, it has also been detected in adults, albeit less frequently. When present, the C3-epimer can be detected at concentrations below 10 ng/mL, though in extreme cases levels as high as 30–50 ng/mL have been found. To date, no physiological role has been attributed to this metabolite, but increased interest exists as to find why some subjects present with such high circulating amounts while others have none [1].

1.9 24(OH)D$_2$ or 1,24(OH)$_2$D$_2$

Widespread vitamin D deficiency has led to increased use of over-the-counter vitamin D supplements (both vitamin D$_3$ and D$_2$), and prescription strength vitamin D$_2$ supplementation (50,000 IU). Alternate metabolites were observed when either a single large dose (1,000,000 IU of vitamin D$_2$) or repeated daily doses (1,000–50,000 IU vitamin D$_2$) were ingested. 24(OH)D$_2$ and 1,24(OH)$_2$D$_2$ were produced via a pathway that resulted in 24-hydroxylation occurring via a liver 25-hydroxylase, presumably the CYP27A1 which prefers vitamin D$_2$ as a substrate over vitamin D$_3$. This alternate pathway has not been observed for vitamin D$_3$ supplements for which the expected 25(OH)D$_3$ and 1,25(OH)$_2$D$_3$ metabolites were produced even at high levels of supplementation. 1,24(OH)$_2$D$_2$ was shown to be physiologically active, and behave similarly to 1,25(OH)$_2$D [21, 22].

1.10   Relation Between Vitamin D, 24(OH)D, and 1,25(OH)₂D

Research in the field has over the years consistently and conclusively shown that 1,25(OH)$_2$D is the biologically active, hormonal form of vitamin D. However, the measurement of inactive 25(OH)D, has commonly been used in studies of disease association with vitamin D. The conversion of inactive 25(OH)D to active 1,25(OH)$_2$D is a tightly regulated step, and circulating levels of 1,25(OH)$_2$D are not directly proportional to the circulating 25(OH)D, but are dependent on physiological states, and respective regulatory stimuli. While small increases in 1,25(OH)$_2$D may result when circulating levels of 25(OH)D increase, due to more substrate availability, much larger changes of 1,25(OH)$_2$D can result from regulation by the physiological state, so that for a given serum level of 25(OH)D, levels of 1,25(OH)$_2$D can vary more than tenfold. Novel methods for a more accurate and precise measurement of 1,25(OH)$_2$D are being developed, and future clinical studies on the effects of vitamin D should include quantification of not only 25(OH)D, but also 1,25(OH)$_2$D the active effector molecule that binds the VDR, and is responsible for physiological responses in target cells.

1.11   Conclusions

Vitamin D as synthesized in the skin or ingested in the diet is inactive, and must undergo two successive hydroxylations to form the active metabolite 1,25(OH)$_2$D. 1,25(OH)$_2$D maintains adequate levels of calcium and phosphorus in the blood by acting on intestine, kidney, and bone, and is responsible for other non-calcemic functions. 1,25(OH)$_2$D carries out its functions through the vitamin D receptor. The 25(OH)D that is produced in the first bio-activation step is inactive, but its measurement in serum or plasma has been adopted as an indicator of an individual's vitamin D status. 25(OH)D levels have also commonly been used in studies of disease association with vitamin D, yet 1,25(OH)$_2$D has dependably been shown to be the biologically active form. The regulation of 1,25(OH)$_2$D is very tight and largely dependent on the physiological state surrounding calcium and phosphorus homeostasis, and thus not directly correlated to the levels of 25(OH)D. Though 25-hydroxyvitamin D, 1,25(OH)$_2$D, and the 24-hydroxylated metabolites are the most important and well-studied, other physiological metabolites of vitamin D exist, and future research may reveal additional physiologically important metabolites.

References

1. Bikle DD. Vitamin D metabolism, mechanism of action, and clinical applications. Chem Biol. 2014;21(3):319–29.
2. Christakos S, et al. Vitamin D: metabolism. Endocrinol Metab Clin North Am. 2010;39(2):243–53.

3. Christakos S, DeLuca HF. Minireview: vitamin D: is there a role in extraskeletal health? Endocrinology. 2011;152(8):2930–6.
4. DeLuca HF. The vitamin D story: a collaborative effort of basic science and clinical medicine. FASEB J. 1988;2(3):224–36.
5. DeLuca HF. Overview of general physiologic features and functions of vitamin D. Am J Clin Nutr. 2004;80(6 Suppl):1689S–96.
6. DeLuca HF. Triennial Growth Symposium – Vitamin D: bones and beyond. J Anim Sci. 2014;92(3):917–29.
7. Deluca HF. History of the discovery of vitamin D and its active metabolites. Bonekey Rep. 2014;3:479.
8. Lo CW, et al. Vitamin D absorption in healthy subjects and in patients with intestinal malabsorption syndromes. Am J Clin Nutr. 1985;42(4):644–9.
9. Speeckaert M, et al. Biological and clinical aspects of the vitamin D binding protein (Gc-globulin) and its polymorphism. Clin Chim Acta. 2006;372(1–2):33–42.
10. Bhan I. Vitamin d binding protein and bone health. Int J Endocrinol. 2014;2014:561214.
11. Yousefzadeh P, Shapses SA, Wang X. Vitamin D binding protein impact on 25-hydroxyvitamin D levels under different physiologic and pathologic conditions. Int J Endocrinol. 2014;2014: 981581.
12. Zhu JG, et al. CYP2R1 is a major, but not exclusive, contributor to 25-hydroxyvitamin D production in vivo. Proc Natl Acad Sci U S A. 2013;110(39):15650–5.
13. Martin A, David V, Quarles LD. Regulation and function of the FGF23/klotho endocrine pathways. Physiol Rev. 2012;92(1):131–55.
14. Renkema KY, et al. Calcium and phosphate homeostasis: concerted interplay of new regulators. Ann Med. 2008;40(2):82–91.
15. Liu S, Quarles LD. How fibroblast growth factor 23 works. J Am Soc Nephrol. 2007;18(6):1637–47.
16. Martin KJ, Gonzalez EA. Long-term management of CKD-mineral and bone disorder. Am J Kidney Dis. 2012;60(2):308–15.
17. Nigwekar SU, Tamez H, Thadhani RI. Vitamin D and chronic kidney disease-mineral bone disease (CKD-MBD). Bonckey Rep. 2014;3:498.
18. Vaziri ND, et al. Impaired intestinal absorption of vitamin D3 in azotemic rats. Am J Clin Nutr. 1983;37(3):403–6.
19. Evans RM, Mangelsdorf DJ. Nuclear receptors, RXR, and the Big Bang. Cell. 2014;157(1): 255–66.
20. St-Arnaud R, et al. Deficient mineralization of intramembranous bone in vitamin D-24-hydroxylase-ablated mice is due to elevated 1,25-dihydroxyvitamin D and not to the absence of 24,25-dihydroxyvitamin D. Endocrinology. 2000;141(7):2658–66.
21. Jones G, et al. Isolation and identification of 24-hydroxyvitamin D2 and 24,25-dihydroxyvitamin D2. Arch Biochem Biophys. 1980;202(2):450–7.
22. Mawer EB, et al. Unique 24-hydroxylated metabolites represent a significant pathway of metabolism of vitamin D2 in humans: 24-hydroxyvitamin D2 and 1,24-dihydroxyvitamin D2 detectable in human serum. J Clin Endocrinol Metab. 1998;83(6):2156–66.

Chapter 2
Epidemiology of Vitamin D Deficiency in Chronic Kidney Disease

Marie Metzger and Bénédicte Stengel

Abstract Vitamin D deficiency is common in both the general population and CKD patients. Currently defined as a circulating 25-dihydroxyvitamin D (25(OH) D) level below 20 ng/mL (50 nmol/L), it is a major risk factor for bone and mineral disorders and has been related to increased risk of non-skeletal health outcomes including mortality, diabetes, and cardiovascular disease. A greater prevalence of this deficiency is expected in patients with CKD because they are older and more likely to have dark skin, obesity, and associated comorbidities such as diabetes and hypertension. In studies of clinical populations, the mean circulating 25(OH)D levels ranged from 18 to 29 ng/mL for patients with non-end-stage CKD and from 12 to 32 ng/mL for those on dialysis. Large population-based and clinical studies, however, describe inconsistent findings about the association between kidney function and vitamin D level. While some studies report significant, positive, and independents associations between glomerular filtration rate and circulating 25(OH)D values, others show low levels only in advanced CKD stages. Still others show no or even an inverse association, with paradoxically higher levels of 25(OH)D in individuals with moderate CKD than in those without CKD. Similarly, it remains unclear whether these discordant relations are direct and causal, or indirect because of confounders. Only a few studies have examined the relations between proteinuria or albuminuria and circulating 25(OH)D levels; they generally report significant negative associations. Potential mechanisms supporting a causal relation between kidney function and damage and vitamin D are discussed at the end of this chapter.

Keywords Chronic kidney disease • Dialysis • Transplantation • Vitamin D deficiency • Recommendations • Epidemiology • Risk factors • Prevalence • Glomerular filtration rate • Albuminuria • Proteinuria

M. Metzger, MD (✉)
Inserm UMR 1018, Centre de Recherches en Épidémiologie et Santé des Populations (CESP),
Villejuif, France
e-mail: marie.metzger@inserm.fr

B. Stengel, MD, PhD
Center for Research in Epidemiology and Population Health (CESP),
Renal and Cardiovascular Epidemiology Team, University Paris-Saclay,
Paris, France
e-mail: benedicte.stengel@inserm.fr

© Springer International Publishing Switzerland 2016   19
P.A. Ureña Torres et al. (eds.), *Vitamin D in Chronic Kidney Disease*,
DOI 10.1007/978-3-319-32507-1_2

2.1 Introduction

Vitamin D deficiency is a global issue affecting nearly a billion people across the globe and across the life span, from childhood to advanced age [1, 2]. According to a 2014 systematic review of vitamin D status in populations worldwide in 2014, 37 % of the 195 studies included from 44 countries reported mean circulating 25-hydroxy vitamin D levels below 50 nmol/mL (20 ng/mL), the most common threshold for defining deficiency [3].

Vitamin D is involved in bone and mineral metabolism; its key role in bone health is consistent with a causal relation [4]. Risks associated with vitamin D deficiency include rickets in children and adolescents [5] and osteomalacia and osteoporosis, which can lead to fractures, in adults and the elderly [6]. Since 2000, many observational studies, reviewed by Theodoratou et al. [7], have also documented vitamin D deficiency as a potentially independent risk factor for non-skeletal outcomes including overall mortality, cancer, cardiovascular disease, autoimmune disease, and several other outcomes. In addition, a recent Cochrane meta-analysis of 56 randomized clinical trials (RCTs) showed that vitamin D supplementation slightly but significantly reduces mortality, especially among the elderly [8]. Several other RCTs on the effects of vitamin D are ongoing [9]. Whether or not vitamin D is causally related to extraskeletal complications, however, is currently debated. Some authors argue that the associations observed may have resulted from confounding or reverse causation [10]. Rather than being a risk factor for these outcomes, vitamin D deficiency may merely be a marker of poor health status associated with malnutrition and sedentary lifestyle.

Vitamin D deficiency is also common in chronic kidney disease (CKD) [11], and its role in the development of secondary hyperparathyroidism (SHPT) and CKD-related bone and mineral disorders (MBD) is well established (see section II of this book). Supplementation with calciferol, as well as with calcitriol or its analogs, has proved to be effective in reducing SHPT in patients with CKD, on dialysis or not [12–14] (but see [15]). Observational studies have also shown associations between vitamin D deficiency and other CKD complications, including anemia [16], insulin resistance [17], and inflammation [18]. Moreover, vitamin D deficiency has been associated with higher risks of overall and cardiovascular mortality in patients with end-stage [19, 20] and non-end-stage CKD [21], as well as with faster decline in the glomerular filtration rate (GFR) and earlier progression to end-stage renal disease (ESRD) [22–25].

This chapter begins with a review of the methods used to assess vitamin D status and a description of the definitions of deficiency used in studies in the general population and among patients with CKD. A brief summary of the main findings about the epidemiology and risk factors of vitamin D deficiency worldwide follows. We then report the prevalence of vitamin deficiency in patients with non-end-stage CKD, those on dialysis, and those living with a kidney transplant. Finally, we discuss whether or not CKD, defined by either increased albuminuria or decreased GFR, is associated with vitamin D deficiency, independently of other established risk factors.

2.2 Assessment of Vitamin D Status and Definition of Vitamin D Deficiency

Vitamin D status is best assessed by the level of its major circulating form, 25-hydroxyvitamin D (25(OH)D), also called calcidiol [4, 26]. Calcitriol or 1,25 dihydroxyvitamin D (1,25(OH)$_2$D$_3$), the active hormonal form of vitamin D, has a very short half-life and its concentration is tightly regulated by PTH, calcium, and phosphate levels (see Chap. 1) and is thus a poor indicator of vitamin D status [1].

Defining normal vitamin D values and comparing mean values or percentages of abnormal values between studies require a standard definition and a reference assay, neither of which currently exists. Normal or reference values for a given biological parameter are usually determined from a large sample of healthy volunteers. However, the production of 25(OH)D depends on sun exposure to UVB and liver 25 hydroxylation, as well as on endogenous factors such as age and skin color (see Chap. 6); because its levels therefore vary strongly according to latitude and season, there is no consensus about this approach. This limitation necessitates caution in the interpretation of variations in the vitamin D estimates between studies, especially in light of the lack of standardized assays for it.

Since 2010, various national or international medical societies and expert groups have published different guidelines for the evaluation, treatment, and prevention of vitamin D deficiency. Experts establishing recommendations for a level sufficient to prevent adverse outcomes have considered primarily its bone and mineral action [6, 27, 28]. Some are based on the relation between the circulating levels of 25(OH)D that reduce PTH level or increase intestinal calcium absorption. Others use findings from RCTs investigating the vitamin D threshold necessary to prevent hip and non-vertebral fractures [29]. The major definitions currently proposed for vitamin D deficiency or insufficiency are summarized in Table 2.1.

The threshold of 10 ng/mL (25 nmol/L) for 25(OH)D has long been used to define low vitamin D values with clinical effects, such as osteomalacia [30, 31]. Most recent guidelines, however, have proposed serum 25(OH)D levels below 20 ng/mL (50 nmol/L) to define vitamin D deficiency in the general population. Debate nonetheless continues about the definition of sufficiency, particularly because of the potentially pleiotropic effects of vitamin D. The Institute of Medicine (IOM) has concluded that values above 20 ng/mL are adequate for all ages and both genders [27]. The Endocrine Society, on the other hand, considers that optimum values should exceed 30 ng/mL and suggested defining deficiency as 25(OH)D below 20 ng/mL and insufficiency by values between 20 and 30 ng/mL (75 nmol/L) [26]. The discrepancies between guidelines for the minimum level of 25(OH)D required to be in "good health" and the need for supplementation reflects the low level of evidence for the extraskeletal effects of vitamin D [32]. Further RCTs are needed [9] to justify raising the vitamin D threshold, in view of the major economic and public health consequences of such an action: the levels of supplementation and/or sun exposure needed to achieve a circulating 25(OH)D concentration ≥30 ng/mL are far greater than those to exceed 20 ng/mL [30]).

Table 2.1 Definitions of vitamin D status based on circulating 25(OH)D levels (in ng/ml) according to scientific societies, healthcare and medical institutions

Reference	Year	Population	Definitions of Vitamin D status		
			Deficient	Insufficient or inadequate	Sufficient or recommended level
International Osteoporosis Foundation [6]	2010	Older adults	NR	NR	>30
Canadian Medical Association Osteoporosis Canada [28]	2010	Adult general population (with exception of pregnant and lactating women)	<10	10–30	>30
US National Academies: Institute of Medicine[27]	2011	General population	NR	<20[a]	20–50[b]
Endocrine Society Clinical practice guidelines [26]	2011	Patients at risk for deficiency	<20	21–29	30–100
French osteoporosis research group [81]	2011	Adult general population	<10	10–29	30–70
National Osteoporosis Society – UK [82]	2013	Adult patients with or at risk of bone disease (excluding those with CKD stage 4–5)	<12	12–20[a]	>20
NICE – UK [83]	2014	General population	<10[c]	NR	NR
KDOQI [35]	2003	CKD patients	<15	15–29	>30
KDIGO [33, 34]	2012	CKD patients	<20	NR	NR

NR not reported
[a]Inadequate
[b]Adequate level in at least 97.5 % of the population of "normal healthy individuals"
[c]Low vitamin D status

Current recommendations from KDIGO 2012 (Kidney Disease: Improving Global Outcomes CKD Work Group) [33] for the evaluation and management of CKD echo those of KDIGO 2009 for the diagnosis, evaluation, prevention, and treatment of CKD-MBD [34]. Both define vitamin D deficiency as a circulating 25(OH)D level below 20 ng/mL, as in the general population, while earlier recommendations from the National Kidney Foundation Kidney Disease Outcomes Quality Initiative (NKF/K-DOQI 2003) defined insufficiency as 25(OH)D values between 15 and 30, and deficiency by values <15 ng/mL [35]. Neither KDIGO guideline reports evidence for setting a threshold for CKD patients different from that of the general population or for adopting different treatment strategies. Many intervention studies have shown the efficacy of vitamin D supplementation in lowering the serum PTH level, particularly in patients on dialysis [12–14], but the target value to be achieved and the type of vitamin D supplementation are left to the discretion of clinicians. Interestingly, in the NephroTest study, a large clinical cohort including 1,700 patients with all-stage CKD not on dialysis or transplanted, the authors showed the rise in PTH accelerates when the circulating vitamin D level was below 20 ng/mL, independent of major risk factors for SHPT. This finding suggests that maintaining vitamin D values above 20 ng/mL is necessary to control PTH [36].

Finally, the IOM recommends that the maximum desirable 25(OH)D value not exceed 50 ng/mL, arguing that no benefits are expected for higher values: observational studies show a U- or reverse-J-shaped relation between 25(OH)Dand mortality, with a higher risk of death associated with high 25(OH)D values [27]. Many experts, however, consider the acceptable upper limit to be well above 50 ng/mL [26]. This acceptable upper limit must not be confused with the threshold for vitamin D intoxication, a rare event that usually follows accidental or intentional absorption of a massive dose of vitamin D. Although this threshold is not fully established, toxicity studies show no cases of hypercalcemia below 150 ng/mL of 25(OH)D [37]. Nonetheless, vitamin D supplementation in CKD patients, on dialysis or not, may be associated with a slight risk of hypercalcemia and hyperphosphatemia [13, 14].

2.3   Worldwide Epidemiology and Risk Factors for Vitamin D Deficiency

It is recognized that vitamin D deficiency is common across the globe, especially among sick people and the institutionalized elderly [2]. However, because of the uncertainty about the definitions of deficiency and insufficiency discussed above, prevalence estimates vary with the vitamin D thresholds used. To overcome this problem and enable meaningful comparisons across studies and between subgroups defined by age, sex, and region, Hilger et al studied continuous values of 25(OH)D in their systematic review of 195 population-based studies worldwide [3]. These studies involving more than 168,000 participants from 44 countries showed considerable variations in mean circulating 25(OH)D levels, ranging from 2 to 54 ng/mL (4.9 to 136.2 nmol/L) with 88.1 % of the studies reporting mean levels below 30 ng/

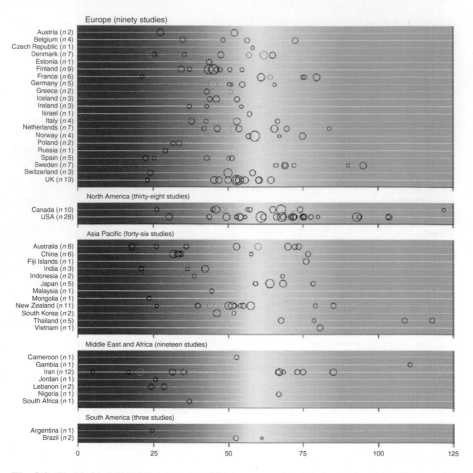

Fig. 2.1 Worldwide 25(OH)D values (nmol/L), by geographical region and country. *Note*: medians are shown in *grey circle* where mean values are not reported; Study size is indicated by *circle size*. The background *colour scheme* is intended to reflect the current uncertainty around the definition of thresholds for deficient, insufficient and adequate circulating 25(OH)D levels. Mean/median values falling within the intensely *red zone* are most consistent with severe vitamin D deficiency; those in the *green zone* reflect adequate vitamin D levels. Values within the *yellow zone* are those thought to be indicative of insufficiency (From Hilger et al. [3]; with permission)

mL (75 nmol/L), 37.3 % below 20 ng/mL (50 nmol/L), and 6.7 % below 10 ng/mL (25 nmol/L) (Fig. 2.1, reprinted from [3]). The highest 25(OH)D values were observed in North America and no sex-related differences were observed in any region. Surprisingly, age was not significantly associated with vitamin D levels in Europe or North America, in contrast to the Asia/Pacific and Middle East/Africa regions (Table 2.2, reprinted from [3]). This study also found that mean 25(OH)D values were lower in the institutionalized than non-institutionalized elderly, especially in Europe and the Asia/Pacific region.

Apart from genetic diseases causing rickets and liver insufficiency, determinants of vitamin D deficiency include factors that reduce or prevent the endogenous production of cholecalciferol, such as dark skin [38], winter season and high latitude [39], or

Table 2.2 Estimated mean circulating 25(OH) vitamin D levels (in ng/ml) (95 % confidence intervals) according to age and region, from the meta-analysis of Hilger et al. [3]

Regions	Estimated mean	(95 % CI)	n (studies)	n (participants)
Europe				
Children/adolescents	20.2	(13.7, 26.7)	6	1,816
Adults	21.2	(18.0, 22.6)	35	28,844
Elderly	20.7	(18.3, 23.1)	30	10,894
North America				
Children/adolescents	31.3	(23.8, 38.9)	3	993
Adults	28.7	(23.1, 34.4)	8	6,201
Elderly	28.7	(25.9, 31.4)	15	5,307
Asia/Pacific				
Children/adolescents	12.8	(10.0, 15.5)[a]	3	899
Adults	27.2	(23.9, 30.5)	13	3,709
Elderly	26.5	(24.9, 28.1)	9	4,965
Middle East/Africa				
Children/adolescents	30.2	(22.6, 37.8)	6	1,913
Adults	13.9	(11.7, 16.0)	6	2,079
Elderly	15.3	(11.7, 18.9)	4	874

See also Fig. 2.1
Ages for children/adolescents group, 1–17 years; adults >17–65 years, elderly >65 years
[a]Values were significantly different from those of the other age groups

lifestyles with low sun exposure or excessive sunblock use [40], and those that reduce the bioavailability of vitamin D, such as obesity [41] (Table 2.3). Although cutaneous synthesis is the main source of vitamin D, it may also come from diet, notably from fatty fish, fish oils, fortified dairy products or fruit juices, and vitamin supplements. The proportion of vitamin D needs met from these sources may vary considerably across populations [1]. Part of the individual variation in circulating 25(OH)D levels and in hormonal response may also be of genetic origin, as pointed by genome-wide association studies and investigations using a candidate gene approach. Both show that 25(OH)D levels are associated with genetic variants in or near genes involved in precursor synthesis, hydroxylation, vitamin D transport (vitamin D binding protein), and the vitamin D receptor [42–44]. Finally, some comorbidities, such as type 2 diabetes or hypertension, are more frequent in individuals with vitamin D deficiency [7].

2.4 Epidemiology of Vitamin D Deficiency in Non-end-Stage Chronic Kidney Disease

The early impairment of vitamin D metabolism in CKD is reflected by the strong decrease in the serum $1,25(OH)_2D$ level and the related SHPT that occur with kidney function decline from its early stages (Fig. 2.2 from [45]). In addition to this reduced kidney function, the decreased substrate available for hydroxylation of 25(OH)D into $1,25(OH)_2D$ may also explain part of the drop in one, $25(OH)_2D$

Table 2.3 Demographic, environmental, and lifestyle risk factors for vitamin D deficiency

Risk factors	Mechanisms
Reducing cutaneous photosynthesis of vitamin D₃	
Aging	Reduction of vitamin D precursor (7-dehydrocholesterol) levels in the skin
Dark skin	Absorption of UVB radiation by skin pigment (melanin)
Winter season and high latitude[a], time of day, air pollution, cloud cover	Reduction or absence of UVB radiation with wavelength 290 to 315 nm
Cultural behavior and clothing, sedentary lifestyle, and limited outdoor activity	Reduction of the exposure to UVB radiation
Sunscreen use	Absorption of UVB radiation by sunscreen
Decreasing vitamin D bioavailability	
Obesity[b]	Sequestration of vitamin D in body fat

Adapted from Refs. [1, 10]
Abbreviation: *VB* solar ultraviolet B
[a]Very little or no production of vitamin D₃ from November to February above 35° north latitude
[b]Inverse association between BMI and circulating 25(OH)D level

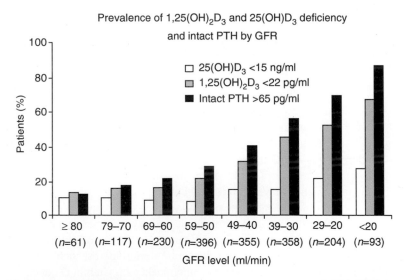

Fig. 2.2 Prevalence of 1,25(OH)₂D₃ and 25(OH)D₃ deficiency, and intact PTH by GFR intervals in the SEEK study (Reproduced with permission from Levin et al. [45])

synthesis in CKD (See Chap. 1). It is not yet known whether the relation of CKD to the decrease in 25(OH)D is direct and causal, or indirect, through potential confounders.

Certainly, individuals with CKD are at least partly at high risk for vitamin D deficiency because they are older and more likely to have dark skin, obesity, or diabetes. Because the nephrotic syndrome increases the risk of vitamin D deficiency due to the loss of both vitamin D binding protein (DBP) and the DBP/vitamin D complex in the urine [1, 35, 46, 47], lower proteinuria levels may also be independently associated with decreased serum vitamin D concentrations. Some authors also suggest a direct relation between the levels of kidney function and 25(OH)D [48]. Several large population-based (Table 2.4) and clinical studies (Table 2.5) have investigated the association between GFR and circulating 25(OH)D levels before and after adjusting for confounders.

Thus, in the US adult population from the National Health and Nutrition Examination Survey (NHANES III), the prevalence of vitamin D insufficiency (15–30 ng/mL) and deficiency (<15 ng/mL) rose significantly although slightly with increasing CKD stage (Fig. 2.3), independently of other risk factors for deficiency (Table 2.4) [11]. In the same study, when the current threshold of 20 ng/mL was applied, the prevalence estimates of vitamin D deficiency were 35.4 % and 30.3 % in participants with eGFR <60 and ≥60 mL/ min/1.73 m², respectively [49]. But after division of the eGFR level into three categories, ≥60, 30–59, and <30 mL/ min/1.73 m², vitamin D insufficiency was found only in the lowest one [17]. Both the Korean National Health and Nutrition Examination Survey (KNAHES IV) [50] and the Australian Diabetes Obesity and Lifestyle Study (AusDiab) showed a similar association, although in AusDiab it was no longer significant after adjustment for confounders. In contrast, the crude prevalence of vitamin D deficiency (<15 ng/mL) was lower in participants with CKD than without CKD in the US Multi Ethnic Study of Atherosclerosis (MESA) [51] and in the Colaus study conducted in the Lausanne region of Switzerland[52], but neither of these studies reported a multivariate analysis of the association between 25(OH)D and GFR. Another population-based study in Switzerland found no association between CKD and vitamin D status, even when the analysis was restricted to individuals receiving neither treatment nor supplementation [53]. The Rancho Bernardo study also found no such association in a community-dwelling elderly population living in southern California, but their prevalence of deficiency was extremely low (3 % with 25(OH) D < 15 ng/mL) [54]. Overall, the available general population studies show conflicting results about the existence of a higher prevalence of vitamin D deficiency in people with CKD; these results are discussed at the end of this chapter.

In clinic-based studies including patients with non-end-stage CKD, the average or median circulating 25(OH)D levels have varied from 18 to 29 ng/mL, and the prevalence of values <15 ng/mL from 9 to 59 % (Table 2.5). Most of these studies have focused on patients without vitamin D supplementation [45, 48, 55–59]. Notable exceptions were the US Chronic Renal Insufficiency Cohort (CRIC) study [60] and the Japanese Osaka study [61], which respectively included 55 % and 30 % of patients receiving supplementation. They are thus difficult to compare with other studies. Comparisons across studies are also difficult because of differences in latitude, study season, participant skin color, and assay methods between studies. However, the values of 25(OH)D have usually been lower in studies conducted in Europe and Asia than in North America, consistent with the global trend described above. Like the studies in the general population, the results of these clinical studies conflict about the existence of an association between kidney function and circulating vitamin D levels. Overall, lower vitamin D levels have been observed with lower

Table 2.4 Circulating vitamin D levels or prevalence of deficiency according to eGFR or albuminuria levels in the general population

Ref, Country, Year	Study/Population/Number	Characteristics	25(OH)D[a]	Association with eGFR[b] Crude	Association with eGFR[b] Adjusted	Association with albuminuria[c]
[11], USA, 1988–1994	National Health and Nutritional Examination Survey (NHANES) III, 15.828 participants, CKD defined by eGFR <60 mL/min/1.73 m² or eGFR ≥60 mL/min/1.73 m² and microalbuminuria (>17 mg/g in men and >25 mg/g in women)	No CKD 86.2 %; CKD stage 1 to 4–5 6.2 %, 3.5 %, 3.8 %, 0.2 %	<15 ng/mL: 8.4 % in participants with no CKD and 14.1 %, 9.1 %, 10.7 %, and 27.2 % in participants with CKD stages 1–5 respectively For distribution of vitamin D status see Fig. 2.2	Yes (+)[d]	Yes (+)[d], adjusted for age, gender, race, BMI, vitamin D intake, health insurance, educational level, family income, month, smoking, hypertension, diabetes, non-HDL cholesterol, CRP, albumin	NR
[64], USA, 1988–1994	National Health and Nutritional Examination Survey (NHANES) III, 15,068 participants	15.3 % with eGFR <60 mL/min/1.73 m², 32 % ≥60 years, 48 % men, 42 % white and 27 % black, 7 % DM	Mean (95 % CI): 28.1 (27.4–28.8) ng/mL vs 29.7 (29.0–30.5) in participants with eGFR <60 mL/min/1.73 m² vs ≥60	Yes (+)	NR	Yes, remain significant after adjustment for age, sex, race, smoking status, BMI, hypertention, diabetes and eGFR
[49], USA, 1988–1994	National Health and Nutritional Examination Survey (NHANES) III, 15,099 participants	No description	<20 ng/mL: 35.4 % vs 30.3 % in participants with eGFR <60 mL/min/1.73 m² vs ≥60 (prevalence estimated from weighted proportion)	Yes (+)	No multivariable analysis	NR

[17], USA, 1988–1994	National Health and Nutritional Examination Survey (NHANES) III, 14,679 participants	eGFR ≥90, 60–89, 30–59 and <30 mL/min/1.73 m²: 66%, 27.9%, 5.8% and 0.3%	Mean adjusted level by eGFR ≥90, 60–89, 30–59, <30 mL/min/1.73 m²: 29.3, 30.9, 30.3 and 24.6 ng/mL	NR	Yes (+), adjusted for age, gender, BMI, race, physical activity, vitamin D supplements, milk consumption, and season.	NR
[51], USA, 2000–2002	Multi Ethnic Study of Atherosclerosis (MESA), 1,370 participants	28.3% with eGFR <60 mL/min/1.73 m², mean age 64 years, 46% men, 41% white and 27% black, 13% DM	<15 ng/mL: 22.6% vs 28.4% In participants with CKD vs without CKD	Yes (−)	No multivariable analysis	No proteinuria or albuminuria reported
[54], USA, 1997–1999	Rancho Bernardo Study, 1,073 participants, community-dwelling older adults (Southern California).	Mean eGFR 74 mL/min/1.73 m², eGFR ≥90, 60–89, <60: 15%, 64%, 22%, mean age 74 years, 38% men, 9% with DM, 21% using vitamin D supplementation	Mean ± SD: 42±14 ng/mL By eGFR level (≥90 60–89<60): 42±11, 42±15, 41±13 <20 ng/mL: 3%	No	NR	NR
[50], South Korea, 2008	Korean National Health and Nutritional Examination Survey IV (KNHANES IV), 6,529 participants	Mean eGFR 84.0 mL/min/1.73 m², eGFR >90, 60–89, 44–60, <45 mL/min/1.73 m²: 33%, 61%, 6%, and 1%, mean age 49 years, 42% men, 9% DM, 9% with proteinuria (dipstick trace or +), 7% with vitamin D supplementation	<15 ng/mL: 31.3%, 29.5%, 24.3%, and 48.3%, in participants with eGFR >90, 60–89, 44–60, <45 mL/min/1.73 m² respectively	Yes (+)	Yes (+), adjusted for age, gender, season, residential area, obesity, smoking, vitamin D supplements, proteinuria, hypertension, diabetes, cardiovascular disease, anemia, hypercholesterolemia, hypertriglyceridemia, and low HDL	Yes, remained significant after adjustment for confounders including eGFR

(continued)

Table 2.4 (continued)

Ref, Country, Year	Study/Population/Number	Characteristics	25(OH)D[a]	Association with eGFR[b] Crude	Association with eGFR[b] Adjusted	Association with albuminuria[c]
[63], Australia, 1999–2000	Australian Diabetes Obesity and Lifestyle Study (Ausdiab), 10,732 participants	Mean eGFR 99.1 mL/min/1.73 m², 2.7 % with eGFR <60 mL/min/1.73 m², mean age 48.2 years, 51.1 % men, 7 % DM, 87 % white, 6.9 % with albuminuria ≥2.5 or 3.5 mg/mmol (in men and women respectively)	Mean: 22.9 and 25.2 ng/mL in participants with eGFR <60 vs >60 mL/min/1.73 m²	Yes (+)	No, adjusted for age, gender, diabetes, cholesterol, triglycerides, body mass index, smoking, race, cardiovascular disease, albuminuria, and systolic blood pressure	Yes, remained significant after adjustment for confounders including eGFR
[84], UK, 2006	Residential care home population, 188 participants, no vitamin D supplementation	Mean eGFR 47.6 mL/min/1.73 m² (stage 3A, 3B, 4: 38 %, 34 %, 10 %), 153 with eGFR <60 mL/min/1.73 m², mean age 85 years, 25 % men, 19 % DM, 100 % white	Median (IQR): 12.5 (8.3–18.6) ng/mL, by CKD stages (≥60 mL/min/1.73 m², 3A, 3B, 4): 10.0 (7.6–18.6), 12.2 (9.4–18.0), 15.1 (8.3–22.2), 10.5 (8.9–13.3) <10 ng/mL: 36 %, 10–30 ng/mL: 56 %	No	No, adjusted for age, gender, body mass index, smoking history, number of medications, length of residence, hemoglobin, diabetes mellitus, and comorbidities	No proteinuria or albuminuria reported.
[52], Switzerland, 2003–2006	CoLaus Study, 4,280 participants	Mean eGFR 85.5 mL/min/1.73 m², 4.3 %(182) with CKD (eGFR <60 mL/min/1.73 m²), mean age 52.5 years, 45.8 % men, 5.4 % DM, mainly white, 5.4 % UACR >30 mg/g	<20 ng/mL: 41.8 % vs 54.4 % in participants with CKD vs without CKD	Yes (−)	No multivariable analysis	No crude association, and no multivariable analysis

| [53], Switzerland, 2010–2011 | Swiss Study on Salt Intake, multicenter, 1,145 participants, CKD defined by eGFR <60 mL/min/1.73 m² or eGFR ≥60 mL/min/1.73 m², and albuminuria >30 mg/24 h | 11.8% (135/1145) with CKD, 48 years, 49% men, 99% white, 3% DM, mean albuminuria 11.9 mg/24 h | <20 ng/mL: 37.2% [34.2–40.3] (95% CI) vs 41.6% [33.4–50.4] in participants with and without CKD | No | No, adjusted for age, gender, BMI, education, latitude and altitude, smoking status, physical activity, alcohol consumption, diabetes and hypertension, vitamin D supplementation. Month-specific tertiles were analyzed. | NR |

CKD chronic kidney disease patients, *NR* not reported, *eGFR* estimated glomerular filtration rate *DM* diabetes mellitus, *UACR* urinary albumin to creatinine ratio

[a]Prevalence of low vitamin D status and/or mean ± SD, mean (95% CI), median(IQR) level of 25(OH)D by eGFR levels or CKD stages were reported

[b]Statistical associations between eGFR and 25(OH)D level or vitamin D status before and after adjusting for confounders: associations are reported as positive (+) when the 25(OH)D level decreased significantly – or prevalence of vitamin D deficiency increased – with decreasing eGFR level or decreasing CKD stages, and as negative (–) when this association was significantly inverse

[c]Crude and adjusted association between albuminuria or proteinuria and 25(OH)D

[d]Association with CKD stages (definition including UACR)

Table 2.5 Circulating vitamin D level or prevalence of deficiency according to eGFR or albuminuria level in clinical studies of patients with CKD

Ref, Country, Year	Study/Population/Number	Characteristics	25(OH)D[a]	Association with eGFR[b]		Association with albuminuria[c]
				Crude	Adjusted	
				Crude	Adjusted	
[55], USA, 2003	Multicenter, cross-sectional study, 201 CKD patients stage 3–4, no vitamin D prescription, none of proteinuria, DM or elevated BP	Mean eGFR 27 mL/min/1.73 m², CKD stages 3–5: 32 %, 56 % and 11 %, mean age 65 years, 64 % men, 17 % black (race available for half the participants)	Mean ± SD: 19.4 ± 13.6 ng/mL, by CKD stage 3–5: 23.3 ± 14.5, 18.6 ± 13.3, 12.0 ± 9.1 ng/mL <10 ng/mL in stage 3 and 4: 14 % and 26 %, 10–30 ng/mL: 57 % and 58 %	Yes (+)	No, adjusted for age, gender, geographic location, calcium, 1,25(OH)D, PTH, and phosphorus	No proteinuria or albuminuria reported
[45], USA, 2004	Study for the Evaluation of Early Kidney disease (SEEK), 1,814 participants with eGFR <60 mL/min/1.73 m², 153 recruitment centers across country, no vitamin D prescription	Mean eGFR 47 mL/min/1.73 m², eGFR >60 mL/min/1.73 m², 30–59, <30: 22 %, 62 %, and 16 %, respectively, mean age 70 years, 48 % men, 12 % black, 48 % DM, 35.6 % with UACR > 30 mg/g	<15 ng/mL by GFR categories (≥60, 30–59, <30): 9.1 %, 13 %, 23 % For distribution of vitamin D deficiency by GFR levels see Fig. 2.3	Yes (+)	No, adjusted for diabetes, UACR, age, sex, race, serum calcium, and phosphorus	NR
[74], USA, 2004	Seattle Kidney Study, subset of 278 CKD patients stage 1–5 not on dialysis	Mean eGFR 45.9 mL/min/1.73 m², mean age 60 years, 83 % men, 19 % black, 55 % DM, UACR 132 mg/g	Mean ± SD: 28.6 ± 14.5 ng/mL	No	No multivariable analysis	NR

[60], USA, 2003–2008	Chronic Renal Insufficiency Cohort study (CRIC), mild to moderate CKD, subset of 1,155 participants (among 3939), 45 % had no vitamin D prescription	Mean eGFR 44.8 mL/min/1.73 m², >60, 30–60 <30 mL/min/1.73 m²: 15 %, 66.5 %, 18.5 %, mean age 64 years, 53 % men, 36 % black, 37 % DM, median proteinuria 0.16 g/24 h	Mean: 21.3 ng/mL <20 ng/mL: 22.7 % of non-blacks and 62.4 % of blacks had no vitamin D supplementation, 3.8 % of non-blacks and 16.5 % of blacks did have vitamin D supplementation (Prevalence or mean level by CKD stages NR)	Yes (+)	Yes (−), adjusted for vitamin D supplementation × race, gender, age, physical activity, season, marital status, socio economic status, smoking status, dietary vitamin D, BMI, and diabetes, proteinuria, serum albumin, cause of CKD	Yes, with proteinuria (>1.5 g/day)
[48], France, 2000–2009	NephroTest, 1026 CKD patients stage 1–5 not on dialysis, subset without vitamin D prescription	Mean measured GFR 39.5 mL/min/1.73 m², CKD stage 1–2, 3a, 3b, 4 and 5: 15 %, 19 %, 31 %, 27 %, and 8 %; mean age 61.7 years, 70 % men, 9 % black, 28 % DM, UACR 89 mg/g	Median (IQR): 17.6 ng/mL (11.0, 26.8), by CKD stages 1–2, 3a, 3b, 4, and 5: 21.2 (14.0, 28.0), 18.4 (11.0, 27.6), 18.0 (11.2, 27.2), 16.0 (9.6, 24.0), 14.9 (10.9, 25.2) ng/mL For distribution of vitamin D. deficiency by CKD stages see Fig. 2.4	Yes (+)	Yes (+) with measured GFR, adjusted for age, gender, race, season, BMI, UACR, albumin, DM, systolic BP, and center	Yes (+), remained significant in the model testing association between 25(OH)D deficiency and mGFR
[21], Germany	LURIC Study, patients referred for coronary angiography but without primary kidney disease, 444 with eGFR <60 mL/min/1.73 m² (among 3316)	CKD stage 3–5: 93 %, 5 %, and 2 %, mean age 70 years, 57 % men, 56 % DM, all white	<20 ng/mL: 74.1 %	Yes (+)	NR	missing urinary measurements

(continued)

Table 2.5 (continued)

Ref, Country, Year	Study/Population/Number	Characteristics	25(OH)D[a]	Association with eGFR[b] Crude	Association with eGFR[b] Adjusted	Association with albuminuria[c]
[57], Spain	Single-center study, 1,836 CKD patients stage 1–5, 205 with 25(OH)D measurements, no vitamin D supplementation	CKD stage 1–5, respectively, 9 %, 19 %, 47 %, 19 %, 6 %; mean age 68 years, 61 % men, 29 % DM (characteristics of all patients)	Mean ± SD by CKD stage 2–5: 24.7 ± 17.8, 29.6 ± 20.7, 26.2 ± 17.9, 23.4 ± 24.3	No	No multivariable analysis	NR
[58], Italy, 2002–2003	168 incident CKD patients stage 2–5, no vitamin D supplementation	Mean eGFR 33.5 mL/min/1.73 m^2, CKD stage 2–5: 9.5 %, 40.5 %, 40.5 % 9.5 % respectively, 63 % men, mean age 70 years, 26 % DM, all white, urinary protein 0.41 g/24 h	Median (IQR): 18.1 (13–26) ng/mL <15 ng/mL: 35 %, by CKD stage 2–5: 25 %, 29 %, 37 %, 56 % 15–29 ng/mL: 46 %	Yes (+)	No multivariable analysis	Yes (−), no multivariate analysis
[61], Japan, 2005–2007	Osaka Vitamin D Study in CKD. 738 CKD patients stage 1–5 not on dialysis, 30 % with vitamin D supplementation	Mean eGFR 35 mL/min/1.73 m^2, mean age 64 years, 64 % men, 19 % DM, 73 % with proteinuria (dipstick trace and more)	Mean: 23.5 ng/mL <30 ng/mL: 83.3 %	Yes (+), below eGFR <20 mL/min/1.73 m^2	No multivariable analysis	NR
[85], Japan, year NR	135 CKD outpatients	Mean eGFR 29.6 mL/min/1.73 m^2, mean age 60 years, 53 % men, 18 % DM, median protein to creatinine ratio 0.57 g/g	Median(IQR) level by CKD stage (30–59, 15–29, <15 mL/min/1.73 m^2): 13.6 (9.5–21.8), 12.9 (7.7–18.3), 13.0 (9.5–20.2) ng/mL <15 ng/mL: 59 %	No	No multivariable analysis testing eGFR	No crude association, no multivariable analysis testing proteinuria

| [59], Thailand, 2010–2012 | 2,895 CKD outpatients with CKD stage 3a–5 not on dialysis, no vitamin D supplementation | Mean eGFR 34.2 mL/min/1.73 m², CKD stage 3a, 3b, 4, and 5: 33.2%, 28.9%, 17.8%, 20.0%, mean age 69 years, 52% male, 39% DM, albuminuria NR | By CKD stage 3a, 3b, 4, and 5: Mean level: 27.8±14.0, 25.9±11.1, 24.1±11.7, 20.8±9.9 ng/mL <30 ng/mL: 66.6%, 70.9%, 74.6%, 84.7% <10 ng/mL: 1.9%, 2.8%, 9.4%, 11.3% | Yes (+) | Yes (+), adjusted for age, gender, hemoglobin, serum albumin, calcium, phosphate, and alkaline phosphatase. | Missing urinary measurements |

CKD Chronic kidney disease patients, *NR* Not reported, *eGFR* Estimated glomerular filtration rate *DM* diabetes mellitus *UACR* urinary albumin to creatinine ratio

[a]Prevalence of low vitamin D status and/or mean ± SD, mean (95 % CI), median(IQR) level of 25(OH)D by eGFR levels or CKD stages were reported

[b]Statistical associations between eGFR and 25(OH)D level or vitamin D status before and after adjustment for confounders: association is reported as positive (+) when 25(OH)D level decreased significantly – or prevalence of vitamin D deficiency increased – with decreasing eGFR level (or decreasing CKD stages), and as negative (–) when this association was significantly inverse.

[c]Crude and adjusted association between albuminuria or proteinuria and 25(OH)D

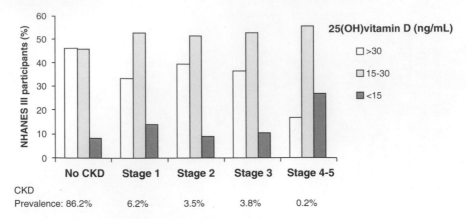

Fig. 2.3 Prevalence of vitamin D deficiency in NHANES III by CKD stage from Mehrotra et al. [11]. *Note*: Definition of stage 1 and 2 used gender-specific threshold for albuminuria: >17 mg/g (25 mg/g) creatinine in men (women)

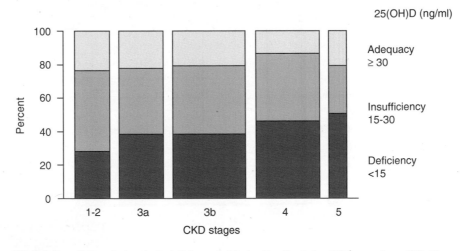

Fig 2.4 Prevalence of vitamin D deficiency in NephroTest Study by CKD stage from [48]. *Note*: Bar widths are proportional to the number of patients in each stage

kidney function [45, 48, 55, 58, 62] (Figs. 2.3 and 2.4). However, after adjusting for potential confounders, this relation remained statistically significant in two studies [48, 59], but was no longer significant in two others [45, 55] and was even significantly reversed in yet another [60].

In the French NephroTest study of 1,026 nondialysis patients with CKD stages 1–5 and no vitamin D supplementation, the prevalence of deficiency (25(OH) D < 15 ng/mL) was inversely associated with GFR measured by 51Cr-EDTA renal clearance (Fig. 2.4). In this study, the prevalence of deficiency was higher in patients of African origin or with obesity, diabetes, hypertension, albuminuria (>300 mg/g or 30 mg/mmol), or hypoalbuminemia, and during winter. After adjusting for these factors and with the reference mGFR value ≥ 60 mL/min/1.73 m^2, the odds ratios for 25(OH)D deficiency increased as mGFR decreased: 1.4 (95 % CI, 0.9–2.3), 1.4 (95 % CI, 0.9–2.1), 1.7 (95 % CI, 1.1–2.7), and 1.9 (95 % CI, 1.1–3.6) for mGFR values of 45–59, 30–44, 15–29, and finally <15 mL/min/1.73 m^2[48]. In contrast, in a subset of 1,155 CKD patients participating in the CRIC study, mean serum 25(OH) D levels were significantly lower – by 13.6 % (5.1–22.6) and 13.7 % (3.2–25.2), respectively – in those with eGFR 30–60 and <30; compared with >60 mL/ min/1.73 m^2, after adjustment for a large number of confounders including supplement use, which was high [60].

In both these CKD cohort studies – NephroTest and CRIC [48, 60] – higher albuminuria (>300 mg/g or 30 mg/mmol) and proteinuria (>1.5 g/day) levels were independently associated with lower circulating vitamin D levels. Similar results were also found in KNAHES IV [50] and AusDiab [63]. All these analyses, however, were cross-sectional and did not allow any conclusion about the chronological direction or causality of these changes. It has also been suggested that kidney damage may be a consequence rather than a cause of 25(OH)D deficiency [24, 64].

Known risk factors including season, race/ethnicity, age, and body mass index have frequently been reported as independent determinants of vitamin D status in individuals with CKD [17]. Diabetes, anemia, hypertension, and hypoalbuminemia have also been described as associated comorbidities. Only two population-based studies have explored whether CKD modifies the associations of vitamin D status with major determinants of deficiency by testing interactions with GFR level. Ausdiab found no interaction by impaired eGFR in the relations of vitamin D deficiency with gender, age, or diabetes mellitus [63]. Similarly, in the Swiss Survey on Salt Intake, there was no interaction between all-stage CKD and age, sex, body mass index, walking activity, or altitude [53].

2.5   Epidemiology of Vitamin D Deficiency in End-Stage Chronic Kidney Disease

Studies of patients on dialysis report average or median circulating levels of 25(OH) D between 12 and 32 ng/mL (Table 2.6), which are quite close to those reported in patients with non-end-stage CKD. These patients, however, are at high risk of vitamin D deficiency because they are more likely to have reduced outdoor activities and sun exposure, as well as dietary restrictions. Moreover, photoproduction of cholecalciferol in the skin was lower in hemodialysis patients than in normal healthy volunteers, probably due to the presence of uremic toxins [65]. Most of these available studies have looked at prevalent hemodialysis patients, except for two US studies of incident patients [66, 67]. Although some of these studies have large sample sizes, including several thousand individuals, none included a reference population to enable a comparison of the prevalence of 25(OH)D deficiency or its level between dialysis and nondialysis patients of similar age and sex. A few studies have included patients with all-stage CKD including a subgroup on dialysis (see [56, 68–70] in

Table 2.6 Circulating vitamin D level or prevalence of low values in adult patients on hemodialysis (HD) or peritoneal dialysis (PD)

Ref, Country, Year	Study/Population/Number	Characteristics	25(OH)D[a]	Risk factors for low vitamin D
[86], USA 2005	Single-center clinical trial, 131 HD patients included	Mean age 59 years, 37 % men, 90 % black, 41 % DM, mean duration on dialysis 5.6 years	Mean ± SD: 16.9 ± 8.5 ng/mL <30 ng/mL: 92 % <15 ng/mL: 51 %	No association with gender, diabetic status or dialysis duration Crude association with race
[66], USA, 2004–2005	Accelerated Mortality on Renal Replacement (ArMORR), prospective cohort of 10,044 incident HD patients, random sample of 907 patients	Mean age 64 years, 53 % men, 32 % black, 43 % with diabetic nephropathy	Median (IQR): 18.2 (11.3–28.0) <30 ng/mL: 79 % <20 ng/mL: 57 % <10 ng/mL: 20 %	Black race, female sex, winter season, and hypoalbuminemia (multivariable analysis using 20 ng/mL cutoff)
[67], USA, 2005–2007	Comprehensive Dialysis Study (CDS), 1432 incident dialysis patients, 192 of them with 25(OH)D measurements, 90 % HD and 10 % PD.	Mean age 62 years, 52 % men, 27 % non-white, 60 % DM.	Median: 12.6 ng/mL 15–30 ng/mL: 33 % <15 ng/mL: 65 % <20 ng/mL: 89 %	Characteristics' associated with low vitamin D after adjustment: younger age, women, winter season, current smoker, higher BMI, PD, lower albumin No association with race, diabetes, or creatinine
[87], Argentina, year NR	Cross-sectional study (2 dialysis units) of 84 HD patients, no vitamin D supplementation 25(OH)D measured at the end of winter	Mean age 59 years, 57 % men, 33 % with "moderately fair skin', 15 % with diabetic nephropathy, mean duration on dialysis 3.4 years	Mean ± SD: 24.4 ng/mL 15 ng/mL: 22.6 % 15–30 ng/mL: 53.5 %	Low sun exposure, high BMI, and female sex (multivariable analysis)
[88], Italy, year NR	Single-center cross-sectional study of 104 HD patients, no vitamin D supplementation	Mean age 53 years, 59 % men, 4 % with diabetic nephropathy, mean duration on dialysis 8 years	Mean ± SD: 32 ± 18.1 ng/mL <15 ng/mL: 14.4 % 16–30 ng/mL: 36.5 %	No association with age

[89], France, 2005–2009	ARNOS prospective cohort (24 dialysis centers in the Rhônes-Alpes region), subset of 648 (of 1348) HD prevalent patients with a 25(OH)D measurement	Mean age 67 years, 60% men, 32% DM, mean duration on dialysis 5.2 years, 22% with vitamin D supplementation	Mean ± SD: 27 ± 18 ng/mL Median: 18 ng/mL <30 ng/mL: 73%	NR
[90], France 2008	PHOTO-GRAPH (French Phosphorus and Calcium Observatory), 130 centers across country, 9,125 HD patients	Mean age 68 years, 58% men, 28% DM, mean duration on dialysis 3.2 years, 32% with native vitamin D	Mean ± SD: 21.7 ± 20 ng/mL	Not associated with age Other associations NR
[20], Netherlands, year	NECOSAD, prospective cohort study of incident dialysis patients, 762 patients (of 1,743) with blood sample available 1 year after inclusion, 64% HD	Mean age 59 years, 61% men, 20% DM	Mean ± SD: 18.2 ± 11.0 ng/mL ≤10.0 ng/mL: 25.3% 10–30 ng/mL: 61.5%	Crude association with diabetes, female sex, and PD No association with age, albumin level, or BMI
[91], Romania, 2010	Prospective cohort study of 600 HD patients from 7 HD centers. N = 600	Median age 56 years, 55% men, 15% DM, median duration on dialysis 2.8 years	In patients with and without DM, median: 21 ng/mL and 15 ng/mL <12 ng/mL: 37% and 24%	Characteristics associated with vitamin D deficiency: older age, DM, and coronary heart disease
[92], Greece and Turkey	Multicenter cross-sectional study of 273 PD patients from 20 centers	Mean age 62 years, 55% men	<15 ng/mL: 92%	Diabetes and older age (multivariable analysis)
[93], Algeria, year NR	Single-center cross-sectional study of 113 HD patients 25(OH)D measured at the end of winter	Mean age 39 years, 48% men, mean duration on dialysis 3.7 years	Median: 19 ng/mL (range 1–68)	NR

(continued)

Table 2.6 (continued)

Ref, Country, Year	Study/Population/Number	Characteristics	25(OH)D[a]	Risk factors for low vitamin D
[94], China, year NR	Single-center longitudinal study of 230 patients receiving PD	Mean age 55 years, 51 % men, 100 % Asian, 24 % with diabetic nephropathy, 30 % with DM, mean duration on dialysis 2.2 years	Median (IQR): 18.3 (14.4–24.3) ng/mL <15 ng/mL: 30 % 15–30 ng/mL: 57 %	Diabetes, female sex, and low residual GFR (multivariable analysis)
[71], Australia, 2002–2005	Single-center cross-sectional study of 242 ESRD patients treated by HD (n = 150) or PD (n = 56) or not on dialysis (n = 36), admitted for kidney transplantation and not treated with native vitamin D	Mean age 43 years, 61 % men, 88 % white and 6 % Asian, 36 % with diabetic nephropathy (mainly type 1), median time on dialysis 1.9 years	Mean ± SD: 26.8 ± 13.6 <15 ng/mL: ~18 % (28 % vs 12 % for patients with vs without DM)	Diabetes, female sex, and patients on PD (multivariable analysis)
Clinical study including hemodialysis patients and non-end-stage chronic kidney disease CKD patients				
[56], USA, year NR	Single-center cross-sectional study of 43 CKD patients stage 1–4 and 103 HD patients, no vitamin D prescription	Mean age 59.1 and 54.6 years, 37 % and 60 % men, 56 % and 85 % African American, 33 % and 39 % with diabetic nephropathy, in CKD stage 1–4 and HD participants respectively (mean duration on dialysis 3.8 years)	Mean ± SD: 18.5 ± 11.2 and 10.7 ± 6.8 ng/mL in participants with CKD stage 1–4 and HD <15 ng/mL: 44 % and 80 %	No crude association between eGFR and 25(OH)D in CKD stage 1–4 However, HD patients were significantly more VD -deficient (<15 ng/mL) than CKD stage 1–4 patients
[70], USA, 2010–2011	Single-center cross-sectional study, 58 HD patients vs 648 CKD patients stage 1–4	Mean age 59 years, 59 % men, 67 % black, 40 % DM, 4 years on HD (characteristics of CKD patients NR)	Mean ± SD: 25.7 ± 13.4 vs 23.6 ± 15.5 ng/mL in CKD stage I–V vs HD patients In HD patients: <30 ng/mL: 96.6 % <20 ng/mL: 70.7 % <10 ng/mL: 20.7 %	25(OH)D level was significantly higher in CKD patients stage 1–4 than in HD patients

| [68], France, 2006–2007 | Single-center longitudinal study, 140 patients with CKD stage 2–5 days | CKD stage 2–5 days: 8 %, 26 %, 26 %, 7 %, 33 %, mean age 67 years, 61 % men, 100 % white, 42 % DM, 36 % vitamin D supplementation | Mean ± SD: 20.5 ± 13.6 Median: 13.6 <15 ng/mL: 42 % | No crude association between CKD stage and 25(OH)D |
| [69], UK, 2007 | Single-center study. 203 CKD patients stage 1–5D (simple random sampling from one center) | Median eGFR 32 mL/min/1.73 m² (CKD stage 1 to 5D: 6 %, 16 %, 33 %, 18 %, 9 % and 18 %) median age 64 years, 64 % men, 88 % white, 20 % DM | Median (IQR): 18 (13–36), by CKD stages 1–5: 19 (15–22), 16 (12–20), 22 (16–29),15 (12–23), 17 (9–21),16 (11–25) <20 ng/mL: 62 % | No crude association between CKD stage and 25(OH)D |

NR not reported, HD hemodialysis, PD peritoneal dialysis, eGFR estimated glomerular filtration rate, DM diabetes mellitus
[a]Prevalence of low vitamin D status and/or mean ± SD, mean (95 % CI), median(IQR) level of 25(OH)D

Table 2.5), but their sample sizes were too small for multivariate analysis. Among them, a single-center study including 103 patients on hemodialysis and 43 with CKD stages 1–4 showed much lower vitamin D levels among the former, but the two groups were not comparable for age, gender, or race [56].

Risk factors for vitamin D deficiency are similar among patients with end-stage and non-end-stage CKD: winter season, race/ethnicity, older age, high BMI, and diabetes (Table 2.5). In the US ArMORR cohort of incident dialysis patients, 57 % of patients had 25(OH)D levels <20 ng/mL, but 100 % of black patients with hypo-albuminemia beginning dialysis in winter had 25(OH)D levels <20 ng/mL [66].

Peritoneal dialysis is likely to be an additional risk factor for vitamin D deficiency because of the potential loss of 25(OH)D through peritoneal fluid [35]. A study of 192 incident dialysis patients, 10 % on peritoneal dialysis, showed that this technique is associated with a 25(OH)D level 20 % lower than in patients on hemodialysis, independent of gender, age, race/ethnicity, body mass index, diabetes, and season of the assay [67]. Other studies found similar overall differences between peritoneal dialysis and hemodialysis [20, 68–71].

Relatively few studies have examined this question among patients living with a kidney transplant (Table 2.7). These patients are usually advised to avoid sun exposure because their immunosuppressive treatments create a high risk of skin cancer. In a British study comparing 31 kidney transplant patients with 31 age- and gender-matched controls without CKD, the median serum 25(OH)D level among the transplant patients was half that of the controls [72].

2.6 Discussion and Conclusions

This review shows that vitamin D deficiency is commonly observed both in CKD patients and the general population. This finding is expected given the high frequency among these patients both of known risk factors for vitamin D deficiency, such as old age, dark skin, and obesity, and of associated comorbidities, such as diabetes. It is uncertain, however, whether the relation between 25(OH)D deficiency and CKD is causal. Epidemiological studies currently provide sparse evidence about the relation between kidney function or damage and circulating 25(OH)D level.

Overall, findings from the general population and clinical studies are inconsistent. Some studies report a significant, positive, and independent association between GFR and 25(OH)D. One potential mechanism suggested to explain this association might be that CKD diminishes the skin's ability to convert 7-dehydrocholesterol into previtamin D3, but thus far this mechanism has been demonstrated only in hemodialysis patients, compared with healthy controls [65]. Another potential mechanism, shown in an experimental study using a uremic animal model [73], involves a reduction in the rate at which the liver converts cholecalciferol into 25(OH)D, mediated by PTH secretion. However, a few studies have also showed no or even an inverse association between GFR and 25(OH)D, with paradoxically higher levels of 25(OH)D in

Table 2.7 Circulating vitamin D level or prevalence of low values in adult kidney transplant recipients

Ref, Country, Year	Study/Population/Number	Population characteristics	25(OH) vitamin D[a]	Risk factors for low vitamin D
[95], Germany, 1992–1993	Single-center study, 129 kidney transplant recipients at 2,3,5,8,12,18, and 24 months after transplantation. Not treated with vitamin D	Mean age 45.4 years, 59 % men	Mean ± SD: 14.1 ± 0.9 ng/mL, 20.3 ± 1.3 and 23.7 ± 1.7 ng/mL, respectively 3, 12 and 24 months after transplantation.	Winter measurement No association with renal function Other association NR
[96], Denmark, 2005–2006	Single-center cross-sectional study of 173 kidney transplant outpatients	Median eGFR 38.9 mL/min/1.73 m². Mean age 53 years, 50 % men, 14 % diabetic nephropathy, 9 % with dark skin, median graft age 7.4 years.	Insufficiency (15–30 ng/mL): 51 % Deficiency (<15 ng/mL): 29 %	Older age, smoking, sun avoidance, high serum albumin, high BMI, low daily intakes
[72], Germany, year NR	Single-center cross-sectional study, 31 kidney transplant outpatients were matched with 31 dermatologic patients without CKD according to age and gender. Not treated with vitamin D	Mean age 52 years, 55 % men, mean graft age of 7 years	Geometric mean (95 %CI): 10.9 (8.2–14.3) ng/mL in kidney transplant recipient vs 20.0 (15.7–25.5) ng/mL in control group	NR
[97], United Kingdom, 1999–2006	Single-center study, 320 kidney transplant recipients of whom 244 were not treated with vitamin D, parathyroidectomy or corticosteroid before transplantation	Mean eGFR 45 mL/min/1.73 m², median age 46 years, 62 % men, mainly white.	<15 ng/mL: 58.2% 15–30 ng/mL: 36.9%	No association with age Other associations NR

(continued)

Table 2.7 (continued)

Ref, Country, Year	Study/Population/Number	Population characteristics	25(OH) vitamin D[a]	Risk factors for low vitamin D
[98]. Spain, year NR	Single-center study, 509 kidney transplant recipients, 378 of whom were treated with vitamin D	Mean eGFR 47.0 mL/min/1.73 m², mean age 45.4 years, 58 % men, mean graft age 9.4 years	Mean ± SD: 20.0 ± 10.6 ng/mL <15 ng/mL: 38.3 % 15–30 ng/mL: 46.9 %	No association with supplementation Women and winter measurement (multivariate analysis in untreated participants)
[99]. Brazil, year NR	Single-center study, 100 kidney transplant recipients without any of DM, impaired graft function and vitamin D supplementation	52 % stage 1–2, 48 % stage 3a, 42 years, 62 % men, mean graft age 1.5 years	<15 ng/mL: 12 % 15–30 ng/mL: 57 %	Winter measurement and high percentage of body fat in multivariate analysis

NR not reported, *eGFR* Estimated glomerular filtration rate
[a]Prevalence of low vitamin D status and/or mean ± SD, mean (95 % CI), median(IQR) level of 25(OH)D

individuals with moderate CKD than in those without CKD [50–52]. In the NHANES III study for example, the adjusted mean level of vitamin D did not differ between participants with GFR >90 and 30–59 mL/min/1.73 m², but it was significantly lower in those with GFR <30 mL/min/1.73 m² [17]. It is established that CKD patients have increased serum FGF23 levels and potentially an increased vitamin D catabolism through the stimulation of 24 hydroxylase activity; paradoxically, a reduced vitamin D catabolism has been proposed to explain the nonlinear association between eGFR and 25(OH)D observed in some studies [53]. Several recent studies have showed lower levels of 24,25-dihydroxyvitamin D, the product of 25(OH)D catabolism, in CKD patients, independent of circulating 25(OH)D level; they suggest that 24-hydroxylase regulation is impaired in patients with reduced kidney function [74–76].

Only a few epidemiological and clinical studies have examined the relations between proteinuria or albuminuria and circulating 25(OH)D levels, and they report significant negative associations [48, 50, 60, 63]. These findings tend to support the hypothesis that subnephrotic levels of proteinuria are associated with low circulating vitamin D levels [11]. Renal hydroxylation of 25(OH)D depends on the process of filtration of the vitamin D-vitamin D binding protein complex in the glomerulus followed by its active reabsorption in the proximal tubule (see Chap. 1). This process might be disturbed by increased albumin filtration and could increase vitamin D loss in urine [64]. Nonetheless, recent clinical studies in children with CKD, which have examined correlations between serum and urinary vitamin D binding protein, and total serum 25(OH)D level [77, 78], appear to have ruled out this hypothesis.

Another possible reason for the cross-sectional association of vitamin D deficiency with GFR decline or kidney damage as assessed by albuminuria is that vitamin D deficiency may be a cause rather than a consequence of CKD progression. Some recent studies have indeed found 25(OH)D and/or 1,25(OH)₂D to be significantly associated with a decline in GFR and/or end-stage renal disease [22, 24, 25, 79], although others failed to find any of these associations [23, 52, 80].

In conclusion, the questions about the relation between kidney damage or function and circulating 25(OH)D levels have yet to be resolved. Further investigations are needed: they should include individuals with and without CKD; they should measure GFR, albuminuria, and circulating level of total 25(OH)D longitudinally, together with 1,25(OH)₂D, 24,25(OH)₂D, PTH and FGF-23; and they should collect information about treatments and dietary, ecological and lifestyle risk factors for vitamin D deficiency. A better understanding of when the impairment of the vitamin D metabolism begins would help to establish evidence-based recommendations for the measurement and treatment of vitamin D deficiency in the early stages of CKD.

References

1. Holick MF. Vitamin D, deficiency. N Engl J Med. 2007;357(3):266–81.
2. Mithal A, Wahl DA, Bonjour JP, Burckhardt P, Dawson-Hughes B, Eisman JA, et al. Global vitamin D status and determinants of hypovitaminosis D. Osteoporos Int. 2009;20(11):1807–20.

3. Hilger J, Friedel A, Herr R, Rausch T, Roos F, Wahl DA, et al. A systematic review of vitamin D status in populations worldwide. Br J Nutr. 2014;111:23–45.
4. Ross AC, Manson JE, Abrams SA, Aloia JF, Brannon PM, Clinton SK, et al. The 2011 report on dietary reference intakes for calcium and vitamin D from the Institute of Medicine: what clinicians need to know. J Clin Endocrinol Metab. 2011;96(1):53–8.
5. Wagner CL, Greer FR. Prevention of rickets and vitamin D deficiency in infants, children, and adolescents. Pediatrics. 2008;122(5):1142–52.
6. Dawson-Hughes B, Mithal A, Bonjour JP, Boonen S, Burckhardt P, Fuleihan GE, et al. IOF position statement: vitamin D recommendations for older adults. Osteoporos Int. 2010;21(7): 1151–4.
7. Theodoratou E, Tzoulaki I, Zgaga L, Ioannidis JP. Vitamin D and multiple health outcomes: umbrella review of systematic reviews and meta-analyses of observational studies and randomised trials. BMJ (Clin Res ed). 2014;1:348–2035.
8. Bjelakovic G, Gluud LL, Nikolova D, Whitfield K, Wetterslev J, Simonetti RG, et al. Vitamin D supplementation for prevention of mortality in adults. Cochrane Database Syst Rev. 2014;1:007470.
9. Meyer HE, Holvik K, Lips P. Should vitamin D supplements be recommended to prevent chronic diseases? BMJ (Clin Res ed). 2015;350:h321.
10. Guessous I. Role of Vitamin D deficiency in extraskeletal complications: predictor of health outcome or marker of health status? BioMed Res Int. 2015;2015:563403.
11. Mehrotra R, Kermah D, Budoff M, Salusky IB, Mao SS, Gao YL, et al. Hypovitaminosis D in chronic kidney disease. Clin J Am Soc Nephrol. 2008;3(4):1144–51.
12. Kandula P, Dobre M, Schold JD, Schreiber Jr MJ, Mehrotra R, Navaneethan SD. Vitamin D supplementation in chronic kidney disease: a systematic review and meta-analysis of observational studies and randomized controlled trials. Clin J Am Soc Nephrol. 2011;6(1):50–62.
13. Palmer SC, McGregor DO, Craig JC, Elder G, Macaskill P, Strippoli GF. Vitamin D compounds for people with chronic kidney disease not requiring dialysis. The Cochrane Database Syst Rev. 2009;(4):CD008175.
14. Palmer SC, McGregor DO, Craig JC, Elder G, Macaskill P, Strippoli GF. Vitamin D compounds for people with chronic kidney disease requiring dialysis. Cochrane Database Syst Rev. 2009;(4):CD005633.
15. Miskulin DC, Majchrzak K, Tighiouart H, Muther RS, Kapoian T, Johnson DS, et al. Ergocalciferol supplementation in hemodialysis patients with vitamin D deficiency: a randomized clinical trial. J Am Soc Nephrol. 2015;27(6):1801–10.
16. Patel NM, Gutiérrez OM, Andress DL, Coyne DW, Levin A, Wolf M. Vitamin D deficiency and anemia in early chronic kidney disease. Kidney Int. 2010;77:715–20.
17. Chonchol M, Scragg R. 25-Hydroxyvitamin D, insulin resistance, and kidney function in the Third National Health and Nutrition Examination Survey. Kidney Int. 2007;71(2):134–9.
18. Isakova T, Gutierrez OM, Patel NM, Andress DL, Wolf M, Levin A. Vitamin D deficiency, inflammation, and albuminuria in chronic kidney disease: complex interactions. J Ren Nutr. 2011;21(4):295–302.
19. Wolf M, Shah A, Gutierrez O, Ankers E, Monroy M, Tamez H, et al. Vitamin D levels and early mortality among incident hemodialysis patients. Kidney Int. 2007;72(8):1004–13.
20. Drechsler C, Verduijn M, Pilz S, Dekker FW, Krediet RT, Ritz E, et al. Vitamin D status and clinical outcomes in incident dialysis patients: results from the NECOSAD study. Nephrol Dial Transplant. 2011;26(3):1024–32.
21. Pilz S, Iodice S, Zittermann A, Grant WB, Gandini S. Vitamin D status and mortality risk in CKD: a meta-analysis of prospective studies. Am J Kidney Dis Off J Natl Kidney Found. 2011;58:374–82.
22. de Boer IH, Katz R, Chonchol M, Ix JH, Sarnak MJ, Shlipak MG, et al. Serum 25-hydroxyvitamin D and change in estimated glomerular filtration rate. Clin J Am Soc Nephrol CJASN. 2011;6:2141–9.
23. O'Seaghdha CM, Hwang SJ, Holden R, Booth SL, Fox CS. Phylloquinone and vitamin D status: associations with incident chronic kidney disease in the Framingham Offspring cohort. Am J Nephrol. 2012;36(1):68–77.

24. Damasiewicz MJ, Magliano DJ, Daly RM, Gagnon C, Lu ZX, Sikaris KA, et al. Serum 25-hydroxyvitamin D deficiency and the 5-year incidence of CKD. Am J Kidney Dis. 2013;62(1):58–66.
25. Hamano T, Nakano C, Obi Y, Fujii N, Matsui I, Tomida K, et al. Fibroblast growth factor 23 and 25-hydroxyvitamin D levels are associated with estimated glomerular filtration rate decline. Kidney Int Suppl. 2013;3(5):469–75.
26. Holick MF, Binkley NC, Bischoff-Ferrari HA, Gordon CM, Hanley DA, Heaney RP, et al. Evaluation, treatment, and prevention of vitamin D deficiency: an endocrine society clinical practice guideline. J Clin Endocrinol Metab. 2011;96:1911–30.
27. Institute of Medicine. Dietery reference intakes for calcium and vitamin D. Washington, DC: The National Academies Press; 2011.
28. Hanley DA, Cranney A, Jones G, Whiting SJ, Leslie WD, Hanley DA, Cranney A, Jones G, Whiting SJ, Leslie WD. Vitamin D in adult health and disease: a review and guideline statement from Osteoporosis Canada (summary). CMAJ Can Med Assoc J J de l'Assoc Med Can. 2010;182(12):1315–9.
29. Bischoff-Ferrari HA, Shao A, Dawson-Hughes B, Hathcock J, Giovannucci E, Willett WC. Benefit-risk assessment of vitamin D supplementation. Osteoporos Int. 2010;21(7):1121–32.
30. Gallagher JC, Sai AJ. Vitamin D insufficiency, deficiency, and bone health. J Clin Endocrinol Metab. 2010;95:2630–3.
31. World Health Organization FAOotUN. Vitamin and mineral requirements in human nutrition. Hong Kong, China: World Health Organization; 2004.
32. Maxmen A. Nutrition advice: the vitamin D-lemma. Nat News. 2011;475(7354):23–5.
33. Kidney Disease: Improving Global Outcomes (KDIGO) CKD Work Group. KDIGO 2012 clinical practice guideline for the evaluation and management of chronic kidney disease. Kidney Inter Supp. 2013;3(1):1–150.
34. Kidney Disease: Improving Global Outcomes (KDIGO) CKD-MBD Work Group. KDIGO clinical practice guideline for the diagnosis, evaluation, prevention, and treatment of chronic kidney disease–mineral and bone disorder (CKD–MBD). Kidney Int. 2009;76 Suppl 113:S1–130.
35. Foundation NK. K/DOQI, clinical practice guidelines for bone metabolism and disease in chronic kidney disease. Am J Kidney Dis. 2003;42 Suppl 3:S1–202.
36. Metzger M, Houillier P, Gauci C, Haymann JP, Flamant M, Thervet E, et al. Relation between circulating levels of 25(OH) vitamin D and parathyroid hormone in chronic kidney disease: quest for a threshold. J Clin Endocrinol Metab. 2013;98:2922–8.
37. Hathcock JN, Shao A, Vieth R, Heaney R. Risk assessment for vitamin D. Am J Clin Nutr. 2007;85(1):6–18.
38. Chen TC, Chimeh F, Lu Z, Mathieu J, Person KS, Zhang A, et al. Factors that influence the cutaneous synthesis and dietary sources of vitamin D. Arch Biochem Biophys. 2007;460(2):213–7.
39. Kroll MH, Bi C, Garber CC, Kaufman HW, Liu D, Caston-Balderrama A, et al. Temporal relationship between vitamin D status and parathyroid hormone in the United States. PLoS One. 2015;10(3):e0118108.
40. Holick MF, Matsuoka LY, Wortsman J. Regular use of sunscreen on vitamin D levels. Arch Dermatol. 1995;131(11):1337–9.
41. Wortsman J, Matsuoka LY, Chen TC, Lu Z, Holick MF. Decreased bioavailability of vitamin D in obesity. Am J Clin Nutr. 2000;72(3):690–3.
42. Wang TJ, Zhang F, Richards JB, Kestenbaum B, van Meurs JB, Berry D, et al. Common genetic determinants of vitamin D insufficiency: a genome-wide association study. Lancet. 2010;376(9736):180–8.
43. Ahn J, Yu K, Stolzenberg-Solomon R, Simon KC, McCullough ML, Gallicchio L, et al. Genome-wide association study of circulating vitamin D levels. Hum Mol Genet. 2010;19(13):2739–45.
44. Levin GP, Robinson-Cohen C, de Boer IH, Houston DK, Lohman K, Liu Y, et al. Genetic variants and associations of 25-hydroxyvitamin D concentrations with major clinical outcomes. JAMA. 2012;308(18):1898–905.
45. Levin A, Bakris GL, Molitch M, Smulders M, Tian J, Williams LA, et al. Prevalence of abnormal serum vitamin D, PTH, calcium, and phosphorus in patients with chronic kidney disease: results of the study to evaluate early kidney disease. Kidney Int. 2007;71(1):31–8.

46. Barragry JM, France MW, Carter ND, Auton JA, Beer M, Boucher BJ, et al. Vitamin-D metabolism in nephrotic syndrome. Lancet. 1977;2(8039):629–32.
47. Schmidt-Gayk H, Grawunder C, Tschope W, Schmitt W, Ritz E, Pietsch V, et al. 25-hydroxy-vitamin-D in nephrotic syndrome. Lancet. 1977;2(8029):105–8.
48. Ureña-Torres P, Metzger M, Haymann JP, Karras A, Boffa J-J, Flamant M, et al. Association of kidney function, vitamin D deficiency, and circulating markers of mineral and bone disorders in CKD. Am J Kidney Dis Off J Natl Kidney Found. 2011;58:544–53.
49. Kramer H, Sempos C, Cao G, Luke A, Shoham D, Cooper R, et al. Mortality rates across 25-hydroxyvitamin D (25[OH]D) levels among adults with and without estimated glomerular filtration rate <60 ml/min/1.73 m2: the third national health and nutrition examination survey. PLoS One. 2012;7:e47458.
50. Oh YJ, Kim M, Lee H, Lee JP, Kim H, Kim S, et al. A threshold value of estimated glomerular filtration rate that predicts changes in serum 25-hydroxyvitamin D levels: 4th Korean National Health and Nutritional Examination Survey 2008. Nephrol Dial Transplant. 2012;27:2396–403.
51. de Boer IH, Kestenbaum B, Shoben AB, Michos ED, Sarnak MJ, Siscovick DS. 25-hydroxyvitamin D levels inversely associate with risk for developing coronary artery calcification. J Am Soc Nephrol. 2009;20(8):1805–12.
52. Guessous I, McClellan W, Kleinbaum D, Vaccarino V, Hugues H, Boulat O, et al. Serum 25-hydroxyvitamin D level and kidney function decline in a Swiss general adult population. Clin J Am Soc Nephrol. 2015;10(7):1162–9.
53. Guessous I, McClellan W, Kleinbaum D, Vaccarino V, Zoller O, Theler JM, et al. Comparisons of serum vitamin D levels, status, and determinants in populations with and without chronic kidney disease not requiring renal dialysis: a 24-hour urine collection population-based study. J Ren Nutr. 2014;24(5):303–12.
54. Jassal SK, Chonchol M, von Muhlen D, Smits G, Barrett-Connor E. Vitamin d, parathyroid hormone, and cardiovascular mortality in older adults: the Rancho Bernardo study. Am J Med. 2010;123(12):1114–20.
55. LaClair RE, Hellman RN, Karp SL, Kraus M, Ofner S, Li Q, et al. Prevalence of calcidiol deficiency in CKD: a cross-sectional study across latitudes in the United States. Am J Kidney Dis. 2005;45(6):1026–33.
56. Gonzalez EA, Sachdeva A, Oliver DA, Martin KJ. Vitamin D insufficiency and deficiency in chronic kidney disease. A single center observational study. Am J Nephrol. 2004;24(5):503–10.
57. Craver L, Marco MP, Martínez I, Rue M, Borràs M, Martín ML, et al. Mineral metabolism parameters throughout chronic kidney disease stages 1–5—achievement of K/DOQI target ranges. Nephrol Dial Transplant. 2007;22:1171–6.
58. Ravani P, Malberti F, Tripepi G, Pecchini P, Cutrupi S, Pizzini P, et al. Vitamin D levels and patient outcome in chronic kidney disease. Kidney Int. 2009;75(1):88–95.
59. Satirapoj B, Limwannata P, Chaiprasert A, Supasyndh O, Choovichian P. Vitamin D insufficiency and deficiency with stages of chronic kidney disease in an Asian population. BMC Nephrol. 2013;14:206.
60. Mariani LH, White MT, Shults J, Anderson CAM, Feldman HI, Wolf M, et al. Increasing use of vitamin D supplementation in the chronic renal insufficiency cohort study. J Ren Nutr Off J Council Ren Nutr Natl Kidney Found. 2014;24:186–93.
61. Nakano C, Hamano T, Fujii N, Matsui I, Tomida K, Mikami S, et al. Combined use of vitamin D status and FGF23 for risk stratification of renal outcome. Clin J Am Soc Nephrol. 2012;7:810–9.
62. Pilz S, Tomaschitz A, Friedl C, Amrein K, Drechsler C, Ritz E, et al. Vitamin D status and mortality in chronic kidney disease. Nephrol Dial Transplant. 2011;26(11):3603–9.
63. Damasiewicz MJ, Magliano DJ, Daly RM, Gagnon C, Lu ZX, Ebeling PR, et al. 25-Hydroxyvitamin D levels and chronic kidney disease in the AusDiab (Australian Diabetes, Obesity and Lifestyle) study. BMC Nephrol. 2012;13:55.
64. de Boer IH, Ioannou GN, Kestenbaum B, Brunzell JD, Weiss NS. 25-Hydroxyvitamin D levels and albuminuria in the Third National Health and Nutrition Examination Survey (NHANES III). Am J Kidney Dis. 2007;50(1):69–77.

65. Jacob AI, Sallman A, Santiz Z, Hollis BW. Defective photoproduction of cholecalciferol in normal and uremic humans. J Nutr. 1984;114(7):1313–9.
66. Bhan I, Burnett-Bowie S-AM, Ye J, Tonelli M, Thadhani R. Clinical measures identify vitamin D deficiency in dialysis. Clin J Am Soc Nephrol CJASN. 2010;5:460–7.
67. Anand S, Kaysen GA, Chertow GM, Johansen KL, Grimes B, Dalrymple LS, et al. Vitamin D deficiency, self-reported physical activity and health-related quality of life: the Comprehensive Dialysis Study. Nephrol Dial Transplant Off Publ Eur Dial Transplant Assoc – Eur Ren Assoc. 2011;26:3683–8.
68. Barreto DV, Barreto FC, Liabeuf S, Temmar M, Boitte F, Choukroun G, et al. Vitamin D affects survival independently of vascular calcification in chronic kidney disease. Clin J Am Soc Nephrol. 2009;4(6):1128–35.
69. Patel S, Barron JL, Mirzazedeh M, Gallagher H, Hyer S, Cantor T, et al. Changes in bone mineral parameters, vitamin D metabolites, and PTH measurements with varying chronic kidney disease stages. J Bone Miner Metab. 2011;29:71–9.
70. Krassilnikova M, Ostrow K, Bader A, Heeger P, Mehrotra A. Low dietary intake of vitamin D and vitamin D deficiency in hemodialysis patients. J Nephrol Ther. 2014;4(3):166.
71. Elder GJ, Mackun K. 25-Hydroxyvitamin D deficiency and diabetes predict reduced BMD in patients with chronic kidney disease. J Bone Miner Res Off J Am Socr Bone Miner Res. 2006;21(11):1778–84.
72. Querings K, Girndt M, Geisel J, Georg T, Tilgen W, Reichrath J. 25-hydroxyvitamin D deficiency in renal transplant recipients. J Clin Endocrinol Metab. 2006;91(2):526–9.
73. Michaud J, Naud J, Ouimet D, Demers C, Petit JL, Leblond FA, et al. Reduced hepatic synthesis of calcidiol in uremia. J Am Soc Nephrol. 2010;21(9):1488–97.
74. Bosworth CR, Levin G, Robinson-Cohen C, Hoofnagle AN, Ruzinski J, Young B, et al. The serum 24,25-dihydroxyvitamin D concentration, a marker of vitamin D catabolism, is reduced in chronic kidney disease. Kidney Int. 2012;82(6):693–700.
75. de Boer IH, Sachs MC, Chonchol M, Himmelfarb J, Hoofnagle AN, Ix JH, et al. Estimated GFR and circulating 24,25-dihydroxyvitamin D3 concentration: a participant-level analysis of 5 cohort studies and clinical trials. Am J Kidney Dis Off J Natl Kidney Found. 2014;64:187–97.
76. Stubbs JR, Zhang S, Friedman PA, Nolin TD. Decreased conversion of 25-hydroxyvitamin D3 to 24,25-dihydroxyvitamin D3 following cholecalciferol therapy in patients with CKD. Clin J Am Soc Nephrol. 2014;9(11):1965–73.
77. Prytula A, Wells D, McLean T, Balona F, Gullett A, Knott C, et al. Urinary and dialysate losses of vitamin D-binding protein in children on chronic peritoneal dialysis. Pediatr Nephrol. 2012;27(4):643–9.
78. Denburg MR, Kalkwarf HJ, de Boer IH, Hewison M, Shults J, Zemel BS, et al. Vitamin D bioavailability and catabolism in pediatric chronic kidney disease. Pediatr Nephrol (Berlin, Germany). 2013;28:1843–53.
79. Kendrick J, Cheung AK, Kaufman JS, Greene T, Roberts WL, Smits G, et al. Associations of plasma 25-hydroxyvitamin D and 1,25-dihydroxyvitamin D concentrations with death and progression to maintenance dialysis in patients with advanced kidney disease. Am J Kidney Dis. 2012;60(4):567–75.
80. de Boer IH, Sachs MC, Cleary PA, Hoofnagle AN, Lachin JM, Molitch ME, et al. Circulating vitamin D metabolites and kidney disease in type 1 diabetes. J Clin Endocrinol Metab. 2012;97(12):4780–8.
81. Benhamou C-L, Souberbielle J-C, Cortet B, Fardellone P, Gauvain J-B, Thomas T. La vitamine D chez l'adulte: recommandations du GRIO. Presse Med. 2011;40(7/8):673–82.
82. Francis R, Aspray T, Fraser W, Gittoes N, Javaid K, MacDonald H, et al. Vitamin D and bone health: a practical clinical guideline for patient management. Natl Osteoporosis Soc [Internet]. 2013.
83. Wood CL, Cheetham TD. Vitamin D: increasing supplement use among at-risk groups (NICE guideline PH56). Arch Dis Child-Educ Prac Ed. 2015:edpract-2015-308299.
84. Carter JL, O'Riordan SE, Eaglestone GL, Delaney MP, Lamb EJ. Bone mineral metabolism and its relationship to kidney disease in a residential care home population: a cross-sectional

study. Nephrol Dial Transplant Off Publ Eur Dial Transplant Assoc – Eur Ren Assoc. 2008;23:3554–65.

85. Echida Y, Mochizuki T, Uchida K, Tsuchiya K, Nitta K. Risk factors for vitamin D deficiency in patients with chronic kidney disease. Intern Med (Tokyo, Japan). 2012;51(8):845–50.

86. Saab G, Young DO, Gincherman Y, Giles K, Norwood K, Coyne DW. Prevalence of vitamin D deficiency and the safety and effectiveness of monthly ergocalciferol in hemodialysis patients. Nephron Clin Pract. 2007;105:c132–8.

87. Del Valle E, Negri AL, Aguirre C, Fradinger E, Zanchetta JR. Prevalence of 25(OH) vitamin D insufficiency and deficiency in chronic kidney disease stage 5 patients on hemodialysis. Hemodial Int Int Symp Home Hemodial. 2007;11(3):315–21.

88. Coen G, Mantella D, Manni M, Balducci A, Nofroni I, Sardella D, et al. 25-hydroxyvitamin D levels and bone histomorphometry in hemodialysis renal osteodystrophy. Kidney Int. 2005; 68(4):1840–8.

89. Jean G, Lataillade D, Genet L, Legrand E, Kuentz F, Moreau-Gaudry X, et al. Impact of hypovitaminosis D and alfacalcidol therapy on survival of hemodialysis patients: results from the French ARNOS study. Nephron Clin Pract. 2011;118(2):c204–10.

90. Pelletier S, Roth H, Bouchet JL, Drueke T, Hannedouche T, London G, et al. Mineral and bone status in French maintenance hemodialysis patients: a comparison of June 2005 and June 2008. Nephrol Ther. 2010;6(1):11–20.

91. Schiller A, Gadalean F, Schiller O, Timar R, Bob F, Munteanu M, et al. Vitamin D deficiency – prognostic marker or mortality risk factor in end stage renal disease patients with diabetes mellitus treated with hemodialysis – a prospective multicenter study. PLoS One. 2015;10(5): e0126586.

92. Taskapan H, Ersoy FF, Passadakis PS, Tam P, Memmos DE, Katopodis KP, et al. Severe vitamin D deficiency in chronic renal failure patients on peritoneal dialysis. Clin Nephrol. 2006;66(4):247–55.

93. Ghazali A, Fardellone P, Pruna A, Atik A, Achard JM, Oprisiu R, et al. Is low plasma 25-(OH) vitamin D a major risk factor for hyperparathyroidism and Looser's zones independent of calcitriol? Kidney Int. 1999;55(6):2169–77.

94. Wang AY, Lam CW, Sanderson JE, Wang M, Chan IH, Lui SF, et al. Serum 25-hydroxyvitamin D status and cardiovascular outcomes in chronic peritoneal dialysis patients: a 3-y prospective cohort study. Am J Clin Nutr. 2008;87(6):1631–8.

95. Reinhardt W, Bartelworth H, Jockenhovel F, Schmidt-Gayk H, Witzke O, Wagner K, et al. Sequential changes of biochemical bone parameters after kidney transplantation. Nephrol Dial Transplant. 1998;13(2):436–42.

96. Ewers B, Gasbjerg A, Moelgaard C, Frederiksen AM, Marckmann P. Vitamin D status in kidney transplant patients: need for intensified routine supplementation. Am J Clin Nutr. 2008;87:431–7.

97. Stavroulopoulos A, Cassidy MJ, Porter CJ, Hosking DJ, Roe SD. Vitamin D status in renal transplant recipients. Am J Transplant Off J Am Soc Transplant Am Soc Transplant Surg. 2007;7(11):2546–52.

98. Marcen R, Ponte B, Rodriguez-Mendiola N, Fernandez-Rodriguez A, Galeano C, Villafruela JJ, et al. Vitamin D deficiency in kidney transplant recipients: risk factors and effects of vitamin D3 supplements. Transplant Proc. 2009;41(6):2388–90.

99. Baxmann AC, Menon VB, Medina-Pestana JO, Carvalho AB, Heilberg IP. Overweight and body fat are predictors of hypovitaminosis D in renal transplant patients. Clin Kidney J. 2015;8:49–53.

Chapter 3
Molecular Biology of Vitamin D: Genomic and Nongenomic Actions of Vitamin D in Chronic Kidney Disease

Adriana S. Dusso

Abstract Chronic kidney disease (CKD) progression is characterized by features of accelerated aging (bone loss, increased propensity for fractures and vascular calcification, hypertension and cardiovascular disease) and a risk of mortality 20- to 30-fold higher than in age- and gender-matched individuals with normal renal function. The progressive loss of renal capacity to maintain the functional integrity of the vitamin D endocrine system is a main determinant of the severe pro-aging features that reduce survival. The goal of this chapter is an update of the progress of the last 5 years in our understanding of the molecular pathophysiology underlying CKD-induced abnormalities in: (a) Systemic and local vitamin D bioactivation to its hormonal form, 1,25-dihydroxyvitamin D or calcitriol; (b) Classical genomic and non-genomic actions of the calcitriol/vitamin D receptor (VDR) complex that compromise survival, and (c) Synergistic VDR activation by calcitriol and its precursor, 25-hydroxyvitamin D, to counteract VDR reductions.

Special focus is directed to the molecular bases supporting the paradigm switch to maximize calcitriol/VDR anti-aging actions. Specifically, from suppression of the PTH gene to attenuate the bone loss predisposing to vascular calcification, to the induction of the FGF23 and α-klotho genes to simultaneously control the pro-aging effects of hyperphosphatemia and of an excess of active vitamin D, while maintaining the plethora of anti-aging/pro-survival actions of renal and circulating klotho. Special attention is also directed into calcitriol/VDR distinct control of Wnt/β--catenin signals to promote mineralization in bone while preventing calcification in the vasculature, and into the emerging fields of calcitriol/VDR regulation of microRNA synthesis and klotho-independent anti-aging actions. This mechanistic knowledge is a mandatory first step to evaluate the accuracy of current biomarkers of disease severity and response to therapy.

Keywords Vitamin D receptor • 1,25-dihydroxyvitamin D • FGF23 • Klotho • Parathyroid hyperplasia • Vascular calcification • Mortality

A.S. Dusso, PhD
Bone and Mineral Research Unit, Instituto Reina Sofía de Investigación Nefrológica,
REDinREN del ISCIII, Hospital Universitario Central de Asturias, Oviedo, Asturias, Spain
e-mail: adriana.dusso@gmail.com; adusso@hca.es

© Springer International Publishing Switzerland 2016
P.A. Ureña Torres et al. (eds.), *Vitamin D in Chronic Kidney Disease*,
DOI 10.1007/978-3-319-32507-1_3

3.1 Introduction

Chronic kidney disease (CKD) affects 11 % of the world population and is a disorder characterized by accelerated aging and by morbidity and mortality rates 20- to 30-fold higher than in gender- and age-matched individuals with normal renal function [1, 2].

CKD-induced pro-aging features include impaired intestinal calcium absorption and renal phosphate excretion, two main contributors to secondary hyperparathyroidism (SHPT) and, consequently, to abnormal bone remodeling and defective mineralization, all of which increase the propensity for bone mass loss, fractures, vascular and soft tissue calcifications [3]. High serum phosphorus is also associated with increases in inflammatory and pro-fibrotic signals causing multiple organ damage [4]. Hypertension, common in these patients, further aggravates the arterial stiffness associated to calcium deposition, as well as renal and cardiovascular damage, thus worsening the already high risk of cardiovascular mortality [5]. Impaired immune function impedes an adequate control of systemic inflammation causing multiple organ damage and also predisposing to viral and bacterial infections, autoimmune diseases and cancer further aggravating the risk for all-cause mortality [6].

CKD, hypertension and systemic inflammation are the main downregulators of renal levels of the longevity gene α-klotho (klotho), the only known gene whose absence is sufficient to accelerate aging and shorten lifespan [7]. Significantly, exclusive ablation of renal klotho fully reproduces the accelerated renal and cardiovascular aging, vascular calcification and high mortality of the global klotho-null mouse [8] and advanced CKD patients [9]. Clearly, strategies directed to maintain renal klotho in CKD should help improve clinical outcomes.

The progressive loss of the capacity of the damaged kidney to maintain the integrity of the vitamin D endocrine system is a main contributor to the pro-aging features that markedly increase mortality rates. In fact, large epidemiological studies in otherwise healthy individuals have demonstrated that vitamin D deficiency is associated with an increased relative risk for cardiovascular and all-cause mortality [10, 11].

The goal of this review is an in depth re-evaluation of our understanding of the abnormalities in vitamin D bioactivation and classical or non-classical genomic and non-genomic vitamin D actions that compromise survival in the course of CKD.

3.2 Abnormalities in Vitamin D Bioactivation in CKD

Vitamin D is not a vitamin, as our body can produce it, but an inactive pro-hormone which exerts its biological actions only upon a two-step bioactivation to the potent calcitropic steroid hormone 1,25-dihydroxyvitaminD (1,25D or calcitriol). As depicted in Fig. 3.1, [12] in mammals, skin exposure to sun light of the ultraviolet B range (UV-B) converts 7-dehydrocholesterol into vitamin D_3 (cholecalciferol) [12],

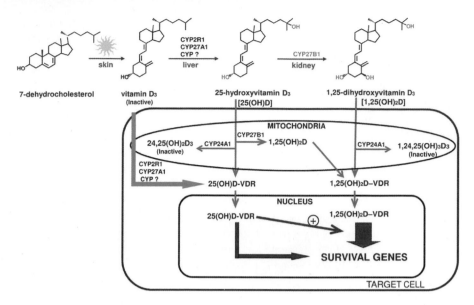

Fig. 3.1 Vitamin D and VDR activation. Systemic and cellular vitamin D activation, degradation and transcriptional regulation by liganded-VDR

a conversion completely prevented by sun blockers [13]. Next, cholecalciferol is 25-hydroxylated mainly in the liver by two cytochromes p450s, mitochondrial CYP27A1 and microsomal CYP2R1. CYP2R1 has emerged as the most critical Vitamin D-25-hydroxylase because mutations in this enzyme, but not in CYP27A1, result in severe vitamin D deficiency [14] (serum 25-hydroxyvitamin D (25(OH)D) levels below 10 ng/ml). Note that serum 25(OH)D and not serum vitamin D levels, are used to estimate vitamin D status. This is because vitamin D measurements require assays too complex for routine biochemistry laboratories. Importantly, 25(OH)D levels accurately estimate vitamin D status because 25-hydroxylases efficaciously convert most circulating vitamin D into 25(OH)D [15]. The tissue distribution and the regulation of 25-hydroxylase expression and activity in health and in CKD are poorly understood. In fact, in 2014, the simultaneous ablation of the CYP27A1 and CYP2R1 genes revealed the existence of a yet unknown 25-hydroxylase, which contributes up to 50 % of circulating 25(OH)D [16].

The 1α-hydroxylation of 25-hydroxyvitaminD [25(OH)D] to produce calcitriol, the most active endogenous vitamin D metabolite, is the most critical and tightly regulated step in vitamin D bioactivation. This step is catalyzed by the mitochondrial cytochrome p450 CYP27B1 [17] and occurs mainly, but not exclusively, in renal proximal tubular cells. Indeed, the kidney is the main, if not the only, contributor to circulating calcitriol, at least under physiological conditions. Therefore, for almost three decades, nephrologists have used oral or intravenous calcitriol therapy to correct the defective renal calcitriol production by a failing kidney.

In addition to the kidney, numerous cell types express CYP27B1 and produce calcitriol in a cell/tissue specific manner. Extrarenal calcitriol production is of high clinical relevance beyond CKD, as the multiple health disorders associated to vitamin D deficiency occur in spite of normal serum calcitriol. The low serum 25(OH) D levels of vitamin D deficiency reduces local calcitriol synthesis by non-renal cyp27B1s, which in turn compromises tissue specific activation of the vitamin D receptor (VDR), a requirement for most vitamin D biological actions. In fact, not only at early CKD stages vitamin D supplementation is sufficient to correct the elevations in serum PTH [18, 19], but also 25(OH)D levels below 23 ng/ml (mild vitamin D insufficiency) in pre-dialysis patients are independently associated with an accelerated CKD progression upon adjustment for all potential confounders [20].

The benefits of an early correction of vitamin D deficiency in CKD patients is that it may suffice to achieve the desired tissue specific activation of the VDR, with minimal, if any, impact on circulating calcitriol. Preventing elevations in serum calcitriol reduce the risks of hypercalcemia and hyperphosphatemia from increased intestinal calcium and phosphorus absorption [12]. Accordingly, current clinical guidelines recommend supplementation with nutritional vitamin D to correct vitamin D deficiency at all CKD stages, prior to any intervention with calcitriol or its analogs (referred to as active vitamin D molecules) [21].

The high incidence of vitamin D deficiency at all stages of CKD [22] has led to the discovery of the crucial role of a normal kidney function to maintain normal serum 25(OH)D: The uptake of 25(OH)D from the urinary ultrafiltrate and its recycling back to the circulation. Briefly, 25(OH)D, a lipid soluble molecule, circulates in the blood bound to its carrier, the vitamin D binding protein (DBP), with a molecular weight similar to that of albumin. The 25(OH)D/DBP complex is filtered through the glomerulus and re-enters proximal tubular cells through a process of endocytosis that requires adequate tubular levels of the endocytosis receptor megalin [23]. In CKD, the early loss of renal megalin [24] contributes to the impaired renal uptake of 25(OH)D to maintain renal and circulating 25(OH)D levels that ensure adequate renal and extrarenal calcitriol production.

The reductions in renal megalin in CKD also contribute to: (a) Proteinuria, by impairing megalin-mediated reabsorption of small molecular weight proteins; (b) Phosphate retention, by impairing megalin-mediated NaPi2a endocytosis from the cell surface in response to PTH or FGF23[25]. Interestingly, vitamin D induces the expression of renal megalin [26]. Thus, the early correction of vitamin D deficiency in CKD may attenuate renal megalin reductions, thereby improving not only renal and extrarenal calcitriol production, but also the adverse cardiovascular effects of proteinuria and the pro-aging actions of hyperphosphatemia.

3.3 Abnormalities in Genomic and Non-genomic Calcitriol/ VDR Actions in CKD

Once calcitriol is synthesized in the kidney or extrarenally, most of its biological actions require calcitriol binding to the VDR, a member of the thyroid/retinoid nuclear receptor superfamily. For the so called "classical" vitamin D/VDR actions

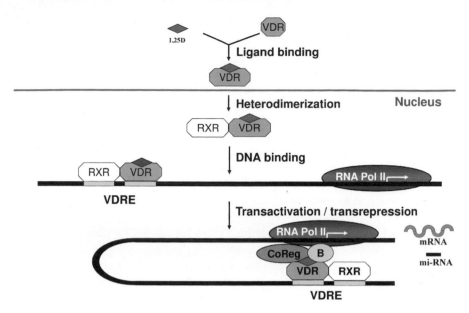

Fig. 3.2 Transcriptional regulation by the calcitriol/VDR complex. Multiple protein-protein and protein-DNA interactions upon ligand binding to the VDR that facilitate the recruitment to the transcriptional initiation complex of basal transcription factors (*B*) and coregulators (*Co-reg*) that mediate vitamin D regulation of mRNA and/or micro RNA (*mi-RNA*) expression

(summarized in Fig. 3.2) upon ligand binding, the VDR molecule undergoes a conformational change that facilitates heterodimerization with the retinoid X receptor (RXR) and the binding of the VDR/RXR complex to vitamin D responsive sequences (VDREs) on the promoter regions of vitamin D responsive genes [27] to induce/repress their expression. There is variability in VDRE sequences, but those associated with the highest affinity for VDR consist in two direct imperfect repeats with a spacer of 3 nucleotides (DR3). Chromosome conformation capture technology has demonstrated multiple simultaneous rather than a single site for binding of the ligand-activated VDR/RXR complex within 100 Kb either 5′ or 3′ from the transcription start site of a target gene [28]. Chromatin looping juxtaposes distal and more proximal VDREs thus facilitating the simultaneous recruitment of basic transcription factors, co-activator and/or co-repressor molecules to multiple VDR-RXR/VDRE complexes, as demonstrated for calcitriol potent induction of the RANKL gene, critical for calcitriol-driven osteoclastogenesis and bone resorption [29].

Similar single or super-complexes of VDR/RXR bound to DNA transcriptionally activate/repress the expression of the 500 to 1,000 genes that regulate a healthy aging, and consequently, the survival benefits of a normal vitamin D status. The most characterized of these calcitriol/VDR genomic actions include the suppression of PTH synthesis, induction of the phosphaturic hormone FGF23, the longevity gene klotho, the calcium channel TRPV6 in enterocytes, the rate limiting step in intestinal calcium absorption, the parathyroid calcium sensing receptor or of the receptor of the canonical Wnt pathway LRP5 in bone, all essential effectors for normal skeletal development and mineralization, as thoroughly reviewed in [27].

In addition, VDRE sequences for VDR/RXR binding have been found in gene promoters that drive the expression of micro RNAs (Fig. 3.2) [30]. Micro RNAs are short (18–25 nucleotides) non-coding RNAs that control the expression of 30 % of the genes in the genome through binding to the 3′ untranslated region (UTRs) of target mRNA decreasing either mRNA stability or protein translation. An example is calcitriol upregulation of microRNA-145 (miR-145), a recently identified mechanism for calcitriol suppression of proliferation in gastric cancer [31]. Importantly, miR-145 is the most abundant microRNA in normal vascular smooth muscle cells and it is downregulated in proliferative vascular diseases [32] suggesting a role for calcitriol induction of miR-145 in the vascular protective actions of calcitriol and analogs.

Additional mechanisms for calcitriol/VDR regulation of microRNA levels include the control of the microRNA processing machinery or of the chromatin opening upon VDR binding to increase the accessibility for transcription factors that induce/repress micro RNA transcription [33]. In fact, calcitriol upregulates KHSRP and TARDBP, two proteins involved in the biogenesis and maturation of micro RNA in colon cancer cells [34].

Several "non-classical" calcitriol/VDR genomic actions involve an indirect control of the expression of an apparent target through the transcriptional control of an essential inducer or repressor. Examples include: (a) Calcitriol induction of the growth suppressor p27 through direct transrepression of p45(Skp2) which bind-sp27to induce its proteosomal degradation [35]; (b) Calcitriol suppression of ADAM17 gene expression to control parathyroid hyperplasia, through the induction of C/EBPβ [36]; (c) Calcitriol 30-fold induction of FGF23, which is markedly attenuated by cycloheximide, an inhibitor of new protein synthesis. This suggests that, in addition to a mild direct induction of the FGF23 gene, calcitriol suppression/induction of a yet unknown mediator is required for the full transactivation of the FGF23 gene [37].

In addition, the calcitriol/VDR complex binds transcriptional regulators and modifies their transcriptional activity, in signaling pathways unrelated to vitamin D biological actions, as demonstrated for VDR inhibition of Wnt activation through physical VDR interactions with β-catenin outside bone [38]. Also, direct protein-protein interactions of calcitriol/VDR complexes with Sirt1 and FOXO proteins, which control aging processes, which modify their cellular function prolonging survival [39].

The calcitriol/VDR complex also affects the rates of mRNA translation. This is a highly needed process when cells need to mount acute responses upon life threatening conditions such as starvation or strong growth signals. These vitamin D actions include both suppression of mTOR as demonstrated in breast cancer [40] and induction of autophagy, through direct upregulation of essential autophagy genes, as demonstrated for VDR protection from immune dysfunction of the intestinal barrier by Paneth cells, thus maintaining the homeostasis of the microbiota [41].

Calcitriol also exerts rapid "non-genomic" actions occurring within minutes of exposure to calcitriol. Some of these less characterized rapid actions also involve the cytosolic VDR, although other potential receptors have been identified [12]. These rapid actions regulate intracellular calcium fluxes, the degree of protein phosphorylation, acetylation and subcellular localization which, by affecting protein function, greatly modify classical and non-classical direct and indirect genomic signals (Reviewed in [12]). An emerging relevant field is the impact of rapid vitamin D actions on pathways regulating the stability and/or processing of microRNAs [34].

For most biological actions, the intracellular levels of both calcitriol and VDR determine the magnitude of calcitriol/VDR complex formation and with it, the efficacy for direct or indirect gene transactivation/transrepression by the 1,25D/VDR complex, and both are reduced in CKD [17]. The development of calcitriol analogs that selectively maintain the benefits of VDR activation with less calcemic or phosphatemic activity [42] has helped therapeutically. They allow compensating the resistance to therapy caused by CKD-induced VDR reductions through safer escalation of analog dosage. However, therapies with high doses of calcitriol or its analogs could reduce the levels of intracellular calcitriol (analog) available to bind VDR by inducing CYP24A1 (See Fig. 3.1). This enzyme, responsible for calcitriol (analog) degradation, is constitutively expressed in the kidney, and strongly induced by either calcitriol or its analogs in every vitamin D target tissue to avoid/reduce the toxicity associated to an excess of active vitamin D [27].

Decreases in cellular levels of the VDR partner for its genomic actions, the retinoid X receptor (RXR), as well as uremic toxin-induced reductions of 1,25D/VDR-RXR binding to DNA, further impair the response of these patients to vitamin D therapy (Reviewed in [43]).

Figure 3.1 also presents a previously unrecognized synergy between 25(OH)D and calcitriol for VDR activation that could be exploited to safely improve clinical outcomes in CKD without increasing calcitriol doses. Studies in the CYP27B1 null mouse [44], which lacks the enzyme that converts 25(OH)D to calcitriol, and also in vitro, using 25(OH)D analogs chemically modified to prevent hydroxylation at carbon 1[45, 46], have demonstrated that 25(OH)D can not only activate the VDR directly, but more importantly, it can synergize with calcitriol activation of the VDR. As will be discussed below, this synergy is sufficient to overcome the parathyroid resistance to low doses of calcitriol (or its analogs) caused by VDR reductions and accumulation of uremic toxins even in advanced CKD [36]. Importantly, this safe synergy can be achieved simply by ensuring normal serum 25(OH)D through nutritional vitamin D supplementation [36].

The ubiquitously distributed 25-hydroxylases are not as tightly regulated as the constitutive renal CYP27B1 and CYP24A1, thus providing a safe alternative to enhance survival by counteracting with local 25(OH)D synthesis the reductions in intracellular levels of the calcitriol/VDR complex induced by CKD. A better understanding of the modulators of the tissue specific expression and activity of 25-hydroxylases in CKD could improve current recommendations to enhance the survival benefits of a normal vitamin D status in these patients.

The next section will update our understanding of the most critical vitamin D actions to attenuate CKD progression and improve clinical outcomes:

1. Suppression of PTH synthesis, parathyroid hyperplasia and the onset of vitamin D resistance;
2. Maintenance of skeletal and vascular integrity unrelated to the attenuation of secondary hyperparathyroidism;
3. Induction of bone FGF23 production and renal klotho content to prevent/attenuate hyperphosphatemia;
4. Downregulation of systemic disorders that reduce renal klotho;
5. Induction of anti-aging actions unrelated to maintenance of renal klotho;

For each of these actions critical for survival, this review will examine:

(a) What is indisputably known on the subject at the molecular level?
(b) What are the findings from the last 5 years that have challenged our current understanding of the pathogenesis of the pro-aging disorder?
(c) How might the new knowledge impact clinical practice regarding both, the safety of current therapeutic strategies with vitamin D and the accuracy of commonly used biomarkers?

3.4 Vitamin D Suppression of PTH Synthesis, Parathyroid Hyperplasia and the Onset of Vitamin D Resistance

Near all patients with end stage renal disease develop SHPT. Because of the severe adverse impact of SHPT on morbidity and mortality, the parathyroid gland is one of the best studied targets of vitamin D actions. Figure 3.3 summarizes the multiple calcitriol/VDR actions involved in the suppression of PTH synthesis and hyperplastic growth.

Hypocalcemia, hyperphosphatemia and vitamin D deficiency are the main causes of SHPT [47]. The calcitriol/VDR complex suppresses PTH synthesis through a direct binding to a "classical" negative VDRE on the PTH gene promoter [27].

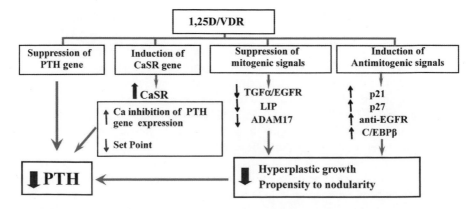

Fig. 3.3 Vitamin D regulation of parathyroid hyper function in CKD

Vitamin D and/or calcitriol deficiency also impair the response of the parathyroid gland to calcium due to reductions in parathyroid content of the calcium sensing receptor (CaSR), as demonstrated in vitamin D deficient rats [48] and CKD patients [49]. In fact, the CaSR gene is directly induced by calcitriol through VDR/RXR binding to VDREs in this gene promoter [50].

Calcitriol induction of FGF23 synthesis in bone cells of the osteoblastic/osteocyte lineage provides an additional indirect mechanism for vitamin D suppression of PTH secretion and parathyroid hyperplasia, provided there is sufficient parathyroid klotho [51], another gene induced by the calcitriol/VDR complex [27].

The prolonged persistence of hypocalcemia or vitamin D deficiency induces parathyroid cell proliferation to meet the requirements for higher serum PTH to normalize serum calcium. Also, hyperphosphatemia directly stimulates parathyroid hyperplasia [52]. The severity of parathyroid cell growth determines not only higher serum PTH but also marked reductions in parathyroid VDR, CaSR, FGF receptors, and cell membrane klotho, which impair PTH suppression by active vitamin D, oral calcium or increases in FGF23.

The reports of increased TGFα in parathyroid adenomas and in diffuse and nodular glands from CKD patients [53] were critical to identify the essential role of TGFα activation of its receptor, the EGF receptor (EGFR), in the severity of parathyroid hyperplasia and VDR reductions [54]. Briefly, as summarized in Fig. 3.4, the release of mature TGFα from its transmembrane precursor by ADAM17, an enzyme essential for parathyroid gland development [36], initiates a powerful

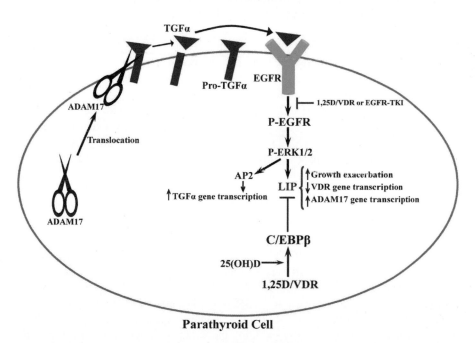

Parathyroid Cell

Fig. 3.4 Pathogenesis of parathyroid hyperplasia and VDR reduction in CKD. The vicious ADAM17/TGFα-EGFR cycle for exacerbated parathyroid growth and VDR reduction is safely and effectively counteracted by synergistic interactions between 25(OH)D and calcitriol through the induction of C/EBPβ

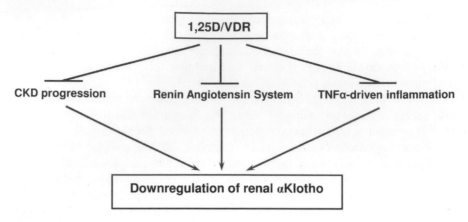

Fig. 3.5 Vitamin D maintenance of renal klotho content in CKD

autocrine loop for excessive TGFα/EGFR-growth signals because TGFα induces its own gene expression [55] and that of the ADAM17 gene [36], in part through increases in AP2 and LIP, respectively. The oncogene LIP is responsible for the suppression of VDR gene expression [54] and may contribute to the transformation of parathyroid growth from diffuse to nodular [56].

The parathyroid phenotype of nephrectomized mice harboring a parathyroid-specific EGFR inactivation has conclusively demonstrated the essential role of EGFR activation in CKD-driven parathyroid hyperplasia, TGFα self-induction and VDR reductions [57]. Interestingly, CKD-induced parathyroid klotho reductions persisted in the transgenic mice despite the absence of parathyroid hyperplasia or VDR reductions suggesting that the calcitriol/VDR complex is not the main determinant of parathyroid klotho content (Fig. 3.5).

The increased parathyroid COX2 expression and prostaglandin E2(PGE2) production reported in the hyperplastic glands of advanced CKD [58] could aggravate EGFR growth signals, as PGE2 transactivates the EGFR [59]. Calcitriol decreases COX2 expression and increases 15-hydroxy prostaglandin dehydrogenase resulting in reduced prostaglandin synthesis through unknown mechanisms [60, 61]. Furthermore, the induction of COX2 expression downstream from EGFR activation in epithelial tumors [62] supports the therapeutic relevance of effectively targeting EGFR signaling.

Different from PTH suppression, or from the induction of the growth suppressors p21 [63] and p27, calcitriol/VDR control of TGFα/EGFR driven hyperplasia involves non "classical" genomic mechanisms including (a) Sequestration of activated EGFR in early endosomes [64]; (b) Induction of C/EBPβ to simultaneously counteract TGFα/EGFR-induction of LIP, ADAM17 and VDR suppression [36].

Calcitriol/VDR suppression of ADAM17 gene expression, a target upstream from EGFR activation, partially explains the synergy between calcitriol and the EGFR-specific tyrosine kinase inhibitor Erlotinib in controlling parathyroid hyperplasia in 5/6 nephrectomized rats fed high dietary phosphorus. Significantly, this Erlotinib/calcitriol synergy that cannot be used in renal patients can be safely mimicked in vivo by the combination of 25(OH)D and the calcitriol analog paricalcitol (Fig. 3.4). In fact, at doses of 25(OH)D that correct vitamin D deficiency but, at doses of either monotherapy insufficient per se to suppress serum PTH or parathyroid cell growth, the 25(OH)D + paricalcitol combination effectively suppressed parathyroid ADAM17 resulting in a 50% reduction of serum PTH [36]. Despite similar serum calcium, this PTH suppression was superior to that of calcitriol/Erlotinib treatment [36]. Mechanistically, both, parathyroid calcitriol synthesis, and the synergy between 25(OH)D and calcitriol for VDR activation reported in in vitro studies, can partly explain the higher efficacy of the combination to inhibit parathyroid ADAM17. The translational message from these findings is that they may explain why the correction of vitamin D deficiency could be insufficient to reduce serum PTH even at early CKD stages [18]. Also, promoting this synergy may also benefit advanced CKD patients whose hypercalcemia or hyperphosphatemia impedes escalating with the dose of active vitamin D. A key therapeutic consideration before extrapolating from these preclinical findings is that oral formulations may not be as safe as the i.p. route used in these studies. The same 25(OH)D/active vitamin D synergy on intestinal VDR could increase calcium and phosphorus absorption aggravating hypercalcemia or hyperphosphatemia.

In view of the efficacy of rapamycin, an mTOR inhibitor, in suppressing parathyroid hyperplasia [65], a role for calcitriol/VDR suppression of mRNA translation in the control of TGF/EGFR induction of LIP synthesis should not be ruled out, as it occurs in breast cancer.

For decades, the safe control of serum PTH by calcitriol (analogs), avoiding hypercalcemia, hyperphosphatemia and PTH oversuppression, has been the treatment of choice for renal osteodystrophy. Indeed, a report from the COSMOS study, a large prospective study with a 3 year follow up of the clinical handling of CKD-5D patients throughout Europe, has provided the optimal range within the U curve for serum PTH that associates with the lowest relative risk of mortality [66] and has also corroborated the survival benefits of correcting serum PTH to achieve values within the optimal range. However, the report that serum levels of the Wnt inhibitor sclerostin were better markers than PTH to reflect poor bone health (assessed by bone biopsies) in CKD patients [67] raised the attention of nephrologists to CKD-induced abnormalities in bone Wnt signals. The next section addresses vitamin D actions to maintain bone health including induction of osteoblastic Wnt signaling and the accuracy of circulating levels of Wnt inhibitors to reflect a poor bone health.

3.5 Vitamin D Maintenance of Skeletal and Vascular Integrity Unrelated to the Attenuation of Secondary Hyperparathyroidism

The essential role of vitamin D for normal skeletal development and mineralization has been known since the discovery that vitamin D deficiency was the cause of rickets, more than a century ago. The combination of vitamin D and/or calcitriol insufficiency and low VDR in bone cells contributes to the wide range of bone disorders in CKD.

Initial studies in the VDR null mouse suggested that VDR was dispensable for the ossification process, as non-visible abnormalities in bone mineral density were observed if there was an adequate supply of calcium and phosphorus by the so called rescue diet [68]. However, comprehensive studies in the VDR null, 1α-hydroxylase null, and PTH null mice and multiple double knock-out combinations demonstrated calcitriol essential actions for a healthy bone. These include the induction of osteoblastogenesis, skeletal anabolism and the appropriate coupling of osteoblastic and osteoclastic activity [69, 70]. Indeed, the calcitriol/VDR complex regulates the expression of genes that control both bone formation, mineralization and remodeling (osteopontin, osteocalcin and, importantly, the Wnt receptor LRP5) as well as osteoclastogenesis and bone resorption genes (RANK ligand and osteoprotegerin) through classical genomic actions (Reviewed in [27]).

In health, the prevalence of bone formation over resorption depends upon the physiological or supraphysiological concentrations of serum calcitriol. Also, comparison of calcitriol and paricalcitol actions in bone, in mouse and rat CKD models, have demonstrated that despite differences in osteoclastogenic potency, both compounds similarly maintained bone anabolism [71, 72]. Indeed, not only high calcitriol potently induces RANK ligand (RANKL) but it also suppresses the expression of its decoy receptor osteoprotegerin (OPG) to amplify resorptive signals. In CKD, defective calcitriol/VDR induction of osteopontin could not only adversely impact ossification and remodeling but also osteoclast recruitment to resorb ectopic bone (reviewed in [27]). Similarly, impaired induction of osteocalcin could negatively affect bone strength and energy metabolism through osteocalcin-mediated insulin release [73]. Calcitriol actions in cells of the osteoblastic lineage also depend on their stage of differentiation being anabolic and anticatabolic in more mature cells, as demonstrated by overexpression of the VDR in mature osteoblasts in vivo [74]. The conflicts regarding net calcitriol actions in bone may result in part from the coexistence of all of these distinct cell maturation stages.

The VDR also induces the LRP5 gene, involved in Wnt pathway activation, a process critical for skeletal development and mineralization. Although LRP5 induction by the VDR appears to occur regardless of calcitriol binding, intracellular calcitriol levels determine cytosolic VDR content, as calcitriol binding protects the VDR from proteosomal degradation [75].

CKD-induced defects in Wnt signaling in osteocytes and osteoblasts have been the focus of intensive research due to the progressive accumulation of the Wnt inhibitors sclerostin and Dkk1 with CKD progression [67] and, more significantly, because of the strong association between impaired Wnt activity, bone loss and increased vascular calcification [76].

Importantly, in CKD, impaired Wnt activation in bone occurs before elevations in serum PTH, as demonstrated in a mouse model of polycystic kidney disease [77]. The early increases in bone sclerostin causing bone loss in these mice could be prevented with an antibody against TGFβ [78], the most abundant cytokine in bone. This suggests an early onset of CKD-induced increases in TGFβ signaling for Wnt inhibition. Studies in 7/8 nephrectomized (NX) rats fed either normal or high phosphorus demonstrated similar bone sclerostin levels at week 8 after NX despite marked differences in serum P, PTH, FGF23 and renal damage between dietary groups, thus corroborating the independence of this early increase in bone sclerostin of the severity of SHPT [79]. Furthermore, in both mouse and rat CKD models, bone sclerostin decreased below the level of sham operated controls as PTH and FGF23 increased, while elevations in bone levels of several Wnt inhibitors other than sclerostin, including Dkk1, parallel the progressive loss of bone mass [77–79]. Accordingly, bone biopsies in CKD patients corroborated Wnt inhibition despite the lower number of osteocytes positive for sclerostin [77]). Undoubtedly, these findings challenge the accuracy of serum sclerostin to reflect the degree of bone Wnt inhibition or even sclerostin levels in bone. More importantly, they provide a previously unrecognized mechanism for the abnormalities in the vitamin D endocrine system in CKD to affect the bone-vasculature axis from early CKD stages: Impaired activation of Wnt signals in bone. Indeed, even disregarding the induction of LRP5 by unliganded VDR, a normal vitamin D status could attenuate the adverse TGFβ/Smad signaling on bone. In fact, VDR signaling antagonizes a range of TGFβ/Smad-dependent transcriptional activation of profibrotic genes through the recruitment of VDR to loci on these genes that prevent/attenuate Smad3 binding [80].

Importantly, vitamin D regulation of Wnt signaling is tissue specific. In contrast to bone, in the kidney and the vasculature, vitamin D inhibits Wnt signals [81, 82] through VDR binding to β-catenin in the cytosol to prevent its translocation to the nucleus [38] thereby attenuating the adverse impact on Wnt activation on the progression of renal damage and vascular calcification.

In addition, calcitriol/VDR transactivation of the FGF23 gene in osteocytes and osteoblasts is an essential pro-survival action, as the dominant role of FGF23 is the renal elimination of phosphorus to prevent hyperphosphatemia and its pro-aging consequences. Indeed, the main features of the FGF23-null mouse are hyperphosphatemia, high circulating calcitriol, ectopic calcifications, premature aging, arteriosclerosis, osteoporosis [83], a phenotype that can be rescued by dietary phosphorus restriction [84–86]. Furthermore, double knockouts of FGF23 and either the VDR [87] or CYP27B1[88] also rescue the adverse pro-aging features of the FGF23 null mice by preventing hyperphosphatemia. Since FGF23 suppresses CYP27B1 and induces CYP24A1 in the kidney [83, 89], it is clear that the capability of FGF23 to simultaneously get rid of excessive phosphorus while tightly preventing elevations in serum calcitriol is essential for its pro-survival effects. However, although renal mRNA levels for CYP27B1 are reduced, 25(OH)D supplementation to hemodialysis patients can normalize serum calcitriol [90]. However, the contribution of extrarenal calcitriol production cannot be fully disregarded as FGF23 increases rather than decrease parathyroid CYP27B1 expression [91]. Similarly, despite the increased CYP24A1 mRNA, serum levels of 24,25-dihydroxyvitamin D in non-supplemented or supplemented patients were persistently lower than normal [92, 93] Clearly, in advanced CKD, the activity of either enzyme fails to reflect FGF23 control of the respective genes, that is, the damaged kidney fails to respond to FGF23 tight control of renal calcitriol production.

There are several putative VDREs for VDR/RXR binding in the FGF23 promoter. Interestingly, FGF23 gene transactivation by calcitriol decreases from 80-fold to four-fold in the presence of inhibitors of new protein synthesis indicating that osteoblasts' full response to calcitriol induction of the FGF23 gene is indirect [37].

The low levels of FGF23 in the VDR null mice and CYP27B1 mice [94] suggest that impaired induction of FGF23 during vitamin D deficiency could contribute to accelerate pro-aging features and mortality. Furthermore, although phosphorus, PTH, calcium and the calcium X phosphorus product are recognized stimulators of circulating FGF23 levels [95–97], in vitro studies have demonstrated that only calcitriol regulates FGF23 gene transcription [98]. Importantly, calcitriol fails to transactivate the FGF23 gene if high calcitriol and hypophosphatemia occur simultaneously, as demonstrated in a transgenic mouse with an ablation in the gene for the phosphorus transporter NPT2a [99]. This supports the prevalent role of phosphorus over calcitriol in the upregulation of FGF23. The COSMOS study has also reported the optimal range for serum phosphorus associated to the lowest risk of mortality in CKD-5D patients and the benefits of correcting serum phosphorus to achieve optimal range [66].

Because FGF23 requires membrane klotho as a co-receptor for its phosphaturic actions [100], and calcitriol also induces the klotho gene [101], it is clear that the maintenance of a normal bone-kidney FGF23/klotho axis is crucial for survival. The next sections examine calcitriol control of renal klotho and its abnormalities in CKD.

3.6 Vitamin D Induction of Bone FGF23 Production and Renal Klotho Content to Prevent/Attenuate Hyperphosphatemia

For decades, the most critical action of the calcitriol/VDR complex in the kidney has been the induction of CYP24A1 to maintain serum calcitriol within normal limits by degrading excessive circulating calcitriol and/or 25(OH)D to prevent hypercalcemia and hyperphosphatemia. Accordingly, CYP24A1 has a 25-fold higher affinity for calcitriol than for 25(OH)D. Induction of CYP24A1 is a classical genomic action of the calcitriol/VDR complex mainly on two proximal VDREs on this gene promoter [27]. The pathophysiological relevance of calcitriol induction of CYP24A1 in almost every vitamin D responsive tissue was conclusively demonstrated by the severe hypercalcemia and nephrocalcinosis of the CYP24A1 null mouse [102] and in children and adults with a loss of function mutation of this gene [103, 104].

At present, calcitriol/VDR induction of the mRNA levels of the longevity gene α-klotho, and the identification of a VDRE in the human klotho promoter [101] provide a potential causal link for the epidemiological association between vitamin

D deficiency and higher risk of all-cause mortality in the general population, a risk markedly aggravated in CKD patients. Indeed, while klotho disruption confers a premature aging like syndrome [7], its overexpression is sufficient to extend lifespan in mice [105].

Klotho is expressed in the kidney, the parathyroid gland and the choroid plexus [106] where it acts as a high affinity receptor for circulating FGF23. In fact, appropriate levels of renal and parathyroid klotho are required for FGF23 phosphaturic and PTH suppressive actions, respectively. Therefore, calcitriol induction of renal klotho should attenuate the pro-aging features of hyperphosphatemia. Accordingly, progressive reductions of renal klotho in CKD patients stages 3–4 were associated with an impaired response to FGF23, reduced fractional excretion of phosphate and with a fourfold higher propensity for abdominal aortic calcification, measured by the Kaupilla index [107], thus supporting the potentiation of FGF23 protective actions in cells harboring klotho.

However, klotho also exists in a soluble form, generated by proteolytic cleavage of the transmembrane klotho, which is found in blood, urine and cerebrospinal fluid [108, 109]. FGF23-independent endocrine actions of soluble klotho (sklotho) include the modulation of the activity of membrane channels, co-transporters and signaling pathways not fully characterized that contribute to its potent survival benefits. Indeed, the systemic administration of recombinant klotho rescues the phenotype of the klotho null mice [110], and the renal and cardiovascular damage associated to acute or chronic renal injury [111–113]. Therefore, maintenance of renal and/or circulating klotho has become a priority in nephrology and so was the need of accurate measurements of sklotho as a biomarker of the severity of CKD and the risk for cardiovascular mortality.

The demonstration that the specific ablation of renal klotho resulted in an 80 % reduction in circulating sklotho supported the main contribution of the kidney to serum sklotho [8]. Furthermore, since the phenotypic features of the mouse with a renal specific klotho ablation recapitulated all of those in the klotho null mice [8], serum sklotho was considered a valuable biomarker of renal klotho content and of mortality risks. Indeed, serum sklotho decreases with age [7], hypertension [110], and systemic inflammation [114], all recognized determinants of renal damage and cardiovascular disease. However, the recent report that the kidney is the main organ for the clearance of circulating klotho into the urine, through a process of transcytosis through tubular cells [115], raised numerous concerns regarding the accuracy of circulating sklotho to reflect renal klotho content and its pro-survival benefits. Indeed, sklotho accumulation in the blood due to an impaired transcytosis by the damage kidney will mask the actual renal klotho reduction. Therefore, upon improvement of currently available assays for serum klotho, it will be important to establish the optimal range for serum sklotho associated with the lowest mortality risk in the course of CKD. It will be also important to identify the optimal range for urinary sklotho, as is in the apical site of the renal tubule where sklotho acts to induce phosphaturia, urinary K excretion and calcium reabsorption (Reviewed in [116]).

Different from the FGF23/klotho complex that decreases phosphate co-transporters at the cell surface [85], sklotho cleaves residues that promote the endocytosis of the sodium-phosphate co-transporter NPT2a, and consequently impedes phosphorus entrance into tubular cells [109]. A similar mechanism appears to mediate sklotho regulation of the function of the potassium (K) channel ROMK to cause urinary K excretion [117]. Since K restriction increases the renin angiotensin system, it is possible that hypertension-driven klotho reductions are directed to K conservation.

In contrast to NPT2a or ROMK, sklotho post-translational modifications on the calcium channel TRVP5 fixes the protein to the cell surface enhancing renal calcium uptake [118] and leading to a positive bone calcium balance [119].

Calcitriol/VDR induction of renal megalin [26] could prevent/attenuate the decreases in urinary sklotho's control of urinary phosphorus and potassium excretion attributable to the reduced renal megalin content, as occurred with the impaired phosphaturic response to PTH upon a kidney specific ablation of the megalin gene [25].

Since vitamin D restriction ameliorates the severe phenotype of the klotho null mouse [120] and klotho suppresses CYP27B1 expression [86], it is clear that the survival effects of the FGF23/calcitriol/soluble klotho axis require a tight control of hyperphosphatemia and excessive levels of vitamin D metabolites. The 25(OH)D/active vitamin D synergy described for the suppression of parathyroid growth could provide a safe approach.

In addition to a direct induction of renal klotho expression, vitamin D attenuates signals from the three main inhibitors of renal klotho reductions CKD, hypertension and systemic inflammation (See Fig. 3.5).

3.7 Vitamin D Downregulation of Pathways that Reduce Renal Klotho

Calcitriol/VDR suppression of the renin gene [121] explains in part the epidemiological association between vitamin D deficiency and hypertension. Furthermore, simultaneous administration of the angiotensin receptor 1 (AT1R) inhibitor Losartan and the calcitriol analog paricalcitol to uremic diabetic rats markedly attenuated Losartan-induced compensatory increases in renin, which resulted in much lower serum angiotensin II [122], a main downregulator of renal klotho [110].

Calcitriol/VDR suppression of ADAM17 [36] could contribute to the prevention of angiotensin-driven renal damage unrelated to hypertension. Lautrette and collaborators have conclusively demonstrated that angiotensin II enhancement of ADAM17 activity at the surface of renal distal tubular cells, and not hypertension, caused tubular hyperplasia, fibrosis, glomerulosclerosis, proteinuria and inflammatory infiltration to the renal parenchyma, through the release of TGFα for EGFR activation [123]. Furthermore, the activation of renal ADAM17/TGFα signals is a critical determinant of renal damage in human CKD of any etiology [124]. The combined suppression of renin and ADAM17 gene expression by calcitriol could contribute to the synergy between paricalcitol and the angiotensin 2 conversion enzyme (ACE) inhibitor enalapril in reducing the inflammatory macrophage infiltration to the renal parenchyma in rat CKD [125].

The release of TNFα to the circulation by the increased renal ADAM17 is sufficient to explain the paricalcitol/enalapril synergy, as TNFα induces ADAM17 gene transcription [126]. This initiates a vicious cycle for increases in renal ADAM17 and TNFα-driven systemic inflammation for klotho reductions and renal inflammatory damage that are independent of angiotensin II, and consequently, no longer responsive to anti-RAS therapy but suppressible by active vitamin D. Indeed, calcitriol is a recognized immunomodulator, known to decrease the antigenicity of antigen presenting cells and the production of pro-fibrotic and pro-inflammatory Th1 cytokines while enhancing the production of anti-inflammatory Th2 cytokines. The combination of several calcitriol/VDR actions on T cells shifts their polarization towards a Th2/regulatory phenotype and stimulates T regulatory lymphocyte development [10, 127]. Therefore, calcitriol/VDR protection from inflammation-driven multiple organ damage could not only attenuate the reductions of renal klotho but the accumulation of damaged DNA induced by excessive oxidative stress.

3.8 Vitamin D Direct Anti-aging Actions Unrelated to Maintenance of Renal Klotho

The calcitriol/VDR complex also contributes to repair damaged DNA. Accumulation of DNA damage is a main determinant of normal cellular aging and premature senescence, which in vascular smooth muscle cells hasten atherosclerosis. Pre Lamin A accumulation contributes to DNA damage and to impaired DNA damage responses that accelerate calcification [128]. The loss of Lamin A in progeria and in laminopaties associates with increases in the protease cathepsin L which, in turn, degrades 53BP1, a protein essential for the early responses to DNA damage. Calcitriol treatment in fibroblast deprived of Lamin A is sufficient to inhibit the activity of the increased cathepsin L [129] and maintain nuclear levels of 53BP1 by preventing its degradation. Therefore, effective reduction of cathepsin L activity is a novel antiaging vitamin D action contributing to multiorgan protection.

Calcitriol upregulation of BRCA1 may also contribute to improve DNA damage repair [130]. Thus, calcitriol/VDR actions not only attenuate the plethora of factors accelerating damaged DNA accumulation in CKD, but also reverse in part the pro-aging features of already adversely affected cells.

3.9 Conclusions

One finding of the last 5 years has ended the 10-year search for the mechanisms underlying vitamin D renal and cardiovascular protection unrelated to the control of SHPT: "Vitamin D induction of the klotho gene" and that the loss of renal klotho fully reproduces the accelerated aging and the short life span of global klotho absence in mice and men. However, the accuracy of serum klotho as a unique biomarker of antiaging potential has been challenged by the identification of a process of renal transcytosis of circulating soluble klotho to the urinary space, through the kidney. Undoubtedly, serum klotho accumulation could reflect an impaired transcytosis through a failing kidney rather than a higher renal klotho content.

The identification that increased osteoblastic Wnt inhibition, responsible for bone mineralization defects that prompt vascular calcifications, occurs even before elevations in serum PTH and associates to increases in TGFβ. Thus, vitamin D induction of Wnt in osteoblasts, suppression of Wnt in the kidney and vasculature, and VDR antagonism of adverse TGFβ/Smad signals add to the mechanisms for vitamin D renal and vascular protection unrelated to the control of SHPT.

Vitamin D simultaneous induction of FGF23, exclusively in hyperphosphatemic states, and of CYP24A1 adds to the induction of klotho and the suppression of PTH to tightly control the development of hyperphosphatemia or of an excess of circulating vitamin D, which could compromise klotho survival actions. However, clinical studies evaluating the impact of high FGF23 on the degradation of vitamin D metabolite showed lower rather than the expected higher degradation, possibly attributable to the lower renal megalin of CKD. Reduced megalin could also compromise soluble klotho induction of urinary phosphorus and potassium excretion. Vitamin D induction of megalin could simultaneously reduce the risk of hyperphosphatemia while preserving sklotho actions.

Finally, we have learned of a 25(OH)D/calcitriol (analog) synergy that can effectively reverse resistant parathyroid hyperplasia and achieve a 50% suppression of PTH without increasing the dosage of active vitamin D, but with the simple correction of vitamin D deficiency through vitamin D supplementation. Importantly, either monotherapy was insufficient per se to suppress PTH or parathyroid growth. Undoubtedly, the safely and efficacy of this therapy to simultaneously maintain renal klotho without hyperphosphatemia should be examined in prospective studies.

We have also learned that simultaneously with all local and systemic attempts to maintain renal klotho (downregulation of hypertension and inflammation), vitamin D induces cellular anti-aging mechanisms by repairing damaged DNA. Furthermore, we have learned about our gap of knowledge of vitamin D control of micro-RNAs, and their diagnostic and therapeutic potential compared to other health areas.

Acknowledgements This work was supported by grants from Plan Estatal de I+D+i 2013–2016, Instituto de Salud Carlos III (ISCIII)-Fondo Europeo de Desarrollo Regional (FEDER) (PI14/01452), Plan de Ciencia, Tecnología e Innovación 2013–2017 del Principado de Asturias (GRUPIN14-028), Fundación para el Fomento en Asturias de la Investigación Científica Aplicada y la Tecnología (FICYT), Instituto Reina Sofía de Investigación Nefrológica, Fundación Renal Íñigo Álvarez de Toledo, Red de Investigación Renal-RedInRen from ISCIII (RD06/0016/1013, RD12/0021/1023), and by Sociedad Asturiana Fomento Investigaciones Metabólicas (SAFIM).

References

1. Ortiz A, Covic A, Fliser D, et al. Epidemiology, contributors to, and clinical trials of mortality risk in chronic kidney failure. Lancet. 2014;383(9931):1831–43.
2. London GM, Guerin AP, Marchais SJ, et al. Arterial media calcification in end-stage renal disease: impact on all-cause and cardiovascular mortality. Nephrol Dial Transplant. 2003; 18(9):1731–40.

3. Hu MC, Kuro-o M, Moe OW. The emerging role of Klotho in clinical nephrology. Nephrol Dial Transplant. 2012;27(7):2650–7.
4. Ellam TJ, Chico TJ. Phosphate: the new cholesterol? The role of the phosphate axis in non-uremic vascular disease. Atherosclerosis. 2012;220(2):310–18.
5. Phan O, Burnier M, Wuezner G. Hypertension in chronic kidney disease – role of arterial calcification and impact on treatment. Eur Cardioil Rev. 2014;9(2):115–20.
6. Kurts C, Panzer U, Anders HJ, et al. The immune system and kidney disease: basic concepts and clinical implications. Nat Rev Immunol. 2013;13(10):738–53.
7. Kuro-o M, Matsumura Y, Aizawa H, et al. Mutation of the mouse klotho gene leads to a syndrome resembling ageing. Nat. 1997;390(6655):45–51.
8. Lindberg K, Amin R, Moe OW, et al. The kidney is the principal organ mediating klotho effects. J Am Soc Nephrol. 2014;25(10):2169–75.
9. Barker SL, Pastor J, Carranza D, et al. The demonstration of alphaKlotho deficiency in human chronic kidney disease with a novel synthetic antibody. Nephrol Dial Transplant. 2015;30(2):223–33.
10. Adams JS, Hewison M. Update in vitamin D. J Clin Endocrinol Metab. 2010;95(2):471–8.
11. Chowdhury R, Kunutsor S, Vitezova A, et al. Vitamin D and risk of cause specific death: systematic review and meta-analysis of observational cohort and randomised intervention studies. BMJ. 2014;348:g1903.
12. Dusso AS, Brown AJ, Slatopolsky E. Vitamin D. Am J Physiol Renal Physio. 2005;289(1):F8–28.
13. Webb AR, Kline L, Holick MF. Influence of season and latitude on the cutaneous synthesis of vitamin D3: exposure to winter sunlight in Boston and Edmonton will not promote vitamin D3 synthesis in human skin. J Clin Endocrinol Metab. 1988;67(2):373–8.
14. Cheng JB, Levine MA, Bell NH, et al. Genetic evidence that the human CYP2R1 enzyme is a key vitamin D 25-hydroxylase. Proc Natl Acad Sci U S A. 2004;101(20):7711–15.
15. Heaney RP, Armas LA, Shary JR, et al. 25-Hydroxylation of vitamin D3: relation to circulating vitamin D3 under various input conditions. Am J Clin Nutr. 2008;87(6):1738–42.
16. Zhu JG, Ochalek JT, Kaufmann M, et al. CYP2R1 is a major, but not exclusive, contributor to 25-hydroxyvitamin D production in vivo. Proc Natl Acad Sci U S A. 2013;110(39):15650–5.
17. Dusso AS, Tokumoto M. Defective renal maintenance of the vitamin D endocrine system impairs vitamin D renoprotection: a downward spiral in kidney disease. Kidney Int. 2011;79(7):715–29.
18. Al-Aly Z, Qazi RA, Gonzalez EA, et al. Changes in serum 25-hydroxyvitamin D and plasma intact PTH levels following treatment with ergocalciferol in patients with CKD. Am J Kidney Dis. 2007;50(1):59–68.
19. Moe SM, Saifullah A, LaClair RE, et al. A randomized trial of cholecalciferol versus doxercalciferol for lowering parathyroid hormone in chronic kidney disease. Clin J Am Soc Nephrol. 2010;5(2):299–306.
20. Nakano C, Hamano T, Fujii N, et al. Combined use of vitamin D status and FGF23 for risk stratification of renal outcome. Clin J Am Soc Nephrol. 2012;7(5):810–19.
21. KDIGO clinical practice guideline for the diagnosis, evaluation, prevention, and treatment of Chronic Kidney Disease-Mineral and Bone Disorder (CKD-MBD). Kidney Int Suppl. 2009;113:S1–130.
22. LaClair RE, Hellman RN, Karp SL, et al. Prevalence of calcidiol deficiency in CKD: a cross-sectional study across latitudes in the United States. Am J Kidney Dis. 2005;45(6):1026–33.
23. Nykjaer A, Dragun D, Walther D, et al. An endocytic pathway essential for renal uptake and activation of the steroid 25-(OH) vitamin D3. Cell. 1999;96(4):507–15.
24. Takemoto F, Shinki T, Yokoyama K, et al. Gene expression of vitamin D hydroxylase and megalin in the remnant kidney of nephrectomized rats. Kidney Int. 2003;64(2):414–20.
25. Bachmann S, Schlichting U, Geist B, et al. Kidney-specific inactivation of the megalin gene impairs trafficking of renal inorganic sodium phosphate cotransporter (NaPi-IIa). J Am Soc Nephrol. 2004;15(4):892–900.
26. Liu W, Yu WR, Carling T, et al. Regulation of gp330/megalin expression by vitamins A and D. Eur J Clin Invest. 1998;28(2):100–7.
27. Haussler MR, Whitfield GK, Kaneko I, et al. Molecular mechanisms of vitamin D action. Calcif Tissue Int. 2013;92(2):77–98.

28. Saramaki A, Diermeier S, Kellner R, et al. Cyclical chromatin looping and transcription factor association on the regulatory regions of the p21 (CDKN1A) gene in response to 1alpha, 25-dihydroxyvitamin D3. J Biol Chem. 2009;284(12):8073–82.

29. Kim S, Yamazaki M, Zella LA, et al. Activation of receptor activator of NF-kappaB ligand gene expression by 1,25-dihydroxyvitamin D3 is mediated through multiple long-range enhancers. Mol Cell Biol. 2006;26(17):6469–86.

30. Giangreco AA, Nonn L. The sum of many small changes: microRNAs are specifically and potentially globally altered by vitamin D3 metabolites. J Steroid Biochem Mol Biol. 2013; 136:86–93.

31. Chang S, Gao L, Yang Y, et al. miR-145 mediates the antiproliferative and gene regulatory effects of vitamin D3 by directly targeting E2F3 in gastric cancer cells. Oncotarget. 2015;6(10):7675–85.

32. Liu X, Cheng Y, Yang J, et al. Flank sequences of miR-145/143 and their aberrant expression in vascular disease: mechanism and therapeutic application. J Am Heart Assoc. 2013; 2(6):e000407.

33. Disanto G, Sandve GK, Berlanga-Taylor AJ, et al. Vitamin D receptor binding, chromatin states and association with multiple sclerosis. Hum Mol Genet. 2012;21(16):3575–86.

34. Cristobo I, Larriba MJ, de los Rios V, et al. Proteomic analysis of 1alpha,25-dihydroxyvitamin D3 action on human colon cancer cells reveals a link to splicing regulation. J Proteomics. 2011;75(2):384–97.

35. Lin R, Wang TT, Miller Jr WH, et al. Inhibition of F-Box protein p45(SKP2) expression and stabilization of cyclin-dependent kinase inhibitor p27(KIP1) in vitamin D analog-treated cancer cells. Endocrinology. 2003;144(3):749–53.

36. Arcidiacono MV, Yang J, Fernandez E, et al. The induction of C/EBPbeta contributes to vitamin D inhibition of ADAM17 expression and parathyroid hyperplasia in kidney disease. Nephrol Dial Transplant. 2015;30(3):423–33.

37. Haussler MR, Whitfield GK, Kaneko I, et al. The role of vitamin D in the FGF23, klotho, and phosphate bone-kidney endocrine axis. Rev Endocr Metab Disord. 2012;13(1):57–69.

38. Egan JB, Thompson PA, Vitanov MV, et al. Vitamin D receptor ligands, adenomatous polyposis coli, and the vitamin D receptor FokI polymorphism collectively modulate beta-catenin activity in colon cancer cells. Mol Carcinog. 2010;49(4):337–52.

39. An BS, Tavera-Mendoza LE, Dimitrov V, et al. Stimulation of Sirt1-regulated FoxO protein function by the ligand-bound vitamin D receptor. Mol Cell Biol. 2010;30(20):4890–900.

40. O'Kelly J, Uskokovic M, Lemp N, et al. Novel Gemini-vitamin D3 analog inhibits tumor cell growth and modulates the Akt/mTOR signaling pathway. J Steroid Biochem Mol Biol. 2006;100(4–5):107–16.

41. Wu S, Zhang YG, Lu R, et al. Intestinal epithelial vitamin D receptor deletion leads to defective autophagy in colitis. Gut. 2015;64(7):1082–94.

42. Dusso AS, Negrea L, Gunawardhana S, et al. On the mechanisms for the selective action of vitamin D analogs. Endocrinol. 1991;128(4):1687–92.

43. Dusso AS. Vitamin D, receptor: mechanisms for vitamin D resistance in renal failure. Kidney Int Suppl. 2003;85:S6–9.

44. Hoenderop JG, Chon H, Gkika D, et al. Regulation of gene expression by dietary Ca2+ in kidneys of 25-hydroxyvitamin D3-1 alpha-hydroxylase knockout mice. Kidney Int. 2004;65(2):531–9.

45. Lou YR, Molnar F, Perakyla M, et al. 25-Hydroxyvitamin D(3) is an agonistic vitamin D receptor ligand. J Steroid Biochem Mol Biol. 2010;118(3):162–70.

46. Munetsuna E, Nakabayashi S, Kawanami R, et al. Mechanism of the anti-proliferative action of 25-hydroxy-19-nor-vitamin D(3) in human prostate cells. J Mol Endocrinol. 2011;47(2):209–18.

47. Slatopolsky E, Brown A, Dusso A. Role of phosphorus in the pathogenesis of secondary hyperparathyroidism. Am J Kidney Dis. 2001;37(1 Suppl 2):S54–7.

48. Brown AJ, Zhong M, Finch J, et al. Rat calcium-sensing receptor is regulated by vitamin D but not by calcium. Am J Physiol. 1996;270(3 Pt 2):F454–60.

49. Kifor O, Moore Jr FD, Wang P, et al. Reduced immunostaining for the extracellular Ca2+-sensing receptor in primary and uremic secondary hyperparathyroidism. J Clin Endocrinol Metab. 1996;81(4):1598–606.
50. Canaff L, Hendy GN. Human calcium-sensing receptor gene. Vitamin D response elements in promoters P1 and P2 confer transcriptional responsiveness to 1,25-dihydroxyvitamin D. J Biol Chem. 2002;277(33):30337–50.
51. Canalejo R, Canalejo A, Martinez-Moreno JM, et al. FGF23 fails to inhibit uremic parathyroid glands. J Am Soc Nephro. 2010;21(7):1125–35.
52. Slatopolsky E, Finch J, Denda M, et al. Phosphorus restriction prevents parathyroid gland growth. High phosphorus directly stimulates PTH secretion in vitro. J Clin Invest. 1996;97(11):2534–40.
53. Gogusev J, Duchambon P, Stoermann-Chopard C, et al. De novo expression of transforming growth factor-alpha in parathyroid gland tissue of patients with primary or secondary uraemic hyperparathyroidism. Nephrol Dial Transplant. 1996;11(11):2155–62.
54. Arcidiacono MV, Sato T, Alvarez-Hernandez D, et al. EGFR activation increases parathyroid hyperplasia and calcitriol resistance in kidney disease. J Am Soc Nephrol. 2008;19(2):310–20.
55. Arcidiacono MV, Cozzolino M, Spiegel N, et al. Activator protein 2{alpha} mediates parathyroid TGF-{alpha} self-induction in secondary hyperparathyroidism. J Am Soc Nephrol. 2008;19:1919–28. doi:10.1681/ASN.2007111216.
56. Zahnow CA, Cardiff RD, Laucirica R, et al. A role for CCAAT/enhancer binding protein beta-liver-enriched inhibitory protein in mammary epithelial cell proliferation. Cancer Res. 2001;61(1):261–9.
57. Arcidiacono MV, Yang J, Fernandez E, et al. Parathyroid-specific epidermal growth factor-receptor inactivation prevents uremia-induced parathyroid hyperplasia in mice. Nephrol Dial Transplant. 2015;30(3):434–40.
58. Zhang Q, Qiu J, Li H, et al. Cyclooxygenase 2 promotes parathyroid hyperplasia in ESRD. J Am Soc Nephrol. 2011;22(4):664–72.
59. Finetti F, Terzuoli E, Giachetti A, et al. mPGES-1 in prostate cancer controls stemness and amplifies epidermal growth factor receptor-driven oncogenicity. Endocr Relat Cancer. 2015;22(4):665–78.
60. Moreno J, Krishnan AV, Swami S, et al. Regulation of prostaglandin metabolism by calcitriol attenuates growth stimulation in prostate cancer cells. Cancer Res. 2005;65(17):7917–25.
61. Thill M, Becker S, Fischer D, et al. Expression of prostaglandin metabolising enzymes COX-2 and 15-PGDH and VDR in human granulosa cells. Anticancer Res. 2009;29(9):3611–18.
62. Popli P, Sirohi VK, Manohar M, et al. Regulation of cyclooxygenase-2 expression in rat oviductal epithelial cells: evidence for involvement of GPR30/Src kinase-mediated EGFR signaling. J Steroid Biochem Mol Biol. 2015;154:130–41.
63. Cozzolino M, Lu Y, Finch J, et al. p21WAF1 and TGF-alpha mediate parathyroid growth arrest by vitamin D and high calcium. Kidney Int. 2001;60(6):2109 17.
64. Cordero JB, Cozzolino M, Lu Y, et al. 1,25-Dihydroxyvitamin D down-regulates cell membrane- and nuclear growth-promoting signals by the epidermal growth factor receptor. J Biol Chem. 2002;277(41):38965–71.
65. Volovelsky O, Cohen G, Kenig A, et al. Phosphorylation of ribosomal protein S6 mediates mammalian target of rapamycin complex 1-induced parathyroid cell proliferation in secondary hyperparathyroidism. J Am Soc Nephrol. 2015;27(4):1091–101.
66. Fernandez-Martin JL, Martinez-Camblor P, Dionisi MP, et al. Improvement of mineral and bone metabolism markers is associated with better survival in haemodialysis patients: the COSMOS study. Nephrol Dial Transplant. 2015;30(9):1542–51.
67. Cejka D, Herberth J, Branscum AJ, et al. Sclerostin and Dickkopf-1 in renal osteodystrophy. Clin J Am Soc Nephrol. 2011;6(4):877–82.
68. Li YC, Amling M, Pirro AE, et al. Normalization of mineral ion homeostasis by dietary means prevents hyperparathyroidism, rickets, and osteomalacia, but not alopecia in vitamin D receptor-ablated mice. Endocrinology. 1998;139(10):4391–6.

69. Panda DK, Miao D, Bolivar I, et al. Inactivation of the 25-hydroxyvitamin D 1alpha-hydroxylase and vitamin D receptor demonstrates independent and interdependent effects of calcium and vitamin D on skeletal and mineral homeostasis. J Biol Chem. 2004;279(16):16754–66.

70. Goltzman D. Use of genetically modified mice to examine the skeletal anabolic activity of vitamin D. J Steroid Biochem Mol Biol. 2007;103(3–5):587–91.

71. Nakane M, Fey TA, Dixon DB, et al. Differential effects of Vitamin D analogs on bone formation and resorption. J Steroid Biochem Mol Biol. 2006;98(1):72–7.

72. Slatopolsky E, Cozzolino M, Lu Y, et al. Efficacy of 19-Nor-1,25-(OH)2D2 in the prevention and treatment of hyperparathyroid bone disease in experimental uremia. Kidney Int. 2003;63(6):2020–7.

73. Oury F, Sumara G, Sumara O, et al. Endocrine regulation of male fertility by the skeleton. Cell. 2011;144(5):796–809.

74. Gardiner EM, Baldock PA, Thomas GP, et al. Increased formation and decreased resorption of bone in mice with elevated vitamin D receptor in mature cells of the osteoblastic lineage. FASEB J. 2000;14(13):1908–16.

75. Wiese RJ, Uhland-Smith A, Ross TK, et al. Up-regulation of the vitamin D receptor in response to 1,25-dihydroxyvitamin D3 results from ligand-induced stabilization. J Biol Chem. 1992;267(28):20082–6.

76. Evenepoel P, D'Haese P, Brandenburg V. Sclerostin and DKK1: new players in renal bone and vascular disease. Kidney Int. 2015;88(2):235–40.

77. Sabbagh Y, Graciolli FG, O'Brien S, et al. Repression of osteocyte Wnt/beta-catenin signaling is an early event in the progression of renal osteodystrophy. J Bone Miner Res. 2012;27(8):1757–72.

78. Liu S, Song W, Boulanger JH, et al. Role of TGF-beta in a mouse model of high turnover renal osteodystrophy. J Bone Miner Res. 2014;29(5):1141–57.

79. Carrillo-López N, Panizo S, Alonso-Montes C, et al. Fgf23 induction of Dkk1 inhibits the osteoblastic Wnt pathway and contributes to bone loss in CKD-MBD. Kidney Int. 2016; 90(1):77–89.

80. Ding N, Yu RT, Subramaniam N, et al. A vitamin D receptor/SMAD genomic circuit gates hepatic fibrotic response. Cell. 2013;153(3):601–13.

81. He W, Kang YS, Dai C, et al. Blockade of Wnt/beta-catenin signaling by paricalcitol ameliorates proteinuria and kidney injury. J Am Soc Nephrol. 2011;22(1):90–103.

82. Al-Aly Z. Arterial calcification: a tumor necrosis factor-alpha mediated vascular Wnt-opathy. Transl Res. 2008;151(5):233–9.

83. Shimada T, Kakitani M, Yamazaki Y, et al. Targeted ablation of Fgf23 demonstrates an essential physiological role of FGF23 in phosphate and vitamin D metabolism. J Clin Invest. 2004;113(4):561–8.

84. Kurosu H, Kuro-o M. The Klotho gene family and the endocrine fibroblast growth factors. Curr Opin Nephrol Hypertens. 2008;17(4):368–72.

85. Razzaque MS, Lanske B. The emerging role of the fibroblast growth factor-23-klotho axis in renal regulation of phosphate homeostasis. J Endocrinol. 2007;194(1):1–10.

86. Yoshida T, Fujimori T, Nabeshima Y. Mediation of unusually high concentrations of 1,25-dihydroxyvitamin D in homozygous klotho mutant mice by increased expression of renal 1alpha-hydroxylase gene. Endocrinology. 2002;143(2):683–9.

87. Hesse M, Frohlich LF, Zeitz U, et al. Ablation of vitamin D signaling rescues bone, mineral, and glucose homeostasis in Fgf-23 deficient mice. Matrix Biol. 2007;26(2):75–84.

88. Renkema KY, Alexander RT, Bindels RJ, et al. Calcium and phosphate homeostasis: concerted interplay of new regulators. Ann Med. 2008;40(2):82–91.

89. Perwad F, Azam N, Zhang MY, et al. Dietary and serum phosphorus regulate fibroblast growth factor 23 expression and 1,25-dihydroxyvitamin D metabolism in mice. Endocrinology. 2005;146(12):5358–64.

90. Dusso A, Lopez-Hilker S, Rapp N, et al. Extra-renal production of calcitriol in chronic renal failure. Kidney Int. 1988;34(3):368–75.

91. Krajisnik T, Bjorklund P, Marsell R, et al. Fibroblast growth factor-23 regulates parathyroid hormone and 1alpha-hydroxylase expression in cultured bovine parathyroid cells. J Endocrinol. 2007;195(1):125–31.
92. Dai B, David V, Alshayeb HM, et al. Assessment of 24,25(OH)2D levels does not support FGF23-mediated catabolism of vitamin D metabolites. Kidney Int. 2012;82(10):1061–70.
93. Bosworth CR, Levin G, Robinson-Cohen C, et al. The serum 24,25-dihydroxyvitamin D concentration, a marker of vitamin D catabolism, is reduced in chronic kidney disease. Kidney Int. 2012;82(6):693–700.
94. Yu X, Sabbagh Y, Davis SI, et al. Genetic dissection of phosphate- and vitamin D-mediated regulation of circulating Fgf23 concentrations. Bone. 2005;36(6):971–7.
95. Ferrari SL, Bonjour JP, Rizzoli R. Fibroblast growth factor-23 relationship to dietary phosphate and renal phosphate handling in healthy young men. J Clin Endocrinol Metab. 2005;90(3):1519–24.
96. Burnett SM, Gunawardene SC, Bringhurst FR, et al. Regulation of C-terminal and intact FGF-23 by dietary phosphate in men and women. J Bone Miner Res. 2006;21(8):1187–96.
97. Quinn SJ, Thomsen AR, Pang JL, et al. Interactions between calcium and phosphorus in the regulation of the production of fibroblast growth factor 23 in vivo. Am J Physiol Endocrinol Metab. 2013;304(3):E310–20.
98. Liu S, Tang W, Zhou J, et al. Fibroblast growth factor 23 is a counter-regulatory phosphaturic hormone for vitamin D. J Am Soc Nephrol. 2006;17(5):1305–15.
99. Miedlich SU, Zhu ED, Sabbagh Y, et al. The receptor-dependent actions of 1,25-dihydroxyvitamin D are required for normal growth plate maturation in NPt2a knockout mice. Endocrinology. 2010;151(10):4607–12.
100. Urakawa I, Yamazaki Y, Shimada T, et al. Klotho converts canonical FGF receptor into a specific receptor for FGF23. Nature. 2006;444(7120):770–4.
101. Forster RE, Jurutka PW, Hsieh JC, et al. Vitamin D receptor controls expression of the anti-aging klotho gene in mouse and human renal cells. Biochem Biophys Res Commun. 2011;414(3):557–62.
102. St-Arnaud R, Arabian A, Travers R, et al. Deficient mineralization of intramembranous bone in vitamin D-24- hydroxylase-ablated mice is due to elevated 1,25-dihydroxyvitamin D and not to the absence of 24,25-dihydroxyvitamin D. Endocrinology. 2000;141(7):2658–66.
103. Jacobs TP, Kaufman M, Jones G, et al. A lifetime of hypercalcemia and hypercalciuria, finally explained. J Clin Endocrinol Metab. 2014;99(3):708–12.
104. Schlingmann KP, Kaufmann M, Weber S, et al. Mutations in CYP24A1 and idiopathic infantile hypercalcemia. N Engl J Med. 2011;365(5):410–21.
105. Kurosu H, Yamamoto M, Clark JD, et al. Suppression of aging in mice by the hormone Klotho. Science. 2005;309(5742):1829–33.
106. Li SA, Watanabe M, Yamada H, et al. Immunohistochemical localization of Klotho protein in brain, kidney, and reproductive organs of mice. Cell Struct Funct. 2004;29(4):91–9.
107. Craver L, Dusso A, Martinez-Alonso M, et al. A low fractional excretion of Phosphate/Fgf23 ratio is associated with severe abdominal Aortic calcification in stage 3 and 4 kidney disease patients. BMC Nephrol. 2013;14:221.
108. Imura A, Iwano A, Tohyama O, et al. Secreted Klotho protein in sera and CSF: implication for post-translational cleavage in release of Klotho protein from cell membrane. FEBS Lett. 2004;565(1-3):143–7.
109. Hu MC, Shi M, Zhang J, et al. Klotho: a novel phosphaturic substance acting as an autocrine enzyme in the renal proximal tubule. FASEB J. 2010;24(9):3438–50.
110. Mitani H, Ishizaka N, Aizawa T, et al. In vivo klotho gene transfer ameliorates angiotensin II-induced renal damage. Hypertension. 2002;39(4):838–43.
111. Hu MC, Shi M, Cho HJ, et al. Klotho and phosphate are modulators of pathologic uremic cardiac remodeling. J Am Soc Nephrol. 2015;26(6):1290–302.
112. Hu MC, Shi M, Zhang J, et al. Klotho deficiency causes vascular calcification in chronic kidney disease. J Am Soc Nephrol. 2011;22(1):124–36.

113. Hu MC, Shi M, Zhang J, et al. Klotho deficiency is an early biomarker of renal ischemia-reperfusion injury and its replacement is protective. Kidney Int. 2010;78(12):1240–51.
114. Izquierdo MC, Perez-Gomez MV, Sanchez-Nino MD, et al. Klotho, phosphate and inflammation/ageing in chronic kidney disease. Nephrol Dial Transplant. 2012;27 Suppl 4:iv6–10.
115. Hu MC, Shi M, Zhang J, et al. Renal production, uptake, and handling of circulating alphaKlotho. J Am Soc Nephrol. 2016;27(1):79–90.
116. Huang CL. Regulation of ion channels by secreted Klotho: mechanisms and implications. Kidney Int. 2010;77(10):855–60.
117. Cha SK, Hu MC, Kurosu H, et al. Regulation of renal outer medullary potassium channel and renal K(+) excretion by Klotho. Mol Pharmacol. 2009;76(1):38–46.
118. Chang Q, Hoefs S, van der Kemp AW, et al. The beta-glucuronidase klotho hydrolyzes and activates the TRPV5 channel. Science. 2005;310(5747):490–3.
119. Alexander RT, Woudenberg-Vrenken TE, Buurman J, et al. Klotho prevents renal calcium loss. J Am Soc Nephrol. 2009;20(11):2371–9.
120. Tsujikawa H, Kurotaki Y, Fujimori T, et al. Klotho, a gene related to a syndrome resembling human premature aging, functions in a negative regulatory circuit of vitamin D endocrine system. Mol Endocrinol. 2003;17(12):2393–403.
121. Li YC, Kong J, Wei M, et al. 1,25-Dihydroxyvitamin D(3) is a negative endocrine regulator of the renin-angiotensin system. J Clin Invest. 2002;110(2):229–38.
122. Zhang Z, Sun L, Wang Y, et al. Renoprotective role of the vitamin D receptor in diabetic nephropathy. Kidney Int. 2008;73(2):163–71.
123. Lautrette A, Li S, Alili R, et al. Angiotensin II and EGF receptor cross-talk in chronic kidney diseases: a new therapeutic approach. Nat Med. 2005;11(8):867–74.
124. Melenhorst WB, Visser L, Timmer A, et al. ADAM17 upregulation in human renal disease: a role in modulating TGF-{alpha} availability. Am J Physiol Renal Physiol. 2009;297(3):F781–90. doi:10.1152/ajprenal.90610.2008.
125. Mizobuchi M, Morrissey J, Finch JL, et al. Combination therapy with an Angiotensin-converting enzyme inhibitor and a vitamin d analog suppresses the progression of renal insufficiency in uremic rats. J Am Soc Nephrol. 2007;18(6):1796–806.
126. Charbonneau M, Harper K, Grondin F, et al. Hypoxia-inducible factor mediates hypoxic and tumor necrosis factor alpha-induced increases in tumor necrosis factor-alpha converting enzyme/ADAM17 expression by synovial cells. J Biol Chem. 2007;282(46):33714–24.
127. Bouillon R, Carmeliet G, Verlinden L, et al. Vitamin D and human health: lessons from vitamin D receptor null mice. Endocr Rev. 2008;29(6):726–76.
128. Warren DT, Shanahan CM. Defective DNA-damage repair induced by nuclear lamina dysfunction is a key mediator of smooth muscle cell aging. Biochem Soc Trans. 2011;39(6):1780–5.
129. Gonzalez-Suarez I, Redwood AB, Grotsky DA, et al. A new pathway that regulates 53BP1 stability implicates cathepsin L and vitamin D in DNA repair. EMBO J. 2011;30(16):3383–96.
130. Campbell MJ, Gombart AF, Kwok SH, et al. The anti-proliferative effects of 1alpha,25(OH)2D3 on breast and prostate cancer cells are associated with induction of BRCA1 gene expression. Oncogene. 2000;19(44):5091–7.

Chapter 4
Vitamin D Receptor and Interaction with DNA: From Physiology to Chronic Kidney Disease

Jordi Bover, César Emilio Ruiz, Stefan Pilz, Iara Dasilva, Montserrat M. Díaz, and Elena Guillén

Abstract The biologically most active vitamin D metabolite, 1,25-dihydroxyvitamin D_3 [calcitriol or $1,25(OH)_2D_3$] exerts the vast majority of its classical actions and attributed "non-traditional" effects by means of interaction with the vitamin D receptor (VDR). Here, we review the VDR structure and function, as well as the molecular actions of vitamin D mediated via this classical endocrine receptor. We also describe the interactions of the $1,25(OH)_2D_3$/VDR complex with the retinoid X receptor, VDR coregulators (coactivators and corepressors) and the vitamin D-response element, whereby the expression of many $1,25(OH)_2D_3$–responsive genes is positively or negatively controlled in many different tissues through complex conformational changes. On the other hand, chronic kidney disease (CKD) may be considered "a disease of dysfunctional receptors" since CKD has been associated with resistance to the action of many hormones including $1,25(OH)_2D_3$. CKD and uremic toxins interfere not only with $1,25(OH)_2D_3$ metabolism but also with various VDR processes such as basal VDR synthesis, binding and function. In view of the ubiquitous nature of VDR, several VDR activators are being developed with the aim of achieving an improved biological profile for a therapeutic application in one of the pleiotropic functions of the natural hormone, while avoiding untoward effects including excessive calcium and phosphate loading. However, randomized clinical trials are required to confirm all the proposed cardiovascular and survival benefits of the old and new VDR activators.

Keywords Vitamin D • Vitamin D receptor • Chronic kidney disease • Calcitriol • Uremia • CKD-MBD • Calcium • Phosphate • Parathyroid hormone • Hyperparathyroidism • Paricalcitol • FGF23 • Klotho • Calcidiol

J. Bover, MD, PhD (✉) • C.E. Ruiz, MD • I. Dasilva, MD • M.M. Díaz, MD, PhD
E. Guillén, MD
Department of Nephrology, Fundaciò Puigvert, IIB Sant Pau, REDinREN, Barcelona, Spain
e-mail: jbover@fundacio-puigvert.es

S. Pilz, MD, PhD
Department of Endocrinology and Metabolism, Medical University of Graz,
Grazy, Styria, Austria

© Springer International Publishing Switzerland 2016

75

P.A. Ureña Torres et al. (eds.), *Vitamin D in Chronic Kidney Disease*,
DOI 10.1007/978-3-319-32507-1_4

4.1   Introduction

Transcriptional regulation is a central process for almost all physiological eukary-
otic actions. Interestingly, gene transcription is repressed in most cases since the
nuclei of eukaryotes contain a complex of genomic DNA and nucleosomes (chromatin) which occludes the binding sites of DNA-binding proteins [1, 2]. *Nuclear*
receptors, currently positioned at the epicenter of the "Big Bang" of molecular
endocrinology [3], are the best characterized representatives of thousands of mammalian proteins that are involved in transcriptional regulation in human tissues [2,
4]. The receptors form a superfamily, the majority of which are activated by small
lipophilic ligands [3, 5]. The subgroup of *endocrine* nuclear receptors bind their
specific ligands such as steroid hormones, sex and adrenal steroids, as well as thyroid hormone, retinoic acid and 1,25-dihydroxyvitamin D_3 (calcitriol or
1,25(OH)$_2$D$_3$), among other intermediate compounds, binding and activating specific intracellular receptors. These transcription factors are now known to function
within the nucleus to regulate (enhancing or suppressing) gene expression and epigenetic changes [6]. Cloning of this nuclear receptor family of genes has contributed to the definition of new biological complexes and progressively known
pathways [6].

The human genome sequence encodes as many as 48 nuclear receptors [7, 8],
and important interrelationships between these receptors have been documented
and will be discussed in this chapter [e.g. vitamin D receptor (VDR) and retinoid X
receptor (RXR)]. On the other hand, different transcriptional effects may reside not
in the genes that are regulated, but in the overlapping but distinct ligand profile (e.g.
the VDR is structurally and functionally closely related to the pregnane X receptor
(PXR) receptor, and it does not respond to vitamin D).

The idea that vitamin D might function as a steroid-like hormone emerged in
1968 [9] and actually predated the documented discovery of 1,25(OH)$_2$D$_3$, the
active hormonal form of vitamin D_3 [6]. The cloning in 1987 of a "binding protein"
[10] present in specific target tissues which mediates the nuclear localization of
1,25(OH)$_2$D$_3$ provided the final confirmation that it was indeed a *steroid-like* hormone capable of regulating gene expression.

4.2   Vitamin D Biology and Ubiquity of the VDR

As previously mentioned in other parts of this book, vitamin D is a prohormone that
is ultimately converted into the biologically most active vitamin D metabolite,
1,25(OH)$_2$D$_3$. The final step in the production of this hormonal form occurs primarily, though not exclusively, in the proximal convoluted tubular cells of the kidney
via tightly regulated 1α-hydroxylation. The cytochrome P450-containing (CYP)
enzymes responsible for catalyzing 25- and 1α-hydroxylations are the microsomal
CYP2R1 and the mitochondrial CYP27B1, respectively. 1,25(OH)$_2$D$_3$ circulates

bound to plasma vitamin D-binding protein (DBP) to a number of target tissues. It has been only shown recently that the VDR present in the apical brush border of the proximal convoluted tubular cells serves to "sense" the level of circulating $1,25(OH)_2D_3$ [11].

The main classical actions [12] of $1,25(OH)_2D_3$ are maintenance of proper calcium (Ca) and phosphate (P) homeostasis: the serum levels of these ions are raised to ensure that the ion concentration is optimal for normal bone mineralization. This is accomplished by way of direct and highly coordinated actions of the hormone on the intestinal tract, kidney and bone and through a feedback inhibition of parathyroid hormone (PTH) production in the parathyroid glands and the induction of fibroblast growth factor 23 (FGF23) from osteocytes of the osteoblastic lineage. Thus, $1,25(OH)_2D_3$ controls the expression of many genes (SPP1 or osteopontin, TRPV6, LRP5, BGP or osteocalcin, RANKL, OPG, CYP24A1, PTH, FGF23, PHEX and klotho, among others) associated with adequacy of bone and mineral homeostasis [16]. $1,25(OH)_2D_3$ also directly promotes osteoblastogenesis via enhanced canonical Wnt signaling (LRP5) [6], prevents osteoblast apoptosis and impacts on bone remodeling by inducing osteoblasts to terminally differentiate into osteocytes and deposit calcified matrix [13], and promotes differentiation of precursor cells into mature osteoclasts in order to maintain an appropriate bone remodeling cycle [14, 15]. Consequently, $1,25(OH)_2D_3$ is involved both in the formation of osteoid matrix and in mineralization, inducing ossification in response to mechano-stress/fracture (e.g. via SPP1) or supplying dietary Ca via transport to build the mineralized skeleton (TRPV6). $1,25(OH)_2D_3$ also regulates the production of receptor activator of nuclear factor kB ligand (RANKL) and osteoprotegerin (OPG) from bone cells, and thus plays an important role in remodeling of normal adult bone. In the intestinal tract and the kidney, many genes regulating Ca and P homeostasis (CYP24A1, calbindin, TRPV6, PMCA1b, CLDN, NPT2a-c, among others) are under the influence of $1,25(OH)_2D_3$ [6]. By inducing TRPV6 and NPT2a-c in the small intestine and kidney, respectively, VDR signaling favors transepithelial transport of Ca and P to generate a fully mineralized skeleton. Through the regulation of SPP1, BGP, LRP5, RANKL, and OPG, VDR ensures the formation of high-volume and fracture-resistant bone with connectivity that is modeled for strength via osteocyte mechano-sensing endocrine cells in the skeleton [16]. Renal megalin (a member of the low-density lipoprotein receptor superfamily that is an endocytic receptor responsible for the renal tubular resorption of albumin and other small molecular weight proteins) also reabsorbs the complex $25(OH)D_3/DBP$, and megalin is induced by the interaction of $1,25(OH)_2D_3$ and VDR [17].

On the other hand, VDR prevents the production of excess $1,25(OH)_2D_3$ and protects against ectopic calcification that is elicited by an excess of Ca or P by the presence of feedback regulatory genes delimiting bone mineralization to the normal skeleton, upregulating CYP24A1, inducing parathyroid calcium-sensing receptor (CaSR), repressing PTH and PHEX, and/or inducing FGF23/klotho system [6, 18]. $1,25(OH)_2D_3$ may also directly or indirectly inhibit vascular calcification or promote osteoclast accumulation for the resorption of ectopic bone (e.g. via SPP1) [6, 19]. CYP24A1 is among the genes most strongly induced by $1,25(OH)_2D_3$ and its catalytic gene product (25-hydroxyvitamin D 24-hydroxylase) is present in all cells expressing VDR [6].

As previously mentioned, PTH and FGF23 are also affected by $1,25(OH)_2D_3$ and the mechanism of FGF23 induction by $1,25(OH)_2D_3$ is partly or entirely due to PHEX repression. Irrespective of the mechanism of FGF23 induction, FGF23 allows osteocytes in bone to communicate with the kidney to govern vitamin D bioactivation and circulating P, and thus to prevent excess $1,25(OH)_2D_3$ function and ectopic calcification as a result of hyperphosphatemia. Interestingly, double knock-outs of FGF23 with either VDR or CYP27B1 [20, 21] essentially rescue the deadly FGF23-null phenotype in mice; this indicates that the ability of FGF23 to function as a counter-regulatory hormone for $1,25(OH)_2D_3$ is one of the key reasons for its benefits in terms of health and longevity. The physiologic activities of $1,25(OH)_2D_3$ appear to promote healthful aging and to prolong life by decreasing the risk of chronic disorders in old age, reducing age-related vascular pathology, inflammation, oxidative stress and atherosclerosis, (e.g. by suppressing NFkB, COX2, the TGF-α/ADAM17/EGFR pathway, protecting against muscle and skin atrophy, organ fibrosis and generally preventing premature aging [16, 22–27].

Many of these pathologies are also a consequence of *hypervita*minosis D [24]. In pharmacological doses or pathological excess, $1,25(OH)_2D_3$ generates a phenotype that is close to that of FGF23-null mice, including ectopic calcification, skin atrophy, vascular disease, and emphysema [14, 16]. This situation is analogous to the excess of the fat-soluble vitamin A and its active retinoic acid metabolite [16]. FGF23 signals via FGFR1 and klotho coreceptors [28]. Klotho is a bona fide longevity gene. When it is inactivated in mice (Kl-/-), the consequence is the generation of a phenotype apparently identical to that of FGF23-null mice [29]. However, klotho can be considered in a class by itself with actions not limited to control of P metabolism [28]. Up-regulation of klotho by $1,25(OH)_2D_3$ is modest but significant [19] and it has been suggested that many health benefits of $1,25(OH)_2D_3$ also may be effected through VDR-mediated enhancement of klotho expression in kidney and perhaps other cell types [16]. Chronic kidney disease (CKD) is now considered a state of klotho-deficiency [30, 31]; consequently, the beneficial pleiotropic effects of $1,25(OH)_2D_3$ may also apply to these complex patients [19]. Appropriate vitamin D concentrations are also associated with longer leukocyte telomere length, a parameter which decreases with each cell cycle, and with increased inflammation, highlighting the potential benefits of $1,25(OH)_2D_3$ with respect to aging and age-related diseases such as CKD [16, 32].

$1,25(OH)_2D_3$ is also a regulator of cellular proliferation, growth and differentiation [33]. $1,25(OH)_2D_3$ affects cell cycle regulators such as p21 (CDKN1A) and p27 (CDKN1B) (the main antiproliferative effect of $1,25(OH)_2D_3$ liganded VDR is the arrest of cells at the G_1 phase by up-regulation of these factors). $1,25(OH)_2D_3$ also modifies cell growth-transcription factors (c-myc and c-fos), represses the Bcl-2 antiapoptotic factor, and induces DNA repair enzymes, among many other actions [16]. This issue highlights potential therapeutic roles for both the hormone and the synthetic vitamin D analogs in cancer, regulation of the immune system and autoimmune diseases, through their action on the differentiation of certain cells in the skin, colon, breast, prostate, hair cycle, etc. $1,25(OH)_2D_3$ also seems to play a role in carbohydrate, lipid and amino acid metabolism, for example by promoting insulin release or improving insulin resistance (e.g. via BGP), and possibly enhancing fatty acid β-oxidation [6, 16, 34]. In the intestinal tract, beyond the previously mentioned genes regulating Ca and P homeostasis, $1,25(OH)_2D_3$ also regulates the metabolic degradation of secondary bile acids, facilitates the transport and metabolism for xenobiotic detoxification (e.g. inducing CYP3A4 – a major target for VDR and PXR in xenobiotically exposed sites such as the skin, intestine and kidney), and controls the proliferation and differentiation of epithelial cells that are prone to fatal malignancies [6].

Interestingly, numerous tissues besides the kidney express the CYP27B1 enzyme (T and other immune cells, pancreas, skin), and consequently these are now recognized as *extrarenal* sites of 1α-hydroxylase action to produce $1,25(OH)_2D_3$ *locally* for *autocrine* and *paracrine* effects, as distinct from the *endocrine* actions on the small intestine and bone [35, 36]. It seems that many of the extraosseous effects of $1,25(OH)_2D_3$ are triggered by this locally produced $1,25(OH)_2D_3$, which appears not to contribute significantly to circulating $1,25(OH)_2D_3$ but is active in a cell- and tissue-specific manner [16]. This also explains the potentially defective local conversion of 25-(OH)D to $1,25(OH)_2D_3$ by "non-renal" cells in states of vitamin D deficiency or vitamin D "resistance", which may affect cell-specific pro-survival actions in spite of the presence of normal serum $1,25(OH)_2D_3$ [37]. Examples include the way in which $1,25(OH)_2D_3$ and its receptor, VDR, appear to have evolved as "specialty" regulators of hair growth, providing physical protection against the harmful UV radiation of the sun, subsequent to their original use by early unicellular organisms for protection of their DNA against UV-B irradiation [38]. $1,25(OH)_2D_3$ also controls, suppresses or tempers the *adaptive* immune system (e.g. repressing IL-17) [39] to lower the incidence of autoimmune disease while boosting the *innate* immune system in order to fight infections, most notably HIV and tuberculosis [40, 41]. A nice example is the role of $1,25(OH)_2D_3$ as a major regulator of the expression of cathelicidin, which is an essential local antimicrobial efector [42]. It also appears that locally produced $1,25(OH)_2D_3$ is capable of benefiting the vasculature (via local extrarenal generation), and the cardiovascular system, in which VDR is expressed in endothelial cells, smooth muscle and cardiac myocytes [16, 43, 44]. On the other hand, beneficial effects of active vitamin D therapy may be achieved indirectly through inhibition of the renin-angiotensin system [45] and/or the tumor necrosis-α-converting enzyme (TACE) or ADAM17-TGF-α/ EGFR pathways [26, 37, 46]. Consequently, $1,25(OH)_2D_3$ may inhibit deleterious angiotensin II-driven TACE activation and this TACE inhibition may contribute not only to bone benefits but also to renal and cardioprotective actions of vitamin D in health or diseases such as CKD [26, 37, 47]. EGFR activation increases parathyroid hyperplasia and calcitriol resistance in kidney disease (see below) [46, 48]. Angiotensin II and kidney disease enhance TACE expression and activity, causing release of mature TGF-α from its transmembrane precursor [37, 49]. This soluble TGF-α binds to and activates EGFR, leading to renal parenchymal lesions [37]. Because EGFR activation stabilizes TACE protein, a vicious cycle is created that may compromise 1,25(OH)$_2$D$_3$-VDR renoprotection through TGF-α/EGFR-driven reductions in renal VDR content, as also demonstrated in the parathyroid glands [46]. Recent results have shown that the described anti-inflammatory actions of VDR activators [50, 51] could depend on the inhibition of TGF-α-ADAM17-EGFR pathway in response to aldosterone, as shown in tubular cells [26].

Genomic studies have also revealed that 1,25(OH)$_2$D$_3$ acts on the Wnt-activated β-catenin pathway. Wnt- molecules bind to transmembrane Frizzled protein and low-density lipoprotein-related protein (LRP) coreceptors to inhibit the β-catenin degradation complex. The result is the accumulation of β-catenin, which translocates into the nucleus, inducing the transcription of several genes. VDR suppresses the transcriptional activity of β-catenin (a proto-oncogene for colorectal cells) in a 1,25(OH)$_2$D$_3$ ligand-dependent manner [16]. On the other hand, VDR is apparently anabolic in bone cells through the enhancement of β-catenin signaling in osteoblasts independently of ligand [16]. This action is consistent with the fact that a sclerostin-1 (SOST-1) inactivating monoclonal antibody [52, 53] is a promising new bone anabolic drug that promotes Wnt/β catenin signaling by removing the soluble, extracellular SOST-1 Wnt antagonist. All the effects of VDR on β-catenin – lowered risk of colon cancer, enhanced bone volume and effective skin protection by hair – indicate that 1,25(OH)$_2$D$_3$ acts as a "fountain of youth" promoting healthy ageing [16]. The regulation of transcription factors such as RUNX2, C/EBP, AP-1 family members, as well as other factors, also influences cell lineage determination (e.g. RUNX2 is an essential osteoblast determining transcription factor which may be induced in smooth muscle vascular cells, leading to active vascular calcification). Comprehensive discussions of vitamin D receptor activation, cardiovascular and vascular calcification and the renal implications have recently been published [54, 55].

4.3 Molecular Actions of Vitamin D: The Vitamin D Receptor

As in tissues that control mineral homeostasis, the underlying central feature of 1,25(OH)$_2$D$_3$ actions in each of these traditional and "non-traditional" tissues is the presence of the vitamin D receptor (VDR), a classical endocrine nuclear receptor and a requirement for cellular response to 1,25(OH)$_2$D$_3$ [6]. The VDR is a chromosomal protein acting as a DNA-binding transcription factor that generates an active signal transduction complex (see below). Inherited mutations in the VDR –defects in the VDR gene on human chromosome 12 such as those found in hereditary hypocalcemic vitamin D resistant rickets (HVDRR) [56]- prevent its expression or compromise its functional activity, resulting in partial or total resistance to the actions of 1,25(OH)$_2$D$_3$ despite the fact that the levels of the hormone are generally very high. A non-genetic, acquired form of resistance to vitamin D is described in uremia (see below) [57].

In 1974 it was firmly established that a protein macromolecule present in the chromatin fraction of the chick intestine was capable of mediating the preferential nuclear uptake of active vitamin D [58, 59]. Subsequent studies [60] demonstrated that this putative receptor was indeed able to bind $1,25(OH)_2D_3$. In addition to their presence in kidney, intestine, bone and parathyroid cells in several species, including mammals, VDRs were also discovered in tissues such as pancreas, placenta, pituitary and mammary gland, ovary, testis and heart [6]. VDRs have also been found in a large series of tumoral cells.

The VDR is expressed in low concentrations in target tissues and cell lines, ranging from a few to thousands of copies per cell. Although the receptor concentration in cells may be a primary determinant of the magnitude of the cellular response to $1,25(OH)_2D_3$, myriad additional factors also play a significant and possibly more important role, including vitamin D-degrading enzymes (such as CYP24A1), the presence and activities of vitamin D-binding protein (DBP) or intracellular vitamin D-binding proteins, specific characteristics of the gene target itself, post-translational modifications of the VDR, vitamin D-response element (VDRE)-binding proteins and finally a mixture of comodulators that act downstream of the VDR but participate directly in the regulation of gene expression. In any case, examples of a strong correlation between cellular VDR levels and biological response are described. VDR abundance is also regulated transcriptionally. As described below, acquired disturbances in the VDR number and/or functionality related to many of these VDR-related processes have been induced in uremic conditions [61].

The most important characteristic of the VDR is its capacity to bind $1,25(OH)_2D_3$ with high affinity and selectivity. The VDR displays an equilibrium dissociation constant (K_D) of ca. 10^{-10} M for the natural ligand $1,25(OH)_2D_3$ and binds its precursors and less active metabolites with significantly lower affinities [6]. Both the 25-hydroxyl and the 1α-hydroxyl group on the $1,25(OH)_2D_3$ molecule contribute to specific and high-affinity binding. In the late 1970s it was discovered that the VDR could bind to DNA [62], and the subsequent identification of specific DNA-binding sites (VDRE's) within gene promoters, enhancers or repressors led to a deeper understanding of such binding. Interestingly, the molecular actions of $1,25(OH)_2D_3$ are largely identical to those of its receptor, but VDR has additional ligand-independent functions [63]. Thus, in addition to increased "affinity" for non-specific DNA following ligand binding, VDR displays "affinity" for DNA in the absence of $1,25(OH)_2D_3$ [6]. VDR may also function unliganded, obviating the need for local generation of $1,25(OH)_2D_3$. For instance, VDR but not vitamin D is required to sustain the mammalian hair cycle [the hairless (Hr) corepressor could function as a surrogate VDR "ligand"], and calbindin induction by VDR does not require vitamin D in brain (unlike in intestine, kidney and bone). However, the ability of VDR to function unliganded is difficult to justify physicochemically and thus it has been suggested that VDR may bind non-vitamin D ligands in order to exert its extraosseous actions [16]. Consequently, several additional nutritional lipids have been identified as candidate low-affinity VDR ligands that may function locally in high concentrations; examples include omega-3 and omega-6 polyunsaturated fatty acids (PUFAs), lithocolic or arachidonic acids, vitamin E derivatives and others [16]. High local concentrations of PUFAs could occur in select cells or tissues and may partially explain the chemoprotective nature of diets rich in PUFAs, plus their cardioprotective and anti-inflammatory influences [16].

Finally, other studies have suggested that the human VDR may comprise several forms, and several polymorphisms have been linked to bone mineral density disorders as well as to various other diseases [6, 64]. Thus, VDR polymorphisms could be involved in the development of secondary hyperparathyroidism in CKD patients or different response patterns secondary to tissue-specific effects of the VDR response to vitamin D metabolites [64, 65]. The BsmI genotype, as well as others such as the ApaI, TaqI and FokI restriction length polymorphisms, can also affect PTH levels, the response of hemodialysis patients to IV $1,25(OH)_2D_3$, and the need for parathyroidectomy [66–69] . Moreover, experimental studies in human primary osteoblasts and human parathyroid glands yielded opposite results with regard to haplotype response to $1,25(OH)_2D_3$ in osteoblasts and parathyroid glands [65]. Overall, the results support the proposed significant role for VDR polymorphisms in bone and parathyroid gland behavior, the observation of different patterns probably being due to tissue-specific effects of the VDR response to $1,25(OH)_2D_3$ [64, 65]. Studies investigating the relationship between VDR genotypes and left ventricular hypertrophy have revealed a highly significant association with the BsmI Bb heterozygous genotype [43]. However, none of these polymorphism-derived data seems particularly robust and no useful direct clinical contribution has been proven [70]. As a matter of fact, none of the VDR polymorphisms showed differences in response to $1,25(OH)_2D_3$ in parathyroid glands in culture [66, 71], and therefore any implications for treatment are still to be considered very preliminary [66]. Consequently, adaptation of treatment algorithms on the basis of the allelic status of the individual patient is not currently recommended since the relevance of VDR polymorphisms are still a matter of debate due to the poorly reproducible clinical correlations [66, 70].

4.4 VDR Structure

The initial cloning of the glucocorticoid and estrogen receptors represented the initial step in the characterization of this intracellular nuclear receptor gene family. Some receptors can act as silencers of transcription in the absence of ligands or the presence of antagonists. Agonists induce an alteration in the structure of the nuclear receptor, which allows interaction with target gene promoters.

These receptors comprise of distinct regions or domains, leading to their designation as A, B, C, D, E and F [72]. The highly conserved DNA-binding domain is designated the C domain. The domain structure of the 427-AA human VDR is depicted in Figs. 4.1 and 4.2 [6, 16], with the two major functional units, the *DNA-binding domain* and *the ligand-binding* domain (LBD). The DNA-binding domain (66 amino acids, from residues 24 to 89) is represented by the N-terminal classical (Cys2-Cys2)2 two Zn-finger motifs, serving for DNA binding within the major groove of genomic DNA. The LBD is represented in the multifunctional C-terminal domain (approximately 200 amino acids). The A/B domains are relatively very short compared with other members of the nuclear receptor family (Fig. 4.1). The C region comprises the highly conserved DNA-binding domain, which mediates binding of

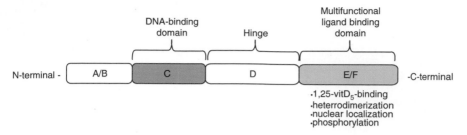

Fig. 4.1 Schematic structure of human VDR

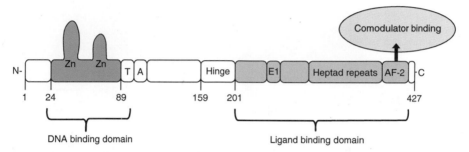

Fig. 4.2 Domains in human VDR. DNA-binding domain with zinc fingers on the *left side*. Ligand-binding domain on the *right side*. AF-2 Activation Function 2 (Adapted from Haussler et al. [16])

VDR to specific regions of the DNA flanking regions of the target genes. The E/F domain contains the ligand $1,25(OH)_2D_3$-binding region of the VDR and serves as an important and highly complex protein-protein interface for a series of additional interacting proteins essential to receptor activity (RXR heterodimerization and transcriptional comodulator binding) (Fig. 4.2) [16]. This region also harbors a highly structured ligand-dependent activation function, termed activation function 2 (AF-2), and hormone binding results in the creation of a functional AF-2 (*see* Fig. 4.2) [16]. The E region of the VDR encodes a multifunctional domain that exerts indirect control over the DNA binding as well as transcription-modifying properties of the VDR. The presumed change in nuclear receptor structure in the AF-2 region that occurs in response to hormone binding appears to play a key role in its ability to attract DNA-binding partners (e.g. it acts as a major interface for dimerization with RXR) and recruit protein complexes (coactivators or corepressors) vital for transcriptional activation (Fig. 4.2) [6, 16, 73]. The F domain is absent in the VDR.

The DNA-binding domain of the VDR is evolutionarily highly homologous to other steroid receptors [74]. This domain comprises two similar modules, each consisting of a Zn-coordinated finger structure. The first Zn finger, the amino-terminal module, is responsible for directing specific DNA binding in the major groove of the DNA-binding site. In order to bind DNA and regulate gene expression, transcription factors require nuclear translocation, and nuclear localization depends on various arrangements of basic amino acids in short stretches within the primary amino acid sequence [75]. The second Zn finger, the carboxy-terminal module,

Fig. 4.3 1,25(OH)$_2$D$_3$
(1,25-dihydroxyvitamin D$_3$
or calcitriol)-induced
heterodimerization
between VDR and the
retinoid X receptor (*RXR*).
1,25(OH)$_2$D$_3$ (ligand)
binds to VDR,
heterodimerizes with the
RXR and binds to a DR-3
type of vitamin D-response
element (*VDRE*) in the
promoter region of
1,25(OH)$_2$D$_3$-responsive
genes (Adapted from
Dowd and MacDonald
[76b])

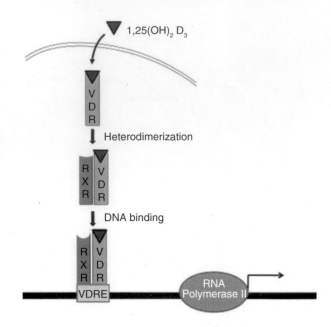

serves as a dimerization interface for interaction with the previously mentioned partner proteins [6, 76] (*see* Fig. 4.2). VDR binding 1,25(OH)$_2$D$_3$ results in the generation of RXR heterodimers for specific DNA binding and coactivator docking for transcriptional activation [8, 16, 76b] (Figs. 4.2 and 4.3). At physiologic receptor concentrations and ionic strength, binding of VDR to VDREs will occur only when both 1,25(OH)$_2$D$_3$ and RXR are present [16, 77]. Furthermore, it has been found that in an in vitro transcription system containing native chromatin, inclusion of RXR is essential for transactivation of 1,25(OH)$_2$D$_3$ via VDR [16, 78]. The key event in this process is the binding of a ligand (e.g. 1,25(OH)$_2$D$_3$) to the VDR (Fig. 4.4) [16].

Several steps are apparently set in motion by the ligand-binding event. The general fold of nuclear receptor LBD comprises a three-layered α-helical sandwich, and LBDs undergo major conformational changes upon ligand binding [79]. The X-ray crystallographic structure of the VDR-LBD was originally considered to consist of 12-α helices (and a set of β-sheets) [80] but recently it has been suggested that it in fact contains 15-α helices [16]. VDR-LBD is a sandwich-like structure that presents VDR surfaces for heterodimerization with RXR as well as for transactivation via interaction with coactivators (*see* Fig. 4.2 and below) [8]. Coactivator interfaces in VDR consist of portions of helices H3, H5 and the previously mentioned H12 (constituting the AF-2 domain), as well as a region immediately N-terminal of the Zn fingers [8, 16] (Fig. 4.2). There is a *pocket* in the middle layer of the sandwich fold [81]. The presence of 1,25(OH)$_2$D$_3$ ligand in the VDR-binding pocket causes a dramatic conformational change in the position of the most carboxy-terminal α-helix at the C-terminus of the VDR. As a result, the ligand-binding pocket is brought, via a "mouse-trap like" intramolecular folding, to the "closed" position, after which it

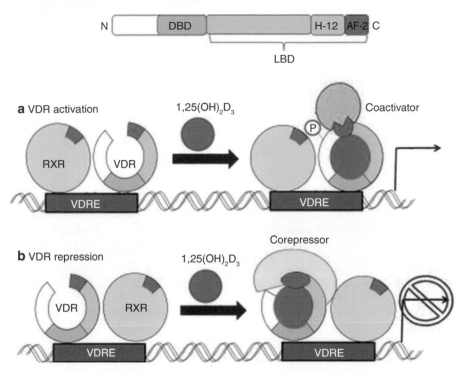

Fig. 4.4 $1,25(OH)_2D_3$ (1,25-dihydroxyvitamin D_3 or calcitriol): potential mechanisms of gene
activation and repression through VDR. (**a**) *Upper panel*: RXR-VDR activation after $1,25(OH)_2D_3$
and coactivator binding, phosphorylation and docking on a positive vitamin D-response element
(*VDRE*) (i.e. osteocalcin gene). (**b**) *Lower panel*: VDR-RXR inactivation after $1,25-(OH)_2 D_3$ and
corepressor binding, dephosphorylation and docking in reverse polarity on a negative vitamin
D-response element (*VDRE*) (i.e. PTH gene) (Adapted from Haussler et al. [16])

can serve in its AF-2 role as part of a platform for coactivator binding [2, 16, 82]
(Fig. 4.4). In other words, H12 folds onto the core of LBD, forming an hydrophobic
cleft together with other surface-exposed residues which accommodate the "nuclear
receptor box" of *coactivators* (see below) [73]. Ligand-intensified heterodimerization, VDRE docking, and coactivator recruitment by VDR appear functionally
inseparable in effecting $1,25(OH)_2D_3$-elicited gene transcription. The binding of
VDR conformationally influences its RXR heteropartner and appears to cause the
RXR-AF2 region to pivot into an active position (Fig. 4.4) [16]. The RXR of the
heterodimer may now be endowed with the potential to bind additional comodulators [16].

   Since the first determination of the crystal structure of the LBD complexed with
$1,25(OH)_2D_3$ was reported in 2000 [80], several dozens of crystal structures accom-
modating various ligands have been presented. Almost all of them display the
canonical active conformation observed in the VDR-LBD/$1,25(OH)_2D_3$ complex,
and they all have quite similar ligand binding pocket architectures within the LBD
described above. The ligand binding pocket refers to the inner surface of the

VDR-LBD forming a cavity that is created by a network of approximately 40 mostly non-polar amino acids [83, 84]. The fact that VDR-LBD has many α-helices and is a densely-packed structure means that its structural modification by ligand binding is difficult [81]. Several analogs modulating this structure are currently opening a new perspective for the development of VDR ligands exhibiting specific biological activities by focusing on the loop region facing the LBP because loop regions in protein tertiary structure are in general more flexible than regions composed of α-helices and/or β-sheets [81].

4.5   Vitamin D Response Elements and VDR Function

In 1989, the sequence elements in the human osteocalcin gene conferring basal activation and inducible response of this gene promoter to hormonal $1,25(OH)_2D_3$ were described [85]. Since then, in addition to classical targets, many genes have been explored for their sensitivity to vitamin D. Recently, at least 50 VDREs residing in or near vitamin D target genes that are directly modulated in their expression by $1,25(OH)_2D_3$ (and possibly other VDR ligands) have been identified [16], although microarray studies suggest that the number of vitamin D-regulated genes is in fact far greater. In some cases VDREs can be even 100 kb and more, either up- or downstream from the transcription start site.

A typical "optimal" VDRE is characterized by a *direct* repeat of two hexanucleotide half-elements (e.g. repeats of AGGTCA resembling the estrogen-responsive element) that are separated by a spacer of three nucleotides (DR3) [2, 16, 86, 87]. Although the sequence of the spacer is not generally conserved, it has recently been suggested that it may modulate DNA binding and transactivation by the VDR in cellular response to natural and synthetic ligands [88]. Thus, the multiple sequence variations in natural VDREs may provide a range of affinities for the VDR/RXR heterodimer, thereby enabling these elements to respond to different concentrations of the receptors or their ligands [2, 16, 88]. It is also possible that other VDRE sequences (e.g. DR4, DR6, everted repeats) induce unique conformations in the VDR/RXR complex, promoting association of the heterodimer with distinct subsets of coactivators or permitting differential actions in the context of diverse tissues [2, 88, 89].

Every transcriptionally responsive primary VDR target gene must contain at least one VDRE in its promoter region and these VDREs are often located relatively close to the transcription start site of these genes (Fig. 4.5) [2]. VDRE clusters are also described (e.g. for CYP24A1, the most responsive known primary $1,25(OH)_2D_3$ target gene), the strong responsiveness being explained by the presence of two DR3 type VDREs that are separated by less than 100 bp and are located in close proximity to the transcription start site (Fig. 4.5) [2]. The concept of multiplicity and remoteness to VDREs has also evolved, leading to the identification of novel VDREs at some distance from the transcription start site [2, 16]. Remote VDREs may be juxtapositioned with more proximal VDREs by way of DNA looping in chromatin, creating a single platform to support the transcription machine [16]. Thus, distal

Fig. 4.5 Schematic
structure of a chromatin unit
(region between two matrix
attachment regions which
often contains only one
gene). DNA looping should
enable DNA sequences
within the same unit to be
located near the basal
transcriptional machinery.
VDRE vitamin D-response
element (Adapted from
Carlberg [2])

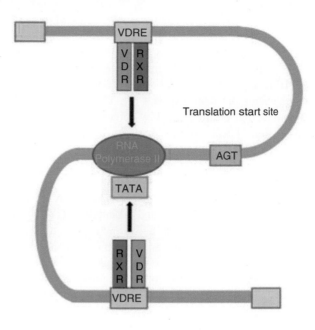

sequences can also serve as VDREs and even sequences downstream of the
transcription start site may act as functional VDR-binding sites [2]. In fact, most
primary VDR target genes use multiple VDREs for full functionality [2]. For
instance, in genes possessing multiple VDREs, such as RANKL, the chromatin
looping permits simultaneous binding of multiple factors in a supercomplex at the
promoter [16]. Typically, these VDREs are arranged in the proximity of binding
sites for other transcription factors into collections of neighboring sites, so-called
modules or enhancers [2]. It has been demonstrated that modules of transcription
factors that act on focused regions are far more effective than individual factors at
isolated locations [2].

1,25(OH)$_2$D$_3$ may also induce *gene repression* to genes encoding, for instance,
PTH, PTHrP and CYP27B1 (also repressed by FGF23). This negative feedback
loop limits the stimulation of CYP27B1 by PTH under low-calcium conditions,
serving to restrict the bone-resorbing effects of PTH in anticipation of 1,25(OH)$_2$D$_3$
increases in intestinal Ca absorption and bone resorption; as a result, hypercalcemia
is prevented. Expression profiling using whole genome microarrays indicates that a
similar number of genes are down- and up-regulated by 1,25(OH)$_2$D$_3$ [90]. Ligand-
dependent repression of gene transcription by VDR/RXR probably shares some
molecular features with induction, but it is evident that it is much more complex
mechanistically since it seems to occur via multiple routes. In general, the mechanisms of *down*-regulation by 1,25(OH)$_2$D$_3$ also appear dependent upon the binding
of a VDR agonist. It is clear that only genes showing basal activity can be down-
regulated and that such genes exhibit basal activity because of other transcription
factors bound to their promoters [2]. Several different models have attempted to

explain the down-regulation of genes, all of which posit that VDR counteracts the activity of specific transcription factors. For instance, for the physiologically important down-regulation of the CYP27B1 gene by $1,25(OH)_2D_3$, a negative VDRE has been proposed to interact directly with a prebound transcriptional activator termed VDIR [2, 6]. The VDR suppresses VDIR-activated expression but active epigenetic mechanisms are also involved [6]. Thus, CYP27B1 is repressed by $1,25(OH)_2D_3$ with a regulation influenced by epigenetic demethylation [91] in order to limit the production of $1,25(OH)_2D_3$. In an outstanding example of a biological counterregulatory feed-back loop, PTH is repressed by $1,25(OH)_2D_3$ and Ca, whereas FGF23 is induced by $1,25(OH)_2D_3$ and P; the consequence is protection of mammals against hypercalcemia and hyperphosphatemia, respectively, avoiding ectopic calcification. Obviously, Ca, P and $1,25(OH)_2D_3$ also inhibit the activities of VDR-dependent enzymes such as CYP27B1 and the catalytic CYP24A1 [92].

In situations in which the activating transcription factors are other nuclear receptors or transcription factors that bind to composite nuclear receptor response elements, VDR might simply compete for DNA-binding sites. Similarly, VDR could compete for binding to partner proteins such as RXR or for common *coactivators* [such as steroid receptor coactivator-1 (SRC-1) or CBP, see below] [2]. The recruitment of nuclear receptor *corepressors* to alter the chromatin structure in the vicinity of the target gene is a further possibility (see below) [16]. Repressor functions may be carried out by "negative VDREs", where liganded VDR is apparently conformed in such a way that it binds corepressors rather than coactivators. Experiments suggest that the DNA binding of the VDR to down-regulated genes such as the PTH gene does not involve RXR [93], although neither is it a uniform mechanism. Because it appears that non-consensus nucleotides in negative VDREs occur in either or both half-elements, it has been proposed that base-pair changes may suffice to drive RXR-VDR into reverse polarity on the negative VDRE [16]. On the other hand, VDR may also be prone to protein-phosphatase rather than protein-kinase activity in this conformation, again favoring corepressor attraction [16, 94]. Furthermore, the regulatory region of primary $1,25(OH)_2D_3$ may contain both negative and positive VDREs (e.g. human *myc* gene) [2]; liganded VDR thus transactivates or represses numerous target genes by binding to positive or negative VDRE present in promoters, enhancers or suppressors of these genes [95, 96]. Finally, it is interesting that classical steroidal nuclear receptors exist as complexes in the cytoplasm with heat shock factor proteins and therefore their transcriptional actions are largely mediated by ligand-induced release from this complex and shuttling into the nucleus [97]. The VDR differs from such receptors by being located in the nucleus even in the absence of ligand and controls gene expression by switching between repressing and activating states, in accordance with availability of ligand [97]. Thus, the distribution of genomic binding sites, or so-called cistrome, of the VDR is biologically significant in both the absence and the presence of even low levels of ligand [97].

A growing number of transcriptional/epigenetic factors that coregulate transcriptional functions of nuclear receptors have been identified, and further novel coregulators, particularly those involved in transrepression, are expected to be found [98].

A review of the regulation of the VDR gene itself by environmental, genetic and epigenetic mechanisms, rather than the way in which VDR regulates other genes, is beyond the scope of this chapter, and we encourage the reader to read recent publications on the subject [99].

4.5.1 Retinoid X Receptor and Coregulators

Nuclear receptor-binding sites can be categorized into three groups: (1) palindromic half-sites that interact with *homodimeric* receptors for the sex-steroids; (2) directly repeated half-sites with variable spacing that interact with *heterodimeric* receptors for 1,25(OH)$_2$D$_3$, retinoic acid, thyroid hormone and other ligands; and (3) single half-sites that mediate the actions of monomeric receptors (e.g. nerve growth factor IB) [100]. The length of the spacer itself is a primary determinant of nuclear receptor selectivity for 1,25(OH)$_2$D$_3$, retinoic acid, etc. Thus, the VDR preferred half-sites are separated by 3 bp (the previously mentioned DR3) [87], in contrast to the retinoic acid receptor (2 or 5 bp) and the thyroid receptor (4 bp). The DR3 percentage differs significantly in the analyzed cellular models, ranging between 38.2 % in macrophages and 9 % in B cells [84]. Interestingly, in every cell type investigated, the top 200 VDR sites show a DR3 rate exceeding 60 %, e.g., DR3 type motifs are found preferentially at highly ligand-responsive VDR loci and may be the first to be addressed by a therapeutic intervention with a synthetic VDR ligand [84].

It has already been mentioned that high-affinity binding of the VDR to DNA in vitro requires the DNA-binding domain and the LBD. Moreover, high-affinity VDRE binding requires the ability of the receptor to form dimers, and in the case of VDR it was a *hetero*dimer with a "nuclear accessory factor", as it was initially termed. This was later identified as the RXR [6, 101], a previously cloned member belonging also to the nuclear receptor family. Both VDR and RXR subunits are necessary not only for high-affinity DNA binding, but also for the activation process itself [8, 16] (*see* Figs. 4.2 and 4.4). Only this liganded VDR/RXR can penetrate the deep groove of DNA and recognize VDREs in the DNA sequence of vitamin-D-regulated genes. Target genes recognized by the combined Zn fingers of the two receptors and their T-box and A-box C-terminal extensions (*see* Fig. 4.2) [8] obviously encode proteins which determine the diverse 1,25(OH)$_2$D$_3$ functions mentioned in this chapter and elsewhere in the book [16].

This binding to the VDRE (DR3-VDRE actually) must follow a defined polarity (RXR binds to the upstream 5′-half-element and the VDR binds to the downstream 3′-half-element of the VDREs oriented in the DNA sense strand) [6] (*see* Fig. 4.3). In this way, the interaction of the liganded VDR/RXR and a VDRE confers target gene selectivity and ultimately exerts an influence on the rate of RNA polymerase II-directed transcription [86]. Moreover, genomic studies have indicated that the VDR is not bound in advance ("prebound") to sites on vitamin D target genes; rather it is induced to bind owing to 1,25(OH)$_2$D$_3$-mediated activation and RXR heterodimerization [6]. On the other hand, significant binding of the VDR and its partner RXR has been observed at various sites (e.g. bone cells) in the absence of $1,25(OH)_2D_3$. Whether the "prebound" VDR/RXR heterodimer manifests activity is unknown [6]. In any case, in the absence of ligand, the VDR/RXR complex associates with *corepressors* (see below) at enhancer and promoter regions to silence gene expression. The binding of ligand induces formation of a *coactivator* complex (see below), leading to target gene transactivation via direct and indirect mechanisms [97].

With respect to the involvement of *coregulators or comodulators* (corepressors and coactivators) in transactivation by the VDR and RXR (*see* Fig. 4.4) [16], it is to be noted that more than 250 published coregulators are known to interact with nuclear receptors and to modify their transactivation potential [86, 102]. Thus, a primary function of the VDR/RXR heterodimer is the recruitment of coregulatory complexes containing enzyme activities essential for the modulation of events associated with gene products. Transactivation requires DNA -binding and ligand-intensified heterodimerization, VDRE docking by recognition of direct repeat responsive elements in the promoters of regulated genes and creation of an intact functional AF-2 domain as part of a platform for coactivator binding (Figs. 4.2 and 4.4) [8, 16]. We have already mentioned that activation of the VDR involves a $1,25(OH)_2D_3$-dependent conformational change in the LBD.

The regulation of VDR-mediated transcription involves a series of temporally coordinated macromolecular interactions between the VDR/RXR heterodimer and other transcription factors [86]. Associations between the liganded VDR/RXR heterodimer and other transcriptional components can be classified into two general categories, namely general transcription factors and the coregulatory proteins [86]. Interaction of VDR with general transcription factors [important examples of which are TATA-binding protein associated factors (TAFs) and basal transcription factors such as TFIIB [16, 86]; (*see* Fig. 4.2) [8] leads to direct contact with the transcriptional preinitiation complex (PIC), which may facilitate assembly or recruitment of the PIC, thereby stimulating transcription by the RNA polymerase II [86]. The liganded VDR is also linked to the transcriptional PIC by the likely *sequential* recruitment of multiple coregulators, proteins which modulate, either positively or negatively, the ability of nuclear receptors to regulate transcription. As mentioned previously, coregulators are classified as *coactivators* and *corepressors*. Coactivator proteins may augment transcription via any of several proposed mechanisms [86]: (1) by acting as macromolecular bridges between the liganded receptor and the transcriptional machinery (by recruiting components of the PIC, assembling the PIC or promoting the stability of the complex); (2) by recruiting *secondary* coactivators which possess chromatin modification or remodeling activities, such as histone acetyl transferase (HAT), histone deacetylase, methyl transferase activities, and other ATP-dependent alterations in plasticity of chromatin structure and rearrangement of nucleosomal arrays [103]; and (3) by increasing the rate of coupling between RNA polymerase II-directed transcription and more downstream events, e.g. transcription elongation and RNA processing [86]. While primary coactivators interact directly with nuclear receptors, secondary coactivators interact with primary coactivators to regulate transcription [86].

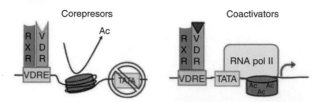

Fig. 4.6 Comodulator activity (coactivators and corepressors) on VDR-mediated expression. The VDR/RXR heterodimer is loosely bound to a vitamin D-response element (*VDRE*) in the absence of ligand, interacting with corepressors which keep gene transcription repressed (partially keeping histone proteins deacetylated). Upon ligand-binding, corepressor is released and replaced by coactivators. Coactivators remodel chromatin and help in the recruitment of RNA polymerase II and other components of the preinitiation complex. *Ac* Acetylation/deacetylation (Adapted from Dowd and MacDonald [76b])

On the other hand, *corepressors* are usually considered to be proteins that interact with unliganded nuclear receptors, thereby repressing the basal expression of hormone-responsive genes. These corepressors are distinct from other transcriptional repressors that interfere with nuclear receptors via different mechanisms. They directly modify histones or recruit modifying enzymes (e.g. histone deacetylases), ensuring that chromatin is maintained in a tightly packed condition, thus silencing transcription from the promoter. They also associate with antagonists bound to the nuclear receptor to inhibit target expression [76b, 86] (Fig. 4.6). At later stages, coregulators may also promote the recruitment or stability of the RNA-processing machinery, enhancing the rate at which mature RNAs are made and subsequently translated [86].

4.5.1.1 Coactivators of VDR

Binding of $1,25(OH)_2D_3$ to the VDR sets in motion a cascade of protein assembly that ultimately leads to transcriptional activation of selected target genes. Ligand-induced coactivator recruitment to the VDR/RXR heterodimer acts as the seed for the assembly of intricate multiprotein complexes. These complexes remodel the chromatin structure and recruit core transcriptional machinery in an orderly and sequential manner [86]. The transfection of many of these factors to cells strongly enhances $1,25(OH)_2D_3$-induced transcription [6], and all are needed for robust VDR-mediated transcription. As mentioned previously, many of the factors (though not all) interact with the same region of VDR, i.e. the C-terminal AF-2 motif [16] (*see* Figs. 4.2 and 4.4). More than 50 nuclear proteins are known to interact with VDR LBD [104]. Chromatin has an intrinsic repressive potential, the purpose of which is conservation of the epigenetic landscape of a differentiated cell, i.e. by default it restricts the access of transcription factors to promoter or enhancer regions, leaving only approximately 50–100,000 accessible chromatin regions per cell type [84, 105]. Stimulation with $1,25(OH)_2D_3$ results in a significant increase in chromatin accessibility [106].

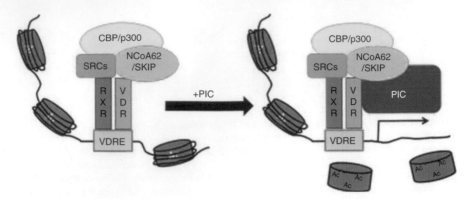

Fig. 4.7 Hypothetical model for comodulator complexes in VDR-activated transcription. *PIC* transcriptional preinitiation complex, *Ac* Acetylation/deacetylation (Adapted from Dowd and MacDonald [76b])

1. ***SRC family of coactivators***

The first nuclear receptor coactivator to be identified was SRC-1 [107], also known as NCoA1. It constitutes the founding member of the p160 or SRC family, which also includes SRC-2 (also known as GRIP-1, TIF-2, and NCoA2) and SRC-3 (also known as p/CIP, RAC3, ACTR, AIB-1, TRAM-1, and NCoA3). These SRCs are thought to prepare target gene promoters, including the VDR, by remodeling the corresponding chromatin. In this way, a template is created that is more accessible to the transcriptional machinery. Such remodeling occurs, for instance, via histone acetylation (HAT activity) since the electrostatic interactions between the positively charged histone tails and the negatively charged P backbone of DNA are weakened by the covalent addition of acetyl groups, thereby inducing local decondensation (relaxation) of the chromatin [73, 86, 108]. Recruitment of other proteins with HAT activity, such as p300/CBP, is also vital and synergistic for transcriptional activation [86, 109, 110]. SRC recruitment is involved in histone methylation and probably also in relaxation of chromatin structure [76b, 86] (Fig. 4.7). Since the cellular concentration of the SRCs is limiting, post-translational changes in phosphorylation, ubiquitinylation, acetylation or methylation are a means of modulating coactivator complex stability, assembly or disassembly [86]. Cell- and time-specific patterns of the relative abundance of coactivators may balance the $1,25(OH)_2D_3$-induced proliferation or differentiation of cells [111]. However, it has not been directly proven that methylation status of the CpG islands (epigenetic silencing) of VDR and CaSR gene promoters are associated with reduced gene expression, at least in parathyroid adenomas [112].

2. *Mediator-D Complex*

In addition to SRCs, a large multiprotein complex designated DRIP (D receptor interacting protein) is a coactivator of VDR and other nuclear receptors. The extensive similarity with other coactivator complexes has led to the proposal of a unified nomenclature using the mammalian mediator complex (MED) as the basis, and DRIP is now referred to as Mediator-D [113]. It has been proposed that

Mediator D interacts with the liganded VDR bound to its enhancer element and recruits RNA polymerase II, thereby establishing a linkage between VDR and the basal transcriptional machinery, thus promoting the formation and function of the preinitiation complex (Fig. 4.7) [76b, 86, 114]. Chromatin immunoprecipitation studies have demonstrated that the entrance of Mediator-D follows the entrance of nuclear receptors and acetylation of histones surrounding the transcriptional start site. The Mediator-D complex comprises a minimum of ten different proteins, as well as numerous subunits anchored by MED1/DRIP205/TRAP220 which interact directly with ligand-activated VDR/RXR heterodimers [86].

3. *NCoA62/SKIP*

NCoA62/SKIP is structurally different from the previously discussed coactivators, and its interaction with VDR is independent of the AF-2 domain, unlike the SRCs and Mediator-D. Furthermore, ligand is not necessary for the interaction in vitro, although it does enhance this interaction. NCoA62/SKIP seems to function at more distal steps of the transactivation process (after the chromatin -remodeling step) and also interacts with basal transcription factors such as TFIIB [86, 115]. Like other coactivators, NCoA62/SKIP may play a role in altering RNA processing (e.g. splicing).

4. *Other coactivators*

Other coactivators interact with VDR, building bridges with TGF-β signal transduction pathways (SMAD3), substrates for PKC signaling, negative regulators of Wnt signaling, etc.[86, 97].

It appears that RXR contributes directly to recruitment of these coactivators since it also contains a functional AF-2 (*see* Fig. 4.4) [16]; RXR thus seems to be a transcriptionally active partner of the VDR rather than a "silent partner" [6, 16, 116]. Genomic studies have demonstrated that $1,25(OH)_2D_3$ induces recruitment of SRC-1, e.g. to the CYP24A1 promoter, and that the recruitment of SRC-2 and SRC-3 follows a temporal pattern. Recruitment of other factors (perhaps an increased presence of MED-1) appears to up-regulate the density of RNA-polymerase II, the enzymatic component essential for the production of RNA transcripts from protein coding and other genes. These studies have also shown that enhancers potentially function as recruitment centers for the RNA polymerase II complex and for the potential synthesis of several types of non-coding RNA transcripts [6, 117, 118]; this offers a completely new future area of research. Recruitment of all the previously mentioned catenin complexes has functional consequences with respect to gene promoter status and transcriptional activity. Furthermore, both nuclear receptors and their coactivator-corepressor complexes cycle on and off the promoter [86], indicating not only that a special and temporal order to the transcriptional process may be necessary for gene regulation but also that the transcriptional process permits better control of the overall process of gene activation [6, 86, 119]. This is an extremely complex and dynamic process that requires a variety of macromolecular machines and coordination of numerous complex pathways and networks [2, 86]. The proposed selectivity of certain vitamin D analogs could be, at least partially, related to various conformational changes induced by different comodulator recruitment, as is discussed below [120].

Finally, the signaling mechanisms of $1,25(OH)_2D_3$ also include non-genomic, rapid, response signaling cascades (within seconds to minutes) which are extranuclear (occur outside the cell nucleus) and therefore do not require transcription of new mRNA, although they may require a functional extranuclear VDR protein [121]. Cross-talk has been described between extranuclear and nuclear vitamin D signaling by: (1) involvement of the cell-specific effect on the VDR phosphorylation state and (2) regulation of cytoplasmic second messengers (such as cAMP, p53, NFkB, IkB, Ca or ERK1) [121]. Even a $1,25(OH)_2D_3$ membrane receptor has been proposed to play an important role in regulating Ca and P transport (the membrane-associated rapid response steroid or MARRS-binding protein [122]. Non-genomic actions of $1,25(OH)_2D_3$ rapidly modulate intestinal Ca transport, intracellular Ca levels and/or the phosphorylation, subcellular localization, and activity of proteins capable of regulating VDR control of gene expression [37]. Interestingly, the VDR molecule has two functionally distinct pockets for ligands that trigger either genomic or non-genomic VDR actions [37, 123].

4.5.2   Corepressors of VDR

Corepressors interact with DNA-bound transcription factors and play key roles in silencing or repressing transcription. Both corepressors and their associated proteins interact with unliganded nuclear receptors and are displaced upon binding of agonist ligands. In the presence of unliganded receptor or antagonist-bound receptor, corepressors generally lower basal promoter activity [86]. In a simplified view of nuclear receptor signaling, in the absence of ligand the receptor interacts with corepressor proteins tightly associated with enzymes that modify histone tails; the modifications include histone deacetylation (leading to chromatin compaction that interferes with gene transcription) and select examples of methylation and ubiquitinylation [2, 86]. As mentioned previously, in the absence of ligand, the VDR/RXR complex associates with corepressors at enhancer and promoter regions to silence gene expression [97]. Ligand binding induces the dissociation of corepressors and the association of coactivators to the receptor. The switch between gene repression and activation is, however, more complex than a simple alternative recruitment of regulatory complexes [124] and, as mentioned above, sequential multiple enzymatic reactions occur and repression and activation are likely promoter- and cell-type specific [2].

Two of the best characterized corepressors are SMRT and NCoR (nuclear receptor corepressor). Both repress basal promoters in systems that are regulated by numerous nuclear receptors, including VDR (although the silencing effects on the latter is weaker than in other systems) [86, 97]. SMRT and NCoR bind to the same hydrophobic cleft on the LBD as SRC coactivators, which makes binding of coactivators and corepressors mutually exclusive. In contrast to SRC coactivators, however, interaction of SMRT/NCoR with the VDR -LBD is independent of the AF-2 domain [86]. SMRT/NCoR are large proteins that additionally serve as platforms for the assembly of multiprotein repression complexes containing histone deacetylases; the latter through deacetylation of core histone proteins, result in a localized region of compact or tightly bound nucleosomal packaging ultimately leading to repressed basal expression of the promoter [86]. Other proteins, such as Hairless (Hr) gene product, TRIP15/Alien and DREAM, may also repress VDR-mediated transcription [16, 86, 97].

These intricate protein-protein interactions with the genome enable the finely tuned control of *epigenetic* states at VDR binding regions and across target gene loci. Such epigenetic events play a central role in the initiation, maintenance and completion of transcription [125]. As mentioned previously, VDR/RXR complex can modulate regional chromatin status in order to regulate transcription, in part via enzymatic control of histone modifications and DNA methylation processes [97]. In the relaxed chromatin state, the VDR complex recruits linking factors (Mediator/DRIP/TRAP complex) and subsequently the basal transcriptional machinery [97]. This is not, however, an indefinite signal as ligand is rapidly metabolized. The VDR itself is also limited in function by proteasome-mediated receptor degradation [126]. In any case, although the structures of the DNA- and LBD binding domains of many nuclear receptors have been determined in great detail, the mechanisms by which they are able to interact and perhaps "communicate" remain a matter of debate [8].

In summary, there are many conformations and coregulator associations that the VDR/RXR heterodimer can achieve while performing its multitude of extraosseous effects to reduce the risk of the chronic diseases of aging or the accelerated aging associated with CKD and uremia [127]. It also offers potential for the development of specific pharmacological targets to differentially affect traditional and non-traditional vitamin D effects in patients with CKD or other chronic diseases [128].

4.6 CKD Affects VDR Function

CKD is associated with resistance to the action of many hormones and is also associated with clinical resistance to the action of $1,25(OH)_2D_3$ [57, 92, 129–131]. Actually it is well known that uremia induces hormonal resistance to other hormones, even in the early stages of renal failure [132–136], and thus uremia could be at least partially considered a "disease of dysfunctional receptors". There is no uniformity to define $1,25(OH)_2D_3$ resistance in dialysis patients [66] but prediction of $1,25(OH)_2D_3$ resistance has been associated, among other factors, to pretreatment FGF23 levels or the maximal longitudinal diameter of the largest parathyroid gland [137, 138].

While resistance to the action of $1,25(OH)_2D_3$ in uremia is essentially undisputed, the underlying mechanisms remain largely unknown, unlike the recognized derangements of vitamin D metabolism in renal failure [130]. Many years ago several studies provided initial evidence that uremic plasma contains compounds that inhibit the interaction of VDR with VDRE [139, 140]. This inhibitory mechanism might account for the end-organ resistance to $1,25(OH)_2D_3$ in renal failure in addition to the decreased number of receptors observed in the parathyroid glands of parathyroidectomized patients, with either primary or secondary hyperparathyroidism [141].

4.6.1   Binding Characteristics of VDR in Renal Failure

While it initially appeared that uremic ultrafiltrate does not impair ligand-VDR binding [142], Hsu and Patel demonstrated that it inhibits the interaction of VDR with DNA by using "classic techniques" such as DNA-cellulose chromatography to model the effect of uremia on this interaction [61, 143]. Preincubation of normal intestinal VDR with uremic ultrafiltrate significantly reduced the VDR interaction with DNA-cellulose. Additionally, the elution profile from DNA-cellulose of $1,25(OH)_2D_3$ labeled intestinal VDR showed that the receptor of subtotally nephrectomized rats eluted as two single peaks whereas that of sham-control rats eluted as a single peak [61, 144]. One of the peaks represented VDR with normal binding while the other represented weak binding characteristics. This weak DNA-cellulose binding VDR was present only in experimental renal failure of at least 5 h' duration: acute renal failure induced by bilateral ureteral obstruction for less than 5 h produced solely the normal binding intestinal VDR [61, 144]. It proved possible to reproduce these binding characteristics of VDR in renal failure in normal rats infused for 24 h with uremic plasma ultrafiltrate [61]. Patel et al. studied the characteristics of binding of the VDR with VDREs in experimental renal failure using the electrophoretic mobility shift assay (EMSA), and obtained results consistent with those acquired with the DNA-cellulose analysis [140]. These authors revealed that the maximal binding capacity, as shown by Scatchard analysis, was reduced in renal failure, and observed that only slightly more than 50 % of the VDR from renal failure rats were capable of binding to the osteocalcin VDRE with a normal Kd [140]. The fact that normal VDR incubated with uremic ultrafiltrate behaved identically and lost approximately 50 % of the maximal binding capacity with a normal Kd, gave rise to the hypothesis that the decreased binding of VDR to the VDREs is attributable to chemical compounds in the uremic plasma ultrafiltrate.

4.6.2   Effect of Uremic Toxins on the VDR-DNA Binding Domain

Hsu and Patel also produced a truncated VDR (amino acids 1–119) lacking the LBD but containing the full Zn fingers and the T and A box domains (*see* Fig. 4.2) [8]. Preincubation of this truncated VDR with uremic ultrafiltrate resulted in a decrease in binding to osteopontin VDRE [61]. As this truncated VDR only contained the short (23 amino acid) amino-terminal domain plus the DNA-binding domain, this finding strongly suggested that uremic toxins interact with the VDR DNA-binding domain; this at least partially explains the presence of potential resistance to vitamin D in uremia even without uremic interaction with the LBD [61]. Finally, reconstituted intestinal nuclei have been used to study the effect of uremic plasma ultrafiltrate on nuclear uptake of the $1,25(OH)_2D_3$-VDR complex in vitro [142]. Patel et al. demonstrated that intestinal VDR isolated from rats with CKD had lower binding affinity for intestinal nuclei. This decreased binding affinity for nuclei (with decreased nuclear uptake of labeled VDR) could be reproduced in normal rats infused with uremic ultrafiltrate. Furthermore, VDR incubated with uremic ultrafiltrate also lost its binding affinity for nuclei [142].

4.6.3   Effect of Uremic Toxins on RXR

Since it is conceivable that uremic toxins could chemically modify not only the VDR but also the RXR, recombinant VDR or RXR were separately preincubated with uremic ultrafiltrate [61, 140]. Such preincubation of VDR inhibited the formation of the VDR/RXR -osteopontin VDRE complex in the case of VDR but not RXR. It therefore appeared that the inhibitory effect of uremic toxins on the formation of the VDR/RXR -VDRE complex was due to a modification on the VDR and not the RXR. Since RXR is a heterodimerization partner for many other nuclear receptors, had RXR been a target for uremic toxins, one could have predicted that this effect would probably have impaired many other nuclear receptors in renal failure [61]. These results also indicate that if uremic toxins are responsible for multiple pathologies at the endocrine level that are associated with renal failure, this effect is probably exerted via direct alteration of other nuclear receptors [61]. Subsequent investigation confirmed the inhibitory effect of uremic solutions on the complex formation of other homo- or heterodimer forming nuclear receptors [145], whereas a monomer binding nuclear receptor did not appear to be affected. These results indicate that VDR is a target of substances in uremic solutions in vitro, but also that other nuclear receptors (e.g., other endocrine signaling systems) may be affected to some extent by renal failure.

The exact chemical reason for this "specificity" is not known as identification of toxic substances associated with this observation is still awaited. It has been reported that compounds that inhibit the function of VDR are likely to contain reactive aldehydes or ketones [61, 146]. These toxins may react with lysine residues in the VDR DNA-binding domain and block the VDR -VDRE interactions [61, 131] through an analogous Schiff base formation mechanism [147]. This suggestion was based on the finding that the VDR and other steroid receptors form Schiff bases with pyridoxal 5'-phosphate or glyoxalate, which weakens the binding of these receptors to the DNA-cellulose [131, 148]. It was later confirmed that uremic solutions derived from ultrafiltrate from hemodialysis patients and dialysate from peritoneal dialysis patients exerted an inhibitory effect on the complex formation and ligand inducibility of VDR/RXR heterodimers on different VDRE types [145]; however, formation of Schiff bases could not be confirmed by point mutagenesis data of different lysine residues in this study [145].

All the previously mentioned negative effects of uremic ultrafiltrate on VDR-VDRE interaction have been shown not only in vitro but also in *cells* incubated in media containing uremic ultrafiltrate [61]. Studies in transfected JEG-3 cells revealed that $1,25(OH)_2D_3$ had an impaired ability to induce the expression of a target gene, suggesting that uremic toxins can not only permeate into cells but also inhibit the interaction of VDR with the VDRE [61, 131]. On the other hand, infusion of uremic plasma ultrafiltrate in rats significantly reduced 24-hydroxylase activity, the synthesis of which is a receptor-mediated process [149]. In rats treated with uremic ultrafiltrate, the administration of a pharmacological dose of $1,25(OH)_2D_3$ failed to normalize the enzymatic activity of 24-hydroxylase [143], indicating a "compensatory" mechanism of decreased $1,25(OH)_2D_3$ degradation in renal failure [143].

4.7   CKD Affects the Expression of VDR

Beyond altered receptor interaction with target genes, decreased VDR concentration might also diminish its biological action [150, 151]. Although it has been reported that the effect of uremic ultrafiltrate in decreasing VDR-VDRE interaction seems not to be attributable to impaired VDR expression [131, 140], it is known that VDR concentration is decreased in renal failure [141]. Reduced density and binding of VDRs have been observed in parathyroid glands of both animals and humans with CKD [141, 152–155]. Merke et al. [154] initially demonstrated that in acute uremia maximal specific binding capacity for $1,25(OH)_2D_3$ in parathyroid glands was diminished, maybe in association with low circulating $1,25(OH)_2D_3$ levels. There was no change of Kd, apparent molecular size (sucrose density gradient) and DNA binding affinity (DNA cellulose chromatography) pointing to intactness of the receptor. Brown et al. [153] examined the $1,25(OH)_2D_3$ receptor in parathyroid glands from normal dogs and dogs with CKD. They demonstrated that the levels of receptor were fourfold lower in parathyroid extracts from uremic dogs than in those from normal dogs. No differences were observed in the binding affinity for $1,25(OH)_2D_3$ or in the sedimentation in sucrose density gradients. In a seminal work, Korkor et al. [152] measured the binding of tritiated $1,25(OH)_2D_3$ to hyperplastic parathyroid glands obtained from seven patients with CKD. These values were compared with those for binding to hyperplastic parathyroid tissue obtained from six patients who had received renal transplants and for binding to parathyroid adenomas removed from five patients who had primary hyperparathyroidism. They found for the first time that Nmax (an estimate of the concentration of $1,25(OH)_2D_3$ receptors) was reduced in patients with CKD as compared with patients with transplanted kidneys and patients with primary hyperparathyroidism. Nmax correlated inversely with the severity of renal dysfunction, the serum level of P, and the logarithm of the serum level of PTH. Fukuda et al. [141] demonstrated later a lower density of VDR in the parathyroid glands showing *nodular* hyperplasia than in those showing *diffuse* hyperplasia. Even in the parathyroid glands showing diffuse hyperplasia, nodule-forming areas were present; these areas were virtually negative for VDR staining. A significant negative correlation was found between VDR density and the weight of the parathyroid glands. Since the biologic response to $1,25(OH)_2D_3$ is proportional to the density of VDR in the cell [156], not only inhibition of the VDR interaction with DNA but also reduction in the number of receptors may diminish the biologic response to $1,25(OH)_2D_3$ in CKD. Thus, reduction in the VDR number renders the parathyroid glands less responsive to the inhibitory action of $1,25(OH)_2D_3$ in renal patients [141, 157, 158].

Various mechanisms (at least three) have been proposed to explain the decrease of VDR in CKD: First, $1,25(OH)_2D_3$ is known to upregulate its own receptor [159–162]; consequently, the low plasma $1,25(OH)_2D_3$ concentration in renal failure could downregulate the VDR in spite of the direct positive effect of FGF23 on VDR [163, 164]. Additionally, it has been found that the VDR content in parathyroid glands of uremic rats is decreased and that the density is correlated with serum $1,25(OH)_2D_3$ levels [165]. On the other hand, replacement of $1,25(OH)_2D_3$ in renal failure appears to restore the receptor concentration [161], perhaps by increasing VDR messenger RNA levels [161] and/or the VDR half-life [161, 166]. Actually, normal serum $1,25(OH)_2D_3$ contributes in maintaining the VDR content in target tissues since $1,25(OH)_2D_3$ binding to the VDR protects the VDR against proteosomal degradation [166]. Finally, treatment with $1,25(OH)_2D_3$ in uremic rats has been found to prevent the decrease in VDR [165], and in a different rat model, administration of $1,25(OH)_2D_3$ to sham-operated rats resulted in an increase in $1,25(OH)_2D_3$ binding capacity in both intestinal mucosa and parathyroid glands. In contrast, Koyama et al. have shown that the VDR content of duodenal cells from uremic animals was unaffected by the administration of $1,25(OH)_2D_3$ [167]. Second, secondary hyperparathyroidism may decrease the concentration of VDR in renal failure, as suggested by the fact that PTH downregulates the VDR and VDR messenger RNA [149] and also blocks $1,25(OH)_2D_3$-induced upregulation of rat intestinal and renal VDR [131, 149]. Furthermore, elevation of PTH secondary to Ca deficiency downregulates renal VDR, despite a high concentration of plasma $1,25(OH)_2D_3$ [168]. Third, infusion of uremic ultrafiltrate in normal rats suppresses VDR synthesis [151], possibly at translational sites [161], and consequently accumulation of uremic toxins in CKD may reduce VDR concentration. This hypothesis is suggested by the low VDR number and high VDR messenger RNA level in CKD and normal rats infused with uremic ultrafiltrate, suggesting an effect at a post-transcriptional level [131, 161]. Consequently, decreased plasma $1,25(OH)_2D_3$, retention of uremic toxins and high plasma PTH could be at least partially responsible for reducing the number of VDR in renal CKD [131].

Calcium has also been shown to regulate the tissue content of VDR, a low Ca level appearing to down-regulate VDR and a high Ca concentration up-regulate VDR [169–171]. Sela-Brown have shown that a decrease in Ca produces an increase in the expression of calreticulin, a cytoplasmatic protein that prevents the binding of VDR-RXR to the PTH VDRE [172]. Moreover, in a model using vitamin D-deficient rats, prevention of secondary hyperparathyroidism by means of large amounts of dietary Ca avoided a decrease in parathyroid VDR expression. Thus, the regulation of VDR by $1,25(OH)_2D_3$ seemed to be mediated principally by serum Ca concentration [164, 169, 170, 173]. Extracellular Ca regulating VDR expression by parathyroid cells, independently of $1,25(OH)_2D_3$, was demonstrated by Garfia et al. [169]. Moreover, these authors also demonstrated that $1,25(OH)_2D_3$ upregulated VDR expression only when serum Ca concentration is elevated, and that the decrease in VDR induced by hypocalcemia may prevent the expected $1,25(OH)_2D_3$ induced reduction of PTH [169]. Thus, the stimulatory effect of $1,25(OH)_2D_3$ on VDR is more evident when adequate amounts of Ca are present [169–171, 174]. These effects of Ca on VDR appeared also to be specific for the parathyroid gland since not uniform results have been observed in other tissues [164, 169, 175]. It has recently been shown that extracellular Ca stimulates VDR expression in parathyroid glands through the elevation of the cytosolic Ca level and the stimulation of the PLA(2)-AA-dependent ERK1/2 pathway [176].

Furthermore, since extracellular Ca regulates VDR expression by parathyroid cells, it is not surprising that a calcimimetic (which potentiates the effects of Ca on the CaSR) results in a dose-dependent stimulatory effect on VDR expression in parathyroid tissue in vitro and in vivo, as well as on VDR protein in a human parathyroid gland with diffuse hyperplasia in vitro [177]. An acute increase in CaSR and VDR in the parathyroid glands of uremic rats treated with a different calcimimetic agent has also been described [170]. The ability of the calcimimetics to increase VDR expression may have potential implications on the combined clinical use of calcimimetics together with vitamin D analogs in the treatment of secondary hyperparathyroidism in dialysis patients [177, 178]. On the other hand, regarding the CaSR, low CaSR expression has been reported to occur in most cases of parathyroid adenoma and hyperplasia, compared with strong expression in normal tissue [179]. In secondary hyperparathyroidism, and similarly to what occurs to VDR, expression of CaSR was often particularly depressed in nodular areas compared with adjacent non-nodular parathyroid tissue [179]. Interestingly, it has also been shown that $1,25(OH)_2D_3$ not only up-regulated the VDR but also the CaSR in parathyroid glands cultured in vitro [173, 180], again with clear implications on the combined use of vitamin D analogs and calcimimetics. $1,25(OH)_2D_3$ did not upregulate kidney CaSR in a different report [181].

It has also been described that FGFR-1 and klotho are present in the parathyroid glands, and that klotho-FGFR1 complex is depressed in uremic conditions [163, 182–185]. In normal parathyroid glands, FGF23 not only decreased PTH secretion but also increased the expression of both CaSR and VDR; by contrast, in hyperplastic parathyroid glands, FGF23 did not produce either a phosphorylation of ERK 1/2 or a significant effect on PTH, cell proliferation, CaSR or VDR [163]. Finally, the $1,25(OH)_2D_3$-VDR complex induces not only CaSR but also klotho gene expression [18, 186], and the reductions in both proteins that occur with parathyroid hyperplasia could therefore be secondary to VDR loss. On the other hand, the importance of preventing EGFR activation to effectively suppress the development of parathyroid hyperplasia and VDR loss in early CKD has recently been demonstrated by Arcidiacono et al. [187, 188].

As is readily appreciated, the intrinsic inter-relationships of all these factors in the regulation of VDR, Ca and PTH, as well as the role of uremia, are complex and not yet completely understood. Additionally, the presence of a myriad of complex inter-relationships among the VDR and other related receptors (CaSR, FGFR/klotho), as well as the non-uniform behavior of these interactions in different tissues [164, 169, 175], complicates the issue further. As an additional example of this complexity, PTH and vitamin D upregulation of VDR and 1α-hydroxylase are deranged in the presence of hyperglycemia in VSMC [189].

In summary, CKD interferes with the metabolism and action of $1,25(OH)_2D_3$ (as reviewed by Dusso in Chap. 3), through decreasing the uptake of 25(OH)D [including non-renal cells expressing 1α-hydroxylase [190], the content of renal megalin available for recycling of 25(OH)D [191], and most notably, at the synthesis and clearance levels of $1,25(OH)_2D_3$, at least partially mediated by FGF-23. Furthermore, CKD also affects various VDR processes such as basal VDR synthesis and number of receptors, $1,25(OH)_2D_3$ binding, the uptake of the $1,25(OH)_2D_3$-VDR complex and the binding of the $1,25(OH)_2D_3$-VDR to VDRE, thereby affecting VDR function [57, 92, 131]. It creates a vicious cycle by which CKD impairs the maintenance of normal $1,25(OH)_2D_3$ metabolism, which in turn impedes vitamin $D/1,25(OH)_2D_3$ cardiovascular and renoprotective actions [37, 55]. In this vicious cycle, CKD may induce the lack of basal inhibition of the renin-angiotensin-aldosterone system, among other systems and pathways, leading to a perpetuation of deleterious protein-uria as well as systemic and renal interstitial inflammation [37, 192]. Recent studies, suggesting that both VDR transgenes are capable of recapitulating basal and regulated expression of the VDR and restore $1,25(OH)_2D_3$ function, may provide a baseline for further dissection of mechanisms integral to VDR gene expression and offer the potential to explore the consequence of selective mutations in VDR proteins in vivo [193].

4.8   Therapeutic Implications: Selective Vitamin D Receptor Activators in CKD

$1,25(OH)_2D_3$ is the active natural ligand of VDR and it is 500–1,000 times more active than its precursor 25-hydroxy-vitamin D [25(OH)D] [37, 101]. Actually, 25(OH)D is a VDR activator also in cells that do not express 1α-hydroxylase, because 25(OH)D can directly bind and activate the VDR especially because it circulates at much higher serum concentrations [101]. On the other hand, we have reviewed in this chapter how the binding of $1,25(OH)_2D_3$ induces conformational changes in the VDR and it seems that synthetic analogs of the natural $1,25(OH)_2D_3$ may induce unique changes that alter their biological function and tissue selectivity. In fact, the final goal of development of VDR activators is to improve their biological profile for a therapeutic application in one of the pleiotropic functions of the natural hormone [84]. Although it was reported that several vitamin D prohormones with low VDR affinity suppressed PTH, even when their activation was inhibited

[194, 195], – raising the possibility that their actions could be VDR independent -, it has also been recently shown in a novel organ culture model that direct suppression of PTH gene expression by doxercalciferol (a selective VDR activator) and 25(OH)D requires the VDR [196].

Since an excessive Ca and P loading is the most undesirable untoward effect of $1,25(OH)_2D_3$, especially in patients with CKD, VDR activators have been developed to reduce the capacity to induce in-vivo hypercalcemia, hyperphosphatemia and hypercalciuria, and thus the concept of *selective* VDR activators has evolved [197]. For instance, paricalcitol and maxacalcitol are considered selective VDR activators because they seem to preferentially effect parathyroid glands by retaining the action on PTH suppression while having less effect on Ca and P intestinal absorption or bone resorption [34, 198–200]. Consequently, these selective VDR activators could possibly avoid deleterious effects derived from serum high levels of Ca and P, including possible passive extraskeletal calcification in vessels or heart valves. Potentially, these differential effects could also have an impact on survival. Experimental studies have shown distinct actions of calcitriol or other VDR activators on extraosseous calcification, the former being a classic dose-dependent inductor of experimental vascular calcification especially in the presence of a high P exposure, or as a result of vitamin-D-induced systemic accumulation of Ca and P rather than a local effect on the arterial wall [162, 201–203]. On the other hand, lower doses of both calcitriol and paricalcitol seemed to be protective probably through restoration of klotho and osteopontin expression [19, 136, 204]. Thus, a bimodal effect of VDR activators has been described with regard to regulation of vascular calcification. This issue is further complicated by the differential expression and regulation of klotho in experimental uremia, and the tissue-dependent effect of a VDR activator such as paricalcitol, recently described [205]. In this study, paricalcitol prevented the decrease of klotho in the kidney, increased expression in the parathyroid, had no effect in the aortic media, but blunted the increase of klotho in the aortic adventitia –probably expressed by fibroblasts [205].

In general, the experimental data supporting less toxicity of some VDR activators compared with calcitriol are not consistent across studies, but they seem to support the claim that there is reduced induction of vascular calcification with different VDR activators, favoring paricalcitol [162, 199, 201, 206, 207]. However, there are no prospective randomized clinical trials that have evaluated the impact of native vitamin D or VDR activators on human vascular calcification. Finally, a robust and consistent survival benefit of VDR activators in hemodialysis patients has been described in several retrospective studies [208, 209], and although it has been questioned [210], the benefit seemed to be more pronounced in the low-dose range and among patients who received *selective* VDR activators [208]. Finally, a recent meta-analysis including 14 observational studies (194,932 patients) has shown that therapies with VDR activators are associated with reduced mortality in CKD patients [211], although another recent meta-analysis and a smaller study in peritoneal dialysis patients do not confirm these previous results [212, 213]. Again, no randomized clinical trial has been performed to prove or rule out this survival hypothesis. Consequently, it is not the time to say that interventions based on vitamin D definitely reduce mortality in patients with CKD, but the opposite cannot be said yet beyond all reasonable doubt [214]. In fact, given the paucity of good quality data, the reliability of the pooled results is still uncertain [214], warranting the need of larger trials on clinically significant hard-outcomes.

The alleged difference among analogs and their effects on different target organs may be related, among other factors, to different pharmacokinetic/pharmacodynamic properties by distinctly interacting with serum-binding proteins (e.g. affinity to circulating DBP) or differential metabolism in a tissue-selective manner. For instance, it has been shown that maxacalcitol has about 400–500 times less binding affinity to DBP than $1,25(OH)_2D_3$ [215], and thus has a shorter half-life and is cleared more rapidly from the circulation. It has also been shown that VDR analogs have a lower affinity for VDR than $1,25(OH)_2D_3$ [216, 217] and differential regulation of 24-hydroxylase in target tissues may also determine the half-life of $1,25(OH)_2D_3$ and analogs [217]. Interestingly, selective VDR activators seem to interact differentially with VDR coregulators and, based on conformational differences induced by these molecules, gene expression may be modified when the VDR/RXR complex binds to the VDRE, causing selectively distinct effects on DNA transcription in different cells and tissues [101, 218, 219]. Thus, the diversity of coregulators and multiple multicomponent complexes help explain receptor, target gene and cell-selective responses to different ligands at the same VDR [73]. As an example, calcitriol has ten times more affinity for binding to the VDR than the selective VDR activator paricalcitol [199, 216]; nevertheless, this difference in binding affinity is not the same for all body tissues, as the affinity of paricalcitol for the VDR in the parathyroid glands is three to four times lower than that of $1,25(OH)_2D_3$. Paricalcitol is less active than $1,25(OH)_2D_3$ in inducing homodimerization (VDR:VD) and heterodimerization of VDR: receptor-associated coactivator 3 (RAC3), and more active than calcitriol in inducing heterodimerization of VDR/RXR and VDR-glucocorticoid receptor interacting protein 1 (DRIP1) [120]. Clinically, it has been shown that selective VDR activators allow synthesis and secretion of PTH to be inhibited more efficiently and with a lower impact on intestinal absorption of Ca and P [199, 220]. Therefore, they are attributed a lower risk of hypercalcemia, hyperphosphatemia, and elevated Ca x P levels. In a five sixths nephrectomized rat model, when paricalcitol is compared with calcitriol, its impact at the same doses is three to four times less than calcitriol on PTH levels and ten times less on Ca and P levels meaning that paricalcitol can act with a larger therapeutic margin for the prevention and treatment of secondary hyperparathyroidism in early stages of CKD, as well as in patients on hemodialysis, and with a lower potential impact on vascular calcification [221, 222]. It has been also shown that switching $1,25(OH)_2D_3$ to *selective* vitamin D receptor activators such as paricalcitol can help controlling previously uncontrolled secondary hyperparathyroidism [223]. On the other hand, although there are no data on this action in humans, Malluche et al. [200] state, based on experimental data, that the vitamin D analogs paricalcitol and maxacalcitol could control PTH levels with a lower suppression of bone remodeling.

The differential effects of selective VDR activators have also been seen on gene expression in various types of cells and tissues, including the expression of molecules involved in the process of vascular calcification. Using DNA microarray technology to evaluate gene expression profiles in VSMC incubated with $1,25(OH)_2D_3$ or paricalcitol, it was shown that, though most of the expression profile was similar, paricalcitol activates and deactivates different genes than $1,25(OH)_2D_3$. These differences are not explained by dissimilar doses; thus, in an experimental model of active vascular calcification induced by uremia and high dietary P, it was shown that comparable doses of $1,25(OH)_2D_3$, paricalcitol and doxercalciferol have significant differences in mRNA expression of Cbfα1 (Runx2) and osteocalcin in aortic tissues, favoring paricalcitol [201, 206]. Paricalcitol, unlike $1,25(OH)_2D_3$, did not increase the expression of transcription factor Cbfα1, which activates one of the signaling pathways for transformation of VSMC into osteoblast-like cells [201, 206, 207]. It has also been shown that paricalcitol prevents the activation of the P-induced Wnt/β-catenin pathway, and also reduces calcification by downregulating the expression of BMP-2 [221, 224]. It is noteworthy that the risk of calciphylaxis was recently reported to be increased in patients treated with calcitriol but not in patients treated with selective vitamin D analogues such as paricalcitol or doxercalciferol [225]. Finally, the combination of nutritional vitamin D supplementation and paricalcitol, at doses ineffective to suppress PTH when given alone, prevented the increases in parathyroid, renal and/or macrophage TACE expression induced by five sixths nephrectomy, thereby markedly reducing parathyroid gland enlargement, proteinuria and aortic calcification [25].

Different VDR agonists also exhibit differential effects on endothelial function and aortic gene expression in five sixths nephrectomized rats, with alfacalcidol exhibiting less of an effect [226]. In patients with stage 3–4 CKD, paricalcitol has been shown to improve endothelium-dependent vasodilation [227], although these results have not been confirmed in patients with type II diabetes and CKD [228]. On the other hand, despite vitamin D deficiency seems to be a risk factor for arterial hypertension, vitamin D supplementation in hypertensive patients with low circulating 25(OH)D levels had no significant effect on blood pressure and several CV risk factors, but it was associated with a significant increase in triglycerides in a recent randomized clinical trial [229]. In contrast to the widely described inverse association between circulating 25(OH)D levels and hypertension risk, calcitriol levels have been recently associated positively with a higher risk of hypertension [230].

Reduction in myocardial VDR expression in rats with renal failure has also been related to myocardial remodeling and an increase in arrhythmogenesis, being reverted by paricalcitol by restoring myocardial VDR levels and prolonging action potentials [231]. VDR activation by different VDR analogs has also been shown to distinctly affect left ventricular hypertrophy, and paricalcitol was the only VDR activator which showed a relevant beneficial effect in the reduction of myocardial fibrosis, a key factor in the myocardial dysfunction in CKD patients [232]. Nevertheless, these apparently positive results are not uniform in all studies [233–235], despite it is now known that VDR may be a negative regulator of the TGF-β/Smad signaling, influences the regulation of T cells and inflammatory cytokines and may ameliorate epithelial-to-mesenchymal transition in different models [236, 237]. Many other studies have also shown positive effects of VDR activation on myocardial structure, left ventricular function or cardiovascular events, including dialysis and pre-dialysis patients [44, 235, 238–241]. However, two prospective RCT's in CKD patients using paricalcitol did not show a significant benefit in their predefined outcomes of left ventricular structure measured by cardiac magnetic resonance and LV function [242, 243], although some positive results (decrease in cardiovascular-related hospitalizations, left atrial volume index, attenuation of BNP rise) were described in secondary or post-hoc analysis [242, 244].

Finally, VS-105, a novel VDR activator, has been recently shown to improve cardiac function in five sixths nephrectomized rats [245]. A thorough review of the different VDR activators that are being developed in different areas, including CKD, heart disease or oncology, is completely beyond the scope of this chapter [73]. However, the current available information underlines the increasing importance of the vitamin D/VDR pleiotropic multifunctional axis, both in health and disease. Nevertheless, it is important to recognize that RCTs are required to confirm all the cardiovascular or survival alleged benefits of the old and these new compounds [34, 44, 219, 220].

References

1. Razin A. CpG methylation, chromatin structure and gene silencing-a three-way connection. EMBO J. 1998;17:4905–8.
2. Carlberg C. Target genes of vitamin D: spatio-temporal interaction of chromatin, VDR, and response elements. In: Vitamin D. 3rd ed. Oxford, UK: Elsevier; 2011. p. 211–26.
3. Evans RM, Mangelsdorf DJ. Nuclear receptors, RXR, and the Big Bang. Cell. 2014;157: 255–66.
4. Maglich JM, Sluder A, Guan X, et al. Comparison of complete nuclear receptor sets from the human, caenorhabditis elegans and drosophila genomes. Genome Biol. 2001;2:RESEARCH0029.
5. Nuclear Receptors Nomenclature Committee. A unified nomenclature system for the nuclear receptor superfamily. Cell. 1999;97:161–63.
6. Pike JW, Meyer MB, Lee SM. The vitamin D receptor: biochemical, molecular, biological and genomic era investigations. In: Vitamin D. 3rd ed. Oxford, UK: Elsevier; 2011. p. 97–135.
7. Robinson-Rechavi M, Carpentier AS, Duffraisse M, et al. How many nuclear hormone receptors are there in the human genome? Trends Genet. 2001;17:554–6.
8. Helsen C, Claessens F. Looking at nuclear receptors from a new angle. Mol Cell Endocrinol. 2014;382:97–106.
9. Norman AW. The mode of action of vitamin D. Biol Rev Camb Philos Soc. 1968;43:97–137.
10. Fraser DR, Kodicek E. Unique biosynthesis by kidney of a biological active vitamin D metabolite. Nature. 1970;228:764–6.
11. Wang Y, Zhu J, DeLuca HF. The vitamin D receptor in the proximal renal tubule is a key regulator of serum 1alpha,25-dihydroxyvitamin D(3). Am J Physiol Endocrinol Metab. 2015;308:E201–5.
12. Rojas-Rivera J, De La Piedra C, Ramos A, et al. The expanding spectrum of biological actions of vitamin D. Nephrol Dial Transplant. 2010;25:2850–65.
13. Owen TA, Aronow MS, Barone LM, et al. Pleiotropic effects of vitamin D on osteoblast gene expression are related to the proliferative and differentiated state of the bone cell phenotype: dependency upon basal levels of gene expression, duration of exposure, and bone matrix competency in norma. Endocrinology. 1991;128:1496–504.

14. Haussler MR, Haussler CA, Whitfield GK, et al. The nuclear vitamin D receptor controls the expression of genes encoding factors which feed the "Fountain of Youth" to mediate healthful aging. J Steroid Biochem Mol Biol. 2010;121:88–97.

15. Bar-Shavit Z, Teitelbaum SL, Reitsma P, et al. Induction of monocytic differentiation and bone resorption by 1,25-dihydroxyvitamin D3. Proc Natl Acad Sci U S A. 1983;80: 5907–11.

16. Haussler MR, Whitfield GK, Haussler CA, Hsieh J-C, Jurutka PW. Nuclear vitamin D receptor: natural lingands, molecular structure-function, and transcriptional control of viral genes. In: Vitamin D. 3rd ed. Oxford, UK: Elsevier; 2011. pp.137–70.

17. Liu W, Yu WR, Carling T, et al. Regulation of gp330/megalin expression by vitamins A and D. Eur J Clin Invest. 1998;28:100–7.

18. Canaff L, Hendy GN. Human calcium-sensing receptor gene. Vitamin D response elements in promoters P1 and P2 confer transcriptional responsiveness to 1,25-dihydroxyvitamin D. J Biol Chem. 2002;277:30337–50.

19. Lau WL, Leaf EM, Hu MC, et al. Vitamin D receptor agonists increase klotho and osteopontin while decreasing aortic calcification in mice with chronic kidney disease fed a high phosphate diet. Kidney Int. 2012;82:1261–70.

20. Hesse M, Frohlich LF, Zeitz U, et al. Ablation of vitamin D signaling rescues bone, mineral, and glucose homeostasis in Fgf-23 deficient mice. Matrix Biol. 2007;26:75–84.

21. Renkema KY, Alexander RT, Bindels RJ, et al. Calcium and phosphate homeostasis: concerted interplay of new regulators. Ann Med. 2008;40:82–91.

22. Cohen-Lahav M, Shany S, Tobvin D, et al. Vitamin D decreases NFkappaB activity by increasing IkappaBalpha levels. Nephrol Dial Transplant. 2006;21:889–97.

23. Moreno J, Krishnan AV, Swami S, et al. Regulation of prostaglandin metabolism by calcitriol attenuates growth stimulation in prostate cancer cells. Cancer Res. 2005;65:7917–25.

24. Keisala T, Minasyan A, Lou Y-R, et al. Premature aging in vitamin D receptor mutant mice. J Steroid Biochem Mol Biol. 2009;115:91–7.

25. Dusso A, Arcidiacono MV, Yang J, et al. Vitamin D inhibition of TACE and prevention of renal osteodystrophy and cardiovascular mortality. J Steroid Biochem Mol Biol. 2010;121: 193–8.

26. Morgado-Pascual JL, Rayego-Mateos S, Valdivielso JM, et al. Paricalcitol inhibits aldosterone-induced proinflammatory factors by modulating epidermal growth factor receptor pathway in cultured tubular epithelial cells. Biomed Res Int. 2015;2015:783538.

27. Husain K, Hernandez W, Ansari RA, et al. Inflammation, oxidative stress and renin angiotensin system in atherosclerosis. World J Biol Chem. 2015;6:209–17.

28. Kuro-o M. Klotho and aging. Biochim Biophys Acta. 2009;1790:1049–58.

29. Kuro-o M, Matsumura Y, Aizawa H, et al. Mutation of the mouse klotho gene leads to a syndrome resembling ageing. Nature. 1997;390:45–51.

30. Hu MC, Kuro-o M, Moe OW. Klotho and chronic kidney disease. Contrib Nephrol. 2013;180: 47–63.

31. Hu MC, Shi M, Zhang J, et al. Klotho deficiency causes vascular calcification in chronic kidney disease. J Am Soc Nephrol. 2010;22:124–36.

32. Richards JB, Valdes AM, Gardner JP, et al. Higher serum vitamin D concentrations are associated with longer leukocyte telomere length in women. Am J Clin Nutr. 2007;86:1420–5.

33. Feldman D, Krishnan AV, Swami S, et al. The role of vitamin D in reducing cancer risk and progression. Nat Rev Cancer. 2014;14:342–57.

34. Cozzolino M, Bover J, Vervloet M, Brandenburg V. A multidisciplinary review of the science of vitamin D receptor activation. Kidney Int Suppl. 2011;1:107–10.

35. Omdahl JL, Morris HA, May BK. Hydroxylase enzymes of the vitamin D pathway: expression, function, and regulation. Annu Rev Nutr. 2002;22:139–66.

36. Adams JS, Singer FR, Gacad MA, et al. Isolation and structural identification of 1,25-dihydroxyvitamin D3 produced by cultured alveolar macrophages in sarcoidosis. J Clin Endocrinol Metab. 1985;60:960–6.

37. Dusso AS, Tokumoto M. Defective renal maintenance of the vitamin D endocrine system impairs vitamin D renoprotection: a downward spiral in kidney disease. Kidney Int. 2011;79:715–29.
38. Holick MF. Vitamin D: evolutionary, physiological and health perspectives. Curr Drug Targets. 2011;12:4–18.
39. Mora JR, Iwata M, von Andrian UH. Vitamin effects on the immune system: vitamins A and D take centre stage. Nat Rev Immunol. 2008;8:685–98.
40. Chun RF, Liu PT, Modlin RL, et al. Impact of vitamin D on immune function: lessons learned from genome-wide analysis. Front Physiol. 2014;5:151.
41. White JH. Vitamin D, signaling, infectious diseases, and regulation of innate immunity. Infect Immun. 2008;76:3837–43.
42. Liu PT, Stenger S, Li H, et al. Toll-like receptor triggering of a vitamin D-mediated human antimicrobial response. Science. 2006;311:1770–3.
43. Santoro D, Lucisano S, Gagliostro G, et al. Vitamin D receptor polymorphism in chronic kidney disease patients with complicated cardiovascular disease. J Ren Nutr. 2015;25: 187–93.
44. Pilz S, Tomaschitz A, Drechsler C, et al. Vitamin D deficiency and heart disease. Kidney Int Suppl. 2011;1:111–5.
45. Li YC, Kong J, Wei M, et al. 1,25-Dihydroxyvitamin D(3) is a negative endocrine regulator of the renin-angiotensin system. J Clin Invest. 2002;110:229–38.
46. Arcidiacono MV, Cozzolino M, Spiegel N, et al. Activator protein 2alpha mediates parathyroid TGF-alpha self-induction in secondary hyperparathyroidism. J Am Soc Nephrol. 2008;19:1919–28.
47. Staab CA, Maser E. 11beta-Hydroxysteroid dehydrogenase type 1 is an important regulator at the interface of obesity and inflammation. J Steroid Biochem Mol Biol. 2010;119:56–72.
48. Cozzolino M, Lu Y, Finch J, et al. p21WAF1 and TGF-alpha mediate parathyroid growth arrest by vitamin D and high calcium. Kidney Int. 2001;60:2109–17.
49. Melenhorst WB, Visser L, Timmer A, et al. ADAM17 upregulation in human renal disease: a role in modulating TGF-alpha availability? Am J Physiol Renal Physiol. 2009;297:F781–90.
50. Donate-Correa J, Dominguez-Pimentel V, Mendez-Perez ML, et al. Selective vitamin D receptor activation as anti-inflammatory target in chronic kidney disease. Mediators Inflamm. 2014;2014:670475.
51. Navarro-González JF, Donate-Correa J, Méndez ML, et al. Anti-inflammatory profile of paricalcitol in hemodialysis patients: a prospective, open-label, pilot study. J Clin Pharmacol. 2013;53:421–6.
52. Shahnazari M, Yao W, Corr M, et al. Targeting the Wnt signaling pathway to augment bone formation. Curr Osteoporos Rep. 2008;6:142–8.
53. Chen D, Li Y, Zhou Z, et al. HIF-1α inhibits Wnt signaling pathway by activating Sost expression in osteoblasts. PLoS One. 2013;8:e65940.
54. London GM. Mechanisms of arterial calcifications and consequences for cardiovascular function. Kidney Int Suppl. 2013;3:442–5.
55. Nigwekar SU, Thadhani R. Vitamin D receptor activation: cardiovascular and renal implications. Kidney Int Suppl. 2013;3:427–30.
56. Labuda M, Fujiwara TM, Ross MV, et al. Two hereditary defects related to vitamin D metabolism map to the same region of human chromosome 12q13–14. J Bone Miner Res. 1992;7:1447–53.
57. Glorieux G, Vanholder R. Blunted response to vitamin D in uremia. Kidney Int Suppl. 2001;78:S182–5.
58. Brumbaugh PF, Haussler MR. 1 Alpha,25-dihydroxycholecalciferol receptors in intestine. I. Association of 1 alpha,25-dihydroxycholecalciferol with intestinal mucosa chromatin. J Biol Chem. 1974;249:1251–7.
59. Lawson DE, Wilson PW. Intranuclear localization and receptor proteins for 1,25-dihydroxycholecalciferol in chick intestine. Biochem J. 1974;144:573–83.

60. Brumbaugh PF, Haussler MR. Specific binding of 1alpha,25-dihydroxycholecalciferol to nuclear components of chick intestine. J Biol Chem. 1975;250:1588–94.
61. Hsu CH, Patel SR. Uremic toxins and vitamin D metabolism. Kidney Int Suppl. 1997;62: S65–8.
62. Pike JW, Haussler MR. Purification of chicken intestinal receptor for 1,25-dihydroxyvitamin D. Proc Natl Acad Sci U S A. 1979;76:5485–9.
63. Polly P, Herdick M, Moehren U, et al. VDR-Alien: a novel, DNA-selective vitamin D(3) receptor-corepressor partnership. FASEB J Off Publ Fed Am Soc Exp Biol. 2000;14: 1455–63.
64. Valdivielso JM, Fernandez E. Vitamin D receptor polymorphisms and diseases. Clin Chim Acta. 2006;371:1–12.
65. Alvarez-Hernandez D, Naves-Diaz M, Gomez-Alonso C, et al. Tissue-specific effect of VDR gene polymorphisms on the response to calcitriol. J Nephrol. 2008;21:843–9.
66. Negri AL, Brandenburg VM. Calcitriol resistance in hemodialysis patients with secondary hyperparathyroidism. Int Urol Nephrol. 2014;46:1145–51.
67. Marco MP, Martinez I, Amoedo ML, et al. Vitamin D receptor genotype influences parathyroid hormone and calcitriol levels in predialysis patients. Kidney Int. 1999;56:1349–53.
68. Marco MP, Martinez I, Betriu A, et al. Influence of Bsml vitamin D receptor gene polymorphism on the response to a single bolus of calcitrol in hemodialysis patients. Clin Nephrol. 2001;56:111–6.
69. Borras M, Torregrossa V, Oliveras A, et al. BB genotype of the vitamin D receptor gene polymorphism postpones parathyroidectomy in hemodialysis patients. J Nephrol. 2003;16: 116–20.
70. Bover J, Bosch RJ. Vitamin D receptor polymorphisms as a determinant of bone mass and PTH secretion: from facts to controversies. Nephrol Dial Transplant. 1999;14:1066–8.
71. Alvarez-Hernandez D, Naves M, Santamaria I, et al. Response of parathyroid glands to calcitriol in culture: is this response mediated by the genetic polymorphisms in vitamin D receptor? Kidney Int Suppl. 2003;63:S19–22.
72. Green S, Walter P, Kumar V, et al. Human oestrogen receptor cDNA: sequence, expression and homology to v-erb-A. Nature. 1986;320:134–9.
73. Natacha Rochel DM. Structural basis for ligand activity in VDR. In: Vitamin D. 3rd ed. Oxford, UK: Elsevier; 2011. p. 171191.
74. Hsu CH, Patel S, Young EW, et al. Production and degradation of calcitriol in renal failure rats. Am J Physiol. 1987;253:F1015–9.
75. Cyert MS. Regulation of nuclear localization during signaling. J Biol Chem. 2001;276:20805–8.
76. Umesono K, Murakami KK, Thompson CC, et al. Direct repeats as selective response elements for the thyroid hormone, retinoic acid, and vitamin D3 receptors. Cell. 1991;65:1255–66; 76b. Dowd DR, MacDonald PN. Coregulators of VDR-mediated gene expression. In: Vitamin D. 3rd ed. Elsevier; 2011, p. 193–210.
77. Thompson PD, Jurutka PW, Haussler CA, et al. Heterodimeric DNA binding by the vitamin D receptor and retinoid X receptors is enhanced by 1,25-dihydroxyvitamin D3 and inhibited by 9-cis-retinoic acid. Evidence for allosteric receptor interactions. J Biol Chem. 1998;273:8483–91.
78. Lemon BD, Fondell JD, Freedman LP. Retinoid X receptor: vitamin D3 receptor heterodimers promote stable preinitiation complex formation and direct 1,25-dihydroxyvitamin D3-dependent cell-free transcription. Mol Cell Biol. 1997;17:1923–37.
79. Greschik H, Moras D. Structure-activity relationship of nuclear receptor-ligand interactions. Curr Top Med Chem. 2003;3:1573–99.
80. Rochel N, Wurtz JM, Mitschler A, et al. The crystal structure of the nuclear receptor for vitamin D bound to its natural ligand. Mol Cell. 2000;5:173–9.
81. Yamamoto K, Anami Y, Itoh T. Development of vitamin D analogs modulating the pocket structure of vitamin D receptor. Curr Top Med Chem. 2014;14:2378–87.
82. Moras D, Gronemeyer H. The nuclear receptor ligand-binding domain: structure and function. Curr Opin Cell Biol. 1998;10:384–91.

83. Molnar F, Perakyla M, Carlberg C. Vitamin D receptor agonists specifically modulate the volume of the ligand-binding pocket. J Biol Chem. 2006;281:10516–26.
84. Carlberg C, Molnar F. Vitamin D receptor signaling and its therapeutic implications: genome-wide and structural view. Can J Physiol Pharmacol. 2015;93:311–8.
85. Kerner SA, Scott RA, Pike JW. Sequence elements in the human osteocalcin gene confer basal activation and inducible response to hormonal vitamin D3. Proc Natl Acad Sci U S A. 1989;86:4455–9.
86. Diane R, Dowd PNM. Corregulators of VDR-mediated gene expression. In: Vitamin D. 3rd ed. Oxford, UK: Elsevier; 2011. p. 193–209.
87. Toell A, Polly P, Carlberg C. All natural DR3-type vitamin D response elements show a similar functionality in vitro. Biochem J. 2000;352(Pt 2):301–9.
88. Van den Bemd G-JCM, Jhamai M, Staal A, et al. A central dinucleotide within vitamin D response elements modulates DNA binding and transactivation by the vitamin D receptor in cellular response to natural and synthetic ligands. J Biol Chem. 2002;277:14539–46.
89. Staal A, van Wijnen AJ, Birkenhager JC, et al. Distinct conformations of vitamin D receptor/retinoid X receptor-alpha heterodimers are specified by dinucleotide differences in the vitamin D-responsive elements of the osteocalcin and osteopontin genes. Mol Endocrinol. 1996;10:1444–56.
90. White JH. Profiling 1,25-dihydroxyvitamin D3-regulated gene expression by microarray analysis. J Steroid Biochem Mol Biol. 2004;89–90:239–44.
91. Kim M-S, Kondo T, Takada I, et al. DNA demethylation in hormone-induced transcriptional derepression. Nature. 2009;461:1007–12.
92. Llach F, Bover J. Renal osteodystrophies. In: Brenner BM, editor. The kidney. 6th ed. Philadelphia: WB Saunders Company; 2000. p. 2013–186.
93. Mackey SL, Heymont JL, Kronenberg HM, et al. Vitamin D receptor binding to the negative human parathyroid hormone vitamin D response element does not require the retinoid x receptor. Mol Endocrinol. 1996;10:298–305.
94. Okazaki T, Nishimori S, Ogata E, et al. Vitamin D-dependent recruitment of DNA-PK to the chromatinized negative vitamin D response element in the PTHrP gene is required for gene repression by vitamin D. Biochem Biophys Res Commun. 2003;304:632–7.
95. Chen LC, Tarone R, Huynh M, et al. High dietary retinoic acid inhibits tumor promotion and malignant conversion in a two-stage skin carcinogenesis protocol using 7,12-dimethylbenz[a]anthracene as the initiator and mezerein as the tumor promoter in female SENCAR mice. Cancer Lett. 1995;95:113–8.
96. Meyer MB, Benkusky NA, Lee C-H, et al. Genomic determinants of gene regulation by 1,25-dihydroxyvitamin D3 during osteoblast-lineage cell differentiation. J Biol Chem. 2014;289:19539–54.
97. Long MD, Sucheston-Campbell LE, Campbell MJ. Vitamin D receptor and RXR in the post-genomic era. J Cell Physiol. 2015;230:758–66.
98. Kozumenko A, Ohtake F, Fujiki R, Kato S. Epigenetic modifications in vitamin D receptor-mediated transrepression. In: Vitamin D. 3rd ed. Oxford, UK: Elsevier; 2011. p. 227–34.
99. Saccone D, Asani F, Bornman L. Regulation of the vitamin D receptor gene by environment, genetics and epigenetics. Gene. 2015;561:171–80.
100. Mangelsdorf DJ, Thummel C, Beato M, et al. The nuclear receptor superfamily: the second decade. Cell. 1995;83:835–9.
101. Dusso AS. Kidney disease and vitamin D levels: 25-hydroxyvitamin D, 1,25-dihydroxyvitamin D, and VDR activation. Kidney Int Suppl. 2011;1:136–41.
102. McKenna NJ, Cooney AJ, DeMayo FJ, et al. Minireview: evolution of NURSA, the nuclear receptor signaling atlas. Mol Endocrinol. 2009;23:740–6.
103. Endo I. Current topics on vitamin D. Combined therapy of anti-resorptive drug and active vitamin D. Clin Calcium. 2015;25:433–8.
104. Molnar F. Structural considerations of vitamin D signaling. Front Physiol. 2014;5:191.
105. Ecker JR, Bickmore WA, Barroso I, et al. The ENCODE Project Consortium. An integrated encyclopedia of DNA elements in the human genome. Nature. 2012;489:57–74.

106. Seuter S, Heikkinen S, Carlberg C. Chromatin acetylation at transcription start sites and vitamin D receptor binding regions relates to effects of 1alpha,25-dihydroxyvitamin D3 and histone deacetylase inhibitors on gene expression. Nucleic Acids Res. 2013;41:110–24.
107. Onate SA, Tsai SY, Tsai MJ, et al. Sequence and characterization of a coactivator for the steroid hormone receptor superfamily. Science. 1995;270:1354–7.
108. Choi JK, Howe LJ. Histone acetylation: truth of consequences? Biochem Cell Biol. 2009;87:139–50.
109. Chakravarti D, LaMorte VJ, Nelson MC, et al. Role of CBP/P300 in nuclear receptor signalling. Nature. 1996;383:99–103.
110. Wang F, Marshall CB, Ikura M. Transcriptional/epigenetic regulator CBP/p300 in tumorigenesis: structural and functional versatility in target recognition. Cell Mol Life Sci. 2013;70: 3989–4008.
111. Oda Y, Sihlbom C, Chalkley RJ, et al. Two distinct coactivators, DRIP/mediator and SRC/ p160, are differentially involved in vitamin D receptor transactivation during keratinocyte differentiation. Mol Endocrinol. 2003;17:2329–39.
112. Varshney S, Bhadada SK, Sachdeva N, et al. Methylation status of the CpG islands in vitamin D and calcium-sensing receptor gene promoters does not explain the reduced gene expressions in parathyroid adenomas. J Clin Endocrinol Metab. 2013;98:E1631–5.
113. Rachez C, Freedman LP. Mediator complexes and transcription. Curr Opin Cell Biol. 2001;13:274–80.
114. Belakavadi M, Fondell JD. Role of the mediator complex in nuclear hormone receptor signaling. Rev Physiol Biochem Pharmacol. 2006;156:23–43.
115. Barry JB, Leong GM, Church WB, et al. Interactions of SKIP/NCoA-62, TFIIB, and retinoid X receptor with vitamin D receptor helix H10 residues. J Biol Chem. 2003;278:8224–8.
116. Pathrose P, Barmina O, Chang C-Y, et al. Inhibition of 1,25-dihydroxyvitamin D3-dependent transcription by synthetic LXXLL peptide antagonists that target the activation domains of the vitamin D and retinoid X receptors. J Bone Miner Res. 2002;17:2196–205.
117. Wang X, Arai S, Song X, et al. Induced ncRNAs allosterically modify RNA-binding proteins in cis to inhibit transcription. Nature. 2008;454:126–30.
118. Wang X, Song X, Glass CK, et al. The long arm of long noncoding RNAs: roles as sensors regulating gene transcriptional programs. Cold Spring Harb Perspect Biol. 2011;3:a003756.
119. Burakov D, Crofts LA, Chang C-PB, et al. Reciprocal recruitment of DRIP/mediator and p160 coactivator complexes in vivo by estrogen receptor. J Biol Chem. 2002;277:14359–62.
120. Issa LL, Leong GM, Sutherland RL, et al. Vitamin D analogue-specific recruitment of vitamin D receptor coactivators. J Bone Miner Res. 2002;17:879–90.
121. Mizwicki MT, Norman AW. Vitamin D sterol/VDR conformational dynamics and nongenomis actions. In: Vitamin D. 3rd ed. Oxford, UK: Elsevier; 2011. p. 271–97.
122. Nemere I, Hintze K. Novel hormone "receptors". J Cell Biochem. 2008;103:401–7.
123. Gallieni M, Kamimura S, Ahmed A, et al. Kinetics of monocyte 1 alpha-hydroxylase in renal failure. Am J Physiol. 1995;268:F746–53.
124. Malinen M, Saramaki A, Ropponen A, et al. Distinct HDACs regulate the transcriptional response of human cyclin-dependent kinase inhibitor genes to trichostatin A and 1alpha,25-dihydroxyvitamin D3. Nucleic Acids Res. 2008;36:121–32.
125. Dobrzynski M, Bruggeman FJ. Elongation dynamics shape bursty transcription and translation. Proc Natl Acad Sci U S A. 2009;106:2583–8.
126. Peleg S, Nguyen CV. The importance of nuclear import in protection of the vitamin D receptor from polyubiquitination and proteasome-mediated degradation. J Cell Biochem. 2010;110:926–34.
127. Cozzolino M, Stucchi A, Rizzo MA, et al. Vitamin D receptor activation and prevention of arterial ageing. Nutr Metab Cardiovasc Dis. 2012;22:547–52.
128. Xu SS, Alam S, Margariti A. Epigenetics in vascular disease - therapeutic potential of new agents. Curr Vasc Pharmacol. 2014;12:77–86.
129. Fukagawa M, Kaname S, Igarashi T, et al. Regulation of parathyroid hormone synthesis in chronic renal failure in rats. Kidney Int. 1991;39:874–81.

130. Helvig CF, Cuerrier D, Hosfield CM, et al. Dysregulation of renal vitamin D metabolism in the uremic rat. Kidney Int. 2010;78:463–72.
131. Hsu CH, Patel SR. Altered vitamin D metabolism and receptor interaction with the target genes in renal failure: calcitriol receptor interaction with its target gene in renal failure. Curr Opin Nephrol Hypertens. 1995;4:302–6.
132. Bover J, Rodriguez M, Trinidad P, et al. Factors in the development of secondary hyperparathyroidism during graded renal failure in the rat. Kidney Int. 1994;45:953–61.
133. Bover J, Jara A, Trinidad P, et al. The calcemic response to PTH in the rat: effect of elevated PTH levels and uremia. Kidney Int. 1994;46:310–7.
134. DeFronzo RA, Alvestrand A, Smith D, et al. Insulin resistance in uremia. J Clin Invest. 1981;67:563–8.
135. Blum WF, Ranke MB, Kietzmann K, et al. Growth hormone resistance and inhibition of somatomedin activity by excess of insulin-like growth factor binding protein in uraemia. Pediatr Nephrol. 1991;5:539–44.
136. Lim K, Lu T-S, Molostvov G, et al. Vascular klotho deficiency potentiates the development of human artery calcification and mediates resistance to fibroblast growth factor 23. Circulation. 2012;125:2243–55.
137. Kazama JJ, Sato F, Omori K, et al. Pretreatment serum FGF-23 levels predict the efficacy of calcitriol therapy in dialysis patients. Kidney Int. 2005;67:1120–5.
138. Vulpio C, Maresca G, Distasio E, et al. Switch from calcitriol to paricalcitol in secondary hyperparathyroidism of hemodialysis patients: responsiveness is related to parathyroid gland size. Hemodial Int. 2011;15:69–78.
139. Manolagas SC, Yu XP, Girasole G, et al. Vitamin D and the hematolymphopoietic tissue: a 1994 update. Semin Nephrol. 1994;14:129–43.
140. Hsu CH, Patel SR, Young EW, et al. The biological action of calcitriol in renal failure. Kidney Int. 1994;46:605–12.
141. Fukuda N, Tanaka H, Tominaga Y, et al. Decreased 1,25-dihydroxyvitamin D3 receptor density is associated with a more severe form of parathyroid hyperplasia in chronic uremic patients. J Clin Invest. 1993;92:1436–43.
142. Patel SR, Ke HQ, Vanholder R, et al. Inhibition of nuclear uptake of calcitriol receptor by uremic ultrafiltrate. Kidney Int. 1994;46:129–33.
143. Walling MW, Kimberg DV, Wasserman RH, et al. Duodenal active transport of calcium and phosphate in vitamin D-deficient rats: effects of nephrectomy, Cestrum diurnum, and 1alpha,25-dihydroxyvitamin D3. Endocrinology. 1976;98:1130–4.
144. Baker LR, Abrams L, Roe CJ, et al. 1,25(OH)2D3 administration in moderate renal failure: a prospective double-blind trial. Kidney Int. 1989;35:661–9.
145. Toell A, Degenhardt S, Grabensee B, et al. Inhibitory effect of uremic solutions on protein-DNA-complex formation of the vitamin D receptor and other members of the nuclear receptor superfamily. J Cell Biochem. 1999;74:386–94.
146. Patel SR, Ke HQ, Vanholder R, et al. Inhibition of calcitriol receptor binding to vitamin D response elements by uremic toxins. J Clin Invest. 1995;96:50–9.
147. Jurutka PW, Hsieh JC, MacDonald PN, et al. Phosphorylation of serine 208 in the human vitamin D receptor. The predominant amino acid phosphorylated by casein kinase II, in vitro, and identification as a significant phosphorylation site in intact cells. J Biol Chem. 1993;268:6791–9.
148. Cake MH, DiSorbo DM, Litwack G. Effect of pyridoxal phosphate on the DNA binding site of activated hepatic glucocorticoid receptor. J Biol Chem. 1978;253:4886–91.
149. Reinhardt TA, Horst RL. Parathyroid hormone down-regulates 1,25-dihydroxyvitamin D receptors (VDR) and VDR messenger ribonucleic acid in vitro and blocks homologous up-regulation of VDR in vivo. Endocrinology. 1990;127:942–8.
150. Chen TL, Li JM, Ye TV, et al. Hormonal responses to 1,25-dihydroxyvitamin D3 in cultured mouse osteoblast-like cells--modulation by changes in receptor level. J Cell Physiol. 1986;126:21–8.
151. Hsu CH, Patel SR, Vanholder R. Mechanism of decreased intestinal calcitriol receptor concentration in renal failure. Am J Physiol. 1993;264:F662–9.

152. Korkor AB. Reduced binding of [3H]1,25-dihydroxyvitamin D3 in the parathyroid glands of patients with renal failure. N Engl J Med. 1987;316:1573–7.
153. Brown AJ, Dusso A, Lopez-Hilker S, et al. 1,25-(OH)2D receptors are decreased in parathyroid glands from chronically uremic dogs. Kidney Int. 1989;35:19–23.
154. Merke J, Hugel U, Zlotkowski A, et al. Diminished parathyroid 1,25(OH)2D3 receptors in experimental uremia. Kidney Int. 1987;32:350–3.
155. De Francisco ALM, Olmos JM, Martinez J. Calcitriol receptors after correction of uremia (Abstract). In: XII international congress of nephrology, Jerusalem; 1993.
156. Hirst M, Feldman D. Regulation of 1,25(OH)2 vitamin D3 receptor content in cultured LLC-PK1 kidney cells limits hormonal responsiveness. Biochem Biophys Res Commun. 1983;116:121–7.
157. Szabo A, Merke J, Thomasset M, et al. No decrease of 1,25(OH)2D3 receptors and duodenal calbindin-D9k in uraemic rats. Eur J Clin Invest. 1991;21:521–6.
158. Szabó A, Ritz E, Schmidt-Gayk H, et al. Abnormal expression and regulation of vitamin D receptor in experimental uremia. Nephron. 1996;73:619–28.
159. Naveh-Many T, Marx R, Keshet E, et al. Regulation of 1,25-dihydroxyvitamin D3 receptor gene expression by 1,25-dihydroxyvitamin D3 in the parathyroid in vivo. J Clin Invest. 1990;86:1968–75.
160. Costa EM, Feldman D. Homologous up-regulation of the 1,25 (OH)2 vitamin D3 receptor in rats. Biochem Biophys Res Commun. 1986;137:742–7.
161. Patel SR, Ke HQ, Hsu CH. Regulation of calcitriol receptor and its mRNA in normal and renal failure rats. Kidney Int. 1994;45:1020–7.
162. Lopez I, Aguilera-Tejero E, Mendoza FJ, et al. Calcimimetic R-568 decreases extraosseous calcifications in uremic rats treated with calcitriol. J Am Soc Nephrol. 2006;17:795–804.
163. Canalejo R, Canalejo A, Martinez-Moreno JM, et al. FGF23 fails to inhibit uremic parathyroid glands. J Am Soc Nephrol. 2010;21:1125–35.
164. Brown AJ, Zhong M, Finch J, et al. The roles of calcium and 1,25-dihydroxyvitamin D3 in the regulation of vitamin D receptor expression by rat parathyroid glands. Endocrinology. 1995;136:1419–25.
165. Denda M, Finch J, Brown AJ, et al. 1,25-dihydroxyvitamin D3 and 22-oxacalcitriol prevent the decrease in vitamin D receptor content in the parathyroid glands of uremic rats. Kidney Int. 1996;50:34–9.
166. Wiese RJ, Uhland-Smith A, Ross TK, et al. Up-regulation of the vitamin D receptor in response to 1,25-dihydroxyvitamin D3 results from ligand-induced stabilization. J Biol Chem. 1992;267:20082–6.
167. Brown AJ, Berkoben M, Ritter CS, et al. Binding and metabolism of 1,25-dihydroxyvitamin D3 in cultured bovine parathyroid cells. Endocrinology. 1992;130:276–81.
168. Goff JP, Reinhardt TA, Beckman MJ, et al. Contrasting effects of exogenous 1,25-dihydroxyvitamin D [1,25-(OH)2D] versus endogenous 1,25-(OH)2D, induced by dietary calcium restriction, on vitamin D receptors. Endocrinology. 1990;126:1031–5.
169. Garfia B, Canadillas S, Canalejo A, et al. Regulation of parathyroid vitamin D receptor expression by extracellular calcium. J Am Soc Nephrol. 2002;13:2945–52.
170. Mendoza FJ, Lopez I, Canalejo R, et al. Direct upregulation of parathyroid calcium-sensing receptor and vitamin D receptor by calcimimetics in uremic rats. Am J Physiol Renal Physiol. 2009;296:F605–13.
171. Russell J, Bar A, Sherwood LM, et al. Interaction between calcium and 1,25-dihydroxyvitamin D3 in the regulation of preproparathyroid hormone and vitamin D receptor messenger ribonucleic acid in avian parathyroids. Endocrinology. 1993;132:2639–44.
172. Sela-Brown A, Russell J, Koszewski NJ, et al. Calreticulin inhibits vitamin D's action on the PTH gene in vitro and may prevent vitamin D's effect in vivo in hypocalcemic rats. Mol Endocrinol. 1998;12:1193–200.
173. Carrillo-Lopez N, Alvarez-Hernandez D, Gonzalez-Suarez I, et al. Simultaneous changes in the calcium-sensing receptor and the vitamin D receptor under the influence of calcium and calcitriol. Nephrol Dial Transplant. 2008;23:3479–84.

174. Kumar R. Abnormalities of the vitamin D receptor in uraemia. Nephrol Dial Transplant. 1996;11 Suppl 3:6–10.
175. Sandgren ME, DeLuca HF. Serum calcium and vitamin D regulate 1,25-dihydroxyvitamin D3 receptor concentration in rat kidney in vivo. Proc Natl Acad Sci U S A. 1990;87:4312–4.
176. Canadillas S, Canalejo R, Rodriguez-Ortiz ME, et al. Upregulation of parathyroid VDR expression by extracellular calcium is mediated by ERK1/2-MAPK signaling pathway. AJP Ren Physiol. 2010;298:F1197–204.
177. Rodriguez ME, Almaden Y, Canadillas S, et al. The calcimimetic R-568 increases vitamin D receptor expression in rat parathyroid glands. Am J Physiol Renal Physiol. 2007;292:F1390–5.
178. Bover J, Ureña P, Ruiz-García C, et al. Clinical and practical use of calcimimetics in dialysis patients with secondary hyperparathyroidism. Clin J Am Soc Nephrol. 2016;11:161–74.
179. Gogusev J, Duchambon P, Hory B, et al. Depressed expression of calcium receptor in parathyroid gland tissue of patients with hyperparathyroidism. Kidney Int. 1997;51:328–36.
180. Carrillo-López N, Fernández-Martín JL, Cannata-Andía JB. The role of calcium, calcitriol and their receptors in parathyroid regulation. Nefrologia. 2009;29:103–8.
181. Piecha G, Kokeny G, Nakagawa K, et al. Calcimimetic R-568 or calcitriol: equally beneficial on progression of renal damage in subtotally nephrectomized rats. Am J Physiol Renal Physiol. 2008;294:F748–57.
182. Ben-Dov IZ, Galitzer H, Lavi-Moshayoff V, et al. The parathyroid is a target organ for FGF23 in rats. J Clin Invest. 2007;117:4003–8.
183. Komaba H, Goto S, Fujii H, et al. Depressed expression of klotho and FGF receptor 1 in hyperplastic parathyroid glands from uremic patients. Kidney Int. 2010;77:232–8.
184. Olauson H, Vervloet MG, Cozzolino M, et al. New insights into the FGF23-Klotho axis. Semin Nephrol. 2014;34:586–97.
185. Latus J, Lehmann R, Roesel M, et al. Analysis of α-klotho, fibroblast growth factor-, vitamin-D and calcium-sensing receptor in 70 patients with secondary hyperparathyroidism. Kidney Blood Press Res. 2013;37:84–94.
186. Forster RE, Jurutka PW, Hsieh J-C, et al. Vitamin D receptor controls expression of the anti-aging klotho gene in mouse and human renal cells. Biochem Biophys Res Commun. 2011;414:557–62.
187. Arcidiacono MV, Yang J, Fernandez E, et al. The induction of C/EBPβ contributes to vitamin D inhibition of ADAM17 expression and parathyroid hyperplasia in kidney disease. Nephrol Dial Transplant. 2015;30:423–33.
188. Arcidiacono MV, Yang J, Fernandez E, et al. Parathyroid-specific epidermal growth factor-receptor inactivation prevents uremia-induced parathyroid hyperplasia in mice. Nephrol Dial Transplant. 2015;30:434–40.
189. Somjen D, Knoll E, Sharon O, et al. Calciotrophic hormones and hyperglycemia modulate vitamin D receptor and 25 hydroxyy vitamin D 1-α hydroxylase mRNA expression in human vascular smooth muscle cells. J Steroid Biochem Mol Biol. 2015;148:210–3.
190. Bachmann S, Schlichting U, Geist B, et al. Kidney-specific inactivation of the megalin gene impairs trafficking of renal inorganic sodium phosphate cotransporter (NaPi-IIa). J Am Soc Nephrol. 2004;15:892–900.
191. Takemoto F, Shinki T, Yokoyama K, et al. Gene expression of vitamin D hydroxylase and megalin in the remnant kidney of nephrectomized rats. Kidney Int. 2003;64:414–20.
192. Andress DL. Adynamic bone in patients with chronic kidney disease. Kidney Int. 2008;73:1345–54.
193. Lee SM, Bishop KA, Goellner JJ, et al. Mouse and human BAC transgenes recapitulate tissue-specific expression of the vitamin D receptor in mice and rescue the VDR-null phenotype. Endocrinology. 2014;155:2064–76.
194. Brown AJ, Ritter CS, Knutson JC, et al. The vitamin D prodrugs 1alpha(OH)D2, 1alpha(OH)D3 and BCI-210 suppress PTH secretion by bovine parathyroid cells. Nephrol Dial Transplant. 2006;21:644–50.
195. Ritter CS, Armbrecht HJ, Slatopolsky E, et al. 25-hydroxyvitamin D(3) suppresses PTH synthesis and secretion by bovine parathyroid cells. Kidney Int. 2006;70:654–9.

196. Ritter CS, Brown AJ. Direct suppression of Pth gene expression by the vitamin D prohormones doxercalciferol and calcidiol requires the vitamin D receptor. J Mol Endocrinol. 2011;46:63–6.
197. Slatopolsky E, Brown AJ. Vitamin D analogs for the treatment of secondary hyperparathyroidism. Blood Purif. 2002;20:109–12.
198. Brown AJ, Finch J, Slatopolsky E. Differential effects of 19-nor-1,25-dihydroxyvitamin D(2) and 1,25-dihydroxyvitamin D(3) on intestinal calcium and phosphate transport. J Lab Clin Med. 2002;139:279–84.
199. Bover J, Dasilva I, Furlano M, et al. Clinical uses of 1,25-dihydroxy-19-nor-vitamin D(2) (Paricalcitol). Curr Vasc Pharmacol. 2014;12:313–23.
200. Malluche HH, Mawad H, Monier-Faugere M-C. Effects of treatment of renal osteodystrophy on bone histology. Clin J Am Soc Nephrol. 2008;3 Suppl 3:S157–63.
201. Lopez I, Mendoza FJ, Aguilera-Tejero E, et al. The effect of calcitriol, paricalcitol, and a calcimimetic on extraosseous calcifications in uremic rats. Kidney Int. 2008;73:300–7.
202. Lomashvili KA, Wang X, O'Neill WC. Role of local versus systemic vitamin D receptors in vascular calcification. Arterioscler Thromb Vasc Biol. 2014;34:146–51.
203. Han T, Rong G, Quan D, et al. Meta-analysis: the efficacy and safety of paricalcitol for the treatment of secondary hyperparathyroidism and proteinuria in chronic kidney disease. Biomed Res Int. 2013;2013:320560.
204. Mathew S, Lund RJ, Chaudhary LR, et al. Vitamin D receptor activators can protect against vascular calcification. J Am Soc Nephrol. 2008;19:1509–19.
205. Ritter CS, Zhang S, Delmez J, et al. Differential expression and regulation of Klotho by paricalcitol in the kidney, parathyroid, and aorta of uremic rats. Kidney Int. 2015;87:1141–52.
206. Mizobuchi M, Finch JL, Martin DR, et al. Differential effects of vitamin D receptor activators on vascular calcification in uremic rats. Kidney Int. 2007;72:709–15.
207. Bover J, Evenepoel P, Urena-Torres P, et al. Pro: cardiovascular calcifications are clinically relevant. Nephrol Dial Transplant. 2015;30:345–51.
208. Teng M, Wolf M, Lowrie E, et al. Survival of patients undergoing hemodialysis with paricalcitol or calcitriol therapy. N Engl J Med. 2003;349:446–56.
209. Vervloet MG, Twisk JWR. Mortality reduction by vitamin D receptor activation in end-stage renal disease: a commentary on the robustness of current data. Nephrol Dial Transplant. 2009;24:703–6.
210. Tentori F, Albert JM, Young EW, et al. The survival advantage for haemodialysis patients taking vitamin D is questioned: findings from the Dialysis Outcomes and Practice Patterns Study. Nephrol Dial Transplant. 2009;24:963–72.
211. Duranton F, Rodriguez-Ortiz ME, Duny Y, et al. Vitamin D treatment and mortality in chronic kidney disease: a systematic review and meta-analysis. Am J Nephrol. 2013;37:239–48.
212. Mann MC, Hobbs AJ, Hemmelgarn BR, et al. Effect of oral vitamin D analogs on mortality and cardiovascular outcomes among adults with chronic kidney disease: a meta-analysis. Clin Kidney J. 2015;8:41–8.
213. Bond TC, Wilson S, Moran J, et al. Mortality rates do not differ among patients prescribed various vitamin D agents. Perit Dial Int. 2015;35:62–9.
214. Morrone LF, Cozzolino M. The beneficial impact of vitamin D treatment in CKD patients: what's next? Clin Kidney J. 2015;8:38–40.
215. Kobayashi T, Okano T, Tsugawa N, et al. Metabolism and transporting system of 22-oxacalcitriol. Contrib Nephrol. 1991;91:129–33.
216. Slatopolsky E, Finch J, Brown A. New vitamin D analogs. Kidney Int Suppl. 2003;62:S83–7.
217. Nakane M, Ma J, Rose AE, et al. Differential effects of vitamin D analogs on calcium transport. J Steroid Biochem Mol Biol. 2007;103:84–9.
218. Carlberg C, Quack M, Herdick M, et al. Central role of VDR conformations for understanding selective actions of vitamin D(3) analogues. Steroids. 2001;66:213–21.
219. Bover J, Egido J, Fernández-Giráldez E, et al. Vitamin D, vitamin D receptor and the importance of its activation in patients with chronic kidney disease. Nefrologia. 2015;35:28–41.

220. Bover J, Cozzolino M. Mineral and bone disorders in chronic kidney disease and end-stage renal disease patients: new insights into vitamin D receptor activation. Kidney Int Suppl. 2011;1:122–9.
221. Martínez-Moreno JM, Muñoz-Castañeda JR, Herencia C, et al. In vascular smooth muscle cells paricalcitol prevents phosphate-induced Wnt/β-catenin activation. Am J Physiol Renal Physiol. 2012;303:F1136–44.
222. Kalantar-Zadeh K. Survival differences between activated injectable vitamin D2 and D3 analogs. Kidney Int. 2007;71:827; author reply 827–8.
223. Llach F, Yudd M. Paricalcitol in dialysis patients with calcitriol-resistant secondary hyperparathyroidism. Am J Kidney Dis. 2001;38:S45–50.
224. Rodriguez M, Martinez-Moreno JM, Rodríguez-Ortiz ME, et al. Vitamin D and vascular calcification in chronic kidney disease. Kidney Blood Press Res. 2011;34:261–8.
225. Nigwekar SU, Bhan I, Turchin A, et al. Statin use and calcific uremic arteriolopathy: a matched case-control study. Am J Nephrol. 2013;37:325–32.
226. Wu-Wong JR, Li X, Chen Y-W. Different vitamin D receptor agonists exhibit differential effects on endothelial function and aortic gene expression in 5/6 nephrectomized rats. J Steroid Biochem Mol Biol. 2015;148:202–9.
227. Zoccali C, Curatola G, Panuccio V, et al. Paricalcitol and endothelial function in chronic kidney disease trial. Hypertension. 2014;64:1005–11.
228. Thethi TK, Bajwa MA, Ghanim H, et al. Effect of paricalcitol on endothelial function and inflammation in type 2 diabetes and chronic kidney disease. J Diabetes Complications. 2015;29:433–7.
229. Pilz S, Gaksch M, Kienreich K, et al. Effects of vitamin D on blood pressure and cardiovascular risk factors: a randomized controlled trial. Hypertension. 2015;65:1195–201.
230. Van Ballegooijen AJ, Gansevoort RT, Lambers-Heerspink HJ, et al. Plasma 1,25-dihydroxyvitamin D and the risk of developing hypertension: the prevention of renal and vascular end-stage disease study. Hypertension. 2015;66:563–70.
231. Diez ER, Altamirano LB, García IM, et al. Heart remodeling and ischemia-reperfusion arrhythmias linked to myocardial vitamin d receptors deficiency in obstructive nephropathy are reversed by paricalcitol. J Cardiovasc Pharmacol Ther. 2015;20:211–20.
232. Panizo S, Barrio-Vázquez S, Naves-Díaz M, et al. Vitamin D receptor activation, left ventricular hypertrophy and myocardial fibrosis. Nephrol Dial Transplant. 2013;28:2735–44.
233. Repo JM, Rantala IS, Honkanen TT, et al. Paricalcitol aggravates perivascular fibrosis in rats with renal insufficiency and low calcitriol. Kidney Int. 2007;72:977–84.
234. Sezer S, Tutal E, Bal Z, et al. Differential influence of vitamin D analogs on left ventricular mass index in maintenance hemodialysis patients. Int J Artif Organs. 2014;37:118–25.
235. Li X-H, Feng L, Yang Z-H, et al. The effect of active vitamin D on cardiovascular outcomes in predialysis chronic kidney diseases: a systematic review and meta-analysis. Nephrology (Carlton). 2015;20:706–14.
236. Zerr P, Vollath S, Palumbo-Zerr K, et al. Vitamin D receptor regulates TGF-β signalling in systemic sclerosis. Ann Rheum Dis. 2015;74:e20.
237. González-Mateo GT, Fernández-Míllara V, Bellón T, et al. Paricalcitol reduces peritoneal fibrosis in mice through the activation of regulatory T cells and reduction in IL-17 production. PLoS One. 2014;9:e108477.
238. Park CW, Oh YS, Shin YS, et al. Intravenous calcitriol regresses myocardial hypertrophy in hemodialysis patients with secondary hyperparathyroidism. Am J Kidney Dis. 1999;33: 73–81.
239. Lemmilä S, Saha H, Virtanen V, et al. Effect of intravenous calcitriol on cardiac systolic and diastolic function in patients on hemodialysis. Am J Nephrol. 1998;18:404–10.
240. Kim HW, Park CW, Shin YS, et al. Calcitriol regresses cardiac hypertrophy and QT dispersion in secondary hyperparathyroidism on hemodialysis. Nephron Clin Pract. 2006;102:c21–9.
241. Bodyak N, Ayus JC, Achinger S, et al. Activated vitamin D attenuates left ventricular abnormalities induced by dietary sodium in Dahl salt-sensitive animals. Proc Natl Acad Sci U S A. 2007;104:16810–5.

242. Thadhani R, Appelbaum E, Pritchett Y, et al. Vitamin D therapy and cardiac structure and function in patients with chronic kidney disease: the PRIMO randomized controlled trial. JAMA. 2012;307:674–84.
243. Wang AY-M, Fang F, Chan J, et al. Effect of paricalcitol on left ventricular mass and function in CKD – the OPERA trial. J Am Soc Nephrol. 2014;25:175–86.
244. Tamez H, Zoccali C, Packham D, et al. Vitamin D reduces left atrial volume in patients with left ventricular hypertrophy and chronic kidney disease. Am Heart J. 2012;164:902–9.e2.
245. Wu-Wong JR, Chen Y-W, Wessale JL. Vitamin D receptor agonist VS-105 improves cardiac function in the presence of enalapril in 5/6 nephrectomized rats. Am J Physiol Renal Physiol. 2015;308:F309–19.

Chapter 5
Measurement of Circulating 1,25-Dihydroxyvitamin D and Vitamin D–Binding Protein in Chronic Kidney Diseases

Etienne Cavalier and Pierre Delanaye

Abstract After providing a short reminder on the physiopathology of vitamin D, we will discuss the potential interest to analyze the different metabolites of vitamin D. Undoubtly, measuring 25(OH) vitamin D is one of the most relevant and frequent dosage in daily clinical practice. Indeed, this is the most interesting measurement to assess global vitamin D status. The number of 25(OH)D determinations has dramatically increased over the last 10 years. This fact has led most of the clinical laboratories to move from the DiaSorin RIA, the most widely used method before twenties, to automated immunoassays or liquid chromatographs coupled with two mass spectrometers in tandem (LC-MS/MS). Anyway, one has to remember that analytical 25(OH)D determination is far from an easy task. Indeed, several important problems have to be overcome to correctly assess this parameter. Among them, the very high lipophilic nature of the molecule and its strong association with vitamin D–binding protein (VDBP) and, to a lesser extent, albumin, necessitates a thorough separation step and, for the one-phase immunoassays, a good equilibrium between the analyte and the antibodies used in the kits. We will also discuss the performance of this measurement in very specific population like pregnant women and chronic kidney diseases patients treated by dialysis among others.

In this chapter, we will also describe potential indications and methods available to measure other vitamin D metabolites like cholecalciferol, 1,25 and 24,25 vitamin D. Finally, we will critically focus on vitamin D binding protein (VDBP) and on the new concept of "free" or "bioavailable" vitamin D.

Keywords Analytical • LCMS/MS • Standardization • 25-OH vitamin D • 24.25(OH)2-vitamin D • 1,25(OH)2-vitamin D

E. Cavalier, PhD (✉)
Department of Clinical Chemistroy, University of Liège, Liège, Belgium
e-mail: etienne.cavalier@chu.ulg.ac.be

P. Delanaye
Department of Nephrology, Dialysis and Transplantion, University of Liege, Liege, Belgium
e-mail: pierre_delanaye@yahoo.fr

© Springer International Publishing Switzerland 2016   117
P.A. Ureña Torres et al. (eds.), *Vitamin D in Chronic Kidney Disease*,
DOI 10.1007/978-3-319-32507-1_5

5.1   Introduction

Patients suffering from chronic kidney diseases (CKD), and particularly those undergoing hemodialysis, are prone to suffer from many diseases, and notably mineral and metabolic bone diseases (MBD). It is also noteworthy that these patients largely suffer from vitamin D deficiency and a chapter of this book will be dedicated to the epidemiology of vitamin D in CKD. Vitamin D plays an important role in the bone and mineral metabolism field, but it has also been suggested that vitamin D deficiency had potential impact on numerous diseases beyond bone pathologies, like cardiovascular diseases, auto-immune diseases, diabetes, malignancies,… [1]. The last version of the Kidney Disease Improving Global Outcome (KDIGO) guidelines, which are followed worldwide to monitor and treat CKD-MBD patients suggests that, in patients with CKD stages 3–5D, circulating 25(OH)D (calcidiol) levels might be measured, and repeated testing determined by baseline values and therapeutic interventions. They also suggest that vitamin D deficiency and insufficiency be corrected using treatment strategies recommended for the general population. Even if these suggestions do not have a high level of evidence (2C), a very large part of nephrologists now supplement their patients with "native" vitamin D and control their 25(OH)D levels routinely whereas this wasn't really the case a few years ago.

In this chapter, we will provide a short reminder on the physiopathology of vitamin D. Then we will discuss the potential interest to analyze the different metabolites of vitamin D and we will insist on some pitfalls that unfortunately happen frequently. Finally, we will critically focus on vitamin D–binding protein (VDBP) and on the new concept of "free" or "bioavailable" vitamin D.

5.2   Physiopathology of Vitamin D

Vitamin D can be found as two forms, namely vitamin D2 (ergocalciferol) from vegetal origin (mainly some mushrooms) and vitamin D3 (cholecalciferol), which is the form synthesized by humans and animals. Vitamin D can be found in some (rare) foods, mainly in fat fish, but the major way for humans to get vitamin D is to expose their skin to the sunlight – or to take supplements. Intestinal diffusion of vitamin D from food or supplements is rather slow and passive and occurs mainly in the proximal part of the small intestine. When human skin is exposed to UVB radiation, the 7-dehydrocholesterol, present in the deep layers of the epidermis gets transformed into vitamin D. This production is quite important as we can estimate that a total fair-skinned body exposition at noon in summer (on a non-cloudy day) during 20 min will lead to the production of up to 15,000 IU of vitamin D. By comparison, 100 g of wild salmon will only provide 600 IU. However, this production will not occur from October to April in Europe and will depend on the age of the individual, use or sun creams, skin pigmentation, pollution and, of course, religious or cultural habits aiming to cover the skin. If intestinal absorption of vitamin D is proportional to the intakes, there will be an auto-limitation of the ability of the skin to produce vitamin D after an important synthesis (by stopping 7-dehydrocholesterol conversion into pre-vitamin D). This explains why there will never be any intoxication after sun-exposure, whereas this can happen – with serious consequences – when large amounts are ingested, i. e. after a dramatic posology error.

Vitamin D3 synthesized by the skin is transported to the liver by VDBP whereas D3 or D2 from intestine absorption is mainly integrated into the chylomicrons. Once in the liver, vitamin D is hydroxylated on the carbon in position 25 to give rise to 25(OH)D or calcidiol. This hydroxylation is weekly regulated and is performed by at least two different 25-hyroxylases, the one encoded by CYP2R1 gene being the main one (mice having normal vitamin D incomes but who are lacking CYP2R1 gene possess circulating 25(OH)D values lower than 50 % compared to wild type, but a normal phenotype) [2]. Calcidiol is finally released in the circulation where it circulates in nanomolar range, tightly bound to VDBP and, for a smaller amount, to albumin.

Half-life of 25(OH)D is about 3 weeks and is actually considered to reflect the vitamin D status. To be completely active (25(OH)D has a very low, but non null activity on the VDR), 25(OH)D must be hydroxylated on the carbon in position 1 by the 1-alpha hydroxylase (an enzyme encoded by the CYP27B1 gene) to give 1,25(OH)2D or calcitriol. Half-life of calcitriol is much shorter than half-life of calcidiol and is about 4–6 h. This hydroxylation classically occurs in the kidney, but we know by now that many other cells also possess a 1-alpha hydroxylase. To be hydroxylated in the kidney, calcidiol bound to VDBP is filtered through the glomerulus and then actively reabsorbed by the proximal tubular cells through different membrane receptors expressed on the luminal membrane, among which megalin is the best known. With the help of a second protein, called cubulin, megalin catches VDBP and internalizes it into the cytoplasm of the proximal cell, where it is further destroyed. Unbound calcidiol is then either transformed by the 1-alpha hydroxylase in the mitochondria or released in the circulation where it is taxied again by a free VDBP. Contrary to the first one, this second step of hydroxylation is tightly regulated, mainly by PTH, fibroblast growth factor 23 (FGF23), phosphate and 1,25(OH)2D itself. Calcitriol is finally released in the circulation in picomolar range where it is also bound (but with a lesser affinity than calcidiol) to VDBP. It is a true hormone which exerts its effects by binding a receptor (vitamin D receptor, or VDR), present in target tissues. These effects can be genomic, like in intestine cells, where VDR-calcitriol complexes – after an association with retinoic acid receptor – bind the DNA to stimulate the synthesis of different protein like calbindin 9 k, TRPV6, claudins 2 and 13 as well as PMCA1 and NCX, involved in active calcium transport from the lumen of the intestine to the circulation. Calcitriol exerts its genomic effects on other targets, like the osteoblast (synthesis of RANKL and osteocalcin), the osteocyte (to stimulate the secretion of FGF23), the kidney (to control the expression of TRPV5) and the parathyroid glands (to control the secretion of parathyroid hormone (PTH)). Next to the genomic effects, calcitriol has also non-genomic effects when binding to membrane-bound VDR, like 1.25-MMARS [3]. This leads to very fast actions like activation of tyrosine kinases or modifications in intracellular calcium flux in muscle or pancreatic cells.

Inactivation of vitamin D is achieved through the hydroxylation of the carbon in position 24 by a 24-hydroxylase, leading to 24,25(OH)2 or 1,24,25(OH)3 vitamin D and finally inactive calcitrioic acid excreted in bile or urine. This enzyme is encoded by the CYP24A1 gene and is present in the proximal tubule, where it is stimulated by FGF23, but also in all the target cells described above which possess a 1-alpha hydroxylase and a VDR. This inactivation pathway is very important since inactivating mutations of the CYP24A1 have been shown to be responsible for a "vitamin D hypersensibility", leading to severe hypercalcemia and nephrocalcinosis [4].

5.3 Measurement of Vitamin D and Its Metabolites: Analytical and Clinical Considerations

The characteristics of vitamin D metabolites described in this section are outlined in Table 5.1.

5.3.1 Cholecalciferol

Cholecalciferol (the non-hydroxylated vitamin D) has been measured with HPLC in the 1990s to evaluate the production of vitamin D after skin exposure to UVB [5] but can be measured nowadays with LCMS/MS methods. This determination is, of course, not performed in routine because, up to now, cholecalciferol has no clinical implications. Nevertheless, cholecalciferol is the substrate for 25(OH)D production. Its half-life is shorter than 25(OH)D (12–24 h), is not stored in the adipose for a later release and is excreted in bile, feces and urine. We have mentioned earlier that 25-hydroxylation was performed in the liver, but extra-hepatic activities of 25-hydroxylase also occur in different other tissues such as kidney and intestine. This contribution is not clear yet, and the physiological implications are likely limited to the autocrine/paracrine functions to regulate tissue specific processes [6]. Posology schemes for vitamin D supplementation are based on daily, weekly and monthly doses and have been shown to be equivalent in terms of 25(OH)D concentrations achievement. The only point that has not been taken into consideration is the steady-state of circulating cholecalciferol that can be obtained with frequent doses, but not with larger, spaced, doses. Since the different enzymes involved in 25-hydroxylation (27A1, 2R1, CYP2J3, CYP2J2, CYP2D25) possess different catalytic properties, it is not known whether the local production of 25(OH)D could be affected by the amount of substrate available for hydroxylation or not. This will probably deserve future investigations. Finally, cholecalciferol measurement could also be used to monitor response to treatment with vitamin, in conjunction with 24.25(OH)2D (see below) [7].

Table 5.1   Analytical characteristics of vitamin D metabolites

Analyte	Determination method	Range of concentration	Pitfalls
Cholecalciferol/ ergocalciferol (vitamin D3/D2)	HPLC, LCMS/ MS	ng/mL	Low concentration. Very lipophilic; difficult to remove from VDBP; short half-life; no standardization; no reference method
Calcifediol (25(OH)D)	ELISA, RIA, automated chemiluminescent analyzers, HPLC, LCMS/MS	ng/mL	Very lipophilic; necessity to displace from VDBP; standardization problems; issues observed in some subgroups of population; can be found as 25(OH)D2 and 25(OH)D3; interference with 24,25(OH)2D with some immune-assays and C3-epimer with some LCMS/MS
Calcitriol (1,25(OH)$_2$D)	ELISA, RIA, automated chemiluminescent analyzers, LCMS/ MS	pg/mL	Very low concentration; short half-life; can be found as 1,25(OH)$_2$D$_2$ and 1,25(OH)$_2$D$_3$; extraction step often needed prior to determination; lack of standardization; no reference method
24,25(OH)2D	LCMS/MS	ng/mL	Low concentration; need to have very good sensitivity to exclude 24-hydroxylase mutation; no standardization; no reference method
Free (or bioavailable) 25(OH)D	ELISA, calculation	pg/mL	Very low concentration. Need to avoid interference by 25(OH)D bound to VDBP or albumin. No reference method, no standardization. Can be found as free/bioavailable 25(OH)D2 or D3. Polymorphism of VDBP. Formula not extensively validated

Abbreviations: *HPLC* high performance liquid chromatography, *LCMS/MS* liquid chromatography mass spectrometry/mass spectrometry, *ELISA* enzyme linked immunosorbent assay, *RIA* radioimmunoassay, *VDBP* vitamin D–binding protein

5.3.2   25(OH)D

The number of 25(OH)D determinations has dramatically increased over the last 10 years. This increasing number of requests has led most of the clinical laboratories to move from the DiaSorin RIA, the most widely used method in the 1990s and early 1920s, to methods presenting a larger throughput, *i. e.* automated immunoassays or liquid chromatographs coupled with two mass spectrometers in tandem (LC-MS/ MS). Anyway, one has to remember that analytical 25(OH)D determination is far from an easy task. Indeed, several important problems have to be overcome to correctly assess this parameter. Among them, the very high lipophilic nature of the molecule and its strong association with vitamin D binding protein (VDBP) and, to a lesser extent, albumin, necessitates a thorough separation step and, for the one-phase immunoassays, a good equilibrium between the analyte and the antibodies used in the kits [8]. VDBP can be present at different concentrations according to some physiological or pathological conditions, like race [9], pregnancy or CKD, which could influence the kinetic of the liberation of the molecule [10, 11]. Vitamin D can be found as vitamin D2 or D3 and the assay should measure both 25(OH)D2 and 25(OH)D3 [12]. Different other metabolites of vitamin D, i.e. C3-epimer or 24,25(OH)2-vitamin D can be present in the serum of the patients at different levels, possibly interfering with either immunoassays or LC-MS/MS methods [13]. Just like any other immunoassays, vitamin D assays are prone to heterophilic antibodies interference, leading to potential spurious results [14]. Last but not least, the standardisation of the different assays remains a major problem. Hopefully, we have now a commonly accepted reference method and an ongoing a worldwide standardisation program, coordinated by the Center of Diseases Control (CDC), the National Institute of Standards and Technology (NIST) and the University of Ghent [15]. All these efforts have globally improved the global concordance of different assays for 25(OH)D determination in the "normal healthy" population, but some issues are still remaining, notably in "special" populations, like pregnant women and African (or Asian) subjects because of their high and low, respectively, concentrations of VDBP .

CKD and patients treated by hemodialysis (HD) or peritoneal dialysis (PD) are also particular populations in whom 25(OH)D determination remain problematic. Indeed, these patients present a serum matrix which is quite different from the general matrix of the "healthy" population. Uremic toxins, present in the samples of CKD patients, but not in the calibrators of the assays, can indeed induce a matrix effect. Protein concentrations can also be quite different in patients suffering from nephrotic syndrome and this can also lead to matrix effects. Proteins are also, to various extents, carbamylated and it remains unknown whether this affects the assays or not. As a result, most of the immunoassays available on the market tend to underestimate 25(OH) in HD and PD patients compared to LCMS, even if they are correctly calibrated [16].

Unfortunately, few manufacturers have taken this issue into consideration, and assays should be improved. In 2012, Heijboer et al. compared 6 routine immunoassays to a LCMS/MS method and shown that, if the slopes ranged from 0.83 (IDS iSYS) to 1.09 (Abbott Architect) in healthy individuals, the slopes observed in HD patients were ranging from 0.50 (Abbott Architect) to 0.82 (DiaSorin RIA). One year later, Depreter et al. showed that the slopes on Abbott Architect were of 0.39 and 0.50, for Roche Modular 0.92 and 0.92 and for IDS iSYS of 0.61 and 0.80 for HD and healthy subjects, respectively compared to a LCMS/MS method. They also concluded that iSYS showed better performance than Modular E170 (Roche) for the HD patients in the 25(OH)D range 10–40 ng/ml, due to a higher number of apparently underestimated concentrations by Modular.

5.3.3   1,25(OH)₂D

As already mentioned, measurement of circulating levels of 1,25(OH)₂D should not be used to evaluate the vitamin D status which is consensually assessed through the measurement of 25(OH)D [17]. However, it is important for the differential diagnosis of several disorders of calcium/phosphorus metabolism, especially in case of hypercalcemia, hypercalciuria, and low serum PTH level [18], or in case of rickets/osteomalacia which persists after vitamin D supplementation [19]. Calcitriol serum levels are modified in many clinical situations, increased for example during pregnancy or primary hyperparathyroidism (PHPT), and decreased in CKD or hypoparathyroidism.

Measurement of $1,25(OH)_2D$ concentration in serum is not an easy task due to its hydrophobic nature and because it circulates at picomolar levels compared to $25(OH)D$ which circulates at a 1,000-fold higher concentration. Currently available $1,25(OH)_2D$ assays are either radio-immunoassays that require time-consuming extraction procedures and long incubation times, semi-automated immunoassays that also require extraction procedures or LCMS/MS methods (that are not available in every lab). The sensitivity of the immunoassays is generally not compatible with the circulating amounts observed in CKD and HD patients. Finally, an interference between very high $25(OH)D$ levels (as seen in intoxications) and 1.25 assays occurs, leading to false positive values [20].

Very recently, a fully automated and rapid method has been launched by DiaSorin on Liaison XL which does not require an extraction step, needs a low sample volume and has very interesting analytical features, among which a very low limit of quantification [21]. With the help of this assay, we found low, but often detectable, $1,25(OH)_2D$ in our cohort of HD patients. Also, the levels of $1,25(OH)_2D$ were significantly increased after 1 year of vitamin D (50.000 IU cholecalciferol/month for 1 year) supplementation versus placebo [22]. An increase in serum $1,25(OH)_2D$ after supplementation with $25(OH)D$ or vitamin D3 in dialysis patients has previously been reported, this is a proof of extra-renal origin of 1-alpha hydroxylase. Another proof is the detectable concentration of $1,25(OH)_2D$ in serum of anephric patients [23].

5.3.4   24,25(OH)2D

The method of choice for the determination of 24,25(OH)2 levels is the LCMS/MS. However, one has to be sure that the method used is i) sensitive enough to differentiate a low value from an undetectable value that should be observed in children suffering from mutations of the CYP24A1 gene ii) specific enough to avoid to consider another metabolic as being 24.25(OH)2D. The quantification of 24.25(OH)2 is also challenging because of its low serum level and low ionization efficiency [24]. Different authors have described LC-MS/MS methods for simultaneous determination of the major vitamin D metabolites, including $25(OH)D$, $1,25(OH)_2D$ and 24,25(OH)2D. The analytical sensitivity of these methods can vary according to the way the authors have estimated it and it is thus difficult to compare their performances and to know if they are suitable for the clinical purposes. For instance, Berg et al. have found that the mean 24.25(OH)2D values (± standard deviation) in community-dwelling White and Black Americans were of 3.6 ± 2.0 and 2.1 ± 1.3 ng/mL, respectively. They present a LOQ of 0.156 ng/mL for their LCMS/MS method, which is quite low, but which has been obtained on four replicates only. In the same vein, de Boer et al. find that 24.25(OH)2D values obtained in 9,596 participants from 5 cohort studies and clinical trials range from 0.8 ± 0.5 to 4.1 ± 2.1 ng/mL [25]. Again, it is difficult to evaluate the performance of the method as the authors only provide a mean CV of 14.6 % which was obtained on a set of 20 samples measured nine times on a spanning period of 6 months Kaufman et al. showed that the CV obtained in 14 days on a sample presenting a value around 2.5 ng/mL was 5–7 %, but no limit of quantification was calculated [26]. If we insist on these analytical details, it is because there is a growing interest on measurement of 24.25(OH)2D, 25(OH)D and 1,25(OH)$_2$D. Kaufman et al. consider that the ratio of 25-OH-D to 24,25-(OH)2D is as a pathophysiologically useful ratio as a novel approach for predicting vitamin D deficiency. The ratio can also be useful for the differential diagnosis between Idiopathic Infantile Hypercalcemia due to loss-of-function CYP24A1 mutations and CYP24A1 defects from hypervitaminosis D during vitamin D intoxication [26]. Binkley has recently suggested that the ratio cholecalciferol 24.25(OH)2D could be used to facilitate "treat-to-target" paradigm and to guide vitamin D supplementation [7]. In CKD patients, Bosworth et al. have found that the 24,25(OH)2D concentration was strongly associated with glomerular filtration rate (GFR) [27]. In their study, non-Hispanic black race, diabetes, albuminuria, and lower serum bicarbonate were also independently and significantly associated with lower 24,25(OH)2D concentrations. The 24,25(OH)2D concentration was more strongly correlated with that of PTH than was 25(OH)D or 1,25(OH)$_2$D. According to these results, the authors concluded that CKD was thus a state of stagnant vitamin D metabolism characterized by decreases in both 1,25(OH)$_2$D production and vitamin D catabolism. Indeed, they suggest that PTH and FGF23 are not the main drivers of vitamin D catabolism in CKD but that, due to a decrease in renal mass, less delivery of 25(OH)D to proximal tubular cells, or lower net metabolic capacity of the proximal tubular cells is the major determinant of renal 24,25(OH)2D production and serum 24,25(OH)2D concentration. Low 24,25(OH)2D may also identify risk of CKD complications as it is strongly associated with hyperparathyroidism, perhaps because 24,25(OH)2D concentration reflects the extent to which vitamin D metabolism is deranged in CKD. Finally, the same team also found that low plasma concentrations of 25(OH)D and 24,25-dihydroxyvitaminD were associated with increased risk of microalbuminuria in type 1 diabetes [28].

5.3.5   Vitamin D–Binding Protein and Free or Bioavailable Vitamin D

The vitamin D binding protein (VDBP) is the major plasma carrier protein of vitamin D and its metabolites. VDBP also exerts several other important biological functions, like actin scavenging, fatty acid transport and macrophage activation. The molecular weight of VDBP is similar to the one of albumin (52–59 kDa). VDBP is in molar excess (5×10^{-6} M), compared to 25(OH)D (5×10^{-8} M) and has a rapid turnover rate. This large molar excess may play an important role in protection against vitamin D intoxication. VDBP has also a much shorter plasma half-life (2.5 days) than 25(OH)D.

An important VDBP polymorphism is observed in humans [29]. Three alleles Gc1F, Gc1S and Gc2 are the mostly known, but more than 120 other rare variants have been identified [17]. VDBP has an interesting geographical distribution: white-skinned individuals have a relatively lower frequency of the Gc1F-allele and a higher frequency (50–60%) of the Gc1S-allele. The Gc1F-allele frequency is mark-edly higher among black Americans and black Africans. The Gc1F- and Gc1S-allele frequencies display a typical geographical cline from Southeast Asia, through Europe and the Middle East, down to Africa [30]. The observed variation in the Gc-allele frequencies in different geographic areas may be correlated with skin pig-mentation and intensity of sun light exposure. Pigmented (black) and keratinized (yellowish) skin types are characterized by a lower rate of UV light penetration and a higher susceptibility to rickets. The higher frequency of Gc1F in dark skinned persons may be explained by its greater affinity for and more efficient transport of vitamin D metabolites.

Regarding affinity, VDBP has a different one for the different metabolites trans-ported: VDBP binds 88% of serum 25(OH)D with high affinity (Ka$=5\times10^8$ M^{-1}), 85% of serum 1,25(OH)$_2$D with a ten-times lower affinity (Ka$=4\times10^7$ M^{-1}), leav-ing 0.40% 'free' and the remainder associated with other serum proteins, mainly albumin [31].

Bioavailable 25OH-D is defined as circulating 25(OH)D not bound to VDBP. The bioavailable fraction consists of albumin-bound 25(OH)D and the free, defined as circulating 25(OH)D bound to neither VDBP nor albumin. To be further metabo-lized or to exert biological activities, 25(OH)D needs to enter target cells. Free 25(OH)D can enter cells passively: this appears to be an ubiquitous mechanism. According to the "free-hormone hypothesis", bound fractions of 25OH-D may be unavailable to enter cells [32]. However, bound 25(OH) (and particularly VDBP-bound 25(OH)D) can be sequestered by cubulin on the cell surface before being internalized by megalin. This megalin cubulin complex of endocytosis is abundant in the proximal tubular epithelium of the kidney and is also expressed in other cells such as osteoblasts.

To date, there are no good assays for the measurement of free or bioavailable vitamin D. Elisa methods have been developed but are lacking sensitivity. LCMS/MS could be the solution, but it remains a technical challenge. Calculation of the free fraction could thus be an alternative to lab measurement. Free 25OH-D can be calculated using specific formula: a simple one was published by Bikle et al. [33] and a more complex one was adapted from Vermeulen's work related to estimation of free testosterone [34]. These formulas are both based on 25(OH)D, albumin and VDBP concentrations, as well as defined binding proteins' affinities for 25(OH)D. Taking the affinity of VDBP for 25(OH)D according to the genotype of the sub-jects, Powe et al. have shown that, if Black Americans had lower VDBP and lower 25(OH)D than their White counterparts, their bioavailable 25(OH)D was similar [9]. Accordingly, the low levels of total 25(OH)D frequently observed in Black Americans does not probably indicate a true vitamin D deficiency and bioavailable

25(OH)D might be more appropriate than total 25(OH)D to detect vitamin D sufficiency. In a population of young healthy subjects, the same authors also demonstrated that bioavailable 25(OH)D levels was independently associated with bone
mineral density (BMD) in multivariate regression models adjusted for age, sex,
body mass index, and race. In this study, free and bioavailable 25(OH)D were more
strongly correlated with BMD than total 25(OH)D [35]. Bhan et al. have studied 94
HD patients in whom 25(OH)D and 1,25(OH)$_2$D had previously been determined
and they measured VDBP and calculated free and bioavailable vitamin D according
to the formula they published in the *New England Journal* [9, 36]. They showed
that, as expected, Black patients, compared to Whites, had lower levels of total
25(OH)D, but not bioavailable vitamin D. However, bioavailable, but not total,
25(OH)D and 1,25(OH)$_2$D were each significantly correlated with serum calcium
and, in univariate and multivariate regression analysis, only bioavailable 25(OH)D
was significantly associated with parathyroid hormone levels. They concluded that
bioavailable vitamin D levels were better correlated with measures of mineral
metabolism than total levels in patients on hemodialysis. This study is not free from
criticisms: indeed, the DiaSorin RIA was used, ant not a LCMS/MS method like in
the New England study. This can definitely have an impact in the values observed in
HD patients. Moreover, the formula has never been validated in HD patients. The
serum matrix of HD subjects is very different than the serum matrix on healthy ones
and this could definitely affect the binding of 25(OH)D with albumin and/or
VDBP. Once again, good analytical methods will be needed to confirm these
conclusions.

References

1. Holick MF. Vitamin D deficiency. N Engl J Med. 2007;357:266–81.
2. Zhu JG, Ochalek JT, Kaufmann M, Jones G, Deluca HF. CYP2R1 is a major, but not exclusive,
   contributor to 25-hydroxyvitamin D production in vivo. Proc Natl Acad Sci USA.
   2013;110:15650–5.
3. Nemere I, Schwartz Z. Identification of a membrane receptor for 1, 25 dihydroxyvitamin D3
   which mediates rapid activation of protein kinase C. J Bone Miner Res. 1998;13:1353–9.
4. Schlingmann KP, Kaufmann M, Weber S, Irwin A, Goos C, John U, Misselwitz J, Klaus G,
   Kuwertz-Bröking E, Fehrenbach H, Wingen AM, Güran T, Bindels RJ, David E, Jones G,
   Konrad M. Mutations in CYP24A1 and idiopathic infantile hypercalcemia. N Engl J Med.
   2011;365:410–21.
5. Matsuoka LY, Wortsman J, Hollis BW. Use of topical sunscreen for the evaluation of regional
   synthesis of vitamin D3. J Am Acad Dermatol. 1990;22:772–5.
6. Zhu J, Deluca HF. Vitamin D 25-hydroxylase - four decades of searching, are we there yet?
   Arch Biochem Biophys. 2012;523:30–6.
7. Binkley N, Lappe J, Singh RJ, Khosla S, Krueger D, Drezner MK, Blank RD. Can vitamin D
   metabolite measurements facilitate a "treat-to-target" paradigm to guide vitamin D supplementation? Osteoporos Int. 2015;26:1655–60.
8. Wallace AM, Gibson S, de la Hunty A, Lamberg-Allardt C, Ashwell M. Measurement of
   25-hydroxyvitamin D in the clinical laboratory: current procedures, performance characteristics and limitations. Steroids. 2010;75:477–88.

9. Powe CE, Evans MK, Wenger J, Zonderman AB, Berg AH, Nalls M, Tamez H, Zhang D, Bhan I, Karumanchi SA, Powe NR, Thadhani R. Vitamin D-binding protein and vitamin D status of black Americans and white Americans. N Engl J Med. 2013;369:1991–2000.
10. Heijboer AC, Blankenstein MA, Kema IP, Buijs MM. Accuracy of 6 routine 25-hydroxyvitamin D assays: influence of vitamin D binding protein concentration. Clin Chem. 2012;58:543–8.
11. Depreter B, Heijboer AC, Langlois MR. Accuracy of three automated 25-hydroxyvitamin D assays in hemodialysis patients. Clin Chim Acta. 2013;415:255–60.
12. Cavalier E, Wallace AM, Carlisi A, Chapelle J-P, Delanaye P, Souberbielle J-C. Cross-reactivity of 25-hydroxy vitamin D2 from different commercial immunoassays for 25-hydroxy vitamin D: an evaluation without spiked samples. Clin Chem Lab Med. 2011;49:555–8.
13. Kobold U. Approaches to measurement of vitamin D concentrations – mass spectrometry. Scand J Clin Lab Invest Suppl. 2012;243:54–9.
14. Cavalier E, Carlisi A, Bekaert A-C, Rousselle O, Chapelle JP. Human anti-animal interference in DiaSorin Liaison total 25(OH)-vitamin D assay: towards the end of a strange story? Clin Chim Acta. 2012;413:527–8.
15. Sempos CT, Vesper HW, Phinney KW, Thienpont LM, Coates PM. Vitamin D status as an international issue: national surveys and the problem of standardization. Scand J Clin Lab Invest Suppl. 2012;243:32–40.
16. Cavalier E, Lukas P, Crine Y, Peeters S, Carlisi A, Le Goff C, Gadisseur R, Delanaye P, Souberbielle JC. Evaluation of automated immunoassays for 25(OH)-vitamin D determination in different critical populations before and after standardization of the assays. Clin Chim Acta. 2014;431:60–5.
17. Holick MF, Binkley NC, Bischoff-Ferrari HA, Gordon CM, Hanley DA, Heaney RP, Murad MH, Weaver CM. Guidelines for preventing and treating vitamin D deficiency and insufficiency revisited. J Clin Endocrinol Metab. 2012;97:1153–8.
18. Kallas M, Green F, Hewison M, White C, Kline G. Rare causes of calcitriol-mediated hypercalcemia: a case report and literature review. J Clin Endocrinol Metab. 2010;95:3111–7.
19. Malloy PJ, Feldman D. Genetic disorders and deficits in vitamin D action. Endocrinol Metab Clin N Am. 2010;39:333–46.
20. Hawkes C, Schnellbacher S, Singh R, Levine M. 25-hydroxyvitamin D can interfere with a common assay for 1,25-dihydroxyvitamin D in vitamin D intoxication. J Clin Endocrinol Metab. 2015;100:2883–9.
21. Van Helden J, Weiskirchen R. Experience with the first fully automated chemiluminescence immunoassay for the quantification of 1α, 25-dihydroxy-vitamin D. Clin Chem Lab Med. 2015;53:761–70.
22. Delanaye P, Weekers L, Warling X, Moonen M, Smelten N, Médart L, Krzesinski J-M, Cavalier E. Cholecalciferol in haemodialysis patients: a randomized, double-blind, proof-of-concept and safety study. Nephrol Dial Transplant. 2013;28:1779–86.
23. Lambert PW, Stern PH, Avioli RC, Brackett NC, Turner RT, Greene A, Fu IY, Bell NH. Evidence for extrarenal production of 1α,25-dihydroxyvitamin D in man. J Clin Invest. 1982;69: 722–5.
24. Aronov PA, Hall LM, Dettmer K, Stephensen CB, Hammock BD. Metabolic profiling of major vitamin D metabolites using Diels-Alder derivatization and ultra-performance liquid chromatography-tandem mass spectrometry. Anal Bioanal Chem. 2008;391:1917–30.
25. De Boer IH, Sachs MC, Chonchol M, Himmelfarb J, Hoofnagle AN, Ix JH, Kremsdorf RA, Lin YS, Mehrotra R, Robinson-Cohen C, Siscovick DS, Steffes MW, Thummel KE, Tracy RP, Wang Z, Kestenbaum B. Estimated GFR and circulating 24,25-dihydroxyvitamin D3 concentration: a participant-level analysis of 5 cohort studies and clinical trials. Am J Kidney Dis. 2014;64:187–97.
26. Kaufmann M, Gallagher JC, Peacock M, Schlingmann KP, Konrad M, DeLuca HF, Sigueiro R, Lopez B, Mourino A, Maestro M, St-Arnaud R, Finkelstein JS, Cooper DP, Jones G. Clinical utility of simultaneous quantitation of 25-hydroxyvitamin D and 24,25-dihydroxyvitamin D by LC-MS/MS involving derivatization with DMEQ-TAD. J Clin Endocrinol Metab. 2014;99:2567–74.

27. Bosworth CR, Levin G, Robinson-Cohen C, Hoofnagle AN, Ruzinski J, Young B, Schwartz SM, Himmelfarb J, Kestenbaum B, de Boer IH. The serum 24,25-dihydroxyvitamin D concentration, a marker of vitamin D catabolism, is reduced in chronic kidney disease. Kidney Int. 2012;82:693–700.

28. De Boer IH, Sachs MC, Cleary PA, Hoofnagle AN, Lachin JM, Molitch ME, Steffes MW, Sun W, Zinman B, Brunzell JD. Circulating vitamin D metabolites and kidney disease in type 1 diabetes. J Clin Endocrinol Metab. 2012;97:4780–8.

29. Constans J, Gouaillard C, Bouissou C, Dugoujon JM. Polymorphism of the vitamin D binding protein (DBP) among primates: an evolutionary analysis. Am J Phys Anthropol. 1987;73:365–77.

30. Speeckaert M, Huang G, Delanghe JR, Taes YEC. Biological and clinical aspects of the vitamin D binding protein (Gc-globulin) and its polymorphism. Clin Chim Acta. 2006;372: 33–42.

31. White P, Cooke N. The multifunctional properties and characteristics of vitamin D-binding protein. Trends Endocrinol Metab. 2000;11:320–7.

32. Chun RF, Peercy BE, Orwoll ES, Nielson CM, Adams JS, Hewison M. Vitamin D and DBP: the free hormone hypothesis revisited. J Steroid Biochem Mol Biol. 2013;144:132–7.

33. Bikle DD, Gee E, Halloran B, Kowalski MA, Ryzen E, Haddad JG. Assessment of the free fraction of 25-hydroxyvitamin D in serum and its regulation by albumin and the vitamin D-binding protein. J Clin Endocrinol Metab. 1986;63:954–9.

34. Vermeulen A, Verdonck L, Kaufman JM. A critical evaluation of simple methods for the estimation of free testosterone in serum. J Clin Endocrinol Metab. 1999;84:3666–72.

35. Powe CE, Ricciardi C, Berg AH, Erdenesanaa D, Collerone G, Ankers E, Wenger J, Karumanchi SA, Thadhani R, Bhan I. Vitamin D-binding protein modifies the vitamin D-bone mineral density relationship. J Bone Miner Res. 2011;26:1609–16.

36. Bhan I, Powe CE, Berg AH, Ankers E, Wenger JB, Karumanchi SA, Thadhani RI. Bioavailable vitamin D is more tightly linked to mineral metabolism than total vitamin D in incident hemodialysis patients. Kidney Int. 2012;82:84–9.

Part II
Classical Mineral and Bone Effects

Chapter 6
Vitamin D and Racial Differences in Chronic Kidney Disease

Orlando M. Gutiérrez

Abstract Compared to Caucasians, African Americans have lower circulating concentrations of 25-hydroxyvitamin D (25(OH)D), the major storage form of vitamin D, leading to the widespread assumption that blacks are at higher risk of vitamin D deficiency. Since low 25(OH)D is associated with adverse cardiovascular and kidney outcomes, this has supported the notion that low 25(OH)D concentrations partly underlie racial disparities in health outcomes, including faster progression of chronic kidney disease (CKD) in blacks vs. whites. However, the finding that blacks maintain better indices of musculoskeletal health than whites throughout their lifespan despite having lower circulating 25(OH)D concentrations suggests that the relationship between vitamin D deficiency and racial health disparities may not be so straight forward. This has been further underscored by epidemiologic studies showing major racial heterogeneity in the association of 25(OH)D with cardiovascular outcomes. When coupled with emerging data showing genetically determined differences in the bioavailability of vitamin D by race, these data suggest that there are important differences in vitamin D metabolism by race which need to inform and perhaps revise our current understanding of the role of vitamin D in racial disparities in CKD outcomes.

Keywords Race and ethnic differences • Chronic kidney disease • Bone mineral density • Vitamin D

6.1 Introduction

Vitamin D is an essential hormone involved in the regulation of numerous physiological systems. While the primary actions of vitamin D involve calcium homeostasis, vitamin D receptors (VDRs) are present in many tissues not explicitly involved

O.M. Gutiérrez
Division of Nephrology, Department of Medicine, School of Medicine; Department of Epidemiology, School of Public Health, University of Alabama, Birmingham, AL, USA
e-mail: ogutierr@uab.edu

© Springer International Publishing Switzerland 2016
P.A. Ureña Torres et al. (eds.), *Vitamin D in Chronic Kidney Disease*,
DOI 10.1007/978-3-319-32507-1_6

in calcium regulation, including cardiac, vascular smooth muscle, endothelial, jux-taglomerular, and immune cells [1]. These data provide biological plausibility for a link between vitamin D deficiency and cardiovascular disease (CVD). Consistent with this, low 25-hydroxyvitamin D (25(OH)D) concentrations have been associated with hypertension, insulin resistance, endothelial dysfunction, and higher risk of CVD events, chronic kidney disease (CKD) and death [2–34]. Since vitamin D deficiency is common in the general population, this has fueled interest for treating vitamin D deficiency as a novel approach to reducing the risk of CVD and CKD.

Enthusiasm for diagnosing and treating vitamin D deficiency has been particularly high in efforts to address racial disparities in CVD and CKD outcomes. This is because the prevalence of 25(OH)D deficiency is substantially higher in individuals of black race than individuals of white race [35, 36]. On the basis of these findings, black individuals have long been assumed to be at increased risk of vitamin D deficiency [1]. When coupled with epidemiologic data linking low 25(OH)D with adverse outcomes, these data support the notion that vitamin D deficiency should be a prime target of therapy for improving health disparities, such as the excess risk of CKD and end-stage renal disease (ESRD) among black individuals.

However, inconsistencies in the relationship between vitamin D and health outcomes in black individuals have raised doubts about these conclusions. Despite having lower circulating 25(OH)D concentrations and lower calcium intake than white individuals, black individuals have markedly lower rates of osteoporosis and skeletal fractures than age- and gender-matched white individuals [37–41]. Similarly, despite a wealth of data showing positive associations of serum 25(OH)D with muscle mass and strength [42–46], black individuals have better indices of muscle health than whites across the life span [47]. Additionally, associations of 25(OH)D and CVD outcomes have been inconsistent in cohorts with large numbers of black participants, with a number of studies showing no association of lower 25(OH)D with CVD risk in blacks whereas a strong association was observed in whites [4, 14, 31, 32, 48]. Why this heterogeneity exists is unclear. However, advances in the understanding of racial differences in vitamin D metabolism have revealed important new insights that may require the development of more refined approaches to the assessment and management of vitamin D status in racially-diverse populations. This is particularly the case in individuals with CKD [49], who are prone to the development of vitamin deficiency, and for whom racial differences in vitamin D metabolism may most strongly inform disparities in outcomes.

6.2 The Case for Vitamin D as a Factor Underlying Racial Disparities in CKD

As mentioned above, the much higher prevalence of 25(OH)D deficiency in blacks than whites has led to the hypothesis that low 25(OH)D concentrations partly underlie racial disparities in a variety of health outcomes, including diabetes, heart disease, CKD progression and cancer [35, 36]. In support of this, studies have shown that suboptimal 25(OH)D concentrations partly explain higher rates of albuminuria, insulin resistance, cancer, hypertension, sleep disorders, peripheral vascular disease and all-cause mortality in blacks as compared to whites [50–57]. Associations of low 25(OH)D with outcomes in CKD also lend credence to the hypothesis that differences in the prevalence of vitamin D deficiency may partly explain racial disparities in outcomes. Low 25(OH)D concentrations have been associated with higher risk of CKD progression and death in individuals with non-dialysis-dependent CKD [58–61]. Perhaps most importantly with respect to racial disparities in CKD outcomes, lower 25(OH)D concentrations were shown to account for a substantial proportion of the increased risk of ESRD in black as compared to white participants of the Third National Health and Nutrition Examination Survey (NHANES) [36]. Moreover, treatment with activated vitamin D analogs was shown to attenuate differences in survival in black vs. white individuals receiving chronic hemodialysis [62] and to be associated with improved survival in black vs. white hemodialysis patients [63], suggesting that vitamin D deficiency at least partly accounts for racial differences in outcomes in ESRD. In the aggregate, these data support the notion that the greater propensity to vitamin D deficiency explains as least some of racial disparities in health outcomes, particularly those in CKD populations.

6.3   Inconsistencies in the Association of Vitamin D with Race Disparities in CKD

6.3.1   Overview of Differences in Vitamin D Metabolism by Race

Before reviewing important inconsistencies in the relationship between vitamin D deficiency and racial disparities in health outcomes, it is first essential to review racial differences in vitamin D metabolism. Vitamin D is obtained through both dietary sources and skin exposure to ultraviolet B radiation [1]. Diet- and sun-derived vitamin D are hydroxylated in the liver to 25(OH)D, the primary circulating form of vitamin D. 25(OH)D is further hydroxylated to $1,25(OH)_2D$ in the kidney and to a lesser extent in peripheral tissues by 1α-hydroxylase (CYP27B1). The primary hormonal regulators of this process are parathyroid hormone (PTH) and fibroblast growth factor 23 (FGF23) [64]. PTH increases $1,25(OH)_2D$ synthesis by inducing the transcription of CYP27B1 and inhibiting that of 24-hydroxylase (CYP24A1) [65], the major catabolic enzyme for 25(OH)D and $1,25(OH)_2D$. In contrast, FGF23 decreases $1,25(OH)_2D$ synthesis by inhibiting CYP27B1 and up-regulating CYP24A1 [65].

Though thresholds to define vitamin D sufficiency are still being debated, 25(OH)D concentrations <30–32 ng/mL and <20 ng/mL are commonly used to categorize insufficient and deficient states, respectively [1]. These conditions are very common, affecting nearly 50% of all US adults according to the most recent estimates [66], and billions more worldwide. Blacks on average have lower 25(OH)D concentrations than whites, with the prevalence of 25(OH)D deficiency in the US being over 80 % in blacks [66]. Since melanin absorbs UV light needed to synthesize vitamin D in the skin, this has historically been attributed to higher melanin skin content in blacks [1]. Prevalence rates of vitamin D deficiency in other populations with high skin pigmentation such as Hispanics and Asian Indians are also higher than their Caucasian counterparts [66, 67], underscoring the disruptive effect of melanin in the cutaneous synthesis of vitamin D. Importantly, however, other biological differences, such as genetically defined differences in vitamin D binding protein (DBP) levels, also play a critical role in explaining racial differences in circulating 25(OH)D concentrations.

Vitamin D is highly lipophilic, similar to steroid and thyroid hormones that require protein carriers to circulate in the serum. As a result, less than 1 % of vitamin D circulates freely [68]. The majority (85–90%) of circulating vitamin D is instead tightly bound to DBP—an abundant circulating α-globulin protein produced by the liver—and the remaining (10–15%) is bound to albumin with much lower affinity (referred to as free or bioavailable vitamin D) [68]. DBP acts as a serum reservoir to stabilize 25(OH)D concentrations [69]. DBP also aids in reabsorption of 25(OH)D filtered by the glomerulus [69]. These findings indicate that the primary roles of DBP are to serve as a serum reservoir for vitamin D and provide an efficient mechanism to prevent urinary losses of filtered, unbound 25(OH)D.

Although over 120 variant forms of DBP have been reported, classically three DBP phenotypes have been described: Gc1S, Gc1F, and Gc2 [70]. Each phenotype variant is characterized by a different combination of two SNPs (rs4588 and rs7041) in the DBP (also known as Gc globulin) gene resulting in amino acid substitutions and differing glycosylation patterns [70]. These phenotypes differ in the associated concentration of DBP in serum, the affinity of DBP for 25(OH)D and possibly other characteristics (Table 6.1 adapted from Ref. [71]). DBP phenotypes strongly influence circulating 25(OH)D concentrations, and show marked differences in prevalence among races with black individuals having a higher prevalence of phenotypes (Gc1F) characterized by very low DBP concentrations than white individuals [72].

The tight affinity of DBP for 25(OH)D has important physiological consequences. This is because the free hormone hypothesis states that hormones liberated from binding proteins or bound to low-affinity carriers such as albumin are free to

Table 6.1 Common phenotypic variants of vitamin D binding protein (DBP) and their effects on DBP concentrations and 25-hydroxyvitamin D (25(OH)D) affinity

Phenotype	DBP concentrations in homozygotes	25(OH)D affinity
Gc1F	Lowest	Highest
Gc1S	Highest	Intermediate
Gc2	Intermediate	Lowest

Adapted from Ref. [71]

The three major DBP phenotypes include GC1F, GC1S, and GC2, defined by SNPs rs7041 and rs4588. The associated nucleotide and amino acid changes are presented, along with known data on DBP levels in homozygotes and affinity for 25-hydroxyvitamin D

enter cells and exert biological activity [73]. Consistent with this, experimental data have shown that DBP inhibits the actions of exogenous vitamin D when added directly to monocytes or osteoblasts in vitro by blocking intracellular transport of vitamin D [69, 74–77]. Chun et al. showed that the induction of cathelicidin expression by 25(OH)D in cultured human monocytes was strongly inhibited by adding DBP to culture media, and that the effects varied according to DBP phenotype, with the Gc1F phenotype showing markedly different responses as compared to Gc1S or Gc2 phenotypes [75]. Additionally, free or bioavailable 25(OH)D (that fraction of 25(OH)D which is not bound to DBP) is more strongly associated with classic measures of vitamin D adequacy such as BMD and PTH than total 25(OH)D (which primarily reflects DBP-bound 25(OH)D) [78, 79]. Collectively, these data indicate that DBP plays a key role in modulating the bioavailability and end-organ responsiveness of 25(OH)D, with critical implications for assessing vitamin D status in humans. Standard 25(OH)D assays do not distinguish between relatively inert 25(OH)D bound to DBP and more biologically active 25(OH)D that is free or loosely bound to albumin. Thus, it is possible that total 25(OH)D reflects total body stores rather than vitamin bioactivity or sufficiency.

6.3.2   The Paradox of Racial Differences in Vitamin D and Outcomes

The classical effects of vitamin D on bone and mineral health and its non-classical effects on cardiovascular function, insulin signaling and immunity support the notion that vitamin D deficiency should be a prime target of therapy for improving health disparities, such as the excess risk of CKD and ESRD in blacks vs. whites. While the breadth of data supporting this viewpoint are compelling, it is instructive to consider racial differences in the association of vitamin D with the physiological system(s) that it is most strongly linked with, namely bone and mineral metabolism. The primary role of vitamin D is to maintain calcium homeostasis (and by extension skeletal health) [1]. Studies have shown that the efficiency of calcium absorption from the intestinal lumen is exquisitely sensitive to vitamin D and that in the absence of sufficient 25(OH)D, intestinal calcium absorption is impaired [80]. When coupled with low dietary calcium intake, this presents the perfect scenario for deficient calcium incorporation into the bone and impaired bone mineralization. Given that black individuals on average have both lower circulating 25(OH)D concentrations and lower dietary calcium intake than whites [66], this would presumably put them at higher risk for bone disease. However, with the notable exception of the higher prevalence of rickets in black as compared to white children [81], quite the opposite has been observed in large, population-based studies.

The vast majority of these studies in fact have shown that black individuals maintain higher BMD than white individuals in both the appendicular and axial skeleton starting in adolescence and continuing through adulthood [66, 82–93]. Further, black individuals have lower risk of osteoporosis compared to their white counterparts

[94]. Similar associations have been noted when examining more sophisticated measures of bone structure and function. Barbour and colleagues examined the associations of 25(OH)D with pQCT-derived indices of bone structure in 446 US white men and 496 men of African descent living in Tobago and found that the associations of 25(OH)D with parameters of bone mass and strength were modified by race [95]. Namely, whereas positive linear trends were noted between increasing 25(OH)D categories (<20 ng/ml, 20–29, and ≥30) and cortical vBMD, total BMC, cortical thickness, and polar and axial strain indexes at the distal radius in white men, increasing 25(OH)D categories were either not associated or were negatively associated with these parameters in men of African descent. Similarly, whereas concentrations of 25(OH)D was linearly associated with BMC and cortical thickness in the tibia of white men, 25(OH)D was not associated with any tibial measures in men of African descent.

Gutiérrez and colleagues examined cross-sectional associations of 25(OH)D and whole body BMD in 4,309 white, 2,025 Mexican-American, and 2,081 black participants of the NHANES from 2003 to 2006 [66]. Analogous to the findings of Barbour et al. the association of 25(OH)D and BMD differed by race—whereas BMD significantly decreased as 25(OH)D concentrations declined among whites and Mexican-Americans, no association of 25(OH)D with whole body BMD was observed among blacks. The relationships between 25(OH)D and PTH were also modified by race. Whereas inverse associations of 25(OH)D and PTH were noted above and below a 25(OH)D cut-point commonly used to define vitamin D deficiency (20 ng/ml) in whites and Mexican-Americans, a significant inverse relationship between 25(OH)D and PTH was only observed when 25(OH)D concentrations were below 20 ng/ml among blacks, with the slope of the relationship being essentially flat above this cut-point. These data suggest that PTH secretion is maximally suppressed at a lower 25(OH)D threshold in blacks as compared to whites or Mexican-Americans. Aloia et al. similarly found that the inflection point of PTH was around a 25(OH)D level of 15 ng/ml among black women vs. 24 ng/ml among white women in an analysis of women between 20 and 80 years of age [96].

van Ballegooijen and colleagues compared the association of 25(OH)D and volumetric trabecular BMD in white, black, Chinese and Hispanic participants of the Multi-Ethnic Study of Atherosclerosis [97]. In line with the findings of Gutiérrez and colleagues, black individuals had the highest mean BMD despite having the lowest 25(OH)D concentrations of any race or ethnic group. Further, lower circulating 25(OH)D concentrations were associated with lower BMD values in white and Chinese participants, but not in black or Hispanic participants. In fact, when 25(OH)D was analyzed on a linear continuous scale, lower 25(OH)D concentrations were associated with higher BMD in black participants, but not in any other race or ethnic group.

Racial differences in the relationship between 25(OH)D and bone outcomes were further highlighted in a case-control study of the associations of 25(OH)D with incident fracture risk in participants of the Women's Health Initiative (WHI) Observational Study [98]. In this study, cases included 381 black, 192 Hispanic, 113 Asian, 46 American Indian, and 400 white women with incident fractures. One control was chosen per case matched on age, race/ethnicity, and blood draw date. Among white participants, women with 25(OH)D concentrations in the highest tertile of 25(OH)D ($\geq$30 ng/mL) had 44 % lower risk of fracture as compared to women in the lowest tertile of 25(OH)D (<20 ng/mL) in multivariable models adjusted for clinical factors, physical activity, calcium intake, previous history of fracture and PTH. In contrast, black women in the highest tertile of 25(OH)D had *higher* risk of fracture as compared to the lowest tertile of 25(OH)D in both unadjusted and fully-adjusted models.

A number of investigators have attempted to explain the paradox of why black individuals have better indexes of bone structure and function and better skeletal outcomes than white individual despite lower 25(OH)D by arguing that black individuals compensate for lower 25(OH)D by increasing the secretion of PTH, the hormone required to convert 25(OH)D to 1,25(OH)$_2$D [35, 99]. While this helps to maintain calcium homeostasis in the short-term, so the argument goes, this compensation becomes maladaptive in the long-term because it comes at the cost of chronically higher PTH concentrations, substantiating the belief that having lower 25(OH)D concentrations (relative to whites) is pathologic in blacks. It is certainly true that black individuals have higher average PTH concentrations than whites and that they tend to have higher 1,25(OH)$_2$D concentrations as a result [100–103]. However, if anything, one would assume that higher PTH and 1,25(OH)$_2$D concentrations would help to keep bone mass similar or only slightly lower, not higher, in blacks than whites if it were solely a maladaptive compensation for lower 25(OH)D concentrations. Furthermore, differences in BMD by race have been observed even in the absence of differences in PTH concentrations [93]. Finally, studies have shown that black individuals manifest skeletal resistance to the bone-resorbing effects of PTH [104, 105], suggesting that higher PTH concentrations may not adversely affect bone strength in black individuals, at least in comparison to whites [106]. Consistent with this, in a prospective study of black and white women from four US centers participating in the Study of Osteoporosis Fractures, the incidence rate of non-spinal fracture was significantly higher in white women as compared to black women irrespective of baseline bone mineral content or density [94]. Further, the relative risk of fracture remained substantially lower in black compared to white women after adjustment for potential confounders (0.43, 95 % confidence interval 0.32–0.57), in line with the findings of other studies [37–41].

When taken together, the results of these studies may have important implications for the concept of vitamin D adequacy in racially-diverse populations. Thresholds of vitamin D sufficiency have most commonly been derived from the mathematical modeling of PTH and/or BMD as a function of 25(OH)D concentrations [107–112] or by determining the 25(OH)D concentration above which fracture risk is minimized [113–116]. However, the results of the studies reviewed above suggest that optimal concentrations of 25(OH)D determined by these criteria may not be the same in white individuals as compared to black individuals.

So how do we best account for this paradox? A number of explanations have been offered including more efficient dietary calcium utilization, better renal calcium conservation (perhaps due to higher basal PTH concentrations), and lower bone turnover in black individuals than white individuals [47, 117]. Even when taking these factors into account, however, the results of these studies suggest that optimal concentrations of 25(OH)D may not be the same in white individuals as compared to black individuals, at least with respect to bone health. Indeed, it is entirely reasonable to conclude from these data that individuals of more recent African descent require lower 25(OH)D concentrations to optimize bone and mineral metabolism as compared to their counterparts of European descent. This in turn begs the question of whether the same is true with respect to the relationships between 25(OH)D and non-skeletal outcomes such as cardiovascular health, glucose metabolism, immune function and, of greatest relevance to this text, kidney disease in black individuals. Though supporting evidence is scarce, important clues may be gleaned from available studies.

In a study of 2,766 non-Hispanic white, 1,736 non-Hispanic black and 1,726 Mexican American participants of NHANES, higher serum concentrations of 25(OH)D were associated with lower odds of diabetes in non-Hispanic whites and Mexican Americans [48]. In contrast, no associations were noted between serum concentrations of 25(OH)D and odds of diabetes among blacks overall—in fact, in some models, higher 25(OH)D was associated with higher odds of diabetes, though these results should be interpreted cautiously because of the low sample size of blacks in higher categories of 25(OH)D. Similarly, despite the observation that 25(OH)D is inversely associated with calcified plaque in population-based studies of European Americans [34, 118], a study showed that 25(OH)D was positively associated with calcified plaque in African Americans with type 2 diabetes, suggesting that higher 25(OH)D may have adverse effects on calcified atherosclerotic lesions in black individuals [119]. In the largest study to examine the association of 25(OH)D with coronary heart disease (CHD), Robinson-Cohen et al. showed that lower total 25D levels were associated with higher risk of CHD in whites but not blacks [32]. Other reports have shown similar racial heterogeneity in the association of total 25D with risk of hypertension, fatal stroke and mortality [4, 14, 31, 48].

The results of these studies should be interpreted in the context of other studies that showed that lower 25(OH)D concentrations in blacks at least partially explained racial disparities in hypertension, albuminuria and ESRD prevalence (reviewed above), supporting the potential mediating role of low vitamin D in disparities in CKD outcomes by race. Nevertheless, while it appears biologically plausible that lower 25(OH)D concentrations (relative to whites) are "bad" for blacks and should be treated, it remains very much unclear at what level of 25(OH)D the excess risk for chronic disease among blacks begins to manifest. That is to say, while blacks can and do become vitamin D deficient at some critical threshold of 25(OH)D, whether that level is the same as for whites remains an open question.

Genetically determined differences in circulating DBP concentrations and, by extension, 25(OH)D bioavailability, may also be key to understanding inconsistencies in the association of vitamin D with health outcomes by race. Epidemiologic studies have shown that estimated bioavailable 25(OH)D concentrations in blacks and whites are similar even though total 25(OH)D concentrations are lower in blacks [72]. A prior study measured total 25(OH)D and DBP concentrations in stored serum samples from black and white subjects enrolled in Healthy Aging in Neighborhoods of Diversity across the Life Span Study, a fixed cohort of community-dwelling black and white adults aged 30–64 [72] and demonstrated that blacks, despite having lower 25(OH)D concentrations than whites, had similar estimated bioavailable 25(OH)D concentrations. This was mostly due to racially-determined genetic variations in DBP which impact both the abundance of DBP in the circulation, and DBP-affinity binding constants for 25(OH)D. Specifically, black participants had a higher prevalence of DBP phenotypes associated with very low DBP levels (Gc1F/1 F) than white participants. These racially-determined variations in DBP explained a large proportion of lower total 25(OH)D concentrations measured in blacks vs whites and helped to explain why BMD in blacks poorly correlated with measures of total 25(OH)D—namely, because low total 25(OH)D concentrations may be a poor marker of true vitamin D deficiency when levels of DBP are also low, such as in many black individuals. In contrast, low 25(OH)D concentrations may be more likely to represent vitamin D deficiency in populations with higher DBP concentrations, such as white individuals (Fig. 6.1). This may explain why low total 25(OH)D concentrations were associated with CVD risk in whites but not blacks in prior studies and raises important questions about whether bioavailable 25(OH)D—which demonstrates much less variability by race—may be a better cross-racial marker of CVD risk.

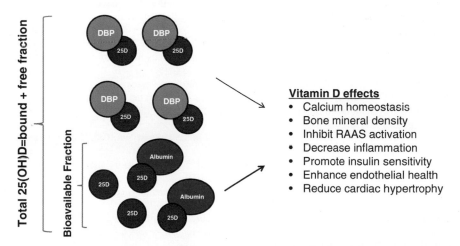

Fig. 6.1 Vitamin D has pleiotropic effects that promote cardiovascular health. Total 25-hydroxyvitamin D (25(OH)D) represents mostly inert 25(OH)D bound to vitamin D binding protein (DBP), which may attenuate vitamin D's physiological effects (*small arrow*). The bioavailable fraction, in term, better represents the biologically active form of vitamin D (*large arrow*). While total 25(OH)D concentrations differ by race, the bioavailable fraction does not seem to differ by race, potentially helping to explain racial heterogeneity in the association of 25(OH)D with bone and cardiovascular outcomes

6.4 Conclusions

Vitamin D deficiency has captured a great deal of attention in the ongoing quest to understand well-known but poorly understood discrepancies in CKD and ESRD risk by race. The basis for this enthusiasm is well-founded in plausible biological pathways linking lower 25(OH)D concentrations with cardiovascular and renal pathology. However, the lingering paradox between lower 25(OH)D concentrations (relative to whites) in blacks and musculoskeletal health should provide a measure of caution in rushing to the conclusion that low average 25(OH)D concentrations are truly detrimental to the overall health of black individuals, especially with respect to CKD outcomes. New insights into genetically determined differences in the bioavailability of vitamin D may provide a window into understanding how and why racial differences in vitamin D metabolism effect disparities in health outcomes by race.

References

1. Holick MF. Vitamin D, deficiency. N Engl J Med. 2007;357:266–81.
2. Resnick LM, Muller FB, Laragh JH. Calcium-regulating hormones in essential hypertension. Relation to plasma renin activity and sodium metabolism. Ann Intern Med. 1986;105: 649–54.
3. Vaidya A, Williams JS. The relationship between vitamin D and the renin-angiotensin system in the pathophysiology of hypertension, kidney disease, and diabetes. Metabolism. 2012;61:450–8.
4. Judd SE, Nanes MS, Ziegler TR, et al. Optimal vitamin D status attenuates the age-associated increase in systolic blood pressure in white Americans: results from the third National Health and Nutrition Examination Survey. Am J Clin Nutr. 2008;87:136–41.
5. Martins D, Wolf M, Pan D, et al. Prevalence of cardiovascular risk factors and the serum levels of 25-hydroxyvitamin D in the United States: data from the Third National Health and Nutrition Examination Survey. Arch Intern Med. 2007;167:1159–65.
6. Hypponen E, Boucher BJ, Berry DJ, et al. 25-hydroxyvitamin D, IGF-1, and metabolic syndrome at 45 years of age: a cross-sectional study in the 1958 British Birth Cohort. Diabetes. 2008;57:298–305.
7. Hintzpeter B, Mensink GB, Thierfelder W, et al. Vitamin D status and health correlates among German adults. Eur J Clin Nutr. 2008;62:1079–89.
8. Pasco JA, Henry MJ, Nicholson GC, et al. Behavioural and physical characteristics associated with vitamin D status in women. Bone. 2009;44:1085–91.
9. Forouhi NG, Luan J, Cooper A, et al. Baseline serum 25-hydroxy vitamin d is predictive of future glycemic status and insulin resistance: the Medical Research Council Ely Prospective Study 1990–2000. Diabetes. 2008;57:2619–25.
10. Gannage-Yared MH, Chedid R, Khalife S, et al. Vitamin D in relation to metabolic risk factors, insulin sensitivity and adiponectin in a young Middle-Eastern population. Eur J Endocrinol. 2009;160:965–71.
11. Forman JP, Giovannucci E, Holmes MD, et al. Plasma 25-hydroxyvitamin D levels and risk of incident hypertension. Hypertension. 2007;49:1063–9.
12. Patel RS, Al Mheid I, Morris AA, et al. Oxidative stress is associated with impaired arterial elasticity. Atherosclerosis. 2011;218:90–5.

13. Al Mheid I, Patel R, Murrow J, et al. Vitamin D status is associated with arterial stiffness and vascular dysfunction in healthy humans. J Am Coll Cardiol. 2011;58:186–92.
14. Melamed ML, Michos ED, Post W, et al. 25-hydroxyvitamin D levels and the risk of mortality in the general population. Arch Intern Med. 2008;168:1629–37.
15. Pilz S, Dobnig H, Fischer JE, et al. Low vitamin d levels predict stroke in patients referred to coronary angiography. Stroke. 2008;39:2611–3.
16. Wang TJ, Pencina MJ, Booth SL, et al. Vitamin D deficiency and risk of cardiovascular disease. Circulation. 2008;117:503–11.
17. Giovannucci E, Liu Y, Hollis BW, et al. 25-hydroxyvitamin D and risk of myocardial infarction in men: a prospective study. Arch Intern Med. 2008;168:1174–80.
18. Dobnig H, Pilz S, Scharnagl H, et al. Independent association of low serum 25-hydroxyvitamin d and 1,25-dihydroxyvitamin d levels with all-cause and cardiovascular mortality. Arch Intern Med. 2008;168:1340–9.
19. Pilz S, Dobnig H, Nijpels G, et al. Vitamin D and mortality in older men and women. Clin Endocrinol (Oxf). 2009;71:666–72.
20. Marniemi J, Alanen E, Impivaara O, et al. Dietary and serum vitamins and minerals as predictors of myocardial infarction and stroke in elderly subjects. Nutr Metab Cardiovasc Dis. 2005;15:188–97.
21. Pilz S, Marz W, Wellnitz B, et al. Association of vitamin D deficiency with heart failure and sudden cardiac death in a large cross-sectional study of patients referred for coronary angiography. J Clin Endocrinol Metab. 2008;93:3927–35.
22. Ginde AA, Scragg R, Schwartz RS, et al. Prospective study of serum 25-hydroxyvitamin D level, cardiovascular disease mortality, and all-cause mortality in older U.S. adults. J Am Geriatr Soc. 2009;57:1595–603.
23. Kilkkinen A, Knekt P, Aro A, et al. Vitamin D status and the risk of cardiovascular disease death. Am J Epidemiol. 2009;170:1032–9.
24. Semba RD, Houston DK, Bandinelli S, et al. Relationship of 25-hydroxyvitamin D with all-cause and cardiovascular disease mortality in older community-dwelling adults. Eur J Clin Nutr. 2010;64:203–9.
25. Anderson JL, May HT, Horne BD, et al. Relation of vitamin D deficiency to cardiovascular risk factors, disease status, and incident events in a general healthcare population. Am J Cardiol. 2010;106:963–8.
26. Cawthon PM, Parimi N, Barrett-Connor E, et al. Serum 25-hydroxyvitamin D, parathyroid hormone, and mortality in older men. J Clin Endocrinol Metab. 2010;95:4625–34.
27. Michaelsson K, Baron JA, Snellman G, et al. Plasma vitamin D and mortality in older men: a community-based prospective cohort study. Am J Clin Nutr. 2010;92:841–8.
28. Hutchinson MS, Grimnes G, Joakimsen RM, et al. Low serum 25-hydroxyvitamin D levels are associated with increased all-cause mortality risk in a general population: the Tromso study. Eur J Endocrinol. 2010;162:935–42.
29. Kestenbaum B, Katz R, de Boer I, et al. Vitamin D, parathyroid hormone, and cardiovascular events among older adults. J Am Coll Cardiol. 2011;58:1433–41.
30. Deo R, Katz R, Shlipak MG, et al. Vitamin D, parathyroid hormone, and sudden cardiac death: results from the Cardiovascular Health Study. Hypertension. 2011;58:1021–8.
31. Michos ED, Reis JP, Post WS, et al. 25-Hydroxyvitamin D deficiency is associated with fatal stroke among whites but not blacks: the NHANES-III linked mortality files. Nutrition. 2012;28:367–71.
32. Robinson-Cohen C, Hoofnagle AN, Ix JH, et al. Racial differences in the association of serum 25-hydroxyvitamin D concentration with coronary heart disease events. JAMA. 2013;310:179–88.
33. de Boer IH, Levin G, Robinson-Cohen C, et al. Serum 25-hydroxyvitamin D concentration and risk for major clinical disease events in a community-based population of older adults: a cohort study. Ann Intern Med. 2012;156:627–34.
34. de Boer IH, Kestenbaum B, Shoben AB, et al. 25-hydroxyvitamin D levels inversely associate with risk for developing coronary artery calcification. J Am Soc Nephrol. 2009;20:1805–12.

35. Harris SS. Vitamin D, and African Americans. J Nutr. 2006;136:1126–9.
36. Melamed ML, Astor B, Michos ED, et al. 25-hydroxyvitamin D levels, race, and the progression of kidney disease. J Am Soc Nephrol. 2009;20:2631–9.
37. Baron JA, Barrett J, Malenka D, et al. Racial differences in fracture risk. Epidemiology. 1994;5:42–7.
38. Farmer ME, White LR, Brody JA, et al. Race and sex differences in hip fracture incidence. Am J Public Health. 1984;74:1374–80.
39. Moldawer M, Zimmerman SJ, Collins LC. Incidence of osteoporosis in elderly whites and elderly Negroes. JAMA. 1965;194:859–62.
40. Silverman SL, Madison RE. Decreased incidence of hip fracture in Hispanics, Asians, and blacks: California Hospital Discharge Data. Am J Public Health. 1988;78:1482–3.
41. Barrett-Connor E, Siris ES, Wehren LE, et al. Osteoporosis and fracture risk in women of different ethnic groups. J Bone Miner Res. 2005;20:185–94.
42. Glerup H, Mikkelsen K, Poulsen L, et al. Hypovitaminosis D myopathy without biochemical signs of osteomalacic bone involvement. Calcif Tissue Int. 2000;66:419–24.
43. Schott GD, Wills MR. Muscle weakness in osteomalacia. Lancet. 1976;1:626–9.
44. Bischoff-Ferrari HA, Dietrich T, Orav EJ, et al. Higher 25-hydroxyvitamin D concentrations are associated with better lower-extremity function in both active and inactive persons aged > or =60 y. Am J Clin Nutr. 2004;80:752–8.
45. Wicherts IS, van Schoor NM, Boeke AJ, et al. Vitamin D status predicts physical performance and its decline in older persons. J Clin Endocrinol Metab. 2007;92:2058–65.
46. Ensrud KE, Ewing SK, Fredman L, et al. Circulating 25-hydroxyvitamin D levels and frailty status in older women. J Clin Endocrinol Metab. 2010;95:5266–73.
47. Aloia JF. African Americans, 25-hydroxyvitamin D, and osteoporosis: a paradox. Am J Clin Nutr. 2008;88:545S–50S.
48. Scragg R, Sowers M, Bell C, et al. Serum 25-hydroxyvitamin D, diabetes, and ethnicity in the Third National Health and Nutrition Examination Survey. Diabetes Care. 2004;27:2813–8.
49. Gutierrez OM, Isakova T, Andress DL, et al. Prevalence and severity of disordered mineral metabolism in Blacks with chronic kidney disease. Kidney Int. 2008;73:956–62.
50. Egan KM, Signorello LB, Munro HM, et al. Vitamin D insufficiency among African-Americans in the southeastern United States: implications for cancer disparities (United States). Cancer Causes Control CCC. 2008;19:527–35.
51. Fiscella K, Winters P, Tancredi D, et al. Racial disparity in blood pressure: is vitamin D a factor? J Gen Intern Med. 2011;26:1105–11.
52. Fiscella KA, Winters PC, Ogedegbe G. Vitamin D and racial disparity in albuminuria: NHANES 2001–2006. Am J Hypertens. 2011;24:1114–20.
53. Reis JP, Michos ED, von Muhlen D, et al. Differences in vitamin D status as a possible contributor to the racial disparity in peripheral arterial disease. Am J Clin Nutr. 2008;88:1469–77.
54. Rostand SG. Ultraviolet light may contribute to geographic and racial blood pressure differences. Hypertension. 1997;30:150–6.
55. Kritchevsky SB, Tooze JA, Neiberg RH, et al. 25-Hydroxyvitamin D, parathyroid hormone, and mortality in black and white older adults: the health ABC study. J Clin Endocrinol Metab. 2012;97:4156–65.
56. Williams SK, Fiscella K, Winters P, et al. Association of racial disparities in the prevalence of insulin resistance with racial disparities in vitamin D levels: National Health and Nutrition Examination Survey (2001–2006). Nutr Res. 2013;33:266–71.
57. Bertisch SM, Sillau S, de Boer IH, et al. 25-hydroxyvitamin D concentration and sleep duration and continuity: multi-ethnic study of atherosclerosis. Sleep. 2015;38:1305–11.
58. Navaneethan SD, Schold JD, Arrigain S, et al. Low 25-hydroxyvitamin D levels and mortality in non-dialysis-dependent CKD. Am J Kidney Dis. 2011;58:536–43.
59. Fernandez-Juarez G, Luno J, Barrio V, et al. 25 (OH) vitamin D levels and renal disease progression in patients with type 2 diabetic nephropathy and blockade of the renin-angiotensin system. Clin J Am Soc Nephrol. 2013;8:1870–6.

60. Shroff R, Aitkenhead H, Costa N, et al. Normal 25-hydroxyvitamin D levels are associated with less proteinuria and attenuate renal failure progression in children with CKD. J Am Soc Nephrol. 2016;27:314–22.
61. de Boer IH, Katz R, Chonchol M, et al. Serum 25-hydroxyvitamin D and change in estimated glomerular filtration rate. Clin J Am Soc Nephrol. 2011;6:2141–9.
62. Wolf M, Betancourt J, Chang Y, et al. Impact of activated vitamin D and race on survival among hemodialysis patients. J Am Soc Nephrol. 2008;19:1379–88.
63. Kalantar-Zadeh K, Miller JE, Kovesdy CP, et al. Impact of race on hyperparathyroidism, mineral disarrays, administered vitamin D mimetic, and survival in hemodialysis patients. J Bone Miner Res. 2010;25:2724–34.
64. Gutierrez OM. Fibroblast growth factor 23 and disordered vitamin D metabolism in chronic kidney disease: updating the "trade-off" hypothesis. Clin J Am Soc Nephrol. 2010;5:1710–6.
65. Bringhurst FR, Demay MB, Kronenberg HM. Williams textbook of endocrinology. 12th ed. Philadelphia: Elsevier Saunders; 2011.
66. Gutierrez OM, Farwell WR, Kermah D, et al. Racial differences in the relationship between vitamin D, bone mineral density, and parathyroid hormone in the National Health and Nutrition Examination Survey. Osteoporos Int. 2011;22:1745–53.
67. Awumey EM, Mitra DA, Hollis BW, et al. Vitamin D metabolism is altered in Asian Indians in the southern United States: a clinical research center study. J Clin Endocrinol Metab. 1998;83:169–73.
68. Bikle DD, Gee E, Halloran B, et al. Assessment of the free fraction of 25-hydroxyvitamin D in serum and its regulation by albumin and the vitamin D-binding protein. J Clin Endocrinol Metab. 1986;63:954–9.
69. Safadi FF, Thornton P, Magiera H, et al. Osteopathy and resistance to vitamin D toxicity in mice null for vitamin D binding protein. J Clin Invest. 1999;103:239–51.
70. Braun A, Bichlmaier R, Cleve H. Molecular analysis of the gene for the human vitamin-D-binding protein (group-specific component): allelic differences of the common genetic GC types. Hum Genet. 1992;89:401–6.
71. Bhan I. Vitamin d binding protein and bone health. Int J Endocrinol. 2014;2014:561214.
72. Powe CE, Evans MK, Wenger J, et al. Vitamin D-binding protein and vitamin D status of black Americans and white Americans. N Engl J Med. 2013;369:1991–2000.
73. Mendel CM. The free hormone hypothesis: a physiologically based mathematical model. Endocr Rev. 1989;10:232–74.
74. Bikle DD, Siiteri PK, Ryzen E, et al. Serum protein binding of 1,25-dihydroxyvitamin D: a reevaluation by direct measurement of free metabolite levels. J Clin Endocrinol Metab. 1985;61:969–75.
75. Chun RF, Lauridsen AL, Suon L, et al. Vitamin D-binding protein directs monocyte responses to 25-hydroxy- and 1,25-dihydroxyvitamin D. J Clin Endocrinol Metab. 2010;95:3368–76.
76. Chun RF, Peercy BE, Adams JS, et al. Vitamin D binding protein and monocyte response to 25-hydroxyvitamin D and 1,25-dihydroxyvitamin D: analysis by mathematical modeling. PLoS One. 2012;7:e30773.
77. Zella LA, Shevde NK, Hollis BW, et al. Vitamin D-binding protein influences total circulating levels of 1,25-dihydroxyvitamin D3 but does not directly modulate the bioactive levels of the hormone in vivo. Endocrinology. 2008;149:3656–67.
78. Powe CE, Ricciardi C, Berg AH, et al. Vitamin D-binding protein modifies the vitamin D-bone mineral density relationship. J Bone Miner Res. 2011;26:1609–16.
79. Bhan I, Powe CE, Berg AH, et al. Bioavailable vitamin D is more tightly linked to mineral metabolism than total vitamin D in incident hemodialysis patients. Kidney Int. 2012;82:84.
80. Christakos S, Dhawan P, Porta A, et al. Vitamin D and intestinal calcium absorption. Mol Cell Endocrinol. 2011;347:25–9.
81. Holick MF. Resurrection of vitamin D deficiency and rickets. J Clin Invest. 2006;116:2062–72.
82. Aloia JF, Vaswani A, Ma R, et al. Comparison of body composition in black and white premenopausal women. J Lab Clin Med. 1997;129:294–9.

83. Bachrach LK, Hastie T, Wang MC, et al. Bone mineral acquisition in healthy Asian, Hispanic, black, and Caucasian youth: a longitudinal study. J Clin Endocrinol Metab. 1999; 84:4702–12.

84. Nelson DA, Jacobsen G, Barondess DA, et al. Ethnic differences in regional bone density, hip axis length, and lifestyle variables among healthy black and white men. J Bone Miner Res. 1995;10:782–7.

85. Aloia JF, Vaswani A, Delerme-Pagan C, et al. Discordance between ultrasound of the calcaneus and bone mineral density in black and white women. Calcif Tissue Int. 1998;62:481–5.

86. Aloia JF, Vaswani A, Yeh JK, et al. Risk for osteoporosis in black women. Calcif Tissue Int. 1996;59:415–23.

87. Bell NH, Shary J, Stevens J, et al. Demonstration that bone mass is greater in black than in white children. J Bone Miner Res. 1991;6:719–23.

88. Harris SS, Wood MJ, Dawson-Hughes B. Bone mineral density of the total body and forearm in premenopausal black and white women. Bone. 1995;16:311S–5S.

89. Looker AC, Wahner HW, Dunn WL, et al. Updated data on proximal femur bone mineral levels of US adults. Osteoporos Int. 1998;8:468–89.

90. Luckey MM, Meier DE, Mandeli JP, et al. Radial and vertebral bone density in white and black women: evidence for racial differences in premenopausal bone homeostasis. J Clin Endocrinol Metab. 1989;69:762–70.

91. Pollitzer WS, Anderson JJ. Ethnic and genetic differences in bone mass: a review with a hereditary vs environmental perspective. Am J Clin Nutr. 1989;50:1244–59.

92. Cauley JA, Gutai JP, Kuller LH, et al. Black-white differences in serum sex hormones and bone mineral density. Am J Epidemiol. 1994;139:1035–46.

93. Meier DE, Luckey MM, Wallenstein S, et al. Calcium, vitamin D, and parathyroid hormone status in young white and black women: association with racial differences in bone mass. J Clin Endocrinol Metab. 1991;72:703–10.

94. Cauley JA, Lui LY, Ensrud KE, et al. Bone mineral density and the risk of incident nonspinal fractures in black and white women. JAMA. 2005;293:2102–8.

95. Barbour KE, Zmuda JM, Horwitz MJ, et al. The association of serum 25-hydroxyvitamin D with indicators of bone quality in men of Caucasian and African ancestry. Osteoporos Int. 2011;22:2475–85.

96. Aloia JF, Chen DG, Chen H. The 25(OH)D/PTH threshold in black women. J Clin Endocrinol Metab. 2010;95:5069–73.

97. van Ballegooijen AJ, Robinson-Cohen C, Katz R, et al. Vitamin D metabolites and bone mineral density: the multi-ethnic study of atherosclerosis. Bone. 2015;78:186–93.

98. Cauley JA, Danielson ME, Boudreau R, et al. Serum 25 hydroxyvitamin (OH)D and clinical fracture risk in a multiethnic Cohort of women: the Women's health initiative (WHI). J Bone Miner Res. 2011;26:2378.

99. Dawson-Hughes B. Racial/ethnic considerations in making recommendations for vitamin D for adult and elderly men and women. Am J Clin Nutr. 2004;80:1763S–6S.

100. Bell NH, Greene A, Epstein S, et al. Evidence for alteration of the vitamin D-endocrine system in blacks. J Clin Invest. 1985;76:470–3.

101. Dawson-Hughes B, Harris S, Kramich C, et al. Calcium retention and hormone levels in black and white women on high- and low-calcium diets. J Bone Miner Res. 1993;8:779–87.

102. Engelman CD, Fingerlin TE, Langefeld CD, et al. Genetic and environmental determinants of 25-hydroxyvitamin D and 1,25-dihydroxyvitamin D levels in Hispanic and African Americans. J Clin Endocrinol Metab. 2008;93:3381–8.

103. Cosman F, Nieves J, Dempster D, et al. Vitamin D economy in blacks. J Bone Miner Res. 2007;22 Suppl 2:V34–8.

104. Cosman F, Morgan DC, Nieves JW, et al. Resistance to bone resorbing effects of PTH in black women. J Bone Miner Res. 1997;12:958–66.

105. Fuleihan GE, Gundberg CM, Gleason R, et al. Racial differences in parathyroid hormone dynamics. J Clin Endocrinol Metab. 1994;79:1642–7.

106. Perry 3rd HM, Horowitz M, Morley JE, et al. Aging and bone metabolism in African American and Caucasian women. J Clin Endocrinol Metab. 1996;81:1108–17.
107. Bischoff-Ferrari HA, Giovannucci E, Willett WC, et al. Estimation of optimal serum concentrations of 25-hydroxyvitamin D for multiple health outcomes. Am J Clin Nutr. 2006;84:18–28.
108. Chapuy MC, Preziosi P, Maamer M, et al. Prevalence of vitamin D insufficiency in an adult normal population. Osteoporos Int. 1997;7:439–43.
109. Holick MF, Siris ES, Binkley N, et al. Prevalence of vitamin D inadequacy among postmenopausal North American women receiving osteoporosis therapy. J Clin Endocrinol Metab. 2005;90:3215–24.
110. Krall EA, Sahyoun N, Tannenbaum S, et al. Effect of vitamin D intake on seasonal variations in parathyroid hormone secretion in postmenopausal women. N Engl J Med. 1989;321:1777–83.
111. Malabanan A, Veronikis IE, Holick MF. Redefining vitamin D insufficiency. Lancet. 1998;351:805–6.
112. Steingrimsdottir L, Gunnarsson O, Indridason OS, et al. Relationship between serum parathyroid hormone levels, vitamin D sufficiency, and calcium intake. JAMA. 2005;294:2336–41.
113. Cauley JA, Lacroix AZ, Wu L, et al. Serum 25-hydroxyvitamin D concentrations and risk for hip fractures. Ann Intern Med. 2008;149:242–50.
114. Cauley JA, Parimi N, Ensrud KE, et al. Serum 25-hydroxyvitamin D and the risk of hip and nonspine fractures in older men. J Bone Miner Res. 2010;25:545–53.
115. Cummings SR, Browner WS, Bauer D, et al. Endogenous hormones and the risk of hip and vertebral fractures among older women. Study of Osteoporotic Fractures Research Group. N Engl J Med. 1998;339:733–8.
116. Looker AC, Mussolino ME. Serum 25-hydroxyvitamin D and hip fracture risk in older U.S. white adults. J Bone Miner Res. 2008;23:143–50.
117. Heaney RP. The importance of calcium intake for lifelong skeletal health. Calcif Tissue Int. 2002;70:70–3.
118. Targher G, Bertolini L, Padovani R, et al. Serum 25-hydroxyvitamin D3 concentrations and carotid artery intima-media thickness among type 2 diabetic patients. Clin Endocrinol (Oxf). 2006;65:593–7.
119. Freedman BI, Wagenknecht LE, Hairston KG, et al. Vitamin d, adiposity, and calcified atherosclerotic plaque in African-Americans. J Clin Endocrinol Metab. 2010;95:1076–83.

Chapter 7
Vitamin D and Parathyroid Hormone Regulation in Chronic Kidney Disease

María E. Rodríguez-Ortiz, Mariano Rodríguez, and Yolanda Almadén Peña

Abstract Parathyroid glands have a predominant role in mineral homeostasis. Calcium and vitamin D are two of the main regulators of the parathyroid function by virtue of the presence of the calcium-sensing receptor and vitamin D receptor in parathyroid cells. FGF23 also modulates parathyroid function. Chronic renal failure is characterized by derangements in factors involved in mineral metabolism that lead to the development of secondary hyperparathyroidism. This chapter reviews in depth the pathophysiology of secondary hyperparathyroidism, the function and regulation of the vitamin D receptor and the calcium-sensing receptor, as well as their roles in the development of parathyroid hyperplasia.

Keywords Calcium • Calcium-sensing receptor • Chronic kidney disease • FGF23 • Hyperplasia • Parathyroid hormone • Phosphorus • Secondary hyperparathyroidism • Vitamin D • Vitamin D receptor

7.1 Physiology of the Parathyroid Gland

Parathyroid glands have a central role in mineral homeostasis. Under physiological conditions, small changes in the level of extracellular calcium (Ca) are detected by the calcium-sensing receptor (CaR) located at the surface of parathyroid cells,

M.E. Rodríguez-Ortiz, PhD
IIS-Fundación Jiménez-Díaz, Madrid, Spain

M. Rodríguez, PhD (✉)
Service of Nephrology, Instituto Maimónides de Investigación Biomédica de Córdoba (IMIBIC), Reina Sofia University Hospital, University of Córdoba, Córdoba, Spain
e-mail: marianorodriguezportillo@gmail.com

Y.A. Peña, PhD
Lipid and Atherosclerosis Unit, Instituto Maimónides de Investigación Biomédica de Córdoba (IMIBIC), Reina Sofia University Hospital/University of Cordoba, Córdoba, Spain

CIBER Fisiopatologia Obesidad y Nutricion (CIBEROBN), Instituto de Salud Carlos III, University of Cordoba, Córdoba, Spain
e-mail: yolandaalmaden@yahoo.es

© Springer International Publishing Switzerland 2016   147
P.A. Ureña Torres et al. (eds.), *Vitamin D in Chronic Kidney Disease*,
DOI 10.1007/978-3-319-32507-1_7

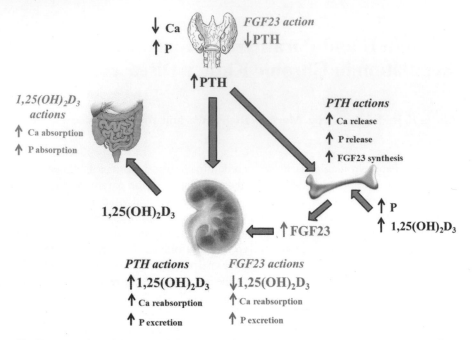

Fig. 7.1 Overview of the elements involved in the maintenance of mineral metabolism, as well as the interconnections among them

which respond with an adequate secretion of parathyroid hormone (PTH). PTH acts on bone promoting the release of Ca and phosphorus (P) ions and on the kidney stimulating the production of calcitriol [1,25(OH)$_2$D$_3$], active metabolite of vitamin D, synthesized from its precursor calcidiol [25(OH)D], through an increase in the activity of the enzyme 1α–hydroxylase. In addition to this action, PTH exerts a phosphaturic activity by decreasing P renal reabsorption. The increase in 1,25(OH)$_2$D$_3$ contributes to the normalization of serum Ca levels by increasing intestinal Ca absorption. Activation of the parathyroid vitamin D receptor (VDR) causes a reduction in PTH production. Fibroblast growth factor 23 (FGF23) is a phosphatonin produced by osteoblasts and osteocytes tightly involved in mineral metabolism. FGF23 regulates mainly P and vitamin D levels by acting on kidney [1] and also has been shown to regulate parathyroid secretion [2]. A scheme of the mechanisms regulating Ca and P metabolism is depicted in Fig. 7.1.

7.2 Regulation of Parathyroid Function by Calcitriol

Vitamin D regulates parathyroid function by acting on the parathyroid VDR and by increasing intestinal absorption of Ca. An early study by Silver et al. [3] was designed to evaluate the effect of 1,25(OH)$_2$D$_3$ and other vitamin D metabolites on

PTH synthesis and secretion. The study was performed in cultured bovine parathyroid cells and the concentration of vitamin D compounds ranged from 10 pM to 0.1 M. All metabolites of vitamin D induced the inhibition of the pre-pro-PTH levels in a reversible manner, but with different intensity.

The effect of a number of vitamin D metabolites has been evidenced in vivo. Intraperitoneal administration of vitamin D reduced parathyroid pre-pro-PTHmRNA levels, being $1,25(OH)_2D_3$ the most potent compound when compared with $24,25(OH)_2D_3$ and 25(OH) [4]. In a later study by Naveh-Many et al. [5], groups of rats were fed with either a normal or a vitamin D-deficient diet for 3 weeks. In vitamin D-deficient rats PTH mRNA expression was twofold increased as compared with controls on a normal diet. The increase in PTH mRNA was not associated with changes in serum Ca concentration and could be reverted by the treatment with exogenous $1,25(OH)_2D_3$.

In dialysis patients, Slatopolsky et al. [6] showed that intravenous administration of $1,25(OH)_2D_3$ produced a reduction in serum PTH level that could not be explained by hypercalcemia. A large number of clinical studies have shown that $1,25(OH)_2D_3$ administration is effective in decreasing serum PTH levels in patients with end-stage renal disease (ESRD), so the use of $1,25(OH)_2D_3$ became a key therapeutic strategy to treat uremic secondary hyperparathyroidism (SHPT).

A large number of dialysis patients are treated with $1,25(OH)_2D_3$ to control SHPT. However, a significant number of dialysis patients exhibit a vitamin D resistance and fail to respond to $1,25(OH)_2D_3$ treatment [7], which may, in part, be explained by a decreased expression of VDR in parathyroid cells from severe hyperplasia [8].

Both Ca and vitamin D are the key physiological factors regulating parathyroid function. Therefore, dysregulation of their levels, as well as a reduced expression of their respective specific receptors, CaR and VDR, has profound effects leading to alteration of the parathyroid function seen in chronic kidney disease (CKD) patients: increased synthesis and secretion of PTH as well as cell proliferation, resulting in gland hyperplasia. Of note, it has been uncovered a complex relationship between Ca and vitamin D, not only at the circulating levels, but also at the receptors levels. $1,25(OH)_2D_3$ renders the parathyroid glands more susceptible to the suppressive action of Ca through modulating the expression of key cellular receptors, such as their own receptors VDR and the CaR.

7.3   The Calcium-Sensing Receptor and Its Implication in the Control of PTH Secretion

The CaR represents a key element in Ca homeostasis that allows cells to detect and respond to small changes in the extracellular Ca concentration. It was firstly identified by Brown and collaborators in 1993 [9] and it belongs to the family C of G-protein coupled receptors (GPCR). In addition to the CaR, the family C also comprises metabotropic glutamate receptors, the gamma-amino-butyric acid (GABA) type B receptors, and the vomeronasal type-2 receptors.

Although Ca is the main agonist of the CaR, other ligands are also capable of activate it. They are classified as a) type I agonists, including other divalent (Mg^{2+}, Sr^{2+}, Ba^{2+}) and trivalent (La^{3+}, Gd^{3+}) cations, and b) type II agonists, as polyamines (putrescine, spermine, spermidine) and amino acids [10]. The ability of these molecules to activate the CaR has prompted the development of calcimimetics, drugs capable of inhibiting the secretion of PTH upon the activation of the receptor.

The human CaR gene is located in the long arm of chromosome 3, at position 13 (3q13) whereas in the rat and mouse it resides on chromosomes 11 and 16, respectively. The protein of CaR has a molecular weight of 120 KDa. It possesses a large N-terminal extracellular domain, a cysteine-rich domain linking the extracellular domain to the first transmembrane helix, a seven transmembrane domain, and an intracellular C-terminal domain. Although it also has been reported a binding site for Ca in the transmembrane region of the receptor, the site located in the extracellular domain is required for the fully activation. The interaction between Ca and the receptor induces a conformational change in its structure, the activation of transduction signals and the mobilization of intracellular Ca.

Mutations in CaR gene are responsible for several disorders. Inactivating mutations cause familial hypocalciuric hypocalcemia (FHH, OMIM 14598) as well as neonatal severe hyperparathyroidism (NSHPT, OMIM 239200), whereas autosomal dominant hypoparathyroidism (ADH, OMIM 601298) is associated to gain-of-function mutations in the CaR gene [11].

The CaR is not only expressed in organs directly involved in mineral homeostasis, such as parathyroid cells, C cells of the thyroid gland, bone or kidney, but also in other tissues as gastrointestinal tract (esophagus, stomach, small intestine, and colon), skin, cardiac and smooth muscle, and nervous system. The presence of the CaR in the surface of parathyroid cells allows them to respond exquisitely to small changes in the concentration of extracellular Ca. The activation of the receptor activates several signaling pathways (phospholipase A_2 and C, protein kinase C, and several mitogen-activated protein kinases) that eventually lead to the inhibition of PTH [12].

The activation of the CaR has also been shown to regulate the synthesis of PTH. Indeed, in a state of hypocalcemia the stability of PTH mRNA is increased by the binding of proteins to the specific region in the 3′-untranslated region (UTR) that protects the transcript from degradation. Naveh-Many et al. identified the A+U-rich element binding factor (AUF1) as a protein that may confer stability to the PTH mRNA transcript [13].

The expression of the CaR is modulated by several factors. Vitamin D augments the expression of the receptor at parathyroid level. In an in vivo study, Brown and collaborators found that administration of $1,25(OH)_2D_3$ in rats fed with diets deficient in vitamin D stimulated the expression of the parathyroid CaR dose-dependently [14]. Of note, the expression of CaR in these vitamin D-deficient animals was already diminished. The effect of vitamin D, as a modulator of the parathyroid CaR, was confirmed in a subsequent work by Canaff and Handy. They identified the transcriptional start sites of promoters P1 and P2 in the CaR and the existence of vitamin D responsive elements (VDREs) in both sites [15].

In addition to vitamin D, other modulators of parathyroid function have also been shown to regulate the CaR expression. For instance, moderately elevated magnesium (Mg) upregulated parathyroid CaR expression in vitro [16]. Similarly, the addition of FGF23 to incubated parathyroid glands produced an increase in the CaR [17].

So far, the results obtained concerning the role of Ca itself as a regulator of the CaR are contradictory. While some authors have not found an independent effect of Ca [18], we observed that high Ca significantly increased the expression of CaR in rat parathyroid glands culture in vitro [17]. On the other hand, several studies have shown that calcimimetics up-regulate the CaR in parathyroid glands from uremic rats, where the expression of the receptor is already decreased [19]. Moreover, this effect appears to be independent of a possible effect on proliferation, as observed in rats shortly after acute administration of calcimimetic [20].

Importantly, a novel mechanism that modulates CaR trafficking from cytosol to the cell membrane has been recently described. The agonist-driven insertional signaling implies that the maturation, trafficking, and insertion of the CaR in the plasma membrane are mediated by the ligand binding [21].

7.4   The Vitamin D Receptor

The biological effects of $1,25(OH)_2D_3$, the most active vitamin D metabolite, are mediated by the VDR. The VDR is a ligand-activated transcription factor belonging to the superfamily of steroid/thyroid hormone receptors nuclear receptor that, when bound to vitamin D, acts as a transcription factor.

The VDR was discovered in 1969 in the intestine of vitamin D–deficient chicks [22]. The VDR protein is composed of different structural regions with a certain degree of variation between species. The primary amino acid sequence of the VDR consists of six functional domains: the variable regions (A and B domains) which include an activator region called AF-1, DNA binding (the C domain) is the most conserved region and responsible for the recognition of the VDRE in the target genes; this region contains two zinc fingers which are absolutely essential to stabilize the binding VDR-DNA. The hinge region (D domain) which gives to VDR an ability of rotation enabling adequate link to VDREs, the ligand-binding region (LBD, E domain) responsible for binding of vitamin D, and transcriptional activation (domain F) is the C-terminal region which contains a site for dimerization and a AF-2 domain with regulatory function of transcription. To date, N terminal isoforms of the receptor have been identified that differ only in the length of their A/B domains [23].

VDR is a DNA-binding transcription factor, which generates an active signaling transduction complex. VDR control of gene transcription is mediated by several stages including binding of vitamin D in the C-terminal portion of VDR, heterodimerization with retinoid X receptor (RXR) and nuclear translocation, binding of VDR–RXR to specific DNA sequences (VDRE) in target gene promoter, and recruitment of VDR-interacting nuclear co-regulators or co-factors resulting in acti-vation or inhibition of gene transcription.

At the parathyroid level, the VDR directly down-regulates the transcription of the gene encoding PTH through binding to VDRE. Negative VDREs have been mapped both in the human and rat PTH promoters, resulting in a reduction of the PTH synthesis [24, 25]. Results from VDR activation in other target tissues will not be commented here.

7.5   Regulation of Vitamin D Receptor in Parathyroid Glands

An homologous regulation of VDR expression by $1,25(OH)_2D_3$ amplifies the effect of circulating $1,25(OH)_2D_3$ on the PTH gene. This effect was described by Naveh-Many et al. [26]: the administration of $1,25(OH)_2D_3$ increased the levels of the VDR mRNA in rat parathyroid glands. Other studies have confirmed this finding. Denda et al. [27] reported that low serum $1,25(OH)_2D_3$ levels were, at least in part, respon-sible for the decrease in VDR content in parathyroid glands of uremic rats and that treatment with $1,25(OH)_2D_3$ prevented this decrease, ameliorating the development of SHPT. In vitro studies also demonstrated a direct effect of $1,25(OH)_2D_3$ to increase VDR expression [18].

Of special importance in the regulation of parathyroid function is the cooperation of Ca and vitamin D on reducing parathyroid function. Several experimental and clinical data suggests that the $1,25(OH)_2D_3$ system is relatively ineffective in con-trolling PTH when serum Ca concentration is low. A study by Naveh-Many et al. [5] showed that the ability of exogenous $1,25(OH)_2D_3$ to inhibit PTH mRNA in vitamin D–deficient rats was largely prevented when serum Ca was low, suggesting that the inhibition of PTH by $1,25(OH)_2D_3$ was not possible if hypocalcemia was present. In another study [28], the administration of calcitriol (CTR) in vitamin D–deficient chickens for 3–6 days increased parathyroid VDR mRNA, and this effect was enhanced when serum Ca levels were normal. In this same study it was observed that 6 days of dietary Ca restriction decreased VDR mRNA and that $1,25(OH)_2D_3$ administration only upregulated VDR expression when chickens were fed a normal Ca diet. In rats fed for 6 weeks with diets containing different vitamin D, Brown et al. [29] did not observe an independent effect of $1,25(OH)_2D_3$, but upregulation of VDR by $1,25(OH)_2D_3$ appeared as being mediated primarily by an increased serum Ca concentration.

A definitive evidence for an independent effect of Ca on parathyroid VDR expression came from in vivo experiments by Garfia et al. [30]. By using a 6-h hypercalcemic or hypocalcemic clamp in rats, it was found that $1,25(OH)_2D_3$ pro-duced an increase in VDR levels only when Ca concentration was elevated; how-ever, $1,25(OH)_2D_3$ did not increase VDR expression in rats maintained with hypocalcemia during a 6-h period. In addition, the downregulation of VDR by hypocalcemia resulted in impairment of the inhibitory action of $1,25(OH)_2D_3$ on parathyroid cell function. $1,25(OH)_2D_3$ administered to rats after the induction of hypocalcemia (when VDR was already downregulated) was not able to reduce PTH mRNA, whereas it was downregulated in rats receiving $1,25(OH)_2D_3$ before the initiation of hypocalcemia. These results were also confirmed in vitro by Cañadillas et al. [31] and by Carrillo et al. [18], who observed in rat parathyroid glands that the higher the Ca, the higher VDR expression. Thus, beside the direct posttranscriptional effect on PTH mRNA, the low Ca may also stimulate PTH levels indirectly through lowering the parathyroid VDR expression which makes $1,25(OH)_2D_3$ less effective. Of note, downregulation of parathyroid VDR caused by low Ca prevents PTH inhibition by $1,25(OH)_2D_3$. This is an important concept in the pathogenesis of SHPT because hypocalcemia may not allow a normal inhibition of parathyroid cells by $1,25(OH)_2D_3$ even when $1,25(OH)_2D_3$ levels are normal.

Finally, Cañadillas et al. [31] characterized in vitro the signaling system responsible for the stimulation of parathyroid VDR by extracellular Ca, which takes place through the elevation of the cytosolic Ca level, and the subsequent stimulation of the PLA2-AA-dependent ERK1/2- pathway. High extracellular Ca also increased the VDR promoter activity through the activation of the Sp1 transcription factor in VDR-transfected HEKCaR cells.

Taken together, the above data support that the tight control of PTH secretion and synthesis by Ca may in part be explained by the fact that high Ca enhances the inhibitory action of vitamin D on parathyroid glands by augmenting VDR expression.

Besides $1,25(OH)_2D_3$ and Ca, several other factors have been reported to regulate VDR expression and/or function. Calcimimetics, such as R-568 and cinacalcet HCl, are allosteric modulators of the CaR, acting by increasing the sensitivity of the parathyroid gland to extracellular Ca. Thus, it was hypothesized that administration of the calcimimetic R-568 may result in increased VDR expression in parathyroid tissue. In in vitro studies with whole rat parathyroid glands, the calcimimetic elicited an increase in VDR mRNA similar to the maximum increase detected with 1.5 mM Ca [32]. Treatment with R-568 also increased VDR protein in normal rat parathyroid glands and, interestingly, in human parathyroid glands with diffuse but not nodular hyperplasia. These results support the convenience of using vitamin D-calcimimetic combinations in the clinical settings. Any increase in VDR would facilitate the inhibitory feedback of vitamin D on the parathyroid glands and would assist in optimization of the positive action of the pharmacological administration of $1,25(OH)_2D_3$ or other vitamin D analogs, which in turn may reduce unwanted side effects as high CaxP products and vascular calcifications.

It is now well-known that FGF23 decreases PTH secretion and PTH mRNA [2]. Furthermore, in normal rat parathyroid glands in vitro, addition of FGF23 to the low-Ca medium increased parathyroid VDR and CaR mRNA and protein expression to levels similar to those observed with a high-Ca concentration [17]. The FGF23-dependent changes in VDR and CaR expression were paralleled by the activation of the ERK1/2 activation. FGF23 also increased VDR and CaR expression and activated ERK1/2 in the parathyroid glands of normal rats in vivo. This upregulation of CaR and VDR may represent another mechanism whereby FGF23 reduces parathyroid function.

In a recent study, the direct effect of Mg in the regulation of the parathyroid function was evaluated [16]; specifically, PTH secretion and the expression of the key parathyroid cell receptors: CaR, VDR and the FGF23 receptor 1 (FGFR1)/klotho system. The results of this study showed that parathyroid glands are sensitive to an inhibitory effect of Mg only when a moderate low Ca concentration is present. Furthermore, the levels of CaR, VDR, FGFR1 and klotho expression, both the mRNA and protein, exhibited a marked increase at a Mg concentration of 2.0 mM when compared with 0.5 mM Mg after 6-h incubation at a Ca concentration of 1.0 mM. The up-regulation of parathyroid receptors may be an additional mechanism whereby Mg inhibits parathyroid gland function. Interestingly, as deduced from these data, Mg would favour the efficiency of therapeutic molecules targeting the parathyroid CaR, VDR, or FGFR1/klotho.

Uremic plasma contains substances that interfere with the action of vitamin D; preincubation of intestinal VDR with uremic ultrafiltrate significantly reduced the interaction of the VDR-hormone complex with DNA [33]. Uremic toxins have been shown to reduce the biological action of $1,25(OH)_2D_3$ by suppressing receptor synthesis. In this regard, Canalejo et al. [34] addressed the role of the uremic milieu on parathyroid VDR function by evaluating in vitro whether uremic toxins had an effect on the regulation of parathyroid cell proliferation by $1,25(OH)_2D_3$. While $1,25(OH)_2D_3$ reduced the number of parathyroid cells entering the S phase of the cell cycle, the addition of total uremic ultrafiltrate prevented this effect. Thus, to avoid the impairment of CTR action trough the parathyroid VDR in CKD patients, dialysis should efficiently remove VDR-targeting uremic toxins.

Figure 7.2 summarizes the signaling pathways regulating the expression of the VDR to facilitate the inhibitory action of $1,25(OH)_2D_3$ on parathyroid cell function.

7.6 Pathophysiology of Secondary Hyperparathyrdism

Normal kidney function is essential for mineral homeostasis. The complex mechanism regulating mineral metabolism is disrupted in CKD patients. In renal failure patients there is an increased load of P that at very early stages of the disease stimulates FGF23 production, which in turn decreases $1,25(OH)_2D_3$ (Fig. 7.3). Both P overload and deficiency of $1,25(OH)_2D_3$ enhance parathyroid gland hyperplasia [35]. Increased levels of FGF23 and PTH help maintain the serum Ca and P within normal levels during CKD 1–3 and even in CKD 4. High serum P concentration directly promotes parathyroid hyperplasia and produces skeletal resistance to the action of PTH; therefore, when P is high, more PTH is required to maintain serum Ca concentration within the normal range. Recent studies have shown that renal klotho expression is reduced early in the development of renal insufficiency [36]. The reduction in klotho may cause resistance to the phosphaturic action of FGF23, and more FGF23 may be produced in an attempt to prevent the accumulation of P. Some authors have proposed that an initial event in the development of SHPT may be the reduction of renal klotho expression, with impairment in the ability of kidneys to excrete the excess of P.

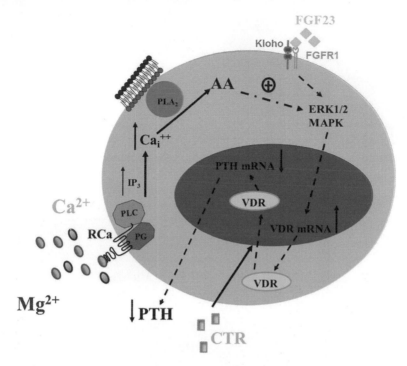

Fig. 7.2 Summary of the signaling pathways involved in the regulation of vitamin D receptor expression promoting the inhibition of parathyroid function by calcitriol

The demand for PTH increases with the progression of the renal disease. At initial stages of renal disease there is parathyroid hyperplasia with a moderate but significant reduction of CaR, VDR and FGFR1-klotho [35]. Therefore, the inhibitory effects of Ca, vitamin D and FGF23 on parathyroid glands are impaired. The expression of these receptors is further reduced in areas of monoclonal parathyroid cell proliferation, which is often observed in severe parathyroid hyperplasia [35, 37].

The term Chronic Kidney Disease-Mineral and Bone Disorder (CKD-MBD) includes the above described abnormalities in mineral metabolism, together with bone disease and calcification of vessels and soft tissues.

7.7   Roles of the Calcium-Sensing Receptor and the Vitamin D Receptor in the Pathophysiology of Secondary Hyperparathyroidism

In order to maintain the biologic effect of $1,25(OH)_2D_3$ on parathyroid cells, it is necessary an adequate level of VDR, as well as of the optimal binding capacity of the VDR to the VDRE in DNA. However, many studies have demonstrated reduced levels of VDR in uremic parathyroid glands from SHPT patients and experimental animals.

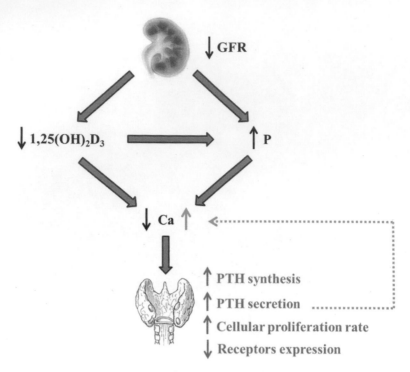

Fig. 7.3 Schematic view of the pathophysiology of secondary hyperparathyroidism. *GFR* glo-merular filtration rate, *1,25(OH)₂D₃* calcitriol, *P* phosphorus, *Ca* calcium, *PTH* parathyroid hormone

Uremic patients develop progressive parathyroid hyperplasia as a consequence of a maintained stimulation of parathyroid function. It is accepted that the progression of parathyroid hyperplasia is enhanced by the decrease in the serum concentrations of $1,25(OH)_2D_3$, the tendency to hypocalcemia and the rise in serum P levels. However, the exact mechanisms that drive parathyroid cells to proliferate are not clear. It is generally accepted that low $1,25(OH)_2D_3$ contributes to the development of parathyroid hyperplasia [38]. $1,25(OH)_2D_3$ is a primary inhibitor of parathyroid cell proliferation by acting on the gene expression of the cell cycle regulator *c-myc* [39]. In vitro and in vivo studies [39–41] indicate that $1,25(OH)_2D_3$ suppress parathyroid hyperplasia.

During the early stages of SHPT, parathyroid growth is polyclonal, giving rise to diffuse hyperplasia (Fig. 7.4). However, at some time point during the late stage in the evolution of SHPT, there is a transformation from diffuse to nodular hyperplasia as a result of monoclonal growth of parathyroid cells. Studies performed in vitro using parathyroid tissue from uremic patients that had required parathyroidectomy demonstrate that in nodular hyperplasia there is blunted response to the inhibitory effect of both Ca [43] and $1,25(OH)_2D_3$ [44]; this is explained by a reduced expression of VDR and CaR [45, 46]. Fukuda et al. [8] firstly showed a lower density of VDR in nodular than in diffuse human parathyroid hyperplasia; similar findings were

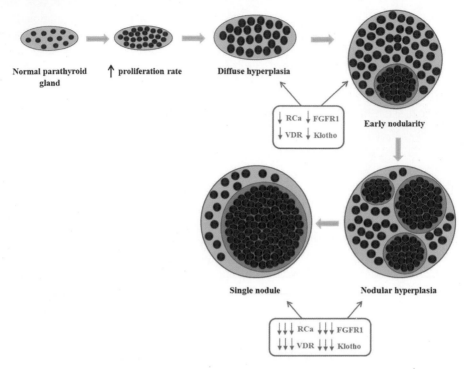

Fig. 7.4 Progression of parathyroid hyperplasia in chronic kidney disease (Adapted from Komaba et al. [42])

reported by Tokumoto et al. [47]. Gogusev et al. [37] showed that CaR is reduced in nodular hyperplasia. This explains, at least in part, the poor control of parathyroid cell proliferation by vitamin D and Ca in patients with markedly advanced SHPT, which is characterized by parathyroid nodular hyperplasia [44]. In parathyroid cells the regulation of activation of the CaR induces the incorporation of CaR to the cell membrane, which results in amplification of the inhibitory signal [21].

Whether the decrease in VDR and CaR occurs at the onset of parathyroid hyperplasia or the reduced expression is a consequence of cell proliferation is controversial. Taniguchi et al. [48] reported that in five-sixth nephrectomized rats on a high P diet (HPD) there was a reduction of parathyroid VDR expression and a simultaneous elevation in p21 (marker of cell proliferation) as early as day 1, while the increase in cell proliferation rate was first observed on day 3. These results suggest that down-regulation of VDR and the elevation of p21 may play a key role in the pathogenesis of SHPT. However, in normal rats the increase in cell proliferation induced by a high phosphorus diet (HPD) was observed on day 1 and preceded a transient down-regulation of VDR expression first observed on day 5; by contrast, an increase in cell proliferation was not seen until day 5 in a low Ca diet (LCD) rats, and coincided with the transient down-regulation of VDR expression. In this experiment, the expression of CaR was no affected by either diet [49].

A number of factors have been suggested to contribute to the down-regulation of VDR in the hyperplasic parathyroid tissue. Firstly, the reduced levels of $1,25(OH)_2D_3$ would prevent the homologous up-regulation of its own receptor. Secondly, as serum Ca has been also established as a key regulator of VDR expression, the hypocalcemia related to SHPT might also contribute to the reduced expression of parathyroid VDR in secondary hyperparathyroidism. Finally, uremic toxins may also reduce the stability of VDR mRNA and then, decrease the expression of VDR protein [50].

7.8   Conclusion

The presence of the vitamin D receptor and the calcium-sensing receptor in parathyroid chief cells enables the parathyroid gland to respond to vitamin D and calcium, two of the main regulators of the parathyroid function.

Calcium and vitamin D have both independent and cooperative effects on parathyroid function inhibition. Besides modulating its own receptor, vitamin D also regulates the calcium-sensing receptor, which makes parathyroid gland more sensitive to the suppressive action of calcium. Vitamin D upregulates vitamin D receptor only if calcium is normal or high. Conversely, vitamin D receptor is downregulated in hypocalcemia and upregulated by activation of the calcium-sensing receptor. Inhibition of parathyroid function by Vitamin D is impaired in the presence of hypocalcemia

In chronic kidney disease, the prolonged stimulation of parathyroid glands promotes parathyroid hyperplasia. If treatment is not applied, severe secondary hyperparathyroidism develops, that may become resistant to medical treatment; such is the case of nodular hyperplasia of the parathyroids. Hyperplasia is accompanied by a decrease in the expression of parathyroid receptors, including FGFR-1 and klotho. Although the exact mechanisms whereby parathyroid hyperplasia is developed are not completely understood, several factors such as the hypocalcemia, the phosphorus retention and the deficiency in vitamin D has been directly associated to an increase in cell proliferation.

References

1. Shimada T, Kakitani M, Yamazaki Y, Hasegawa H, Takeuchi Y, Fujita T, et al. Targeted ablation of Fgf23 demonstrates an essential physiological role of FGF23 in phosphate and vitamin D metabolism. J Clin Invest. 2004;113:561–8. doi:10.1172/JCI200419081.
2. Ben-Dov IZ, Galitzer H, Lavi-Moshayoff V, Goetz R, Kuro-o M, Mohammadi M, et al. The parathyroid is a target organ for FGF23 in rats. J Clin Invest. 2007;117:4003–8. doi:10.1172/JCI32409.
3. Silver J, Russell J, Sherwood LM. Regulation by vitamin D metabolites of messenger ribonucleic acid for preproparathyroid hormone in isolated bovine parathyroid cells. Proc Natl Acad Sci U S A. 1985;82:4270–3.

4. Silver J, Naveh-Many T, Mayer H, Schmeizer HJ, Popovtzer MM. Regulation by vitamin D metabolites of parathyroid hormone gene transcription in vivo in the rat. J Clin Invest. 1986;78:1296–01.
5. Naveh-Many T, Silver J. Regulation of parathyroid hormone gene expression by hypocalcemia, hypercalcemia and vitamin D in the rat. J Clin Invest. 1990;86:1313–9.
6. Slatopolsky E, Weerts C, Thielan J, Horst R, Harter H, Martin KJ. Marked suppression of secondary hyperparathyroidism by intravenous administration of 1,25-dihydroxycholecalciferol in uremic patients. J Clin Invest. 1984;74:2136–43.
7. Fukagawa M, Kitaoka M, Kurokawa K. Resistance of the parathyroid glands to vitamin D in renal failure: implications for medical management. Kidney Int. 1997;52:60–4.
8. Fukuda N, Tanaka H, Tominaga Y, Fukagawa M, Kurokawa K, Seino Y. Decreased 1,25-dihydroxyvitamin D receptor density associated with a more severe form of parathyroid hyperplasia in chronic uremic patients. J Clin Invest. 1993;92:1436–43.
9. Brown EM, Gamba G, Riccardi D, Lombardi M, Butters R, Kifor O, et al. Cloning and characterization of an extracellular Ca^{2+}-sensing receptor from bovine parathyroid. Nature. 1993;366:575–80. doi:10.1038/366575a0.
10. Brown EM, MacLeod J. Extracellular calcium sensing and extracellular calcium signaling. Physiol Rev. 2001;81:239–97.
11. Ward BK, Magno AL, Walsh JP, Ratajczak T. The role of the calcium-sensing receptor in human disease. Clin Biochem. 2012;45:943–53. doi:10.1016/j.clinbiochem.2012.03.034.
12. Brown EM. Clinical lessons from the calcium-sensing receptor. Nat Clin Pract Endocrinol Metab. 2007;3:122–33. doi:10.1038/ncpendmet0388.
13. Naveh-Many T, Bell O, Silver J, Kilav R. Cis and trans acting factors in the regulation of parathyroid hormone (PTH) mRNA stability by calcium and phosphate. FEBS Lett. 2002;529:60–4. doi:10.1016/S0014-5793(02)032529-3.
14. Brown AJ, Zhong M, Finch J, Ritter C, McCracken R, Morrisey J, et al. Rat calcium-sensing receptor is regulated by vitamin D but not by calcium. Am J Physiol. 1996;270:F454–60.
15. Canaff L, Hendy GN. Human Calcium-sensing receptor gene. Vitamin D response elements in promoters P1 and P2 confer transcriptional responsiveness to 1,25-dihydroxyvitamin D. J Biol Chem. 2002;277:30337–50. doi:10.1074/jbc.M201804200.
16. Rodríguez-Ortiz ME, Canalejo A, Herencia C, Martínez-Moreno JM, Peralta-Ramírez A, Perez-Martínez P, et al. Magnesium modulates parathyroid hormone secretion and upregulates parathyroid receptor expression at moderately low calcium concentration. Nephrol Dial Transplant. 2014;29:282–9. doi:10.1093/ndt/gft400.
17. Canalejo R, Canalejo A, Martínez-Moreno JM, Rodríguez-Ortiz ME, Estepa JC, Mendoza FJ, et al. FGF23 fails to inhibit uremic parathyroid glands. J Am Soc Nephrol. 2010;21:1125–35. doi:10.1681/ASN.2009040427.
18. Carrillo-López N, Alvarez-Hernández D, González-Suárez I, Román-García P, Valdivielso JM, Fernández-Martín JL, et al. Simultaneous changes in the calcium-sensing receptor and the vitamin D receptor under the influence of calcium and calcitriol. Nephrol Dial Transplant. 2008;23:3479–84. doi:10.1093/ndt/gfn338.
19. Mizobuchi M, Hatamura I, Ogata H, Saji F, Uda S, Shiizaki K, et al. Calcimimetic compound upregulates decreased calcium-sensing receptor expression level in parathyroid glands of rats with chronic renal insufficiency. J Am Soc Nephrol. 2004;15:2579–87. doi:10.1097/01. ASN.0000141016.20133.33.
20. Mendoza FJ, Lopez I, Canalejo R, Almaden Y, Martin D, Aguilera-Tejero E, et al. Direct upregulation of parathyroid calcium-sensing receptor and vitamin D receptor by calcimimetics in uremic rats. Am J Physiol Renal Physiol. 2009;296:F605–13. doi:10.1152/ajprenal.90272.2008.
21. Grant MP, Stepanchick A, Cavanaugh A, Breitwieser GE. Agonist-driven maturation and plasma membrane insertion of calcium-sensing receptors dynamically control signal amplitude. Sci Signal. 2011;4:ra78. doi:10.1126/scisignal.2002208.
22. Haussler MR, Norman AW. Chromosomal receptor for a vitamin D metabolite. Proc Natl Acad Sci U S A. 1969;62:155–62.

23. Sunn KL, Eisman JA, Gardiner EM, Jans DA. FRAP analysis of nucleocytoplasmic dynamics of the vitamin D receptor splice variant VDRB1: preferential targeting to nuclear speckles. J Biochem. 2005;388:509–14. doi:10.1042/BJ20042040.

24. Demay MB, Kiernan MS, DeLuca HF, Kronenberg HM. Sequences in the human parathyroid hormone gene that bind the 1,25-dihydroxyvitamin D3 receptor and mediate transcriptional repression in response to 1,25-dihydroxyvitamin D3. Proc Natl Acad Sci U S A. 1992;89:8097–01.

25. Russell J, Ashok S, Koszewski NJ. Vitamin D receptor interactions with the rat parathyroid hormone gene: synergistic effects between two negative vitamin D response elements. J Bone Miner Res. 1999;14:1828–37. doi:10.1359/jbmr.1999.14.11.1828.

26. Naveh-Many T, Marx R, Keshet E, Pike JW, Silver J. Regulation of 1,25 dihydroxyvitamin D3 receptor gene expression by 1,25-dihydroxyvitamin D3 in the parathyroid in vivo. J Clin Invest. 1990;86:1968–75.

27. Denda M, Finch J, Brown AJ, Nishii Y, Kubodera N, Slatopolsky E. 1,25-dihydroxyvitamin D3 and 22-oxacalcitriol prevent the decrease in vitamin D receptor content in the parathyroid glands of uremic rats. Kidney Int. 1996;50:34–9.

28. Russell J, Bar A, Sherwood LM, Hurwitz S. Interaction between calcium and 1,25 -dihydroxyvitamin D3 in the regulation of preparathyroid hormone and vitaminD receptor messenger ribonucleic acid in avian parathyroids. Endocrinology. 1993;132:2639–43. doi:10.1210/endo.132.6.8389284.

29. Brown AJ, Zhong M, Finch J, Ritter C, Slatopolsky E. The roles of calcium and 1,25-Dihydroxyvitamin D3 in the regulation of vitamin D receptor expression by rat parathyroid glands. Endocrinology. 1995;136:1419–25. doi:10.1210/endo.136.4.7895652.

30. Garfia B, Cañadillas S, Canalejo A, Luque F, Siendones E, Quesada M, et al. Regulation of parathyroid vitamin D receptor expression by extracellular calcium. J Am Soc Nephrol. 2002;13:2945–52. doi:10.1097/01.ASN.0000037676.54018.CB.

31. Cañadillas S, Canalejo R, Rodriguez-Ortiz ME, Martinez-Moreno JM, Estepa JC, Zafra R, et al. Upregulation of parathyroid VDR expression by extracellular calcium is mediated by ERK1/2-MAPK signaling pathway. Am J Physiol Renal Physiol. 2010;298:F1197–204. doi:10.1152/ajprenal.00529.2009.

32. Rodriguez ME, Almaden Y, Cañadillas S, Canalejo A, Siendones E, Lopez I, et al. The calcimimetic R-568 increases vitamin D receptor expression in rat parathyroid glands. Am J Physiol Renal Physiol. 2007;292:F1390–5. doi:10.1152/ajprenal.00262.2006.

33. Patel SR, Ke HQ, Vanholder R, Koenig RJ, Hsu CH. Inhibition of calcitriol receptor binding to vitamin D response elements by uremic toxins. J Clin Invest. 1995;96:50–9. doi:10.1172/JCI118061.

34. Canalejo A, Almadén Y, De Smet R, Glorieux G, Garfia B, Luque F, et al. Effects of uremic ultrafiltrate on the regulation of the parathyroid cell cycle by calcitriol. Kidney Int. 2003;63:732–7. doi:10.1046/j.1523-1755.2003.00785.x.

35. Cunningham J, Locatelli F, Rodriguez M. Secondary hyperparathyroidism: pathogenesis, disease progression, and therapeutic options. Clin J Am Soc Nephrol. 2011;6:913–21. doi:10.2215/CJN.06040710.

36. Kuro-o M. Phosphate and Klotho. Kidney Int. 2011;79:S20–3. doi:10.1038/ki.2011.26.

37. Gogusev J, Duchambon P, Hory B, Giovannini M, Goureau Y, Sarfati E, Drüeke TB. Depressed expression of calcium receptor in parathyroid gland tissue of patients with hyperparathyroidism. Kidney Int. 1997;51:328–36.

38. Naveh-Many T, Rahamimov R, Livni N, Silver J. Parathyroid cell proliferation in normal and chronic renal failure rats. The effects of calcium, phosphate, and vitamin D. J Clin Invest. 1995;96:1786–93. doi:10.1172/JCI118224.

39. Kremer R, Bolivar I, Goltzman D, Hendy GN. Influence of calcium and 1,25-dihydroxycholecalciferol on proliferation and hyperplasia in uremic rats precedes downregulation of the calcium proto-oncogene expression in primary cultures of bovine parathyroid cells. Endocrinology. 1989;125:935–41. doi:10.1210/endo-125-2-935.

40. Szabo A, Merke J, Beier E, Mall G, Ritz E. 1,25(OH)2 vitamin D3 inhibits parathyroid cell proliferation in experimental uremia. Kidney Int. 1989;35:1045–56.
41. Fukagawa M, Kaname S-Y, Igarashi T, Ogata E, Kurokawa K. Regulation of parathyroid hormone synthesis in chronic renal failure in rats. Kidney Int. 1991;39:874–81.
42. Komaba H, Koizumi M, Fukagawa M. Parathyroid resistance to FGF23 in kidney transplant recipients: back to the past or ahead to the future? Kidney Int. 2010;78(10):953–5.
43. Wallfelt C, Gylfe E, Larsson R, Ljunghall S, Rastad J, Akerström G. Relationship between external and cytoplasmic calcium concentrations, parathyroid hormone release and weight of parathyroid glands in human hyperparathyroidism. J Endocrinol. 1988;116:457–64.
44. Canalejo A, Almadén Y, Torregrosa V, Gomez-Villamandos JC, Ramos B, Campistol JM, et al. The in vitro effect of calcitriol on parathyroid cell proliferation and apoptosis. J Am Soc Nephrol. 2000;11:1865–72.
45. Merke J, Hugel U, Zlotkowski A, Szabo A, Bommer J, Mall G, et al. Diminished parathyroid 1,25-(OH)2D3 receptors in experimental uremia. Kidney Int. 1987;32:350–3.
46. Brown AJ, Dusso A, Lopez-Hilker S, Lewis-Finch J, Grooms P, Slatopolsky E. 1,25-(OH)2D3 receptors are decreased in parathyroid glands from chronically uremic dogs. Kidney Int. 1989;35:19–23.
47. Tokumoto M, Tsuruya K, Fukuda K, Kanai H, Kuroki S, Hirakata H. Reduced p21, p27 and vitamin D receptor in the nodular hyperplasia in patients with advanced secondary hyperparathyroidism. Kidney Int. 2002;62:1196–07. doi:10.1111/j.1523-1755.2002.kid585.x.
48. Taniguchi M, Tokumoto M, Matsuo D, Tsuruya K, Hirakata H, Iida M. Parathyroid growth and regression in experimental uremia. Kidney Int. 2006;69:464–70. doi:10.1038/sj.ki.5000090.
49. Canalejo A, Canalejo R, Rodriguez ME, Martinez-Moreno JM, Felsenfeld AJ, Rodríguez M, et al. Development of parathyroid gland hyperplasia without uremia: role of dietary calcium and phosphate. Nephrol Dial Transplant. 2010;25:1087–97. doi:10.1093/ndt/gfp616.
50. Patel SR, Ke HQ, Hsu CH. Regulation of calcitriol receptor and its mRNA in normal and renal failure rats. Kidney Int. 1994;45:1020–7.

Chapter 8
The Parathyroid Type I Receptor and Vitamin D in Chronic Kidney Disease

Pablo A. Ureña Torres, Jordi Bover, Pieter Evenepoel, Vincent Brandenburg, Audrey Rousseaud, and Franck Oury

Abstract Parathyroid hormone (PTH) regulates mineral and bone metabolism through its specific type I receptor (PTH1R). In the kidney, PTH inhibits proximal tubular reabsorption of phosphate, stimulates the synthesis of $1,25(OH)_2D_3$, and enhances calcium reabsorption in the thick ascending limb of Henle's loop. In the skeleton, the physiological action of PTH is more complex. PTH has a paradoxical anabolic/catabolic effect and combines the simultaneous modulation of resorption and formation of bone tissue, and ultimately of bone remodeling rate. This paradoxical anabolic/catabolic effect relies on its mode of administration. Intermittent or pulsatile PTH has a bone anabolic effect, while chronic administration or excessive production of PTH, as in case of primary and secondary hyperparathyroidism, is detrimental for the skeleton due to stimulation of bone resorption. The PTH1R is an 84-kDa glycosylated protein that belongs to the seven transmembrane domains G protein-coupled receptors family. It activates two intracellular signaling pathways, protein kinase A and phospholipase C, through the stimulation of Gs and Gq proteins. The differential use of one or another of these two signaling pathways

P.A. Ureña Torres, MD, PhD (✉)
Ramsay-Générale de Santé, Service de Néphrologie et Dialyse, Clinique du Landy, Saint Ouen, France

Department of Renal Physiology, Necker Hospital, University of Paris V, René Descartes, Paris, France
e-mail: urena.pablo@wanadoo.fr

J. Bover, MD, PhD
Department of Nephrology, Fundaciò Puigvert, IIB Sant Pau, REDinREN, Barcelona, Spain

P. Evenepoel, MD
Division of Nephrology, Dialysis and Renal Transplantation, Department of Medicine, University Hospital Leuven, Leuven, Belgium

V. Brandenburg
Department of Cardiology and Center for Rare Diseases (ZSEA), RWTH University Hospital Aachen, Aachen, Germany

A. Rousseaud • F. Oury, MD
Institut National de la Santé et de la Recherche Médicale (INSERM) U115, Institut Necker Enfants Malades (INEM), Université Paris Descartes, Paris, France

© Springer International Publishing Switzerland 2016
P.A. Ureña Torres et al. (eds.), *Vitamin D in Chronic Kidney Disease*,
DOI 10.1007/978-3-319-32507-1_8

163

depends on the connection of PTH1R with the sodium-dependent hydrogen exchanger regulatory factor-1 (NHERF-1). In early chronic kidney disease (CKD), PTH1R is down-regulated in bone and kidney, which may favor the development of secondary hyperparathyroidism and CKD-mineral and bone disorders (CKD-MBD). In contrast, vitamin D deficiency is able to up-regulate renal and skeletal PTH1R in subjects with normal renal function. However, daily and intermittent administration of active vitamin D inhibits PTH1R expression and function in bone cells. This chapter reviews basic and clinical data regarding PTH1R and its physiological actions, as well as resistance to PTH hypercalcemic action and PTH1R implications in CKD-MBD.

Keywords CKD-MBD • Calcium • Phosphate • PTH • Bone • Cholecalciferol • Adynamic bone disease • Fracture

8.1 Introduction

The parathyroid hormone (PTH) is a polypeptide produced by the chief cells of the parathyroid glands and stored in secretory granules. Many years ago, PTH was identified as one of the major regulators of the calcium (Ca^{2+})/phosphate homeostasis in vertebrates, with bone and kidney as the main target organs [1, 2]. In the kidney level, PTH has three major physiological functions which are essential for the maintenance of the (Ca^{2+})/phosphate homeostasis. First, PTH stimulates calcium reabsorption in the thick ascending limb of Henle's loop [2, 3]. Second, it inhibits proximal tubular reabsorption of phosphate in blocking sodium-dependent phosphate co-transport by reducing the amount of the Npt2a and Npt2c proteins on the cell surface [4–6]. Third, PTH will also promote the synthesis of active vitamin D ($1,25(OH)_2D_3$ or calcitriol), that will enhance calcium and phosphate absorption by the intestine. In the bone, PTH leads to the release of calcium and phosphate. However, the physiological actions of PTH on bone metabolism are more complex and only partially understood. PTH has a paradoxical anabolic/catabolic effect that relies on its mode of administration. Excessive production of PTH observed in primary hyperparathyroidism or chronic administration of PTH leads to an increase in bone resorption by modulating osteoclast number and activity. In contrast, intermittent administration or pulsatile secretion of PTH leads to an increase of bone formation [7, 8].

In turn, Ca^{2+} is the most important regulator of circulating PTH levels. Via its binding to- and the activation of the calcium sensing receptor (CaSR) in the chief cells of the parathyroid glands, Ca^{2+} modulates PTH secretion and biosynthesis, PTH gene expression and parathyroid cellular proliferation. Indeed, hypocalcemia will induce, while hypercalcemia will decrease PTH secretion.

In mammals, PTH functions are mediated by two known receptors that belong to the G protein-coupled receptor family: PTH1R and PTH2R. PTH1R is the classical PTH receptor involved in regulating mineral ion homeostasis and playing an essential role in the clinical and biological manifestations of the secondary hyperparathyroidism (SHPT) observed in chronic kidney disease (CKD). In addition to PTH, PTH1R possesses also the property to bind the paracrine factor PTHrP (parathyroid hormone-related protein) with nearly equal affinity [1, 9]. In contrast, PTH-related functions of the second receptor, PTH2R, are less known. Moreover, PTH2R does not recognize PTHrP but presents a high affinity profile to another ligand, the neuropeptide tuberoinfundibular peptide of 39 amino acid residues (Tip39) [10].

In this chapter will review the basic and clinical data regarding PTH1R and its physiological actions, as well as resistance to PTH, hypercalcemic action and PTH1R implications in CKD-MBD.

8.2 Parathyroid Related Peptide

PTHrP was initially identified in the course of investigating the cause of tumors associated with humoral hypercalcemia of malignancy [11]. The human *PTHrP* gene is a complex transcriptional unit located on chromosome 3 (3p21.1–p24.2). Importantly, PTH and PTHrP evolve presumably from a common ancestry precursor after gene duplication event in the beginning of vertebrate diversification [12]. What remains from this common heritage is a limited region of amino acid sequence homology in the N terminus regions, a feature that enable these two molecules to bind and activate a common receptor, PTH1R, a member of the G-protein coupled receptor family B.

In contrast to PTH, which is only physiologically produced by the parathyroid glands, PTHrP is made in various tissues, both at embryonic and adult stages. Indeed, although initially discovered in malignancies, PTHrP is expressed in a large variety of other organs, such as the kidney, bone, central nervous system, endocrine pancreas, fetal parathyroid glands or placenta, where it can modulate cell growth and differentiation in an autocrine/paracrine [13–16].

Numerous studies have clearly documented the indispensable biological importance of PTHrP/PTH1R signaling which is involved in: (i) the regulation of smooth muscle cells contraction and relaxation, namely in the bladder, uterus, intestine and vessels [17, 18]; (ii) the trans-epithelial mineral ion transport in the mammary glands, placenta and kidney [19]; (iii) the skeletal fetal development, in particular, endochondral bone ossification [20]; and (iv) the control of the epithelial/mesenchymal interaction in the skin and the mammary glands. In vitro studies have also shown that PTHrP displays other functions largely relating to intracrine signaling in the nucleus/nucleolus [21–23]. Some tumors, including epidermal, renal and urothelial tumors, go along with excessive PTHrP production, which may spill over to the circulation and extent distant PTH-like effects such as increased calcium bone release, underlying the phenomenon of malignancy hypercalcemia [17, 24–26].

8.3 Tuberoinfundibular Peptide 39

Tuberoinfundibular peptide 39 (TIP39) is a 39-amino acid molecule member of the PTH and PTHrP family of peptide hormones that exerts its function by interacting, at least in part, with the PTH type 2 receptor (PTH2R). TIP39 is mainly expressed in the hypothalamus and in other distinct areas of the central nervous system. Recent studies suggested that the interaction between PIT39 and PTH2R in the brain modulate the regulatory network of nociception and response to the fear (16–17). Importantly, TIP39 and PTH2R are also expressed in other tissues, including testis, seminiferous tubules, liver, kidney and chondrocytes, suggesting that it might have other physiological actions. For instance and as expected, in chondrocyte cells TIP39 is an efficient PTH2R activator whereas it is a potent antagonist of the PTH1R. In such way that TIP39/PTH2R signaling inhibits cell proliferation and alters differentiation of chondrocytes through the modulation of *SOX9* gene expression [27]. Circulating TIP39 is measurable and its concentration has been associated with functional parameters and fertilizing capacity of spermatozoa in animals [28], however, to the best of our knowledge there is no clinical data reporting serum TIP39 levels in CKD nor if TIP39/PTH2R are modulated by vitamin D.

8.4 Biochemical and Functional Characteristics of the PTH1R

PTH and PTHrP can bind and activates the PTH receptor type I (PTH1R) with the same affinity. The PTH1R is an 84-kDa glycosylated protein, which belong to the large family of G protein-coupled receptors also known as seven transmembrane domain receptors. After binding to its receptor, PTH stimulates one of the G proteins, in the occurrence, the Gs protein (composed of three subunits α, β and γ), which activates adenylate cyclase and increases intracellular cAMP in target cells [1, 9]. PTH is also capable of increasing intracellular free calcium concentration by at least three mechanisms: (1) firstly by stimulating phospholipase C (PLC)/diacylglycerol/inositide-triphosphate pathway and activating protein kinase C (PKC) [29]. The coupling between PTH1R and PLC is ensured by the protein Gq; (2) secondly, by stimulating the release of stored ionized calcium from intracellular compartments independently of the activation of PLC; and (3) thirdly, by stimulating an inward calcium flux through the activation of calcium channels [2, 3, 30].

The differential use and activation of one or another intracellular signaling pathways by PTH depends on the connection of PTH1R with the adaptative and regulatory protein NHERF-1 (sodium-dependent hydrogen exchanger regulatory factor-1) [31]. In case of activation of the PKC signaling pathway by PTH, NHERF-1 is the only protein allowing the interaction between PTH1R and PLCβ. This implies that the presence or the absence of NHERF-1 in a given cell type will determine the intracellular signaling pathway chosen by PTH to exert its specific biological action [31].

The PTH1R may also require another important adapter protein, Dvl (Dishevelled), which is implicated in the complex formed by frizzled receptor/ LRP5-6 (low-density lipoprotein-related protein) and the activation of the Wnt (Wingless)/beta-catenin signaling pathway in bone cells. Indeed, the binding of PTH to PTH1R activates beta-catenin pathway by directly recruiting Dvl, independent of Wnt or LRP5-6, and thereby modulates osteoblast differentiation and osteoclastogenesis [32].

PTH acts on bone by inducing the phosphorylation of its receCptor PTH1R and activates both the protein kinase A (PKA) and Wnt pathways [33]. PTH also increases FGF23 mRNA levels through both the PKA and Wnt pathways [34]. Activation of PKA by the activated PTH1R increases the orphan nuclear receptor Nurr1 mRNA levels to induce FGF23 transcription [35, 36].

The cloning of the PTH1R in 1992 provided essential insights regarding its molecular structure [1, 9]. The gene is located on chromosome 11 and contains at least 15 exon-coding regions, which give rise to an amino acid sequence with seven putative transmembrane domains, and several conserved cysteine residues that are required for the receptor function and where the receptor can be glycosylated. Three promoters have been identified on the PTH1R gene, which might be selectively utilized in distinct organs such as kidney and bone [37]. The PTH1R belongs to the class II subgroup of G protein-coupled receptor family together with the receptors for calcitonin, secretin, glucagon, glucagon-like peptide (GLP), gastric inhibitor peptide (GIP), pituitary adenylate cyclase-activating peptide (PACAP), and vasointestinal peptide (VIP). The PTH1R cloning also allowed to definitively answer three historical questions: (1) the PTH receptor expressed in the kidney and in bone cells was the same one; (2) the PTH1R was capable of activating the two intracellular signaling pathways already known to be stimulated by PTH; and (3) PTH and PTHrP bind with the same affinity and activate with the same potency the PTH1R. Finally, the identification of the PTH1R demonstrated that this receptor plays a crucial role in endochondral bone development and growth.

8.5 Specific Features of PTH1R

PTH1R was the first receptor identified for PTH, which also indistinctly recognizes PTHrP [1, 9]. A second receptor was then identified and called PTHR2 because of its amino acids similarity with PTH1R. This receptor binds to TIP39 and PTH, but does not recognize PTHrP [38]. PTHR2 is mainly expressed in the brain and in somatostatin-producing cells in pancreatic islets, and does not appear to participate in mineral and bone metabolism as PTH does [39]. Its human gene is located on chromosome 2 (2q33) [40]. A third nucleotide sequence has been identified, which has a great similarity with the two other PTH receptors [41]. This receptor is present in zebrafish, seabream, and chicken and shows a stronger affinity for PTHrP than for other members of the PTH receptors family [42–44], however, this receptor has not yet been identified in human. There are also biochemical and functional evidences of the existence of another receptor (PTHR3) that recognizes C-terminal fragments of PTH (53–84 PTH), and that is detectable in osteoblast lineages as well as in osteoclast cells [45, 46]. Another receptor, that exclusively recognizes PTHrP and is expressed in the supra-optic nucleus, skin, and in the placenta has also been suggested [24, 47], however, those receptors have not been yet cloned (Table 8.1).

The susceptibility of menopausal women to develop severe osteoporosis has been demonstrated to be associated with the presence of polymorphisms on several genes including VDR, collagen type I, and apolipoprotein-E (Apo-E). It is thus plausible that polymorphisms or mutations in the PTH1R gene could also explain some cases of osteoporosis, such as CKD patients with inappropriately low serum PTH levels and severe clinical and histological manifestations of osteoporosis. Indeed, a frequent PTH1R gene polymorphism in exon M7 has been identified and associated with the extent of bone mass reduction in primary hyperparathyroidism [48]. Likewise, another polymorphism in the P3 promoter of the PTH1R gene has been associated with adult height, and urinary pyridinoline excretion, a marker of bone resorption, in Caucasians [49]. Finally, as an intronic PTH1R gene polymorphism (Van91) has also been associated with a greater urinary cAMP response to PTH in healthy Japanese volunteers [50].

Table 8.1 Characteristics of parathyroid receptors

	PTH1R	PTH2R	PTH3R
Natural ligand	PTH; PTHrP	TIP39	cPTH
Ligand specificity	Inhibited by TIP39	Inhibited by PTH	Low response to PTH-L
		Does not recognize PTHrP	
Intracellular signaling	cAMP, PLC, ERK ½	cAMP, PLC	cAMP
	Inositol triphosphate		
Tissue expression	Kidney	Pancreas	Osteoblast
	Bone	Brain, hypothalamus	Osteoclast
	Liver		
	Heart		
	Testes		
	Brain		
Function	Mineral and bone metabolism	Nociception, memory	Mineral and bone metabolism
	Embryo development	Affection, anxiety	
	Placental ions transport	Depression	
	Lactation		
	Smooth muscle relaxation		

PTH parathyroid hormone, *PTH1R* PTH type 1 receptor, *PTH2R* PTH type 2 receptor, *PTH3R* PTH type 3 receptor, *cPTH* C-terminal PTH fragments, *PTHrP* PTH-related peptide, *PTH-L* PTH-like peptide, *cAMP* cyclic adenosine monophosphate, *PLC* phospholipase C, *ERK* extracellular signal-regulated kinases

8.6 Expression and Function of the PTH1R in Chronic Kidney Disease

It has been recognized since the 1960s [51] that CKD is associated with a skeletal resistance to the hypercalcemic action of PTH [52, 53]. This resistance is multifactorial, and it is at least in part due to the down-regulation of PTH1R mRNA and its protein in osteoblasts and in proximal convolute tubular cells [54, 55]. Besides the reduced number of PTH1R at the surface of these cells, resulting from its low mRNA, the uremic state may also alter the intracellular signaling pathway through the reduction of adenylate cyclase activation by Gs protein [54, 55].

Three principal factors were thought to be involved in the PTH1R down-regulation observed in CKD: increased circulating PTH concentrations, high serum phosphate levels, and increased intracellular free calcium concentration [54–56]. The implication of the first two factors, high PTH and phosphate, can now be excluded, since total parathyroidectomy did not prevent the renal PTH1R down-regulation in uremic rats [57]. Inversely, the increase of intracellular calcium induced by high PTH seems to be the principal mechanism leading to the PTH1R down-regulation [56, 58]. Moreover, such an increase in the basal intracellular calcium concentration in subjects and animals with CKD is mainly due to two PTH-dependent mechanisms: an increase in the inward calcium transport, and a decrease in the calcium flux exit. Indeed, PTH activates verapamil sensitive calcium channels and the entry of calcium to the cell. As high PTH continuously stimulates this pathway it leads to a reduction in the intracellular concentration of ATP and the activity of Na^+/K^+ ATPase, the Ca^{2+}ATPase, and the Na/Ca^{2+} exchanger, which contribute to the reduced calcium extrusion. In order to reduce its intracellular calcium concentration, the cell would utilize the PTH1R down-regulation, and would protect itself against an accelerated apoptosis and death. The mechanisms by which ionized calcium decreases the PTH1R mRNA expression are still unknown, but it could act on the PTH1R gene promoter and inhibit its transcription or stimulate PTH1R mRNA degradation [56].

8.7 Implication of the PTH1R in the Pathogenesis of Secondary Hyperparathyroidism and Adynamic Osteopathy

The PTH1R can be implicated in the pathophysiology of SHPT from the earlier CKD stages. Indeed, its renal down-regulation certainly explains the decreased tubular calcium reabsorption, urinary phosphate excretion, and 1α-hydroxylase activity. The low calcitriol synthesis contributes to less intestinal calcium absorption [55]. All together, these alterations stimulate parathyroid cell proliferation, PTH synthesis and secretion, and the development of SHPT. As the parathyroid cells do not seem to express PTH1R, there is no negative feedback loop by which PTH could regulate its own production. In addition, the PTH1R down-regulation in bone cells accentuates the negative calcium balance by impeding the resorptive and hypercalcemic action of PTH.

As regards of the adynamic osteopathy, a CKD-MBD complication that has long times been recognized, numerous contributing factors have been proposed including age, race, diabetes, excessive calcium and phosphate loading, calcitriol deficiency and excess as well, accumulation of PTH fragments that antagonize PTH1R, high serum osteoprotegerin (OPG) levels, decreased circulating bone morphogenetic proteins, high leptin, decreased PTH pulsatility, and PTH1R down-regulation in bone cells [53, 55, 59–64]. The skeletal PTH1R down-regulation is certainly one of the major players as it has been related to the skeletal resistance to the resorptive and hypercalcemic action of PTH. For these reasons, and to overcome the reduced number of PTH1R in uremic bone cells, it is actually recommended to maintain a serum PTH concentration above two times the upper limit of normal values in CKD patients (KDIGO) [65]. In case of very low serum PTH levels, the scarce PTH1R number that could be stimulated by such a low PTH would be insufficient to maintain a normal bone turnover rate [66, 67]. In addition, as vitamin D down-regulates the PTH1R in osteoblast cells [66, 68], it is likely that this phenomenon is implicated in the cases of adynamic osteopathy observed in uremic children treated by peritoneal dialysis and high doses of active vitamin D derivatives [69–71].

The anabolic effect of PTH on bone is mediated, at least partly, by down-regulating SOST gene expression and the resulting amount of sclerostin production by osteocyte and osteoblast cells, which frees the Wnt signaling pathway [72, 73]. Consequently, sclerostin over-expression reduces PTH-associated bone gain in experimental animals [73]. PTH, through the PTH1R, has also sclerostin-independent bone anabolic activities, which are mediated by Wnt10b produced by T-cell [74]. Accordingly, dysregulation of the osteocyte Wnt/β-catenin signaling pathway, the major skeletal anabolic principle of the postnatal skeleton, seems to be also involved in the pathophysiology of CKD-MBD [72].

8.8   Diseases Associated with PTH1R Mutations

Constitutively activating mutations of the PTH1R have been described in subjects with Jansen's disease, an autosomal dominant methaphyseal chondrodysplasia characterized by dwarfism, severe cartilage conjugation, hypercalcemia, and hypophosphatemia in the presence of paradoxically low PTH and PTHrP [75]. In contrast, inhibiting mutations of the PTH1R have also been identified in lethal forms of autosomal recessive chondrodysplasia characterized by a premature endochondral ossification [76]. These activating and inhibiting mutations illustrate the crucial role played by this PTH1R in the development of endochondral bone, where it slows down PTHrP-induced differentiation of pre-hypertrophic chondrocytes in hypertrophic chondrocytes [13].

8.9   Vitamin D Regulates Renal and Bone PTH1R

Vitamin D deficiency is associated with up-regulation of the renal and skeletal PTH1R in subjects with normal renal function. However, daily and intermittent administration of calcitriol, for the treatment of SHPT in uremic children, inhibits PTH1R expression and function in bone cells [68]. As previously mentioned in this chapter, PTH1R down-regulation in bone cells plays a central role in the skeletal resistance to PTH action and the development of a low bone turnover disease in CKD [54, 66, 69, 70].

PTH and vitamin D ($1,25(OH)_2D_3$) stimulate calcium reabsorption in the renal distal convoluted tubules (DCT), and vitamin D further stimulates this phenomenon by increasing PTH-stimulated calcium transport by DCT cells. It has now been shown that vitamin D exerts this effect by considerably increasing the PTH1R mRNA expression in DCT cells. This up-regulation is specific since $1,25(OH)_2D_3$ does not change mRNA expression for other genes including the adrenergic receptor and the sodium-hydrogen exchanger (Na^+/H^+). Of note, the inactive vitamin D form, $25(OH)D_3$ did not have any effect on the PTH1R mRNA expression level [77]. Vitamin A, through the retinoid X receptor (RXR), and the vitamin D/VDR complex, may also modulate PTH1R expression. In combination with the putative RXR ligand, 9-cis-retinoic acid, $1,25(OH)_2D_3$ increases PTH1R mRNA expression by fourfold in DCT cells, however, 9-cis-retinoic acid alone did not have any effect. Likewise, the putative ligand for the retinoic acid receptor (RAR), all-trans-retinoic acid, either alone or in combination with $1,25(OH)_2D_3$, increases PTH1R mRNA expression in DCT cells. Altogether, these findings indicate that $1,25(OH)_2D_3$ up-regulates the PTH1R in renal cells in a manner consistent with VDR/RXR heterodimers binding to a VDRE in the promoter region and trans-activating the PTH1R gene [77].

8.10   Other Factors Regulating PTH1R

Extremely and continuously high levels of circulating PTH down-regulate renal and bone PTH1R [78]. Thus, it was thought that parathyroidectomy could correct such a down-regulation; however, several experimental animal models have not been able to demonstrate any improvement of skeletal PTH1R expression by parathyroidectomy, in particular in cases of CKD [57]. Nevertheless, blocking calcium channels with verapamil in uremic rats normalized intracellular calcium concentration and returned PTH1R expression to normal levels in cardiomyocytes; despite of the marked elevation of serum PTH levels [56].

PTHrP can also down-regulate renal PTH1R as shown in rats over-producing PTHrP by bearing the Walker carcinoma tumor [79]. This regulation is tissue-specific and pamidronate, which partially corrected hypercalcemia and high circulating PTH levels in this model, also normalized the PTH1R mRNA expression in the kidney but not in tumors [79]. Breast cancer cells express both PTHrP and PTH1R and the PTH1R expression can be modulated by substrates present in the extracellular matrix as well as by hydrocortisone [80], supporting the active participation of stromal collagen composition in the regulation of PTHrP production and probably carcinogenesis [80]. In choriocarcinoma JAR cells, the PTH1R is up-regulated by epidermal growth factor (EGF), estradiol (E2) and dexamethasone, but active vitamin D (1,25-dihydroxyvitamin D) down-regulated PTH1R in the same cells and may act as an anti-proliferative agent [81].

Glucocorticosteroids and transforming growth factor beta (TGFβ) have distinct tissular effects; they up-regulate the PTH1R expression in osteoblastic cells whereas the same compounds down-regulate PTH1R expression in renal cells [78].

The renin-angiotensin-aldosterone system plays a crucial role in systemic blood pressure control as well as regulating renal blood flow and glomerular filtration rate. In addition, increased plasma aldosterone concentration, as well as the aldosterone to renin ratio, has been shown to be independently associated with circulating PTH levels. And, exclusively in patients with high circulating PTH levels, plasma aldosterone levels are independently associated with an increased risk of cardiovascular mortality [82]. In CKD, angiotensin II participates in the pathogenesis of kidney damage, and PTHrP, a known vasodilator and proliferating agent, is up-regulated by angiotensin II in renal tubules, glomeruli and renal vessels in case of renal injury [83]. The PTH1R mRNA expression is also increased by angiotensin II in these renal structures. The blockage of angiotensin II action by AT1 (antagonists of type 1 angiotensin receptor), but not by AT2 antagonists, significantly reduced angiotensin II-induced renal PTHrP and PTH1R overexpression and decreased tubular damage and renal fibrosis [84–87]. Locally produced PTHrP exerts its vasodilating action by binding and activating the PTH1R in vascular smooth muscle cells (VSMC). In these cells, angiotensin II also stimulates PTHrP production, which is followed by a rapid desensitization of PTHrP-related cAMP response due to PTH1R down-regulation. Contrarily to bone cells where the PTH1R down-regulation and desensitization are mediated by a protein kinase pathway, in VSMC the activation of this signaling pathway does not seem to be involved, which suggests that such diversity in the PTH1R regulatory mechanisms provides a means for restricting the length and duration of the cellular response to PTH and PTHrP in a tissular specific manner [88].

8.11 Conclusions and Perspectives

Although several PTH receptors have been identified in vertebrates, but PTH1R appears to be the principal mediator of PTH actions and regulator of mineral and bone metabolism. PTH1R expression is down-regulated in bone and kidney at early stages of CKD and represent a determinant factor for the development of SHPT and CKD-MBD. The mechanisms responsible for this down-regulation remain largely elusive. From a clinical point of view, the identification of these mechanisms and mode of action represents an important challenge to improve uremic SHPT prevention. Use of supra-physiological doses of active vitamin D analogs to treat uremic SHPT may contribute to the development of low bone turnover disease, adynamic osteopathy, and longitudinal growth retardation in uremic children, through the down-regulation of the skeletal PTH1R. PTH1R gene polymorphisms or mutations might explain some cases of severe osteoporosis and renal osteodystrophy in CKD subjects with inappropriately low serum PTH levels and severe clinical and histological manifestations of bone loss. Finally, the accumulation of truncated PTH fragments in CKD may compete with the bioactive whole (1–84) PTH and act as inhibitors of the PTH1R, favoring then favor the skeletal resistance to PTH hypercalcemic action.

References

1. Abou-Samra AB, Juppner H, Force T, et al. Expression cloning of a common receptor for parathyroid hormone and parathyroid hormone-related peptide from rat osteoblast-like cells: a single receptor stimulates intracellular accumulation of both cAMP and inositol trisphosphates and increases intracellular free calcium. Proc Natl Acad Sci U S A. 1992;89:2732–6.
2. Urena P, Abou Samra AB, Juppner H, et al. Mode of action of parathyroid hormone (PTH) and PTH-related peptide (PTHrP) in target organs. Ann Endocrinol. 1994;55:133–41.
3. Segre GV, Abou-Samra AB, Juppner H, et al. Characterization of cloned PTH/PTHrP receptors. J Endocrinol Invest. 1992;15:11–7.
4. Nissenson RA, Diep D, Strewler GJ. Synthetic peptides comprising the amino-terminal sequence of a parathyroid hormone-like protein from human malignancies. Binding to parathyroid hormone receptors and activation of adenylate cyclase in bone cells and kidney. J Biol Chem. 1988;263:12866–71.
5. Orloff JJ, Wu TL, Stewart AF. Parathyroid hormone-like proteins: biochemical responses and receptor interactions. Endocr Rev. 1989;10:476–95.
6. Stewart AF, Horst R, Deftos LJ, Cadman EC, Lang R, Broadus AE. Biochemical evaluation of patients with cancer-associated hypercalcemia: evidence for humoral and nonhumoral groups. N Engl J Med. 1980;303:1377–83.
7. Funk JL, Migliati E, Chen G, et al. Parathyroid hormone-related protein induction in focal stroke: a neuroprotective vascular peptide. Am J Physiol Regul Integr Comp Physiol. 2003;284:R1021–30.
8. Weir EC, Brines ML, Ikeda K, Burtis WJ, Broadus AE, Robbins RJ. Parathyroid hormone-related peptide gene is expressed in the mammalian central nervous system. Proc Natl Acad Sci U S A. 1990;87:108–12.
9. Juppner H, Abou-Samra AB, Freeman M, et al. A G protein-linked receptor for parathyroid hormone and parathyroid hormone-related peptide. Science. 1991;254:1024–6.
10. Usdin TB, Hoare SR, Wang T, Mezey E, Kowalak JA. TIP39: a new neuropeptide and PTH2-receptor agonist from hypothalamus. Nat Neurosci. 1999;2:941–3.
11. Strewler GJ, Nissenson RA. Hypercalcemia in malignancy. West J Med. 1990;153:635–40.
12. Schipani E, Jensen GS, Pincus J, Nissenson RA, Gardella TJ, Juppner H. Constitutive activation of the cyclic adenosine 3',5'-monophosphate signaling pathway by parathyroid hormone (PTH)/PTH-related peptide receptors mutated at the two loci for Jansen's metaphyseal chondrodysplasia. Mol Endocrinol. 1997;11:851–8.
13. Kronenberg HM, Chung U. The parathyroid hormone-related protein and Indian hedgehog feedback loop in the growth plate. Novartis Found Symp. 2001;232:144–52; discussion 52–7.
14. Lee K, Brown D, Urena P, et al. Localization of parathyroid hormone/parathyroid hormone-related peptide receptor mRNA in kidney. Am J Physiol. 1996;270:F186–91.

15. Lee K, Deeds JD, Bond AT, Juppner H, Abou-Samra AB, Segre GV. In situ localization of PTH/PTHrP receptor mRNA in the bone of fetal and young rats. Bone. 1993;14:341–5.
16. Urena P, Kong XF, Abou-Samra AB, et al. Parathyroid hormone (PTH)/PTH-related peptide receptor messenger ribonucleic acids are widely distributed in rat tissues. Endocrinology. 1993;133:617–23.
17. Clemens TL, Cormier S, Eichinger A, et al. Parathyroid hormone-related protein and its receptors: nuclear functions and roles in the renal and cardiovascular systems, the placental trophoblasts and the pancreatic islets. Br J Pharmacol. 2001;134:1113–36.
18. Massfelder T, Helwig JJ. The parathyroid hormone-related protein system: more data but more unsolved questions. Curr Opin Nephrol Hypertens. 2003;12:35–42.
19. Kovacs CS, Chafe LL, Fudge NJ, Friel JK, Manley NR. PTH regulates fetal blood calcium and skeletal mineralization independently of PTHrP. Endocrinology. 2001;142:4983–93.
20. Lanske B, Amling M, Neff L, Guiducci J, Baron R, Kronenberg HM. Ablation of the PTHrP gene or the PTH/PTHrP receptor gene leads to distinct abnormalities in bone development. J Clin Invest. 1999;104:399–407.
21. de Miguel F, Fiaschi-Taesch N, Lopez-Talavera JC, et al. The C-terminal region of PTHrP, in addition to the nuclear localization signal, is essential for the intracrine stimulation of proliferation in vascular smooth muscle cells. Endocrinology. 2001;142:4096–105.
22. Fiaschi-Taesch N, Takane KK, Masters S, Lopez-Talavera JC, Stewart AF. Parathyroid-hormone-related protein as a regulator of pRb and the cell cycle in arterial smooth muscle. Circulation. 2004;110:177–85.
23. Henderson JE, Amizuka N, Warshawsky H, et al. Nucleolar localization of parathyroid hormone-related peptide enhances survival of chondrocytes under conditions that promote apoptotic cell death. Mol Cell Biol. 1995;15:4064–75.
24. Kovacs CS, Lanske B, Hunzelman JL, Guo J, Karaplis AC, Kronenberg HM. Parathyroid hormone-related peptide (PTHrP) regulates fetal-placental calcium transport through a receptor distinct from the PTH/PTHrP receptor. Proc Natl Acad Sci U S A. 1996;93:15233–8.
25. Lanske B, Divieti P, Kovacs CS, et al. The parathyroid hormone (PTH)/PTH-related peptide receptor mediates actions of both ligands in murine bone. Endocrinology. 1998;139:5194–204.
26. Massfelder T, Saussine C, Simeoni U, Enanga B, Judes C, Helwig JJ. Evidence for adenylyl cyclase-dependent receptors for parathyroid hormone (PTH)-related protein in rabbit kidney glomeruli. Life Sci. 1993;53:875–81.
27. Panda D, Goltzman D, Juppner H, Karaplis AC. TIP39/parathyroid hormone type 2 receptor signaling is a potent inhibitor of chondrocyte proliferation and differentiation. Am J Physiol Endocrinol Metab. 2009;297:E1125–36.
28. Selvaraju S, Somashekar L, Krishnan BB, et al. Relationship between seminal plasma tuberoinfundibular peptide of 39 residues and sperm functional attributes in buffalo (Bubalus bubalis). Reprod Fertil Dev. May 5, 2015, DOI: 10.1071/RD15008.
29. Iida-Klein A, Guo J, Xie LY, et al. Truncation of the carboxyl-terminal region of the rat parathyroid hormone (PTH)/PTH-related peptide receptor enhances PTH stimulation of adenylyl cyclase but not phospholipase C. J Biol Chem. 1995;270:8458–65.
30. Abou-Samra AB, Juppner H, Kong XF, et al. Structure, function, and expression of the receptor for parathyroid hormone and parathyroid hormone-related peptide. Adv Nephrol Necker Hosp. 1994;23:247–64.
31. Mahon MJ, Segre GV. Stimulation by parathyroid hormone of a NHERF-1-assembled complex consisting of the parathyroid hormone I receptor, phospholipase Cbeta, and actin increases intracellular calcium in opossum kidney cells. J Biol Chem. 2004;279:23550–8.
32. Romero G, Sneddon WB, Yang Y, Wheeler D, Blair HC, Friedman PA. Parathyroid hormone receptor directly interacts with dishevelled to regulate beta-Catenin signaling and osteoclastogenesis. J Biol Chem. 2010;285:14756–63.
33. Maeda A, Okazaki M, Baron DM, et al. Critical role of parathyroid hormone (PTH) receptor-1 phosphorylation in regulating acute responses to PTH. Proc Natl Acad Sci U S A. 2013;110:5864–9.

34. Lavi-Moshayoff V, Wasserman G, Meir T, Silver J, Naveh-Many T. PTH increases FGF23 gene expression and mediates the high-FGF23 levels of experimental kidney failure: a bone parathyroid feedback loop. Am J Physiol Ren Physiol. 2010;299:F882–9.
35. Fan Y, Bi R, Densmore MJ, et al. Parathyroid hormone 1 receptor is essential to induce FGF23 production and maintain systemic mineral ion homeostasis. FASEB J Off Pub Fed Am Soc Exp Biol. 2016;30:428–40.
36. Meir T, Durlacher K, Pan Z, et al. Parathyroid hormone activates the orphan nuclear receptor Nurr1 to induce FGF23 transcription. Kidney Int. 2014;86:1106–15.
37. Frohlich LF, Gensure RC, Schipani E, Juppner H, Bastepe M. Haplotype frequencies and linkage disequilibrium analysis of four frequent polymorphisms at the PTH/PTH-related peptide receptor gene locus. Mol Cell Probes. 2004;18:353–7.
38. Usdin TB, Gruber C, Bonner TI. Identification and functional expression of a receptor selectively recognizing parathyroid hormone, the PTH2 receptor. J Biol Chem. 1995;270:15455–8.
39. Usdin TB, Bonner TI, Harta G, Mezey E. Distribution of parathyroid hormone-2 receptor messenger ribonucleic acid in rat. Endocrinology. 1996;137:4285–97.
40. Usdin TB, Modi W, Bonner TI. Assignment of the human PTH2 receptor gene (PTHR2) to chromosome 2q33 by fluorescence in situ hybridization. Genomics. 1996;37:140–1.
41. Bergwitz C, Klein P, Kohno H, et al. Identification, functional characterization, and developmental expression of two nonallelic parathyroid hormone (PTH)/PTH-related peptide receptor isoforms in Xenopus laevis (Daudin). Endocrinology. 1998;139:723–32.
42. Pinheiro PL, Cardoso JC, Power DM, Canario AV. Functional characterization and evolution of PTH/PTHrP receptors: insights from the chicken. BMC Evol Biol. 2012;12:110.
43. Rubin DA, Hellman P, Zon LI, Lobb CJ, Bergwitz C, Juppner H. A G protein-coupled receptor from zebrafish is activated by human parathyroid hormone and not by human or teleost parathyroid hormone-related peptide. Implications for the evolutionary conservation of calcium-regulating peptide hormones. J Biol Chem. 1999;274:23035–42.
44. Rubin DA, Juppner H. Zebrafish express the common parathyroid hormone/parathyroid hormone-related peptide receptor (PTH1R) and a novel receptor (PTH3R) that is preferentially activated by mammalian and fugufish parathyroid hormone-related peptide. J Biol Chem. 1999;274:28185–90.
45. Divieti P, Inomata N, Chapin K, Singh R, Juppner H, Bringhurst FR. Receptors for the carboxyl-terminal region of pth(1-84) are highly expressed in osteocytic cells. Endocrinology. 2001;142:916–25.
46. Divieti P, Lanske B, Kronenberg HM, Bringhurst FR. Conditionally immortalized murine osteoblasts lacking the type 1 PTH/PTHrP receptor. J Bone Miner Res. 1998;13:1835–45.
47. Orloff JJ, Kats Y, Urena P, et al. Further evidence for a novel receptor for amino-terminal parathyroid hormone-related protein on keratinocytes and squamous carcinoma cell lines. Endocrinology. 1995;136:3016–23.
48. Kanzawa M, Sugimoto T, Kobayashi T, Kobayashi A, Chihara K. Association between parathyroid hormone (PTH)/PTH-related peptide receptor gene polymorphism and the extent of bone mass reduction in primary hyperparathyroidism. Horm Metab Res Horm StoffwechselforschungHorm Metab. 2000;32:355–8.
49. Minagawa M, Yasuda T, Watanabe T, et al. Association between AAAG repeat polymorphism in the P3 promoter of the human parathyroid hormone (PTH)/PTH-related peptide receptor gene and adult height, urinary pyridinoline excretion, and promoter activity. J Clin Endocrinol Metab. 2002;87:1791–6.
50. Heishi M, Tazawa H, Matsuo T, Saruta T, Hanaoka M, Tsukamoto Y. A novel Van91 I polymorphism in the 1st intron of the parathyroid hormone (PTH)/PTH-related peptide (PTHrP) receptor gene and its effect on the urinary cAMP response to PTH. Biol Pharm Bull. 2000;23:386–9.
51. Evanson JM. The response to the infusion of parathyroid extract in hypocalcaemic states. Clin Sci. 1966;31:63–75.
52. Llach F, Bover J. Renal osteodystrophies. In: Brenner BM, editor. The kidney. 6th ed. Philadelphia: W. B. Saunders Company; 2000. p. 2103–86.

53. Slatopolsky E, Finch J, Clay P, et al. A novel mechanism for skeletal resistance in uremia. Kidney Int. 2000;58:753–61.
54. Urena P, Ferreira A, Morieux C, Drueke T, de Vernejoul MC. PTH/PTHrP receptor mRNA is down-regulated in epiphyseal cartilage growth plate of uraemic rats. Nephrol Dial Transplant. 1996;11:2008–16.
55. Urena P, Kubrusly M, Mannstadt M, et al. The renal PTH/PTHrP receptor is down-regulated in rats with chronic renal failure. Kidney Int. 1994;45:605–11.
56. Smogorzewski M, Tian J, Massry SG. Down-regulation of PTH-PTHrP receptor of heart in CRF: role of [Ca2+]i. Kidney Int. 1995;47:1182–6.
57. Urena P, Mannstadt M, Hruby M, et al. Parathyroidectomy does not prevent the renal PTH/PTHrP receptor down-regulation in uremic rats. Kidney Int. 1995;47:1797–805.
58. Smogorzewski M, Islam A. Parathyroid hormone stimulates the generation of inositol 1,4,5-triphosphate in brain synaptosomes. Am J Kidney Dis. 1995;26:814–7.
59. Bover J, Rodriguez M, Trinidad P, et al. Factors in the development of secondary hyperparathyroidism during graded renal failure in the rat. Kidney Int. 1994;45:953–61.
60. Bover J, Urena P, Brandenburg V, et al. Adynamic bone disease: from bone to vessels in chronic kidney disease. Semin Nephrol. 2014;34:626–40.
61. Coen G, Mantella D, Manni M, et al. 25-hydroxyvitamin D levels and bone histomorphometry in hemodialysis renal osteodystrophy. Kidney Int. 2005;68:1840–8.
62. Divieti P, John MR, Juppner H, Bringhurst FR. Human PTH-(7-84) inhibits bone resorption in vitro via actions independent of the type 1 PTH/PTHrP receptor. Endocrinology. 2002;143:171–6.
63. Massry SG, Smogorzewski M. The mechanisms responsible for the PTH-induced rise in cytosolic calcium in various cells are not uniform. Miner Electrolyte Metab. 1995;21:13–28.
64. Reichel H, Esser A, Roth HJ, Schmidt-Gayk H. Influence of PTH assay methodology on differential diagnosis of renal bone disease. Nephrol Dial Transplant. 2003;18:759–68.
65. KDIGO. KDIGO clinical practice guideline for the diagnosis, evaluation, prevention, and treatment of Chronic Kidney Disease-Mineral and Bone Disorder (CKD-MBD). Kidney Int Suppl. 2009;113:S1–S130.
66. Picton ML, Moore PR, Mawer EB, et al. Down-regulation of human osteoblast PTH/PTHrP receptor mRNA in end-stage renal failure. Kidney Int. 2000;58:1440–9.
67. Kuwahara M, Inoshita S, Nakano Y, Terada Y, Takano Y, Sasaki S. Expression of bone type 1 PTH receptor in rats with chronic renal failure. Clin Exp Nephrol. 2007;11:34–40.
68. Gonzalez E, Martin K. Coordinate regulation of PTH/PTHrP receptors by PTH and calcitriol in UMR 106-01 osteoblast-like cells. Kidney Int. 1996;50:63–70.
69. Kuison B, Goodman W, Jüppner H, et al. Diminished linear growth during intermittent calcitriol therapy in children undergoing CCPD. Kidney Int. 1998;53:205–11.
70. Kuizon B, Salusky I. Intermittent calcitriol therapy and growth in children with chronic renal failure. Miner Electrolyte Metab. 1998;24:290–5.
71. Salusky IB, Ramirez JA, Oppenheim W, Gales B, Segre GV, Goodman WG. Biochemical markers of renal osteodystrophy in pediatric patients undergoing CAPD/CCPD. Kidney Int. 1994;45:253–8.
72. Ferreira JC, Ferrari GO, Neves KR, et al. Effects of dietary phosphate on adynamic bone disease in rats with chronic kidney disease – role of sclerostin? PLoS One. 2013;8:e79721.
73. Kramer I, Loots GG, Studer A, Keller H, Kneissel M. Parathyroid hormone (PTH)-induced bone gain is blunted in SOST overexpressing and deficient mice. J Bone Miner Res. 2010;25:178–89.
74. Li JY, Walker LD, Tyagi AM, Adams J, Weitzmann MN, Pacifici R. The sclerostin-independent bone anabolic activity of intermittent PTH treatment is mediated by T-cell-produced Wnt10b. J Bone Miner Res. 2014;29:43–54.
75. Schipani E, Langman CB, Parfitt AM, et al. Constitutively activated receptors for parathyroid hormone and parathyroid hormone-related peptide in Jansen's metaphyseal chondrodysplasia. N Engl J Med. 1996;335:708–14.

76. Jobert AS, Zhang P, Couvineau A, et al. Absence of functional receptors for parathyroid hormone and parathyroid hormone-related peptide in Blomstrand chondrodysplasia. J Clin Invest. 1998;102:34–40.
77. Sneddon WB, Barry EL, Coutermarsh BA, Gesek FA, Liu F, Friedman PA. Regulation of renal parathyroid hormone receptor expression by 1, 25-dihydroxyvitamin D3 and retinoic acid. Cell Physiol Biochem Int J Exp Cell Phys Biochem Pharmacol. 1998;8:261–77.
78. Urena P, Iida-Klein A, Kong XF, et al. Regulation of parathyroid hormone (PTH)/PTH-related peptide receptor messenger ribonucleic acid by glucocorticoids and PTH in ROS 17/2.8 and OK cells. Endocrinology. 1994;134:451–6.
79. Yaghoobian J, Morieux C, Denne MA, Bouizar Z, Urena P, de Vernejoul MC. Pamidronate corrects the down-regulation of the renal parathyroid hormone (PTH)/PTH-related peptide (PTHrP) receptor mRNA in rats bearing Walker tumors. Horm Metab Res Horm StoffwechselforschungHorm Metab. 1998;30:249–55.
80. Luparello C, Santamaria F, Schilling T. Regulation of PTHrP and PTH/PTHrP receptor by extracellular Ca2+ concentration and hormones in the breast cancer cell line 8701-BC. Biol Chem. 2000;381:303–8.
81. Alokail MS. Potential regulation of PTH/PTHrP receptor expression in choriocarcinoma cells. Saudi Med J. 2004;25:615–20.
82. Tomaschitz A, Pilz S, Rus-Machan J, et al. Interrelated aldosterone and parathyroid hormone mutually modify cardiovascular mortality risk. Int J Cardiol. 2015;184:710–6.
83. Romero M, Ortega A, Olea N, et al. Novel role of parathyroid hormone-related protein in the pathophysiology of the diabetic kidney: evidence from experimental and human diabetic nephropathy. J Diabetes Res. 2013;2013:162846.
84. Bosch RJ, Ortega A, Izquierdo A, Arribas I, Bover J, Esbrit P. A transgenic mouse model for studying the role of the parathyroid hormone-related protein system in renal injury. J Biomed Biotechnol. 2011;2011:290874.
85. Esbrit P, Santos S, Ortega A, et al. Parathyroid hormone-related protein as a renal regulating factor. From vessels to glomeruli and tubular epithelium. Am J Nephrol. 2001;21:179–84.
86. Lorenzo O, Ruiz-Ortega M, Esbrit P, et al. Angiotensin II increases parathyroid hormone-related protein (PTHrP) and the type 1 PTH/PTHrP receptor in the kidney. J Am Soc Nephrol. 2002;13:1595–607.
87. Ortega A, Romero M, Izquierdo A, et al. Parathyroid hormone-related protein is a hypertrophy factor for human mesangial cells: implications for diabetic nephropathy. J Cell Physiol. 2012;227:1980–7.
88. Okano K, Wu S, Huang X, et al. Parathyroid hormone (PTH)/PTH-related protein (PTHrP) receptor and its messenger ribonucleic acid in rat aortic vascular smooth muscle cells and UMR osteoblast-like cells: cell-specific regulation by angiotensin-II and PTHrP. Endocrinology. 1994;135:1093–9.

Chapter 9
Vitamin D and Klotho in Chronic Kidney Disease

Hirotaka Komaba and Beate Lanske

Abstract Klotho, originally identified as an aging suppressor, forms a complex with the fibroblast growth factor (FGF) receptor and functions as an obligatory co-receptor for FGF23, a bone-derived hormone that regulates phosphate and vitamin D metabolism. The identification and characterization of the klotho-FGF23 axis has considerably advanced our understanding of chronic kidney disease-mineral and bone disorder (CKD-MBD). By acting as a co-factor for FGFR in FGF23 signaling, klotho plays a central role in the pathogenesis of disturbances of phosphate and vitamin D metabolism in CKD. Klotho also exists as a soluble circulating protein, which is produced by cleavage of the extracellular region. Although the detailed mechanism remains to be determined, soluble klotho has been shown to possess multiple functions. Accumulating data suggest that both transmembrane and soluble form of klotho is deficient in patients with CKD and such klotho deficiency contributes to the pathogenesis of secondary hyperparathyroidism, vascular calcification, left ventricular hypertrophy, and worsening of kidney injury. In this chapter, we present recent insights into the role of the klotho-FGF23 axis in the altered metabolism of phosphate and vitamin D in CKD. We also discuss the reported multifunctional roles of soluble klotho and their potential involvement in the pathophysiology of CKD-MBD.

Keywords FGF23 • Klotho • Vitamin D • CKD-MBD • Secondary hyperparathyroidism

H. Komaba, MD, PhD (✉)
Division of Nephrology, Endocrinology and Metabolism, Tokai University School of Medicine, Shimo-Kasuya, Isehara, Japan
e-mail: Hirotaka_Komaba@hsdm.harvard.edu

B. Lanske, MD
Department of Oral Medicine, Infection & Immunity, Harvard School of Dental Medicine, Boston, MA, USA
e-mail: beate_lanske@hsdm.harvard.edu

© Springer International Publishing Switzerland 2016
P.A. Ureña Torres et al. (eds.), *Vitamin D in Chronic Kidney Disease*,
DOI 10.1007/978-3-319-32507-1_9

9.1 Introduction

Klotho was originally identified by Kuro-o and co-workers while attempting to create a rodent model of hypertension when the transgene accidentally generated a phenotype resembling premature-aging syndromes. Mice homozygous for the transgene (*kl/kl* mice) develop complex phenotypes resembling human aging, including growth arrest, soft-tissue calcifications, osteopenia, generalized tissue atrophy, and short life-span [1].

The *klotho* gene encodes a single-pass transmembrane protein and is expressed primarily in the kidney, the parathyroid gland, and the choroid plexus in the brain. The principal function of klotho is to regulate phosphate and vitamin D metabolism through acting as a co-receptor for bone-derived fibroblast growth factor 23 (FGF23) [2, 3]. Loss of klotho hampers the binding of FGF23 to FGF receptors (FGFRs) and results in severe hyperphosphatemia and hypervitaminosis D, which is considered to explain the most part of the premature-aging features in *kl/kl* mice [4–7]. Beside its physiological roles, accumulating evidences have demonstrated the critical role of klotho-FGF23 axis in the pathogenesis of chronic kidney disease-mineral and bone disorder (CKD-MBD) [8].

In this chapter, we present recent insights into the role of klotho and FGF23 in the altered metabolism of phosphate and vitamin D in CKD. We also discuss the reported multifunctional roles of soluble form klotho and their potential involvement in the pathophysiology of CKD-MBD.

9.2 Klotho as a Co-receptor for FGF23

The major function of klotho to regulate mineral metabolism has been uncovered by the identification of FGF23 as a regulator of phosphate and vitamin D metabolism [2, 3]. The *Fgf23* gene was first cloned in mice as a new member of the FGF family [9] and subsequently identified as a causative humoral factor for autosomal dominant hypophosphatemic rickets/osteomalacia (ADHR) [10] and tumor-induced osteomalacia (TIO) [11]. FGF23 induces urinary phosphate excretion by suppressing the expression of the sodium-phosphate cotransporter [12]. FGF23 also suppresses $1,25(OH)_2D$ via inhibition of the 1α-hydroxylase (CYP27B1) that converts 25-hydroxyvitamin D [25(OH)D] to $1,25(OH)_2D$ and stimulation of the 24-hydroxylase (CYP24) that converts $1,25(OH)_2D$ to inactive metabolites in the proximal tubule of the kidney [12]. Depletion of FGF23 has been shown to induce hyperphosphatemia, excessive levels of $1,25(OH)_2D$, soft tissue calcification, and short life-span [13], which are also observed in klotho-deficient (*kl/kl*) mice [1].

The strikingly similar phenotypes between *Fgf23*-null and klotho-deficient mice implicate that the premature aging-like features may be partly regulated through a common signaling pathway involving both FGF23 and klotho. This speculation led to the identification of klotho as a co-factor for FGF23 and its receptor interactions [2, 3]. FGF23 has been shown to bind to multiple FGFRs, including FGFR1c, FGFR3c, and FGFR4 [3]. Among these FGFRs, FGFR1c is likely to be the physiologically relevant target for FGF23, because klotho-dependent FGF23 signaling defined by upregulation of the gene *early growth-responsive 1 (Egr-1)* is enhanced only through interaction with FGFR1c but not with other FGFRs [2]. Structural analysis of FGF23 protein found that the N-terminal region of FGF23 binds to and activates FGFR whereas the C-terminal region of FGF23 is necessary for the interaction with klotho [14].

The functional importance of klotho as a co-receptor for FGF23 has been evidenced in several in vivo studies. Genetic inactivation of *klotho* in either *Hyp* mice, a murine homolog of X-linked hypophosphatemic rickets (XLH) [15], or *FGF23* transgenic mice [16] has been shown to reverse the phenotype to the one identical to *Fgf23*-null mice. Furthermore, an exogenous injection of bioactive FGF23 into either *klotho* knockout mice or *Fgf23/klotho* double knockout mice did not produce any obvious changes in phosphate and vitamin D metabolism [17]. These observations strongly support the in vivo importance of klotho in FGF23 action, although it remains to be determined why FGF23-mediated phosphate and vitamin D metabolism takes place in the proximal tubules, despite the predominant expression of klotho in the distal tubular epithelial cells. One previous study has detected robust induction of phosphorylated ERK1 (a marker of FGF23 bioactivity) only within klotho-expressing distal tubules following FGF23 injection [18], suggesting that FGF23-mediated signaling might be initiated in the distal tubule. However, a recent study has shown that proximal tubular cells also express klotho and that FGF23 directly downregulates NaPi-2a in the proximal tubule through activation of ERK1/2 and serum/glucocorticoid-regulated kinase-1 (SGK1) [19]. Furthermore, the targeted deletion of klotho in the distal tubule yielded only minor phenotypes compared to klotho-deficient mice [20]. Collectively, these data suggest interdependency between proximal and distal tubular cells for mediating FGF23 action but further research is needed to confirm this possibility.

Given the critical role of klotho in regulating phosphate and vitamin D metabolism, the premature-aging phenotype of klotho-deficient mice has been explained by its dramatic changes in mineral metabolism. Indeed, it has been shown that low phosphate diet [4] and vitamin D-deficient diet [5] both rescue several aging-like phenotypes in klotho-deficient mice, together with restoration of mineral disturbance. Furthermore, genetic ablation of *Cyp27b1* [6] or *NaPi2a* [7] has also been shown to attenuate the premature aging-phenotype of klotho-deficient mice. These data have provided compelling evidence that the premature aging syndrome caused by klotho deficiency is due to retention of phosphate, calcium, and/or $1,25(OH)_2D$, but still cannot completely eliminate the possibility of unique functions of klotho as discussed below.

9.3 The Role of Klotho-FGF23 Axis in CKD-MBD

The identification and characterization of klotho-FGF23 axis has reshaped our understandings of the pathogenesis of CKD-MBD [8]. In patients with CKD, circulating FGF23 levels increase progressively as kidney function declines [21, 22], presumably to maintain neutral phosphate balance by promoting urinary phosphate excretion. However, this compensation results in suppression of renal 1,25(OH)$_2$D production and thereby triggers the early development of secondary hyperparathyroidism (Fig. 9.1). This concept has recently been supported by an experimental study in a rat model of CKD, which showed that treatment with neutralizing anti-FGF23 antibodies normalized 1,25(OH)$_2$D levels and thereby decreased PTH levels, but with the trade-off of overt hyperphosphatemia [23].

Interestingly, a recent study by Andrukhova et al. has shown that FGF23 increases renal Na$^+$ reabsorption by upregulating the Na$^+$:Cl$^-$ cotransporter NCC in the distal renal tubules through klotho-dependent activation of the ERK1/2-SGK1-WNK4 (with-no lysine kinase-4) signaling pathway. This could lead to volume expansion, hypertension, and heart hypertrophy [24]. Another recent study by Faul and co-workers has demonstrated that FGF23 directly acts on the heart independently of klotho, which induces left ventricular hypertrophy through activation of the calcineurin-NFAT (nuclear factor of activated T cells) signaling pathway [25] (Fig. 9.1). Thus, elevated FGF23 not only plays a role in the pathogenesis of CKD-MBD but also could cause cardiac hypertrophy through mechanisms dependent or independent of klotho, which may explain the association of FGF23 with cardiovascular risk in patients with CKD.

Before patients reach end-stage renal disease (ESRD), normophosphatemia is maintained by the action of FGF23 and PTH to augment phosphaturia, but progression of CKD leads to a reduction in the ability of the kidney to excrete urinary phosphate, which finally overcomes the compensatory effects of these phosphaturic hormones. This process results in an increase in serum phosphate and progressive

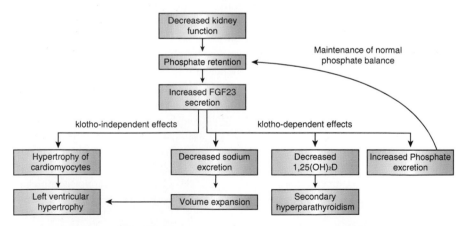

Fig. 9.1 Klotho-dependent and klotho-independent effects of FGF23 in CKD. In patients with CKD, FGF23 secretion is increased to maintain neutral phosphate balance, but this leads to suppression of renal 1,25(OH)$_2$D production and thereby triggers the development of secondary hyperparathyroidism. FGF23 also increases renal Na+ reabsorption in a klotho-dependent manner, which leads to volume expansion, hypertension, and left ventricular hypertrophy. Excess FGF23 also cause left ventricular hypertrophy by directly acting on cardiomyocytes in a klotho-independent manner. Abbreviations: *1,25(OH)$_2$D* 1,25-dihydroxy vitamin D, *CKD* chronic kidney disease, *FGF23* fibroblastic growth factor 23

reduction in 1,25(OH)$_2$D levels, both of which further stimulate PTH secretion [8]. Patients with ESRD thus commonly manifest hyperphosphatemia, decreased levels of 1,25(OH)$_2$D, and secondary hyperparathyroidism. Interestingly, the renal expression of klotho has been shown to decrease in patients with ESRD [26] as well as rodent models of CKD [27], which may partly contribute to the resistance to FGF23 and subsequent inability to promote phosphaturia (Fig. 9.2). The precise mechanism for the decreased klotho expression in CKD is not well understood but may be due to kidney damage per se or the inhibitory effects of increased FGF23 and decreased 1,25(OH)$_2$D on klotho expression, because FGF23 [28] and 1,25(OH)$_2$D [5] can downregulate and upregulate klotho expression, respectively. Several other factors may also be involved in the dysregulation of klotho in CKD, including inflammation, oxidative stress, and uremic toxins [29]. Conversely, several kinds of medications, such as statin, renin-angiotensin system (RAS) blockers, and peroxisome proliferator-activated receptor (PPAR)-γ agonists, have been shown to enhance klotho expression [29].

Importantly, klotho is also expressed in the parathyroid gland, and mediates the effect of FGF23 to negatively regulate PTH synthesis and secretion [30]. However, in ESRD patients undergoing dialysis, PTH secretion remains elevated despite extremely high FGF23 levels. Recent data suggest that this parathyroid resistance to FGF23 may be caused by decreased expression of klotho-FGFR1 complex in the parathyroid gland [31] (Fig. 9.2), in analogy to the downregulation of calcium-sensing receptors

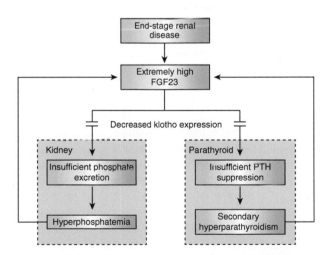

Fig. 9.2 Resistance to FGF23 due to decreased klotho expression in ESRD. In patients with ESRD, circulating FGF23 levels markedly increase in response to chronic phosphate load, active vitamin D therapy, and PTH hypersecretion. In this setting, increased FGF23 fails to stimulate phosphate excretion due to kidney dysfunction and decreased expression of klotho. FGF23 also fails to inhibit PTH secretion due to downregulation of the parathyroid klotho. The resultant hyperphosphatemia and secondary hyperparathyroidism further stimulates FGF23 secretion by bone cells. Abbreviations: *ESRD* end-stage renal disease, *FGF23* fibroblastic growth factor 23, *PTH* parathyroid hormone

and vitamin D receptors in hyperplastic parathyroid glands. Indeed, experimental studies have demonstrated that FGF23 fails to decrease PTH secretion in both in vitro cultures of parathyroid cells from rats with CKD and in vivo rat models of CKD, as a result of downregulation of this receptor complex [32, 33]. Of interest, a recent genetic study by Olauson and co-workers demonstrated that parathyroid-specific deletion of klotho did not affect mineral metabolism including PTH secretion, and the researchers proposed a novel, klotho-independent signaling pathway, which is mediated through the calcineurin-NFAT pathway [34]. However, why such a klotho-independent pathway is not activated by FGF23 in the kidney in klotho-deficient mice remains to be determined, and additional studies would be needed to confirm this hypothesis.

A recent study by Lim et al. also found klotho expressions in human arteries and demonstrated that FGF23 attenuated vascular calcification in isolated human vascular smooth muscle cells in a klotho-dependent manner [35]. However, many other researchers could not detect klotho in the vasculature [36, 37] and the presence and functions of klotho in arterial cells remains unclear.

Klotho is also reported to be present in bone cells in a recent study by Rhee et al. [38]. This study demonstrated increased expressions of *Egr-1* and *Egr-2*, downstream targets of FGF23 signaling, in osteocytes from mice with osteocyte-specific constitutive activation of PTH receptor signaling that exhibit elevated FGF23 levels. This observation suggests that bone is another target organ for FGF23 with klotho acting as a co-receptor. Because disordered bone structure is one of the characteristic features of klotho-deficient mice [1], it is intriguing to speculate whether klotho in bone cells plays a role in the bone metabolism and skeletal growth.

9.4 Soluble Form of Klotho

The klotho protein is composed of a large extracellular domain with two internal repeats (KL1 and KL2), a transmembrane domain, and a very short intracellular domain (10 amino acids). The extracellular domain is subject to ectodomain shedding and the entire extracellular region (approximately 120–130 kDa) can be released into the extracellular space including blood, urine, and cerebrospinal fluid [39]. This ectodomain cleavage is known to be mediated by α-secretase, ADAM (a disintegrin and metalloprotease) 10 and 17, and β-secretase, β-APP cleaving enzyme 1 [40] (Fig. 9.3). This molecule is called soluble klotho, secreted klotho, cleaved klotho, or cut klotho (Table 9.1). Another form of soluble klotho exists, which is generated from the klotho gene through alternative splicing. This molecule only encodes the N-terminal half of klotho with its extracellular domain (KL1) and has a molecular weight of approximately 65–70 kDa (Fig. 9.3). This molecule is also called soluble klotho or secreted klotho (Table 9.1). However, this small, soluble form cannot be detected in blood [39] and its physiological role remains unclear. Thus, soluble klotho or secreted klotho is generally used to indicate the cleaved form of klotho with a molecular weight of approximately 120–130 kDa.

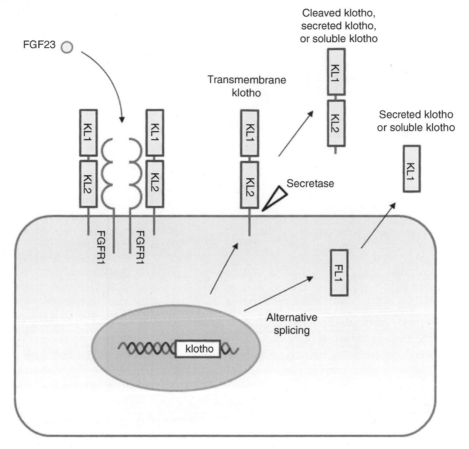

Fig. 9.3 Transmembrane and secreted forms of klotho. Transmembrane klotho forms a complex with FGFR1 and functions as a co-receptor for FGF23 signaling. The extracellular domain (KL1+KL2) can be released into the extracellular space through ectodomain shedding by secretase. Secreted klotho (KL1) is also generated through alternative RNA splicing, but this small molecule cannot be detected in the circulation and the physiological role remains unclear. Abbreviations: *FGF23* fibroblastic growth factor 23, *FGFR* fibroblastic growth factor receptor

Because the kidney is the principal organ expressing klotho [1], it has been postulated that the kidney is the main source of circulating klotho. This expectation has been confirmed by a recent genetic study by Lindberg and co-workers showing that targeted-deletion of klotho in the total kidney resulted in a marked reduction in serum klotho levels [41]. Of note, these kidney-specific *klotho* knockout mice resemble the premature-aging phenotype of systemic *klotho* knockout mice. This finding suggests that klotho synthesized in the kidney is the principle contributor for the antiaging traits, which could be mediated either by the transmembrane form, soluble form, or both. A more recent study by Hu et al. further demonstrated that serum klotho levels were higher in suprarenal compared with infrarenal inferior vena and these levels dropped precipitously after bilateral nephrectomy [42].

Table 9.1 Characteristics of transmembrane and secreted forms of klotho

Popular name	Other names	Structure	Molecular weight	Comments
Transmembrane klotho	Klotho, membrane-bound klotho	KL1, KL2, transmembrane domain, intracellular domain	130 kDa	Acting as a co-receptor for FGF23
Cleaved klotho	Soluble klotho, secreted klotho, circulating klotho, cut klotho	KL1, KL2	120–130 kDa	Released by the ectodomain cleavage of transmembrane klotho. Reported to possess multifunctional bioactivities. Specific receptor unknown
Secreted klotho	Soluble klotho, circulating klotho	KL1	65–70 kDa	Generated through alternative splicing. Physiological role unclear

Collectively, these data provide evidence that the kidney is the principal source of soluble klotho production. This notion is in line with the clinical observations that unilateral nephrectomy in living donors reduced serum soluble klotho levels [43], whereas surgical removal of parathyroid glands, another potential source of soluble klotho production, resulted in only transient and modest reduction in soluble klotho levels [44].

The metabolism of soluble klotho has been unclear until a recent discovery that the kidney also serves as a portal of clearance of circulating klotho [42]. This study demonstrated that klotho is excreted from the blood into the urinary lumen through transcytosis-mediated trafficking from the basal to the apical side of the proximal tubule and that the serum half-life of exogenous klotho in anephric rats was four- to fivefold longer than that in normal rats. This finding may explain why serum soluble klotho is decreased after kidney transplantation and why inconsistent results exist regarding serum soluble klotho levels in patients with CKD and ESRD (as discussed below).

The regulation of soluble klotho secretion and clearance is largely unknown, but a recent rodent study found that serum and urinary levels of soluble klotho were increased after administration of calcitriol or its analog paricalcitol [45]. Surprisingly, there was no significant upregulation of klotho expression in the kidney as well as other organs, suggesting that the increased levels of soluble klotho were caused by accelerated shedding of klotho without change in klotho synthesis. Although the detailed mechanism of increased soluble klotho by active vitamin D remains to be determined, this finding fits the clinical observations that serum soluble klotho levels increased progressively during periods of active calcitriol administration after parathyroidectomy for severe secondary hyperparathyroidism [44] whereas these levels did not change markedly by cinacalcet treatment with a fixed dose of active vitamin D [46]. Clearly, further research is needed to determine how the secretion and clearance of klotho is regulated by active vitamin D and other possible factors.

9.5   Multiple Functions of Soluble Klotho

Because the main function of membrane-bound klotho is to mediate FGF23 bioactivity, it has been of interest whether secreted klotho also possesses such a property. Previous studies have demonstrated binding of cleaved klotho (KL1+KL2) to FGF23 and FGFR1, which renders this possibility [2, 3]. This question was addressed by a mechanistic study by Farrow et al. [18]. This study found enhanced *Egr-1* expression and phosphorylated ERK1/2 activity by FGF23 treatment in cells stably expressing membrane klotho, but such a robust signaling by FGF23 was not observed by adding cleaved klotho (KL1+KL2) or secreted klotho (KL1). These data provide plausible evidence that only transmembrane klotho determines the ligand specificity of FGFR1. However, several other researchers reported enhanced downstream signaling of FGFR1 by adding cleaved klotho (KL1+KL2) together with FGF23 [47, 48], still leaving the possibility that cleaved klotho can form the FGF23-FGFR1 interaction. This possibility however seems unlikely under physiological conditions, because in such circumstance almost every tissue could be a target for FGF23, which would disrupt normal endocrine homeostasis.

Recent studies also demonstrated that soluble klotho functions as an endocrine factor by modulating ion channels and transporters. One of such biological actions is to regulate renal calcium transport by modulating TRPV5, a calcium-permeable channel essential for the transcellular calcium reabsorption in the distal tubule. Chang and co-workers first demonstrated that soluble klotho increases cell-surface abundance of TRPV5 by entrapping the channel in the plasma membrane. Mutation of a single asparagine for N-glycosylation prevents the effect of soluble klotho, which suggested that soluble klotho stabilizes TRPV5 on the cell surface by hydrolysis of its extracellular N-linked oligosaccharides [49]. Cha and co-workers further investigated the sugar substrates of the N-glycans of TRPV5 for soluble klotho. They found that secreted klotho has sialidase activity which removes α2,6-sialic acids from the N-glycan chains on TRPV5 and exposes underlying N-acetyl-D-lactosamine for binding to galectin-1. This binding of TRPV5 to galectin-1 prevents internalization and endocytosis leading to accumulation of the channels on the cell surface [50]. Thus, theoretically, soluble klotho should enhance calcium reabsorption in the distal nephron by increasing TRPV5; however, in vivo effects of soluble klotho on systemic calcium metabolism have not been sufficiently examined and their physiological significance remains to be determined.

Another function of soluble klotho is to increase urinary phosphate excretion by suppressing Napi-2a, which was first reported by Hu and co-workers [51]. They demonstrated that soluble klotho inhibits NaPi-2a and causes phosphaturia and hypophosphatemia. This effect was also observed in *Fgf23*-null mice, suggesting that the phosphaturic action of soluble klotho is independent from FGF23. Additional cell culture studies suggested that the direct inhibition of NaPi-2a by soluble klotho includes inhibition of transporter activity, induction of proteolytic degradation, and internalization from the apical membrane, which are likely mediated through the β-glucuronidase activity of soluble klotho. However, the substrate of NaPi-2a on which soluble klotho acts as a glycan-modifying enzyme is not known. Furthermore, β-glucuronidase activity of soluble klotho is known to be very weak [52]. Thus, additional research is needed to determine the mechanism of soluble klotho action on phosphate metabolism.

Besides inhibiting NaPi-2a, soluble klotho also inhibits phosphate transport through NaPi-3 isoforms Pit-1 and Pit-2 in vascular smooth muscle cells [27]. This phosphate transport inhibition prevents calcification and osteogenic transformation induced by high phosphate. In addition, exogenous injection of recombinant soluble klotho into klotho-deficient mice has been shown to attenuate vascular calcification. However, the detailed mechanisms how soluble klotho inhibits Pit-1 and Pit-2 is completely unknown. Similarly to soluble klotho, transmembrane klotho was also shown to inhibit vascular calcification by mediating FGF23 signaling [35]. However, many other researches could not detect klotho in the vasculature and this issue remains controversial [36, 37]. Clearly, additional research is needed to determine whether and how klotho, either the transmembrane or soluble form, could inhibit vascular calcification.

Interestingly, a recent study by Smith and co-workers has shown that soluble klotho directly regulates FGF23 production and secretion [48]. The researchers injected adeno-associated virus producing soluble klotho (KL1+KL2) into mice and found that these mice manifested hypophosphatemia and severe osteomalacia together with markedly enhanced FGF23 production. Because the adeno-associated virus does not produce transmembrane klotho, it is suggested that soluble klotho, produced by infected organs, circulates in blood to bone and stimulates FGF23 production through still unknown mechanism. However, such findings have not been reported in mice injected with recombinant soluble klotho or transgenic mice that overexpress klotho [53]. Furthermore, marked FGF23 production is one of the characteristic features of klotho-deficient mice, indicating that soluble klotho is not indispensable for the production of FGF23. Further research is needed to determine the physiological role of soluble klotho in the regulation of FGF23 production.

Soluble klotho has also been shown to possess other multiple functions beyond mineral metabolism [29]. One of the most attractive functions is the renoprotective effect. In a variety of kidney disease models, transgenic overexpression of klotho or exogenous injection of soluble klotho has been shown to improve kidney function and renal fibrosis [29, 54]. Soluble klotho has been shown to suppress activity of insulin, insulin-like growth factor-1 (IGF-1), Wnt, and transforming growth factor-β1 (TGF-β1), which may in part contribute to the renoprotective action of soluble klotho [29]. Recent experimental studies also demonstrated that soluble klotho protects against cardiac hypertrophy through downregulation of TRPC6 channels in the heart [55]. Because both acute and chronic kidney disease are reported to be a state of klotho deficiency [27, 54], supplementation of soluble klotho shows promise for the treatment of kidney disease. However, it should be stressed that no specific receptor for soluble klotho has been identified and the basic mechanism of the pleiotropic effects of soluble klotho remains unclear. Furthermore, a recent study has shown little or no predictivity of serum soluble klotho on the occurrence of death or initiation of renal replacement therapy [56], posing a question on the therapeutic use of soluble klotho for CKD patients. Much further work must be undertaken before any clinical application can be considered.

9.6   Soluble Klotho in CKD

In accordance with the reductions in transmembrane klotho in the kidney and the parathyroid gland in CKD [26, 31], Hu and co-workers have shown that circulating soluble klotho levels decrease in rodents and humans with CKD [27]. They established a semiquantitative method combining immunoprecipitation and immunoblotting and found that serum soluble klotho starts to decline in early CKD. Based on these findings, the researchers claim that soluble klotho serves as an early biomarker for CKD.

However, such findings have not been consistently reproduced when serum soluble klotho was measured by a sandwich ELISA that was recently provided by Immuno-Biological Laboratories, Co, Ltd [57]. This assay detects circulating soluble klotho by using two monoclonal antibodies that specifically recognize the extracellular domain of klotho. Using this assay, Pavik and co-workers found that serum soluble klotho started to decrease at early CKD stages [58]. However, a subsequent larger study by Seiler et al. found no significant association of serum soluble klotho with kidney function [56]. Another study by Akimoto et al. also found no meaningful changes in serum soluble klotho during course of CKD [59]. Furthermore, several recent studies have shown that serum soluble klotho levels do not decrease so markedly even in patients with ESRD [44, 46, 60]. Collectively, it remains controversial whether serum soluble klotho is actually deficient in patients with CKD. Several studies have shown progressive reductions in urinary soluble klotho in CKD [59], but these data should be interpreted with caution because soluble klotho is highly unstable in urine [61].

One possible explanation for these inconsistent results is that the kidney has dual roles in soluble klotho homeostasis, producing and clearing from the blood into the urine [42]. It is possible that in patients with ESRD, serum soluble klotho is accumulated due to decreased renal clearance even though the renal production is decreased. A recent clinical observation that serum soluble klotho is decreased after kidney transplantation supports this possibility [43].

Given the lack of sufficient evidence regarding the status of serum soluble klotho in CKD, it may be too early to determine whether soluble klotho contributes to the pathogenesis of CKD-MBD. However, if soluble klotho is depleted in CKD, this should theoretically contribute to alterations in mineral metabolism. In this instance,

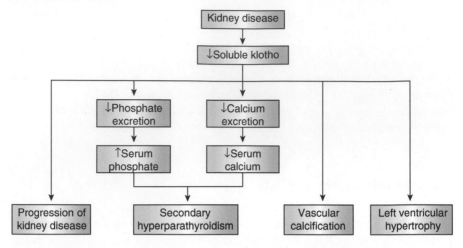

Fig. 9.4 Putative role of soluble klotho in the pathogenesis of CKD-MBD. If soluble klotho is depleted in CKD, this may lead to decreased urinary phosphate excretion and renal calcium reabsorption, which can aggravate hyperphosphatemia and secondary hyperparathyroidism. Decreased soluble klotho may also cause progression of vascular calcification, worsening of kidney function, and development of left ventricular hypertrophy. However, conflicting results exist regarding the status of serum soluble klotho in CKD, and further research is needed to confirm this hypothetical scenario. Abbreviations: *CKD* chronic kidney disease, *CKD-MBD* chronic kidney disease-mineral and bone disorder

decreased soluble klotho may lead to decreased urinary phosphate excretion and renal calcium reabsorption, which can aggravate hyperphosphatemia and secondary hyperparathyroidism. In addition, decreased soluble klotho may also cause progression of vascular calcification and worsening of kidney function, which further accelerates the progression of CKD-MBD (Fig. 9.4). Thus, supplementation of soluble klotho may have a potential to halt or even reverse the progression of CKD-MBD. However, this concept is still hypothetical and further research is needed to determine the role of soluble klotho in the pathogenesis of CKD-MBD.

9.7 Conclusions

The recent identification of klotho as a physiological regulator of phosphate and vitamin D metabolism has considerably advanced our understanding of CKD-MBD. By acting as a co-factor for FGFR in FGF23 signaling, klotho plays a central role in the pathogenesis of disturbances of phosphate and vitamin D metabolism in CKD. Recent work also demonstrated that both the transmembrane and soluble form of klotho is deficient in patients with CKD and ESRD and such klotho deficiency is likely to contribute to the pathogenesis of secondary hyperparathyroidism, vascular calcification, left ventricular hypertrophy, and worsening of kidney injury. Future research should determine whether klotho deficiency is universal phenomena in patients with CKD and whether treatments to induce klotho or supplementation of soluble klotho have a therapeutic potential to improve the progression of CKD-MBD.

References

1. Kuro-o M, Matsumura Y, Aizawa H, Kawaguchi H, Suga T, Utsugi T, et al. Mutation of the mouse Klotho gene leads to a syndrome resembling ageing. Nature. 1997;390:45–51.
2. Kurosu H1, Ogawa Y, Miyoshi M, Yamamoto M, Nandi A, Rosenblatt KP, et al. Regulation of fibroblast growth factor-23 signaling by Klotho. J Biol Chem. 2006;281:6120–3.
3. Urakawa I, Yamazaki Y, Shimada T, Iijima K, Hasegawa H, Okawa K, et al. Klotho converts canonical FGF receptor into a specific receptor for FGF23. Nature. 2006;444:770–4.
4. Morishita K, Shirai A, Kubota M, Katakura Y, Nabeshima Y, Takeshige K, et al. The progression of aging in klotho mutant mice can be modified by dietary phosphorus and zinc. J Nutr. 2001;131:3182–8.
5. Tsujikawa H, Kurotaki Y, Fujimori T, Fukuda K, Nabeshima Y. Klotho, a gene related to a syndrome resembling human premature aging, functions in a negative regulatory circuit of vitamin D endocrine system. Mol Endocrinol. 2003;17:2393–403.
6. Ohnishi M, Nakatani T, Lanske B, Razzaque MS. Reversal of mineral ion homeostasis and soft-tissue calcification of klotho knockout mice by deletion of vitamin D 1alpha-hydroxylase. Kidney Int. 2009;75:1166–72.
7. Ohnishi M, Nakatani T, Lanske B, Razzaque MS. In vivo genetic evidence for suppressing vascular and soft-tissue calcification through the reduction of serum phosphate levels, even in the presence of high serum calcium and 1,25-dihydroxyvitamin d levels. Circ Cardiovasc Genet. 2009;2:583–90.
8. Komaba H, Fukagawa M. The role of FGF23 in CKD–with or without Klotho. Nat Rev Nephrol. 2012;8:484–90.
9. Yamashita T, Yoshioka M, Itoh N. Identification of a novel fibroblast growth factor, FGF-23, preferentially expressed in the ventrolateral thalamic nucleus of the brain. Biochem Biophys Res Commun. 2000;277:494–8.
10. ADHR Consortium. Autosomal dominant hypophosphataemic rickets is associated with mutations in FGF23. Nat Genet. 2000;26:345–8.
11. Shimada T, Mizutani S, Muto T, Yoneya T, Hino R, Takeda S, et al. Cloning and characterization of FGF23 as a causative factor of tumor-induced osteomalacia. Proc Natl Acad Sci U S A. 2001;98:6500–5.
12. Shimada T, Hasegawa H, Yamazaki Y, Muto T, Hino R, Takeuchi Y, et al. FGF-23 is a potent regulator of vitamin D metabolism and phosphate homeostasis. J Bone Miner Res. 2004;19:429–35.
13. Shimada T, Kakitani M, Yamazaki Y, Hasegawa H, Takeuchi Y, Fujita T, et al. Targeted ablation of Fgf23 demonstrates an essential physiological role of FGF23 in phosphate and vitamin D metabolism. J Clin Invest. 2004;113:561–8.
14. Shimada T, Muto T, Urakawa I, Yoneya T, Yamazaki Y, Okawa K, et al. Mutant FGF-23 responsible for autosomal dominant hypophosphatemic rickets is resistant to proteolytic cleavage and causes hypophosphatemia in vivo. Endocrinology. 2002;143:3179–82.
15. Nakatani T, Ohnishi M, Razzaque MS. Inactivation of klotho function induces hyperphosphatemia even in presence of high serum fibroblast growth factor 23 levels in a genetically engineered hypophosphatemic (Hyp) mouse model. FASEB J. 2009;23:3702–11.
16. Bai X, Dinghong Q, Miao D, Goltzman D, Karaplis AC. Klotho ablation converts the biochemical and skeletal alterations in FGF23 (R176Q) transgenic mice to a Klotho-deficient phenotype. Am J Physiol Endocrinol Metab. 2009;296:E79–88.

17. Nakatani T, Sarraj B, Ohnishi M, Densmore MJ, Taguchi T, Goetz R, et al. In vivo genetic evidence for klotho-dependent, fibroblast growth factor 23 (Fgf23) -mediated regulation of systemic phosphate homeostasis. FASEB J. 2009;23:433–41.
18. Farrow EG, Davis SI, Summers LJ, White KE. Initial FGF23-mediated signaling occurs in the distal convoluted tubule. J Am Soc Nephrol. 2009;20:955–60.
19. Andrukhova O, Zeitz U, Goetz R, Mohammadi M, Lanske B, Erben RG. FGF23 acts directly on renal proximal tubules to induce phosphaturia through activation of the ERK1/2-SGK1 signaling pathway. Bone. 2012;51:621–8.
20. Olauson H, Lindberg K, Amin R, Jia T, Wernerson A, Andersson G, et al. Targeted deletion of Klotho in kidney distal tubule disrupts mineral metabolism. J Am Soc Nephrol. 2012;23: 1641–51.
21. Shigematsu T, Kazama JJ, Yamashita T, Fukumoto S, Hosoya T, Gejyo F, et al. Possible involvement of circulating fibroblast growth factor 23 in the development of secondary hyperparathyroidism associated with renal insufficiency. Am J Kidney Dis. 2004;44:250–6.
22. Gutierrez OI, Isakova T, Rhee E, Shah A, Holmes J, Collerone G, et al. Fibroblast growth factor-23 mitigates hyperphosphatemia but accentuates calcitriol deficiency in chronic kidney disease. J Am Soc Nephrol. 2005;16:2205–15.
23. Hasegawa H, Nagano N, Urakawa I, Yamazaki Y, Iijima K, Fujita T, et al. Direct evidence for a causative role of FGF23 in the abnormal renal phosphate handling and vitamin D metabolism in rats with early-stage chronic kidney disease. Kidney Int. 2010;78:975–80.
24. Andrukhova O, Slavic S, Smorodchenko A, Zeitz U, Shalhoub V, Lanske B, et al. FGF23 regulates renal sodium handling and blood pressure. EMBO Mol Med. 2014;6:744–59.
25. Faul C, Amaral AP, Oskouei B, Hu MC, Sloan A, Isakova T, et al. FGF23 induces left ventricular hypertrophy. J Clin Invest. 2011;121:4393–408.
26. Koh N, Fujimori T, Nishiguchi S, Tamori A, Shiomi S, Nakatani T, et al. Severely reduced production of klotho in human chronic renal failure kidney. Biochem Biophys Res Commun. 2001;280:1015–20.
27. Hu MC, Shi M, Zhang J, Quiñones H, Griffith C, Kuro-o M, et al. Klotho deficiency causes vascular calcification in chronic kidney disease. J Am Soc Nephrol. 2011;22:124–36.
28. Dai B, David V, Martin A, Huang J, Li H, Jiao Y, et al. A comparative transcriptome analysis identifying FGF23 regulated genes in the kidney of a mouse CKD model. PLoS One. 2012;7:e44161.
29. Hu MC, Kuro-o M, Moe OW. αKlotho and vascular calcification: an evolving paradigm. Curr Opin Nephrol Hypertens. 2014;23:331–9.
30. Ben-Dov IZ, Galitzer H, Lavi-Moshayoff V, Goetz R, Kuro-o M, Mohammadi M, et al. The parathyroid is a target organ for FGF23 in rats. J Clin Invest. 2007;117:4003–8.
31. Komaba H, Goto S, Fujii H, Hamada Y, Kobayashi A, Shibuya K, et al. Depressed expression of Klotho and FGF receptor 1 in hyperplastic parathyroid glands from uremic patients. Kidney Int. 2010;77:232–8.
32. Galitzer H, Ben-Dov IZ, Silver J, Naveh-Many T. Parathyroid cell resistance to fibroblast growth factor 23 in secondary hyperparathyroidism of chronic kidney disease. Kidney Int. 2010;77:211–8.
33. Canalejo R, Canalejo A, Martinez-Moreno JM, Rodriguez-Ortiz ME, Estepa JC, Mendoza FJ, et al. FGF23 fails to inhibit uremic parathyroid glands. J Am Soc Nephrol. 2010;21:1125–35.
34. Olauson H, Lindberg K, Amin R, Sato T, Jia T, Goetz R, et al. Parathyroid-specific deletion of Klotho unravels a novel calcineurin-dependent FGF23 signaling pathway that regulates PTH secretion. PLoS Genet. 2013;9:e1003975.
35. Lim K, Lu TS, Molostvov G, Lee C, Lam FT, Zehnder D, et al. Vascular Klotho deficiency potentiates the development of human artery calcification and mediates resistance to fibroblast growth factor 23. Circulation. 2012;125:2243–55.
36. Scialla JJ, Lau WL, Reilly MP, Isakova T, Yang HY, Crouthamel MH, et al. Fibroblast growth factor 23 is not associated with and does not induce arterial calcification. Kidney Int. 2013;83:1159–68.

37. Lindberg K, Olauson H, Amin R, Ponnusamy A, Goetz R, Taylor RF, et al. Arterial klotho expression and FGF23 effects on vascular calcification and function. PLoS One. 2013;8:e60658.
38. Rhee Y, Bivi N, Farrow E, Lezcano V, Plotkin LI, White KE, et al. Parathyroid hormone receptor signaling in osteocytes increases the expression of fibroblast growth factor-23 in vitro and in vivo. Bone. 2011;49:636–43.
39. Imura A, Iwano A, Tohyama O, Tsuji Y, Nozaki K, Hashimoto N, et al. Secreted Klotho protein in sera and CSF: implication for post-translational cleavage in release of Klotho protein from cell membrane. FEBS Lett. 2004;565:143–7.
40. Bloch L, Sineshchekova O, Reichenbach D, Reiss K, Saftig P, Kuro-o M, et al. Klotho is a substrate for alpha-, beta- and gamma-secretase. FEBS Lett. 2009;583:3221–4.
41. Lindberg K, Amin R, Moe OW, Hu MC, Erben RG, Östman Wernerson A, et al. The kidney is the principal organ mediating klotho effects. J Am Soc Nephrol. 2014;25:2169–75.
42. Hu MC, Shi M, Zhang J, Addo T, Cho HJ, Barker SL, et al. Renal production, uptake, and handling of circulating αKlotho. J Am Soc Nephrol. 2016;27(1):79–90.
43. Kimura T, Akimoto T, Watanabe Y, Kurosawa A, Nanmoku K, Muto S, et al. Impact of renal transplantation and nephrectomy on urinary soluble klotho protein. Transplant Proc. 2015;47:1697–9.
44. Takahashi H, Komaba H, Takahashi Y, Sawada K, Tatsumi R, Kanai G, et al. Impact of parathyroidectomy on serum FGF23 and soluble Klotho in hemodialysis patients with severe secondary hyperparathyroidism. J Clin Endocrinol Metab. 2014;99:E652–8.
45. Lau WL, Leaf EM, Hu MC, Takeno MM, Kuro-o M, Moe OW, et al. Vitamin D receptor agonists increase klotho and osteopontin while decreasing aortic calcification in mice with chronic kidney disease fed a high phosphate diet. Kidney Int. 2012;82:1261–70.
46. Komaba H, Koizumi M, Tanaka H, Takahashi H, Sawada K, Kakuta T, et al. Effects of cinacalcet treatment on serum soluble Klotho levels in haemodialysis patients with secondary hyperparathyroidism. Nephrol Dial Transplant. 2012;27:1967–9.
47. Medici D, Razzaque MS, Deluca S, Rector TL, Hou B, Kang K, et al. FGF-23-Klotho signaling stimulates proliferation and prevents vitamin D-induced apoptosis. J Cell Biol. 2008;182:459–65.
48. Smith RC, O'Bryan LM, Farrow EG, Summers LJ, Clinkenbeard EL, Roberts JL, et al. Circulating αKlotho influences phosphate handling by controlling FGF23 production. J Clin Invest. 2012;122:4710–5.
49. Chang Q, Hoefs S, van der Kemp AW, Topala CN, Bindels RJ, Hoenderop JG. The beta-glucuronidase klotho hydrolyzes and activates the TRPV5 channel. Science. 2005;310:490–3.
50. Cha SK, Ortega B, Kurosu H, Rosenblatt KP, Kuro-O M, Huang CL. Removal of sialic acid involving Klotho causes cell-surface retention of TRPV5 channel via binding to galectin-1. Proc Natl Acad Sci U S A. 2008;105:9805–10.
51. Hu MC, Shi M, Zhang J, Pastor J, Nakatani T, Lanske B, et al. Klotho: a novel phosphaturic substance acting as an autocrine enzyme in the renal proximal tubule. FASEB J. 2010;24:3438–50.
52. Tohyama O, Imura A, Iwano A, Freund JN, Henrissat B, Fujimori T, et al. Klotho is a novel beta-glucuronidase capable of hydrolyzing steroid beta-glucuronides. J Biol Chem. 2004;279:9777–84.
53. Kurosu H, Yamamoto M, Clark JD, Pastor JV, Nandi A, Gurnani P, et al. Suppression of aging in mice by the hormone Klotho. Science. 2005;309:1829–33.
54. Hu MC, Shi M, Zhang J, Quiñones H, Kuro-o M, Moe OW. Klotho deficiency is an early biomarker of renal ischemia-reperfusion injury and its replacement is protective. Kidney Int. 2010;78:1240–51.
55. Xie J, Cha SK, An SW, Kuro-O M, Birnbaumer L, Huang CL. Cardioprotection by Klotho through downregulation of TRPC6 channels in the mouse heart. Nat Commun. 2012;3:1238.
56. Seiler S, Wen M, Roth HJ, Fehrenz M, Flügge F, Herath E, et al. Plasma Klotho is not related to kidney function and does not predict adverse outcome in patients with chronic kidney disease. Kidney Int. 2013;83:121–8.

57. Yamazaki Y, Imura A, Urakawa I, Shimada T, Murakami J, Aono Y, et al. Establishment of sandwich ELISA for soluble alpha-klotho measurement: age-dependent change of soluble alpha-klotho levels in healthy subjects. Biochem Biophys Res Commun. 2010;398:513–8.
58. Pavik I, Jaeger P, Ebner L, Wagner CA, Petzold K, Spichtig D, et al. Secreted Klotho and FGF23 in chronic kidney disease Stage 1 to 5: a sequence suggested from a cross-sectional study. Nephrol Dial Transplant. 2013;28:352–9.
59. Akimoto T, Yoshizawa H, Watanabe Y, Numata A, Yamazaki T, Takeshima E, et al. Characteristics of urinary and serum soluble Klotho protein in patients with different degrees of chronic kidney disease. BMC Nephrol. 2012;13:155.
60. Yokoyama K, Imura A, Ohkido I, Maruyama Y, Yamazaki Y, Hasegawa H, et al. Serum soluble α-klotho in hemodialysis patients. Clin Nephrol. 2012;77:347–51.
61. Adema AY, Vervloet MG, Blankenstein MA, Heijboer AC. α-Klotho is unstable in human urine. Kidney Int. 2015;88(6):1442–4.

Chapter 10
Vitamin D and FGF23 in Chronic Kidney Disease

Dominique Prié

Abstract The Fibroblast Growth Factor 23 (FGF23) has been identified less than 20 years ago. It rapidly appeared that FGF23 was not only the hormone that control phosphate homeostasis but also the metabolism of the active form of vitamin D, calcitriol. FGF23, by contrast with many other FGF belongs to the small hormone-like FGF sub-family with FGF15/19 and FGF21. FGF23 is secretes by osteocytes and osteoblasts in response to high phosphate or calcitriol levels. FGF23 inhibits the expression of renal sodium phosphate transporters, which augments phosphate excretion in urine. FGF23 also stimulates the expression of the enzyme that inactivates calcitriol, the CYP24A1, and lowers the expression of CYP27B1, which converts 25(OH) vitamin D into calcitriol. Hence FGF23 controls calcitriol levels in plasma. By decreasing calcitriol levels FGF23 indirectly diminishes intestinal phosphate absorption. Calcitriol directly stimulates FGF23 production in osteocytes. The physiological action of FGF23 requires the expression at the cell surface of a FGFR and the co-receptor αklotho. αKlotho is mainly expressed in the kidney, brain, and in the muscle. Calcitriol stimulates αklotho expression. αKlotho can be released from the cell surface by cleavage producing a circulating protein the role of which is insufficiently delineated, see previous chapter. FGF23 concentration increases at the early steps of renal insufficiency to maintain plasma phosphate concentration within normal range. This participates to the genesis of secondary hyperparathyroidism. High concentrations of FGF23 induce cardiac hypertrophy despite the absence of klotho in cardiac tissue. The decrease in calcitriol concentration induced by FGF23 may contribute to its deleterious effect on heart.

Keywords Phosphate • Calcitriol • Heart

D. Prié, MD
INSERM U845, Centre de Recherche Croissance et Signalisation,
Université Paris Descartes, Hôpital Necker Enfants Malades, Paris, France
e-mail: dominique.prie@inserm.fr

© Springer International Publishing Switzerland 2016
P.A. Ureña Torres et al. (eds.), *Vitamin D in Chronic Kidney Disease*,
DOI 10.1007/978-3-319-32507-1_10

10.1 Introduction

Fibroblast Growth Factor 23 (FGF23) has been identified less than 20 years ago by studying two disorders combining low plasma phosphate concentration and inappropriately low concentration of calcitriol (1,25(OH)$_2$vitamin D) [1, 2]. It became rapidly evident that FGF23 plays a major role not only in phosphate homeostasis but also in the control of calcitriol concentration [3]. FGF23 has a special place among the FGF family. The FGF family comprises 22 members (human FGF19 being the ortholog of mouse FGF15) [4]. Most FGFs are intracrine or paracrine factors. FGF23 belongs with FGF15/19 and FGF21 to the small hormone-like FGF sub family and differs from all other FGF by at least two characteristics: first the sequence of its carboxy terminal tail, which shows low sequence analogy with any other FGF, and second its unique ability to bind specifically to its co-receptor αklotho. By contrast with other FGFs, FGF23 exhibits all the features of a hormone: it is secreted in blood, it has action at distance of its secretion site on specific targets, it controls parameters that exert a feedback on its production and secretion. The reciprocal control of FGF23 and vitamin D and its consequences during chronic kidney disease have been clarified during the last decade showing new possibilities of therapeutic strategies to treat calcium and phosphate disorders.

10.2 Main Properties and Characteristics of FGF23

Under physiological conditions FGF23 is secreted mainly by osteocytes and osteoblast. FGF23 mRNA was also detected in the brain. In the liver and the kidneys expression of FGF23 become detectable in liver cirrhosis [5] or renal insufficiency [6]. FGF23 is released in plasma as a 32 kDa protein that, after the removal of its signal peptide, contains 226 amino acids. This intact form of FGF23 is considered as the active form of the molecule [7]. In different circumstances FGF23 can be cleaved between amino acids 176 and 179, at a RXXR/S180 subtilisin-like proprotein convertase motif, releasing a N-terminal and a C-terminal peptide. The enzymes responsible for this cleavage in vivo have not been clearly identified. It is also uncertain if the cleavage takes place only in cells, before FGF23 secretion, or also in other locations after FGF23 release in the plasma. The proper glycosylation of FGF23 at specific sites protects FGF23 from cleavage. One of the enzymes responsible for the glycosylation of FGF23 is the UDP-N-acetyl-α-D-galactosamine/polypeptide N-acetylgalactosaminyl transferase3 (GalNAc transferase 3 or GALNT3). Inactivating mutations of this enzyme, as well as FGF23 mutation at specific glycosylation sites, make FGF23 very sensitive to cleavage resulting in a decrease in, or even the absence of, circulating intact FGF23, while the N-terminal and C-terminal fragments represent the main forms of FGF23 in the plasma in these disorders [8]. Phosphorylation of ser180 by the Family with sequence similarity 20, member C (Fam20C) protein inhibits O-glycosylation of FGF23 by GALNT3 and promotes FGF23 cleavage and inactivation [9]. A role for FGF23 cleavage to control FGF23 concentration and its effects has been reported in anemia secondary to iron defi-ciency. In this condition an overproduction of cleaved FGF23 is observed while plasma intact FGF23 concentration remains normal [10].

Intact FGF23 has low affinity for the FGFRs and seems unable to activate sig-naling pathways at common plasma concentration in the absence of its co-receptor αklotho [11, 12]. αKlotho is a 1012 or 1014–amino acid–long protein depending on the species. It is expressed at the cell surface and is bound to the plasma membrane by a one-span trans-membrane domain. Its short intracellular tail is less than 15 amino acids long. αklotho expression is restricted to a small number of tissues including kidneys, parathyroid glands, brain, and skeletal muscles. Intriguingly the main site of expression of αklotho in the kidney is the distal tubule, whereas FGF23 exerts most of its renal action on the proximal tubule. A circulating or soluble form of αklotho is also present in the plasma and in urine and the cerebrospinal fluid [13]. This form is thought to originate from the shedding of the full-length protein expressed at the cell surface but it might also come from an intracellular processing of αklotho leading to the secretion of this slightly shorter form. Enzymes belonging to the A Disintegrin and Metalloproteinase (ADAM) family (ADAM 10 and 17) can cleave and release αklotho from the cell surface [14]. The β-secretase β-APP cleaving enzyme 1 (BACE1) can also participate to αklotho shedding. It is unknown however if under normal conditions these enzymes participate to the release of circulating αklotho. The physiologic role of the circulating form of αklotho remains also to be established. However the role of the full length-trans-membrane αklotho as a co-receptor of FGF23 is strongly supported first by the identical phenotype of FGF23 and αklotho knock-out mice while in the later plasma FGF23 concentration is increased and second by the modest effect of the injection of soluble αklotho on the phenotype of αklotho deficient-mice [15, 16]. Calcitriol plasma concentration is similarly elevated in FGF23 or αklotho deficient mice, supporting that FGF23 effects on vitamin D metabolism requires the presence of αklotho [17].

10.3   FGF23 Controls Vitamin D Metabolism

The roles of FGF23 have been revealed by the study of animal models and human diseases with primary alteration of FGF23 expression [1, 2, 18, 19]. Disruption of the FGF23 gene in mice induces an increase in plasma phosphate and calcitriol concentrations. Elevated plasma phosphate concentration is secondary to inappro-priate phosphate reabsorption in the renal proximal tubule due to the lack of inhibi-tion of the renal phosphate transporters by FGF23. The high level of calcitriol, by stimulating the expression of the intestinal sodium-phosphate co-transporter NPT2b expression, participates to the elevated plasma phosphate concentration. High cal-citriol concentration also stimulates intestinal calcium absorption leading to high plasma plasma levels with low parathyroid hormone (PTH) concentration. In FGF23 knock-out mice, the absence of FGF23 is responsible for high calcitriol concentra-tion despite low plasma PTH concentration, which emphasizes the predominant role of FGF23 on the regulation of calcitriol metabolism independently of PTH. A similar phenotype is observed in humans with inappropriately low plasma intact FGF23 concentration [20–22].

In the absence of FGF23 elevated plasma calcitriol levels are secondary to the simultaneous increase in the mRNA expression of the 25-hydroxyvitamin D 1α-hydroxylase (1α-hydroxylase, CYP27B1) and inhibition of the mRNA expression of CYP24A1, the enzyme that inactivates calcitriol [15]. All these effects take place in the renal proximal tubule, which is the main site of production and release of calcitriol in the plasma. The control of calcitriol levels is due to intact FGF23. In humans, mutations in the FGF23 or GALNT3 genes leading to the absence of intact or low levels of intact FGF23 in the plasma, is associated with high plasma calcitriol, despite the presence of high levels of the c-terminal, and N-terminal fragments FGF23.

The overexpression of intact FGF23 in mice or in human mirrors the defect. FGF23 overexpression induces hypophosphatemia with inappropriately low concentration of calcitriol while PTH concentration is moderately increased. This effect is due to the stimulation of CYP24A1 expression and the decrease in CYP27B1 activity in the kidney.

The signaling pathways involved in the control of the expression of CYP24A1 and CYP27B1 by intact FGF23 are partially understood. FGF23 can activate multiple intracellular signals. In the presence of αklotho and a FGFR, FGF23 mainly activates the MAPkinase and the AKT pathways [23]. When FGF23 concentration increases beyond normal concentration, as observed when the renal function is impaired, FGF23 can also stimulate FGFR in organs that do not express αklotho. In these situations FGF23 stimulates the PLCγ and NFAT pathways unraveling new properties [24]. Several lines of evidence show that the effects of FGF23 on calcitriol metabolism require the stimulation of a FGFR in the presence of αklotho. Indeed, injection of a FGFR inhibitor in mice increases calcitriol concentration despite the augmentation of intact FGF23 level [25, 26]. Also, as previously mentioned, in the absence of αklotho, high concentrations of intact FGF23 are unable to control calcitriol concentration. The requirement of both αklotho and a FGFR suggests that the MAPK or AKT pathways mediate the decrease in calcitriol production by the kidney. Indeed the pharmacologic inhibition of the MAPK pathway abolishes the FGF23-induced suppression of CYP27B1 expression in the kidney [23]. By contrast, in the parathyroid gland, FGF23 stimulates CYP27B1 expression, which increase local synthesis of calcitriol that inhibits PTH secretion. The opposite effects of FGF23 on CYP27B1 in the renal proximal tubule and in the parathyroid cells may be due to the activation of different signaling pathways. Indeed specific disruption of αklotho expression in the parathyroid tissue does not abolish FGF23 effects on PTH secretion while cyclosporine A, an inhibitor of the calcineurin NFAT pathway abolishes FGF23 effects [27].

In summary, when phosphate intake increases FGF23 maintains plasma phosphate concentration within the normal range by inhibiting renal phosphate reabsorption, calcitriol production and indirectly phosphate intestinal absorption. When phosphate intake is low FGF23 concentration decreases, which augments renal

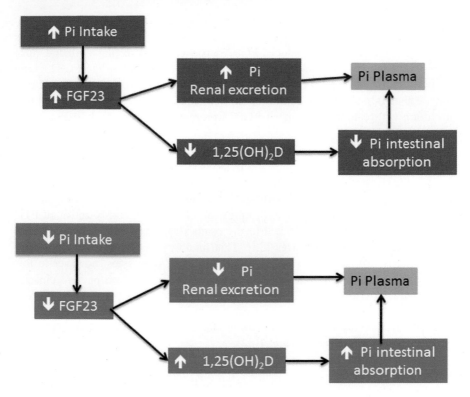

Fig. 10.1 Mechanisms by which plasma phosphate concentration is kept within the normal range when phosphate intakes vary

phosphate reabsorption, calcitriol production and indirectly phosphate intestinal absorption (Fig. 10.1).

10.4   Calcitriol Controls FGF23 Production

Mainly three parameters control FGF23 concentration: phosphate intake and/or plasma phosphate concentration, PTH and calcitriol levels.

Calcitriol seems to be the most efficient factor to stimulate production of intact FGF23 by osteocytes. Injection of calcitriol in mice or in human markedly and transiently increases plasma intact FGF23 concentration within a few hours. Calcitriol-induced FGF23 increase does not require the presence of PTH since it is observed in patients with hypoparathyroidism, in a murine model of genetic ablation of PTH gland and in thyroparathyroidectomized rats and mice [28, 29]. The expression of the vitamin D receptor (VDR) is mandatory for the calcitriol-induced FGF23 synthesis. Indeed VDR knock-out mice exhibit low plasma FGF23 concentrations that were not modified by calcitriol injections even when plasma phosphate concentration was controlled by diet to prevent phosphate-mediated inhibition of FGF23 production [30]. In another model, targeted-VDR-inactivation in chondrocytes markedly reduced calcitriol-induced FGF23 production suggesting a direct control of FGF23 synthesis by calcitriol on osteocytes [31]. Analysis of the FGF23 gene promoter revealed the presence of several vitamin D responsive elements (VDRE) that are able to bind VDR in cultured bone cells [32]. Treatment of various cell line in culture with calcitriol enhanced FGF23 promoter activity and FGF23 mRNA expression.

The effect of PTH on FGF23 concentration is complex and different studies have yielded conflicting results: on one hand by decreasing plasma phosphate concentration PTH can lower FGF23 production on the other hand PTH can directly stimulates FGF23 production by osteocytes. PTH could also stimulate FGF23 synthesis by stimulating calcitriol production Expression of a spontaneously activated PTH type 1 receptor (PTH1R) restricted to the osteocytes in mice markedly increases FGF23 production by osteocytes [33]. This finding supports the view that PTH could directly stimulate intact FGF23 production by osteocytes, however in this model calcitriol concentration was also increased. In hemodialysis patients cinacalcet, which decreases plasma PTH concentration, also lowers plasma FGF23 concentration [34, 35].

In summary FGF23 lowers calcitriol production and calcitriol exerts a positive feedback on FGF23 synthesis (Fig. 10.2).

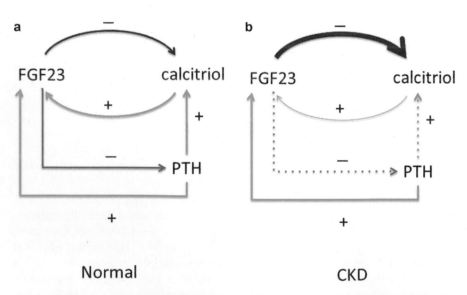

Fig. 10.2 Mutual control of calcitriol and FGF23 production when renal function is normal (**a**) or markedly altered (**b**). In CKD the inhibiting effect of FGF23 on calcitriol production in the kidney overwhelm the stimulatory effect of PTH

10.5   Modifications of FGF23 and Calcitriol When the Glomerular Filtration Rate Declines

Clinical and experimental studies constantly showed that plasma intact FGF23 concentration increases when GFR diminishes. This is an early modification that appears for slight decrease in GFR and that precedes modifications of PTH and plasma phosphate concentrations [36, 37]. Analyses of clinical observational data and experimental studies performed in animal has led to the conclusion that the early increase in FGF23 aims at controlling plasma phosphate concentration. When GFR declines the amount of phosphate filtered at the glomerulus decreases in parallel (Fig. 10.3). To prevent an accumulation of phosphate its reabsorption in the proximal tubule must be lowered. By a still undiscovered mechanism this undetectable accumulation of phosphate stimulates FGF23 production that inhibits renal phosphate reabsorption and also reduces intestinal absorption by lowering calcitriol production. When GFR further declines FGF23 concentration increases and clinical studies report strong negative correlations between FGF23 and GFR values. When FGF23 concentration increases its powerful inhibitory effect on calcitriol synthesis leads to insufficient intestinal calcium absorption that triggers the release of PTH to prevent a fall of plasma calcium concentration. The increase in plasma PTH levels is unable to reverse the powerful inhibitory effect of FGF23 on calcitriol metabolism (Fig. 10.2b). When GFR is still above 30 ml/min/1.73 m^2 the rise in plasma PTH concentration participate to the control of phosphate levels by diminishing renal phosphate reabsorption. Clinical observation report that plasma phosphate concentration increases lately during CKD evolution, preceded first by FGF23 increase, then calcitriol lowering and PTH rising [36]. However when GFR is low (below 30 ml/min/1.73 m^2), the amount of phosphate released from the bone by

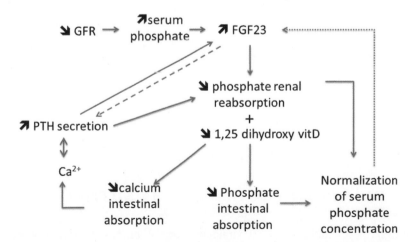

Fig. 10.3 Mechanisms leading to the increase in FGF23 concentration and the genesis of secondary hyperparathyroidism when GFR declines

PTH exceeds the capacity of the kidney to eliminate phosphate. Subsequently plasma phosphate concentration augments, aggravating FGF23 production that further decreases calcitriol levels and worsens secondary hyperparathyroidism. This mechanism is supported by experimental data. In rats with CKD, injection of antibodies blocking the action of FGF23 induced a rapid and significant increase in plasma calcitriol concentration, associated to a rise of calcium levels that reduces PTH production. The consequence is a rise of plasma phosphate concentration and the increase in vascular and tissue calcification and in mortality of the animals [38, 39]. In many but not all studies, a decline of αklotho expression paralleled the rise of plasma FGF23 concentration. This additional aftermath may contribute to the augmentation of FGF23 [40].

In summary during CKD, phosphate accumulation is the poison, FGF23 is the antidote and the decrease in calcitriol and the secondary hyperparathyroidism, and potentially the decrease in αklotho expression, are the side effects of the antidote.

Contributions of FGF23 and calcitriol to adverse outcomes in CKD.

High circulating FGF23 concentrations are associated with increased mortality in CKD patients and have deleterious cardiac effects. Experimental studies showed that at elevated concentration FGF23 could directly stimulate FGFR in the absence of αklotho on cardiomyocytes, inducing heart hypertrophy, and alteration of cardiac functions [41]. Low plasma vitamin D levels have been associated with similar adverse cardiovascular outcomes in CKD patients. It is unclear if low calcitriol levels have deleterious effects on heart independently of FGF23 in CKD patients. Studies assessing the effects of treatment with vitamin D analogs on cardiovascular mortality or morbidity led to conflicting results in CKD patients before or during dialysis. These discrepancies between studies could depend on the consequences of vitamin D treatment on FGF23 and αklotho levels. We can hypothesize, on the basis of the findings mentioned above, that beneficial impacts on survival could be observed mainly in patients with no further increase in FGF23 plasma concentration or with significant stimulation of αklotho expression. Indeed, many experimental and observational data suggest that low levels of αklotho expression have deleterious consequences on heart function. The identification of parameters that could predict a beneficial effect of vitamin D treatment would permit to target a subpopulation of CKD patients.

Low vitamin D or αklotho levels or high FGF23 plasma concentrations have been also associated with susceptibility to infection, modifications of the immune system, insulin resistance, or anemia. The relative weight of each factor when considered altogether has not yet been assessed in particular in CKD.

10.6   Perspectives for the Treatments of CKD Patients

Based on these findings several strategies can be proposed to control FGF23 and prevent secondary hyperparathyroidism. Treatment with calcitriol, or its analogs, has been used for decades. Calcitriol is efficient to prevent secondary hyperparathyroidism however it also stimulates FGF23 production. The ideal calcitriol analog for the treatment of secondary hyperparathyroidism in CKD should be able to stimulate intestinal calcium absorption and αklotho expression without stimulating intestinal phosphate absorption and FGF23 production. Such an analog has not been identified to date. A more promising possibility is blocking of FGF23 effect in patients on dialysis. In these patients the lack of calcitriol production by the kidneys is very likely more due to FGF23 overproduction than to the destruction of the renal parenchyma. By contrast to the situation before dialysis, FGF23 does not participate anymore to phosphate elimination by the kidney in dialysis patients. In this condition high FGF23 has deleterious consequences without beneficial effects. Consequently the use of anti-FGF23 antibodies or FGFR antagonists in patients on dialysis might be able to increase calcitriol production and reverse secondary hyperparathyroidism. Anti-FGF23 antibodies are already on trials in human with X-linked hypophosphatemic rickets and are efficient to hinder FGF23 effects [42].

In non-dialysis CKD patients, diminishing FGF23 production to tackle low plasma calcitriol concentration and secondary hyperparathyroidism might be achieved by combining several approaches: decreasing intestinal phosphate absorption, preventing calcitriol-induced phosphate absorption in the intestine, increasing phosphate excretion in urine. Phosphate binders have shown interesting but limited results on plasma FGF23 and vitamin D concentrations on dialysis patients. This might be due to the fact that any diminution in FGF23, following the reduction of phosphate absorption, induces a slight increase in calcitriol secretion that stimulates intestinal phosphate absorption that in turn triggers FGF23 production. Inhibitors of the intestinal sodium-phosphate co-transporter could prevent the calcitriol-induced increase of phosphate reabsorption in this context. Nicotinamide is already available and pharmacological inhibitors could be designed for use in human in a near future. Inhibition of renal sodium- phosphate co-transporters can be also interesting. The diminution of renal phosphate reabsorption could lower plasma FGF23 concentration and consequently stimulate calcitriol synthesis. Again the association to molecules that inhibits intestinal sodium phosphate co-transporters would prevent a subsequent increase in intestinal phosphate absorption. These inhibitors however are not yet available for clinical use.

References

1. ADHR Consortium. Autosomal dominant hypophosphataemic rickets is associated with mutations in FGF23. Nat Genet. 2000;26(3):345–8.
2. Shimada T. Cloning and characterization of FGF23 as a causative factor of tumor-induced osteomalacia. Proc Natl Acad Sci. 2001;98(11):6500–5.
3. Saito H. Human fibroblast growth factor-23 mutants suppress Na+ -dependent phosphate co-transport activity and 1alpha,25-dihydroxyvitamin D3 production. J Biol Chem. 2002;278(4):2206–11.
4. Itoh N, Ohta H. Pathophysiological roles of FGF signaling in the heart. Front Physiol. 2013;4:247.

5. Prié D, Forand A, Francoz C, Elie C, Cohen I, Courbebaisse M, Eladari D, Lebrec D, Durand F, Friedlander G. Plasma fibroblast growth factor 23 concentration is increased and predicts mortality in patients on the liver-transplant waiting list. PLoS ONE. 2013;8(6):e66182.

6. Zanchi C, Locatelli M, Benigni A, Corna D, Tomasoni S, Rottoli D, Gaspari F, Remuzzi G, Zoja C. Renal expression of FGF23 in progressive renal disease of diabetes and the effect of ace inhibitor. PLoS ONE. 2013;8(8):e70775.

7. Shimada T, Muto T, Urakawa I, Yoneya T, Yamazaki Y, Okawa K, Takeuchi Y, Fujita T, Fukumoto S, Yamashita T. Mutant FGF-23 responsible for autosomal dominant hypophosphatemic rickets is resistant to proteolytic cleavage and causes hypophosphatemia in vivo. Endocrinology. 2002;143(8):3179–82.

8. Ichikawa S, Sorenson AH, Austin AM, Mackenzie DS, Fritz TA, Moh A, Hui SL, Econs MJ. Ablation of the Galnt3 gene leads to low-circulating intact fibroblast growth factor 23 (Fgf23) concentrations and hyperphosphatemia despite increased Fgf23 expression. Endocrinology. 2009;150(6):2543–50.

9. Tagliabracci VS, Engel JL, Wiley SE, Xiao J, Gonzalez DJ, Nidumanda Appaiah H, Koller A, Nizet V, White KE, Dixon JE. Dynamic regulation of FGF23 by Fam20C phosphorylation, GalNAc-T3 glycosylation, and furin proteolysis. Proc Natl Acad Sci U S A. 2014;111(15):5520–5.

10. Imel EA, Peacock M, Gray AK, Padgett LR, Hui SL, Econs MJ. Iron modifies plasma FGF23 differently in autosomal dominant hypophosphatemic rickets and healthy humans. J Clin Endocrinol Metab. 2011;96(11):3541–9.

11. Kurosu H. Regulation of fibroblast growth factor-23 signaling by Klotho. J Biol Chem. 2006;281(10):6120–3.

12. Urakawa I, Yamazaki Y, Shimada T, Iijima K, Hasegawa H, Okawa K, Fujita T, Fukumoto S, Yamashita T. Klotho converts canonical FGF receptor into a specific receptor for FGF23. Nature. 2006;444(7120):770–4.

13. Imura A, Iwano A, Tohyama O, Tsuji Y, Nozaki K, Hashimoto N, Fujimori T, Nabeshima Y-I. Secreted Klotho protein in sera and CSF: implication for post-translational cleavage in release of Klotho protein from cell membrane. FEBS Lett. 2004;565(1–3):143–7.

14. Chen CD, Podvin S, Gillespie E, Leeman SE, Abraham CR. Insulin stimulates the cleavage and release of the extracellular domain of Klotho by ADAM10 and ADAM17. Proc Natl Acad Sci. 2007;104(50):19796–801.

15. Shimada T. Targeted ablation of Fgf23 demonstrates an essential physiological role of FGF23 in phosphate and vitamin D metabolism. J Clin Investig. 2004;113(4):561–8.

16. Yoshida T, Fujimori T, Nabeshima Y. Mediation of unusually high concentrations of 1,25-dihydroxyvitamin D in homozygous klotho mutant mice by increased expression of renal 1alpha-hydroxylase gene. Endocrinology. 2002;143(2):683–9.

17. Tsujikawa H. Klotho, a gene related to a syndrome resembling human premature aging, functions in a negative regulatory circuit of vitamin D endocrine system. Mol Endocrinol. 2003;17(12):2393–403.

18. Shimada T, Hasegawa H, Yamazaki Y, Muto T, Hino R, Takeuchi Y, Fujita T, Nakahara K, Fukumoto S, Yamashita T. FGF-23 is a potent regulator of vitamin D metabolism and phosphate homeostasis. J Bone Miner Res. 2003;19(3):429–35.

19. Bai X. Transgenic mice overexpressing human fibroblast growth factor 23 (R176Q) delineate a putative role for parathyroid hormone in renal phosphate wasting disorders. Endocrinology. 2004;145(11):5269–79.

20. Araya K, Fukumoto S, Backenroth R, Takeuchi Y, Nakayama K, Ito N, Yoshii N, Yamazaki Y, Yamashita T, Silver J, Igarashi T, Fujita T. A novel mutation in fibroblast growth factor 23 gene as a cause of tumoral calcinosis. J Clin Endocrinol Metab. 2005;90(10):5523–7.

21. Benet-Pages A, Orlik P, Strom TM, Lorenz-Depiereux B. An FGF23 missense mutation causes familial tumoral calcinosis with hyperphosphatemia. Hum Mol Genet. 2005;14(3):385–90.

22. Larsson T, Yu X, Davis SI, Draman MS, Mooney SD, Cullen MJ, White KE. A novel recessive mutation in fibroblast growth factor-23 causes familial tumoral calcinosis. J Clin Endocrinol Metab. 2005;90(4):2424–7.

23. Yamashita T. Fibroblast growth factor (FGF)-23 inhibits renal phosphate reabsorption by activation of the mitogen-activated protein Kinase pathway. J Biol Chem. 2002;277(31):28265–70.
24. Faul C, Amaral AP, Oskouei B, Hu M-C, Sloan A, Isakova T, Gutiérrez OM, Aguillon-Prada R, Lincoln J, Hare JM, Mundel P, Morales A, Scialla J, Fischer M, Soliman EZ, Chen J, Go AS, Rosas SE, Nessel L, Townsend RR, Feldman HI, St. John Sutton M, Ojo A, Gadegbeku C, Di Marco GS, Reuter S, Kentrup D, Tiemann K, Brand M, Hill JA, Moe OW, Kuro-o M, Kusek JW, Keane MG, Wolf M. FGF23 induces left ventricular hypertrophy. J Clin Investig. 2011;121(11):4393–408.
25. Wöhrle S, Bonny O, Beluch N, Gaulis S, Stamm C, Scheibler M, Müller M, Kinzel B, Thuery A, Brueggen J, Hynes NE, Sellers WR, Hofmann F, Graus-Porta D. FGF receptors control vitamin D and phosphate homeostasis by mediating renal FGF-23 signaling and regulating FGF-23 expression in bone. J Bone Miner Res. 2011;26(10):2486–97.
26. Yanochko GM, Vitsky A, Heyen JR, Hirakawa B, Lam JL, May J, Nichols T, Sace F, Trajkovic D, Blasi E. Pan-FGFR inhibition leads to blockade of FGF23 signaling, soft tissue mineralization, and cardiovascular dysfunction. Toxicol Sci Off J Soc Toxicol. 2013;135(2):451–64.
27. Olauson H, Lindberg K, Amin R, Sato T, Jia T, Goetz R, Mohammadi M, Andersson G, Lanske B, Larsson TE. Parathyroid-specific deletion of Klotho Unravels a Novel Calcineurin-Dependent FGF23 signaling pathway that regulates PTH secretion. PLoS Genet. 2013;9(12):e1003975.
28. Saito H. Circulating FGF-23 is regulated by 1,25-Dihydroxyvitamin D3 and phosphorus in vivo. J Biol Chem. 2004;280(4):2543–9.
29. Collins MT, Lindsay JR, Jain A, Kelly MH, Cutler CM, Weinstein LS, Liu J, Fedarko NS, Winer KK. Fibroblast growth factor-23 is regulated by 1alpha,25-dihydroxyvitamin D. J Bone Mineral Res: Off J Am Soc Bone Mineral Res. 2005;20(11):1944–50.
30. Yu X, Sabbagh Y, Davis S, Demay M, White K. Genetic dissection of phosphate- and vitamin D-mediated regulation of circulating Fgf23 concentrations. Bone. 2005;36(6):971–7.
31. Masuyama R, Stockmans I, Torrekens S, Van Looveren R, Maes C, Carmeliet P, Bouillon R, Carmeliet G. Vitamin D receptor in chondrocytes promotes osteoclastogenesis and regulates FGF23 production in osteoblasts. J Clin Invest. 2006;116(12):3150–9.
32. Haussler MR, Whitfield GK, Kaneko I, Forster R, Saini R, Hsieh JC, Haussler CA, Jurutka PW. The role of vitamin D in the FGF23, klotho, and phosphate bone-kidney endocrine axis. Rev Endocr Metab Disord. 2012;13(1):57–69.
33. Rhee Y, Bivi N, Farrow E, Lezcano V, Plotkin LI, White KE, Bellido T. Parathyroid hormone receptor signaling in osteocytes increases the expression of fibroblast growth factor-23 in vitro and in vivo. Bone. 2011;49(4):636–43.
34. Moe SM, Chertow GM, Parfrey PS, Kubo Y, Block GA, Correa-Rotter R, Drueke TB, Herzog CA, London GM, Mahaffey KW, Wheeler DC, Stolina M, Dehmel B, Goodman WG, Floege J. Evaluation of cinacalcet HTtLCETI. Cinacalcet, fibroblast growth factor-23, and cardiovascular disease in hemodialysis: the evaluation of cinacalcet HCl therapy to lower cardiovascular events (EVOLVE) trial. Circulation. 2015;132(1):27–39.
35. Sprague SM, Wetmore JB, Gurevich K, Da Roza G, Buerkert J, Reiner M, Goodman W, Cooper K. Effect of cinacalcet and vitamin D analogs on fibroblast growth factor-23 during the treatment of secondary hyperparathyroidism. Clin J Am Soc Nephrol: CJASN. 2015;10(6):1021–30.
36. Isakova T, Wahl P, Vargas GS, Gutiérrez OM, Scialla J, Xie H, Appleby D, Nessel L, Bellovich K, Chen J, Hamm L, Gadegbeku C, Horwitz E, Townsend RR, Anderson CAM, Lash JP, Hsu C-y, Leonard MB, Wolf M. Fibroblast growth factor 23 is elevated before parathyroid hormone and phosphate in chronic kidney disease. Kidney Int. 2011;79(12):1370–8.
37. Larsson T, Nisbeth U, Ljunggren O, Juppner H, Jonsson KB. Circulating concentration of FGF-23 increases as renal function declines in patients with chronic kidney disease, but does not change in response to variation in phosphate intake in healthy volunteers. Kidney Int. 2003;64(6):2272–9.
38. Hasegawa H, Nagano N, Urakawa I, Yamazaki Y, Iijima K, Fujita T, Yamashita T, Fukumoto S, Shimada T. Direct evidence for a causative role of FGF23 in the abnormal renal phosphate

handling and vitamin D metabolism in rats with early-stage chronic kidney disease. Kidney Int. 2010;78(10):975–80.

39. Shalhoub V, Shatzen EM, Ward SC, Davis J, Stevens J, Bi V, Renshaw L, Hawkins N, Wang W, Chen C, Tsai M-M, Cattley RC, Wronski TJ, Xia X, Li X, Henley C, Eschenberg M, Richards WG. FGF23 neutralization improves chronic kidney disease–associated hyperparathyroidism yet increases mortality. J Clin Investig. 2012;122(7):2543–53.

40. Olauson H, Larsson TE. FGF23 and Klotho in chronic kidney disease. Curr Opin Nephrol Hypertens. 2013;22(4):397–404.

41. Faul C. Fibroblast growth factor 23 and the heart. Curr Opin Nephrol Hypertens. 2012;21(4):369–75.

42. Fukumoto S. Anti-fibroblast growth factor 23 antibody therapy. Curr Opin Nephrol Hypertens. 2014;23(4):346–51.

Chapter 11
Wnt/Sclerostin and the Relation with Vitamin D in Chronic Kidney Disease

Mugurel Apetrii and Adrian Covic

Abstract The skeleton, while strong, isn't made of static tissue. It is a highly dynamic organ that constantly undergoes changes and regeneration. A continuous change is taking place, as osteoclasts degrade bone and osteoblasts rebuild new bone. This ongoing skeletal adaptation is greatly influenced by the amount of mechanical strain that the skeleton senses as a result of everyday movement and physical activity. However, many burning questions were, at least until recently, without an answer. In particular, was how does the skeleton "feel" mechanical strain and maybe most importantly how does it turn this information into the act of making more or less bone?

Keywords Bone • Osteoporosis • Sclerosteosis • Calcium • Phosphate • BMD • Vascular calcification • Vitamin D • FGF23

11.1 Introduction

The skeleton, while strong, isn't made of static tissue. It is a highly dynamic organ that constantly undergoes changes and regeneration. A continuous change is taking place, as osteoclasts degrade bone and osteoblasts rebuild new bone. This ongoing skeletal adaptation is greatly influenced by the amount of mechanical strain that the skeleton senses as a result of everyday movement and physical activity. However, many burning questions were, at least until recently, without an answer. In particular, was how does the skeleton "feel" mechanical strain and maybe most importantly how does it turn this information into the act of making more or less bone?

The answer to this question seems to be related to the nerve-like osteocyte network embedded throughout bone acting as a mechano sensor that allows the skeleton

M. Apetrii, MD, PhD (✉)
Nephrology Unit, Dr CI Parhon University Hospital, Iasi, Romania
e-mail: mugurelu_1980@yahoo.com

A. Covic, MD, PhD, FRCP (London), FERA
Nephrology and Internal Medicine, University "Grigore T. Popa", Iasi, Romania
e-mail: acccovic@gmail.com

© Springer International Publishing Switzerland 2016   207
P.A. Ureña Torres et al. (eds.), *Vitamin D in Chronic Kidney Disease*,
DOI 10.1007/978-3-319-32507-1_11

to "feel" and respond to mechanical strain. This network produces a powerful and cryptic inhibitory signal which most likely represents a master regulator of the skeleton. This master regulatory molecule, called sclerostin, is a glycoprotein (22 kDa) product of the SOST gene, which is localized at chromosome region 17q 12-p21 [1]. Inactivating mutations of this gene lead to a rare genetic disease characterized by high bone mass, namely sclerosteosis. The tremendous increase in bone mass and bone mineral density (BMD) that is observed in these patients is similar to what is seen in another autosomal recessive, inherited high bone mass disorder, Van Buchem disease. In the Van Buchem disease *SOST* itself is not mutated; however, there is a 52-kb deletion in the downstream region of the SOST gene that results in the absence of postnatal sclerostin production. Thus, both sclerosteosis and Van Buchem disease are causes by sclerostin deficiency, leading to the conclusion that sclerostin must be a natural brake for bone formation, preventing the body from making too much bone. When mechanical forces are applied to the bone, the osteocytes stop secreting sclerostin and bone formation is initiated on the bone surface.

Wnt/B-catenin signaling pathway is a critical regulator of skeletal development and mass, working in part through the stimulation of Runx2 gene expression. Activation of the canonical Wnt signaling involves the formation of a complex between Wnt proteins, frizzled and low density lipoprotein receptor-related protein 5 (LRP5) or LRP6 receptors. Osteocytes are the predominant cellular source of the Wnt antagonist sclerostin, a limiting factor for osteoblast generation and bone mass accrual that mediates the homeostatic adaptation of bone to mechanical loading. Sclerostin is a negative regulator of Wnt signaling. It binds to both LRP5 and LRP6 and prevents activation of the Wnt receptor complex, resulting in inhibition of bone formation. In addition to sclerostin, the DKK family members, particularly DKK-1 (Dickkopf-1), inhibit the Wnt pathway by binding to the LPR-5/6 receptor. Wnt signaling can also be blocked by other proteins, such as soluble frizzled-related protein, that bind to Wnt ligands.

Osteocytes effectively act as mechanoreceptors for bone formation, and sclerostin was shown to play a key role in the development of osteoporosis associated with lack of mechanical stimulation, as observed in weightless astronauts or in patients confined to bed for a long period of time. Most studies, in both the general and the osteoporotic populations, sustain this hypothesis by reporting a positive association between circulating sclerostin levels and bone mineral density (BMD).

Several clinical and biological variables have been described as determinants of sclerostin secretion. Among the most important of them, age and CKD have been found to be directly associated with increased circulating sclerostin concentrations, whereas an inverse correlation has been observed between circulating sclerostin and parathyroid hormone (PTH) levels and other bone biomarkers [2].

11.2   Sclerostin in CKD

In the setting of CKD, circulating sclerostin concentrations clearly increase as glomerular filtration rate (GFR) decreases reaching an almost four times higher serum sclerostin level in predialysis patients with CKD stage V than in participants with normal renal function [3]; whether this is due to reduced renal clearance, increased skeletal production, or both is still a subject of debate. Recently, Cejka et al. showed that excretion of sclerostin increases with declining renal function [4] thus invalidating the hypothesis that increasing serum levels of sclerostin in CKD patients are related only to renal retention. The reason for increased circulating levels of sclerostin is therefore linked to an increase in its production; this hypothesis has been also suggested by previous research of Sabbagh et al. using immunohistochemical staining of sclerostin in bone biopsies from CKD patients [5]. Thus, in an experimental study of mice experiencing progressive CKD, the repression of the Wnt/b-catenin pathway and its inhibitor sclerostin was associated with increased osteoclast activity and repression of bone formation suggesting a possible implication in pathogenesis of renal osteodystrophy [5]. However, the exact underlying mechanism of increased production of sclerostin in CKD is still a matter of debate. It has been suggested that PTH, which is a known repressor of SOST gene expression and an inhibitor of sclerostin production in normal situations [6] might have a role. Indeed, it is well known that uremia is associated with a renal and skeletal resistance to the actions of PTH [7], which may in some extent be related to the increased production of sclerostin in CKD patients. This finding may open new possible therapeutic strategies in which anti-sclerostin antibodies which are currently in development [8], might ameliorate bone formation rates especially in elderly osteoporotic subjects with some degree of renal impairment.

However, the PTH-sclerostin correlation is not consistent through all the studies. Thus, Kanbay et al. suggest a possible role of other factors including phosphorus and FGF23 in the regulation of sclerostin through a PTH-independent mechanism in CKD patients treated by hemodialysis (HD) [9]. Moreover, sclerostin at least partly regulates bone matrix mineralization through a signaling pathway involving phosphate regulators—the phosphate regulating neutral endopeptidase on chromosome X (PHEX) and the matrix extracellular phosphoglycoprotein (MEPE) axis [10]. However, the mechanism underlying the positive association between serum sclerostin levels and serum phosphate levels remains unclear. They seem to interact via another phosphate regulator like FGF23, PHEX or MEPE and thus regulating bone turnover, bone mineralization, and renal mineral homeostasis [10, 11].

In peritoneal dialysis patients, as in HD patients, there is also a higher than normal serum level of sclerostin which is inversely correlated with the degree of bone formation rate [12]. According to the KDIGO (Kidney Disease Improving Global Outcome) guidelines [13] and other studies [12], the most frequent pattern of renal osteodystrophy in PD is characterized by a low bone turnover, with the leading entity being adynamic bone disease. Sclerostin is therefore one potential "actor" that may play a role in the pathophysiology of adynamic bone disease.

In renal transplanted patients, sclerostin acknowledge a rapid decrease to normal or even subnormal values shortly after transplantation in contrast with the persistent elevation of PTH and FGF23 [14]. This decrease of sclerostin is probably due to the improvement of renal function, increased physical activity and use of glucocorticoids. Subsequently, in the first year after renal transplantation there is a gradual increase in serum sclerostin levels towards normal values; this rise is not influenced by the GFR, but paralleled the reduction of PTH and the normalization of serum calcium, phosphate and vitamin D concentrations [14].

Although preliminary data suggest that sclerostin may be a promising biomarker in assessing bone health in CKD patients, it is not clear whether it has any added value compared with existing bone biomarkers in predicting bone turnover and/or BMD. Its clinical utility in determining hard clinical end points such as fracture is unknown. Indeed, given that global bone strength is determined both by qualitative changes in bone (for instance, mineralization and turnover) and by quantitative changes in bone volume and density it is perhaps unrealistic to expect a single bio-marker to predict such outcomes. Therefore the biological significance and interpretation of circulating sclerostin levels in CKD remain uncertain.

11.3   Sclerostin and Vascular Calcification in CKD

Vascular calcifications (VCs) are recognized as a strong predictor of all-cause and cardiovascular mortality in CKD patients [15]. The discovery of CKD bone-vascular axis, addressing the complex interactions between bone and vessel which share similar underlying mechanisms, let bone turnover inhibitors emerge as potential risk factors for VC. More recently, attention has focused on sclerostin, a novel candidate for the bone-vascular axis.

Vascular smooth muscles cells undergo osteo/chondrogenic transdifferentiation in a pro-calcifying environment. In the late phase of VC, sclerostin is expressed. This can be interpreted as a defensive response that aims to block the Wnt pathway in order to reduce the mineralization in the vascular tissue. Sclerostin may spill over to the circulation and may reciprocally inhibit bone metabolism [16].

Several studies report a positive association between sclerostin and VC [15, 17] (Table 11.1); furthermore, expression of sclerostin has also been demonstrated in the vascular wall, in the calcification site [18]. However, once again other authors reported discordant results describing an inverse correlation between sclerostin and VC. Thus, in a cohort of hemodialyzed patients, those with more severe aortic calcifications had significantly lower serum sclerostin levels. In addition, low levels of sclerostin remained a significant predictor of cardiovascular outcome even after adjusting for age and gender, suggesting that Wnt/β-catenin signaling plays an additional role in uremic VC beyond aging [19].

11.4   Sclerostin and Mortality in CKD

Even if experimental and clinical studies suggest that the Wnt pathway may also play a role in atherosclerosis and vascular calcification, the association between sclerostin and mortality in CKD patients remains so far inconsistent (Table 11.2). In a post-hoc analysis in 100 prevalent HD patients, Viaene et al. [16], found a positive association between higher circulating sclerostin levels (defined as values superior to the median) and survival after a median follow-up time of 637 days.

Table 11.1 Association between sclerostin with vascular calcification

Trial, (year)	Study patients	Scl as independent determinant in vascular calcification
Qureshi et al. (2015) [31]	ESRD	Yes (Higher sclerostin levels were found with epigastric and coronary artery calcification)
Claes et al. (2013) [32]	Predialysis CKD	Yes (Patients with aortic calcifications had higher sclerostin levels, but in multivariate analysis, the association became inverse)
Desjardins et al. (2014) [33]	CKD stages 2-5D	No
Balci et al. (2015) [34]	Prevalent HD	Yes (Sclerostin level was significantly important in AVF calcification but it was not independent predictor of AVF dysfunction
Yang et al. (2015) [19]	Prevaent HD	Yes (Lower sclerostin levels were associated with the severity of aortic calcification)
Pelletier et al. (2015) [35]	Prevalent HD	Yes (Serum sclerostin was associated with a 33 % increase of severe AAC risk for each 0.1 ng/ml rise in serum sclerostin, $p < 0.001$)
Kim et al. (2011) [36]	Prevalent HD	Yes (Sclerostin and FGF-23 were independently associated with AAC)
Delanaye et al. (2014) [21]	Prevalent HD	No (The clinical interest of sclerostin to assess vascular calcifications in HD is limited, no association between sclerostin and calcification score in the univariate analysis, but association became significant and negative in the multivariate model)

The authors link this survival benefit to the possible attenuation of the progression of VC in the setting of high sclerostin [16]. However, within a fully adjusted model including bone-specific alkaline phosphatase the association between survival and sclerostin lost statistical significance [16]. In the same line, a very recent prospective study, from The (Netherlands) (the NECOSAD cohort), Drechsler et al. found that high or intermediate levels of circulating sclerostin were strongly associated with lower risk factor for future all-cause and cardiovascular mortality in 637 incident dialysis patients, particularly in the short term follow-up (18 months) [20]. The results were quite impressive, cardiovascular mortality being 70 % lower in patients of the highest tertile of sclerostin within 18 months when compared with patients of the lowest tertile. In addition, compared with Viaene et al. study, these results remained consistent even in the fully adjusted model. In contrast with the results previously reported, our group [9] found in 173 non-dialyzed patients with CKD stages 3–5 that higher sclerostin values were associated with fatal and non-fatal cardiovascular events after a mean follow-up of 26 months even after multiple

Table 11.2 Studies reporting the correlation between circulating sclerostin levels and mortality

Trial, (year)	Type	Patients number	Age (mean), (year)	Renal status and dialysis duration, (time)	Follow up (time)	Scl as independent determinant in CV events	Scl as independent determinant in CV mortality	Scl as independent determinant in all-cause mortality
Gonçalves et al. (2014) [37]	Cohort-single center-prospective	91	42±19	Hemodialysis	10 years	N/A	Yes	Yes
Viaene et al. (2013) [16]	Cohort-single center-prospective	100	68±13	Hemodialysis	637 days	N/A	N/A	Yes
Nowak et al. (2015) [22]	Cohort-multicenter-prospective	239	68±14	Hemodialysis	1461 days	N/A	No	No
Drechsler et al. (2015) [20]	Cohort-multicenter-prospective	673	63±14	Hemodialysis (93%) Peritoneal dialysis (7%)	4 years	N/A	Yes	Yes
Kanbay et al. (2014) [9]	Cohort-single center-prospective	173	47 (38–59)	CKD (nondialysis)	26 months	Yes	No	Yes
Desjardins et al. (2014) [33]	Cohort-single center-prospective	140	67±12	CKD (2–5 including 5D)	829 days	N/A	N/A	Yes

adjustments [9]. The discrepancy with previous studies might be related first of all with the different study population (hemodialysed vs. non-dialysed CKD patients) with different serum vitamin D, PTH, or calcium levels and thus with possible different underlying bone disease. Unfortunately neither study performed direct bone histomorphometry in order to confirm this hypothesis. To further complicate the understanding of the impact of sclerostin on mortality, Delanaye et al. [21] and Nowak et al. [22] found no correlation between serum sclerostin level and mortality in hemodialysis patients.

The potential reasons for these differences remain somewhat unclear. Some possible explanations are related to the heterogeneity of patients includes in those studies. Thus, the study of Viaene et al. included a higher proportion of diabetics and had an overall shorter dialysis vintage in the hemodialysis; the NECOSAD study by Drechsler et al. included incident (and not prevalent) patients of younger age; meanwhile, Kanbay et al. enrolled non-dialyzed CKD patients. Moreover, it is highly probable that all the patients included in the aforementioned studies had different medication like vitamin D or phosphate binders and different cardiovascular comorbidities which may thus confer a different impact on survival. Furthermore, different assays were used to measure the circulating sclerostin levels; even in healthy individuals these kits are not in perfect agreement; possible binding of sclerostin fragments may occur, and this could partly explain different values obtained.

11.5 Vitamin D and Sclerostin

Vitamin D is of paramount importance to skeletal development, integrity and health. Vitamin D homeostasis is typically deranged in a number of chronic conditions, of which CKD is one of the most important. The vitamin D or calcitriol receptor is not the classic, membrane-bound type, but rather a member of the nuclear receptor family located within the cytoplasm of the cell, and when activated by its ligand, travels into the nucleus and activates specific areas on the genome. Other members of this family include the steroid, sex hormone, retinoid, and thyroid hormone receptors. What makes these nuclear receptors unique is that each tissue containing these receptors has its own mix of regulatory proteins that repress or activate the receptor once it has been engaged by the ligand, causing it to change shape. The final conformational change induced by the natural ligand or its analogues will determine whether or not the receptor is active or inactive in that tissue. This is one of the reasons why the different analogues of active vitamin D will have different effects on various tissues from that of calcitriol and each other.

The effects of vitamin D on bone tissue as a whole are not yet fully understood but are likely due to a combination of direct effects via VDREs, downstream effects of the induced gene expression and effects at specific stages of bone cell proliferation and differentiation. One direct action that has been clearly demonstrated is the ability of plasma 1,25 vitamin D to stimulate bone resorption by the activation of osteoclast [23]. Furthermore, 1,25 vitamin D is capable of regulating osteoblast gene transcription, proliferation, differentiation and mineralization as was shown in in vitro studies [24, 25].

Vitamin D may also modulate the bone homeostasis by affecting key osteocytic genes and thus interfere with the sclerostin secretion. While it has not been studied in detail, it is likely that osteocytes are responsible for the majority of osteocalcin synthesis, which may be under the control of 1,25 vitamin D. The direct regulatory effect of 1,25 vitamin D on sclerostin was demonstrated by several studies. Thus, in one of them, treatment of human primary osteoblasts, including cells differentiated to an osteocyte-like stage, with 1,25 vitamin D resulted in the dose-dependent increased expression of SOST mRNA which may in turn increase the secretion of sclerostin [26]. The association between sclerostin and vitamin D was also reported in a cohort of patients suffering from hypercalciuria in which a positive correlation between sclerostin expression by osteocytes and serum 1,25D levels was depicted [27]. However, other in-vivo study reported a decrease in serum sclerostin level after vitamin D3 treatment in vitamin D-deficient young adult females [28]. This inconsistency with previous studies might be attributable to the fact that vitamin D deficiency affects osteocytes and thus alters serum sclerostin levels. Understanding the effects of vitamin D on serum sclerostin may improve knowledge of bone physiology; future studies should further investigate this complex physiological relationship.

11.6   Conclusions and Future Perspectives

In the last years, the Wnt/sclerostin pathway has been the focus of intense basic and clinical research in the bone field because of its importance in skeletal development and maintenance of bone mass. Disturbances in Wnt/sclerostin pathway can be added to the whole spectrum of changes associated with the CKD-MBD progression. However, the relative impact of this pathway on the progression of cardiovascular calcification and importantly on cardiovascular mortality requires additional investigation.

Growing evidence confers sclerostin a central role in the pathogenesis of CKD-MBD. This fact, all along with the rather disappointing results of current therapeutic strategies on hard-outcomes in CKD-MBD opens new perspectives for targeted therapy, including pharmacological neutralization of sclerostin or DKK1 by monoclonal antibodies. In the next years, sclerostin inhibition will probably become a possible approach in the bone anabolic treatment of osteoporosis. This is supported by several experimental studies in which anti-sclerostin antibodies were associated with improved bone properties [29] and decreased vascular calcification in combination with phosphate binders [30]. A potential concern is that the use of therapies to promote bone anabolism might have a negative impact on the cardiovascular disease. Conversely, improvement of bone health may reduce other risk factors that have higher impact on cardiac disease such as serum phosphate and FGF23. Additional studies are thus required to define determinants of Wnt inhibitors in

CKD and to evaluate the efficacy and safety of recently introduced pharmaceuticals inhibitors. Other questions related to the normal range of sclerostin through the different stages of CKD, to the standardization of current laboratory testing methods or to the effect of dialysis or other concurrent medication on sclerostin serum level need a definite answer before introducing sclerostin into day-by-day clinical practice.

References

1. Poole KE, et al. Sclerostin is a delayed secreted product of osteocytes that inhibits bone formation. FASEB J. 2005;19(13):1842–4.
2. Robling AG, et al. Mechanical stimulation of bone in vivo reduces osteocyte expression of Sost/sclerostin. J Biol Chem. 2008;283(9):5866–75.
3. Pelletier S, et al. The relation between renal function and serum sclerostin in adult patients with CKD. Clin J Am Soc Nephrol. 2013;8(5):819–23.
4. Cejka D, et al. Renal elimination of sclerostin increases with declining kidney function. J Clin Endocrinol Metab. 2014;99(1):248–55.
5. Sabbagh Y, et al. Repression of osteocyte Wnt/beta-catenin signaling is an early event in the progression of renal osteodystrophy. J Bone Miner Res. 2012;27(8):1757–72.
6. Keller H, Kneissel M. SOST is a target gene for PTH in bone. Bone. 2005;37(2):148–58.
7. Llach F, et al. Skeletal resistance to endogenous parathyroid hormone in patients with early renal failure. A possible cause for secondary hyperparathyroidism. J Clin Endocrinol Metab. 1975;41(2):339–45.
8. Padhi D, et al. Single-dose, placebo-controlled, randomized study of AMG 785, a sclerostin monoclonal antibody. J Bone Miner Res. 2011;26(1):19–26.
9. Kanbay M, et al. Serum sclerostin and adverse outcomes in nondialyzed chronic kidney disease patients. J Clin Endocrinol Metab. 2014;99(10):E1854–61.
10. Atkins GJ, et al. Sclerostin is a locally acting regulator of late-osteoblast/preosteocyte differentiation and regulates mineralization through a MEPE-ASARM-dependent mechanism. J Bone Miner Res. 2011;26(7):1425–36.
11. Asamiya Y, et al. Associations between the levels of sclerostin, phosphate, and fibroblast growth factor-23 and treatment with vitamin D in hemodialysis patients with low intact PTH level. Osteoporos Int. 2015;26(3):1017–28.
12. de Oliveira RA, et al. Peritoneal dialysis per se is a risk factor for sclerostin-associated adynamic bone disease. Kidney Int. 2015;87(5):1039–45.
13. Kidney Disease: Improving Global Outcomes (KDIGO) CKD-MBD Work Group. KDIGO clinical practice guideline for the diagnosis, evaluation, prevention, and treatment of Chronic Kidney Disease-Mineral and Bone Disorder (CKD-MBD). Kidney Int Suppl. 2009;(113): S1–130.
14. Bonani M, et al. Sclerostin blood levels before and after kidney transplantation. Kidney Blood Press Res. 2014;39(4):230–9.
15. Haas MH. The risk of death in patients with a high coronary calcification score: does it include predialysis patients? Kidney Int. 2010;77(12):1057–9.
16. Viaene L, et al. Sclerostin: another bone-related protein related to all-cause mortality in haemodialysis? Nephrol Dial Transplant. 2013;28(12):3024–30.
17. Hampson G, et al. The relationship between inhibitors of the Wnt signalling pathway (Dickkopf-1(DKK1) and sclerostin), bone mineral density, vascular calcification and arterial stiffness in post-menopausal women. Bone. 2013;56(1):42–7.
18. Didangelos A, et al. Extracellular matrix composition and remodeling in human abdominal aortic aneurysms: a proteomics approach. Mol Cell Proteomics. 2011;10(8):M111.008128.

19. Yang CY, et al. Circulating Wnt/beta-catenin signalling inhibitors and uraemic vascular calcifications. Nephrol Dial Transplant. 2015;30(8):1356–63.
20. Drechsler C, et al. High levels of circulating sclerostin are associated with better cardiovascular survival in incident dialysis patients: results from the NECOSAD study. Nephrol Dial Transplant. 2015;30(2):288–93.
21. Delanaye P, et al. Clinical and biological determinants of sclerostin plasma concentration in hemodialysis patients. Nephron Clin Pract. 2014;128(1–2):127–34.
22. Nowak A, et al. Sclerostin quo vadis? – is this a useful long-term mortality parameter in prevalent hemodialysis patients? Kidney Blood Press Res. 2015;40(3):266–76.
23. Suda T, et al. Vitamin D and bone. J Cell Biochem. 2003;88(2):259–66.
24. Atkins GJ, et al. RANKL expression is related to the differentiation state of human osteoblasts. J Bone Miner Res. 2003;18(6):1088–98.
25. Matsumoto T, et al. Stimulation by 1,25-dihydroxyvitamin D3 of in vitro mineralization induced by osteoblast-like MC3T3-E1 cells. Bone. 1991;12(1):27–32.
26. Wijenayaka AR, et al. 1alpha,25-dihydroxyvitamin D3 stimulates human SOST gene expression and sclerostin secretion. Mol Cell Endocrinol. 2015;413:157–67.
27. Menon VB, et al. Expression of fibroblast growth factor 23, vitamin D receptor, and sclerostin in bone tissue from hypercalciuric stone formers. Clin J Am Soc Nephrol. 2014;9(7):1263–70.
28. Cidem M, et al. Serum sclerostin is decreased following vitamin D treatment in young vitamin D-deficient female adults. Rheumatol Int. 2015;35(10):1739–42.
29. Moe SM, et al. Anti-sclerostin antibody treatment in a rat model of progressive renal osteodystrophy. J Bone Miner Res. 2015;30(3):499–509.
30. Fang Y, et al. CKD-induced wingless/integration1 inhibitors and phosphorus cause the CKD-mineral and bone disorder. J Am Soc Nephrol. 2014;25(8):1760–73.
31. Qureshi AR, et al. Increased circulating sclerostin levels in end-stage renal disease predict biopsy-verified vascular medial calcification and coronary artery calcification. Kidney Int. 2015;88:1356–64.
32. Claes KJ, et al. Sclerostin: Another vascular calcification inhibitor? J Clin Endocrinol Metab. 2013;98:3221–8.
33. Desjardins L, et al. Uremic toxicity and sclerostin in chronic kidney disease patients. Nephrol Ther. 2014;10:463–70.
34. Balci M, et al. Sclerostin as a new key player in arteriovenous fistula calcification. Herz. 2015;40:289–97.
35. Pelletier S, et al. Serum sclerostin: the missing link in the bone-vessel cross-talk in hemodialysis patients? Osteoporos Int. 2015;26:2165–74.
36. Kim KI, et al. A novel biomarker of coronary atherosclerosis: serum DKK1 concentration correlates with coronary artery calcification and atherosclerotic plaques. J Korean Med Sci. 2011;26:
37. Goncalves FL, et al. Serum sclerostin is an independent predictor of mortality in hemodialysis patients. BMC Nephrol. 2014;15:190.

Chapter 12
Vitamin D and Bone in Chronic Kidney Disease

Martine Cohen-Solal and Pablo A. Ureña Torres

Abstract The metabolic bone disorders induced by CKD have a major impact on bone fragility as illustrated by the high incidence of fractures in patients with CKD. These are the results of altered bone structure and mineralization both impairing the competence of bone to mechanical loading. Several mechanisms are involved such as the levels of bone remodeling and the production of hormones and soluble factors such as FGF23 and sclerostin. The main hormones are however parathyroid hormone (PTH) and vitamin D that closely regulate bone metabolism and structure. The levels of both native (Calcidiol or 25OH vitamin D) or active (Calcitriol or 1,25(OH)$_2$ vitamin D) are low in patients with CKD. The failure of 1α hydroxylation in patients with CKD is responsible for low 1,25(OH)$_2$ vitamin D levels that increase PTH levels and contribute to bone fractures. Administration of Calcitriol of derivatives reduces PTH levels, but insufficient data are available on the impact on bone mineral density and fractures. In contrast, Calcidiol fails to reduce PTH levels in end-stage renal disease, but contribute to ameliorate the mineralization and subsequently the bone capacity and pain. CKD-MBD is a complex disease involving several confounding factors that each contribute to the bone fragility. Improving the knowledge of the pathophysiology of CKD-MBD and the development of new tools are needed to identify patients at risk of fractures and improve their quality of life.

Keywords CKD-MBD • Fractures • Vitamin D • PTH • Osteoporosis • Renal osteodystrophy • Calcium • Phosphate • Bone mineral density

M. Cohen-Solal, MD, PhD (✉)
Rheumatology Department, Hospital Lariboisiere, Inserm U1132 and University Paris-Diderot, Paris, France
e-mail: Martine.cohen-solal@inserm.fr

P.A. Ureña Torres, MD, PhD
Ramsay-Générale de Santé, Service de Néphrologie et Dialyse, Clinique du Landy, Saint Ouen, France

Department of Renal Physiology, Necker Hospital, University of Paris V, René Descartes, Paris, France

© Springer International Publishing Switzerland 2016   217
P.A. Ureña Torres et al. (eds.), *Vitamin D in Chronic Kidney Disease*,
DOI 10.1007/978-3-319-32507-1_12

12.1   Introduction

Metabolic bone disorders in chronic kidney disease (CKD) are the results of altered mineral and bone metabolism (MBD) due to impaired renal function [1]. The bone pattern are secondary to multiple metabolic abnormalities such as decreased synthesis of 1,25-dihydroxyvitamin D, hypocalcemia, hyperphosphatemia, metabolic acidosis, decreased klotho, increased fibroblast growth factor 23 (FGF23) and sclerostin, and insufficiently inhibited parathyroid hormone (PTH) by calcium, vitamin D and FGF23 because of the reduced expression of the calcium-sensing receptor, vitamin D receptor (VDR) and klotho in uremic parathyroid cells [2–4]. In addition, there is an insensitivity of bone cells to PTH because of the downregulation of its receptor in osteoblast cells [5]. Bone diseases which are induced by these abnormalities are highly variable from one patient to another and influence the metabolism of calcium and phosphate through bone tissue which is the main mineral reservoir. Moreover, the bone diseases related to CKD are linked to major extraskeletal complications such as vascular calcifications, making the regulation of the mineral disorder an important target to avoid other tissues alterations [6]. In this chapter, we will review the clinical effect of vitamin D on bone and the potential impact use for therapies. The identification of bone mineral mechanisms related to CKD will provide elements in order to prevent mineral disorders and fractures.

12.2   Metabolism of Vitamin D in CKD

Vitamin D is provided by diet (ergocalciferol or D2 and cholecalciferol or D3) or synthetized by the skin (D3) [7]. Cholecalciferol is then transported by vitamin D binding protein (DBP) to the liver where it is converted to 25-hydroxivitamin D (calcidiol) by the enzyme 25-hydroxylase. This native form is stored in the lipid tissues and available to progressively generate an active metabolite. The 1α hydroxylase then converts calcidiol to 1,25 dihydroxivitamin D (calcitriol) in the kidney. Calcitriol is the active form and acts as a hormone with several endocrine and immune functions. The synthesis of calcitriol is regulated by PTH, calcium, phosphate, and FGF23 whereas PTH increases 1 α hydroxylase activity. Anomalies of vitamin D metabolism are one of the most important factors in the pathogenesis of secondary hyperparathyroidism and features of CKD-MBD. In addition, many observational studies have shown an association with vitamin D disturbance, i.e. low circulating levels of vitamin D in CKD and cardiovascular disease [8].

Patients with CKD have low circulating calcidiol levels [9]. The levels of 25(OH)D are inversely associated with the glomerular filtration rate (GFR) in a dose-dependent manner. The low levels are observed at early stages of CKD, beginning before other mineral metabolism disturbances [10]. The prevalence of vitamin D deficiency (25(OH)D <15 ng/ml) in the population with CKD is higher than in the general population, ranging from 28 % for a GFR of 60 ml/mn to 51 % for a GFR below

15 ml/mn. The serum 25(OH)D levels are influenced by other known risk factor such as ethnicity, diabetes, hypertension and albuminuria [9]. In contrast, there is an association between bone disease in CKD and calcidiol level in small series that used bone biopsies. However, optimal 25(OH)D3 levels are required to allow the deposition of minerals in bone and prevent osteomalacia [11, 12]. Therefore, calcidiol might have a direct impact on bone mineralization by promoting the deposition of calcium.

Calcitriol levels are also low in CKD. Its production is stimulated by PTH and by low calcium while it is reduced by high phosphate and FGF23. The binding of 1α-25-dihydroxyvitamin D3 to its receptor induces gut absorption of calcium and phosphate, decreases PTH synthesis and stimulates FGF23. Calcitriol levels are low in CKD patients as the results of reduced renal 1a hydroxylase activity and low stock of its substrate calcidiol. This latter are the common causes shared with non-CKD patients such as low sun exposure or diet restriction which further decreased the generation of calcitriol in end-stage renal disease (ESRD). The raise in FGF23 levels occurs in early stages of CKD and precedes the decrease in calcitriol. The administration of low doses of calcitriol reduces serum PTH levels. A Renal Cochrane group assessed the impact of various active vitamin D compounds such as calcitriol in 894 patients with CKD on biomarkers [13]. Supplementation with active forms of vitamin D did not change the risk of mortality nor did postpone the need for dialysis. However, a 30 % reduction of serum PTH was achieved allowing a reduction of other treatment that targeted calcium and phosphate. All those metabolic effects influence the rate of bone turnover and subsequently bone mineral density, bone fragility and the risk of skeletal fracture (Fig. 12.1).

12.3   Different Forms of Renal Osteodystrophy in CKD-MBD

The classification of different forms of CKD-MBD has evolved in recent years. Several parameters has been included that are interrelated and participate to the bone fragility such as the levels of bone turnover, bone density and bone mineralization [14]. All these factors separately or synergistically contribute to skeletal fragility and the high risk of fractures in CKD [15]. However, these indices are poorly correlated because they measure different aspects of bone such as structure or mineral deposition in addition that some of them are variable during the course of CKD. Therefore, bone biopsy remains the gold standard for classifying different forms of renal osteodystrophy (RO) although more rarely done. The rate of bone turnover assessed by cycline double labeling and the thickness of osteoid are the main parameters that define the forms of RO [12, 16–18]. These indices allow separating high bone turnover forms from the low bone turnover ones including osteomalacia, which is characterized by a mineralization defect and adynamic bone disease mainly defined by a low bone remodeling rate. Using this definition, the prevalence of each bone disease has changed the last decades, adynamic bone diseases being the most common in contrast to a high frequency of high bone

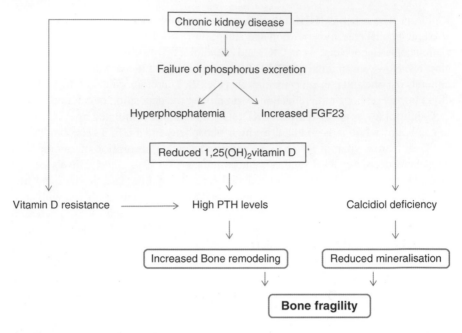

Fig. 12.1 Metabolic effects influencing the rate of bone turnover and subsequently bone mineral density, bone fragility and the risk of skeletal fracture

remodeling types that were observed in the late 1980s [19]. This illustrates the effort made by the nephrologists to reduce PTH secretion and to keep controlled secondary hyperparathyroidism. This new profile could however reflect moderately the current prevalence because of several biases. Bone biopsies are generally performed in symptomatic patients or at the inclusion of patients participating in clinical trials, which may not reflect the whole CKD population and may be limited by the presence of many confounding factors. Interestingly, the bone volume parameter has been added to the criterion of CKD-MBD in addition to bone remodeling rate, which clearly illustrates the interest for osteoporosis, an outgrowing bone complication that can lead to fractures.

The accuracy of serum PTH levels to predict or diagnose a given type of RO is low, which has led the experts of the Kidney Disease Improving Global Outcomes (KDIGO) to change the recommendations of the PTH target value in CKD, which is now targeting levels between two and nine times the upper normal value of the assays [15]. In non CKD patients, bone biomarkers are useful tools to assess the level of bone remodeling, which is a good predictive factor of bone fragility. Total and bone-specific alkaline phosphatase serum levels are the most used biomarkers on bone metabolism in addition to PTH. However, the sensitivity and the specificity of these two biomarkers are modest regarding the prediction of the type of RO. Indeed, the sensitivity and the specificity do not exceed 80 % for PTH value of 200 pg/ml in order to differentiate patients with high and low bone turnover diseases [20]. However, a significant number of patients with serum PTH levels between two and four times the upper normal values have adynamic bone disease [21]. Serum total and bone-specific alkaline phosphatases have quite comparable sensitivity value to that of serum PTH to predict high bone turnover disease. However, serum total and bone-specific alkaline phosphatases do not have a good sensitivity to predict adynamic osteopathy, hence less than 60 % of subjects with bone-specific alkaline phosphatase value lower than 20 g/ml have histological signs of low bone turnover disease [20]. This was confirmed in 492 patients in whom PTH and alkaline phosphatase alone and in combination discriminated the extremes low or high bone remodeling diseases, as defined histologically and despite of their low sensitivity and specificity [22].

New circulating bone biomarkers could have an additive value for the prediction of bone fragility. FGF23 is synthesized by osteocytes and subjects with normal renal function and high levels of FGF23 have mineralization defects mainly attributed to hypophosphatemia. In contrast, in CKD patients treated by in dialysis, serum phosphate levels are high despite the extremely increased levels of circulating FGF23. No significant relationship could be demonstrated between biomarkers of bone turnover or bone mineral density (BMD) with serum FGF23 levels, suggesting that FGF23 had no direct effect on BMD in adult dialyzed CKD subjects [23], whereas serum FGF23 levels are inversely correlated with histomorphometric parameters of mineralization in CKD children tretaed by peritoneal dialysis [24]. Sclerostin and Dickkopf-1 (Dkk-1), Wingless integration site (Wnt) inhibitors that reduce bone formation, could also play a role in bone diseases related to CKD and might explain the low bone formation observed in some uremic forms [4]. Serum sclerostin levels were higher in CKD patients than in normal women [25]. Serum sclerostin levels are negatively correlated to PTH but not with bone-specific alkaline phosphatases or DKK-1. Surprisingly, serum sclerostin levels are positively correlated with BMD, bone microarchitecture, and histomorphometric parameters of bone turnover. In addition, high serum sclerostin levels have been associated with reduced risk of mortality in CKD patients treated by dialysis [25–27]. Basal serum levels of sclerostin and tartrate resistant acid phosphatase (TRAP), a marker of bone resorption, are good predictors of bone loss in CKD patients as measured by DEXA or QCT [28]. Overall, these biomarkers could reflect the severity of the bone disease, which may also partly explain the increased risk of the mortality.

12.4   Bone Fragility in CKD

Fractures are more common in patients with CKD than in the age and gender-matched peoples from the general population. They are dramatic events since they increase the rate of mortality and the length of hospital stay [29–32]. Data obtained from the United Stated and French registers with large number of patients showed that the risk of hip fracture is at least four times higher in subjects with CKD [32–34]. These skeletal fractures maily affect peripheral bones and vertebrae although this latter site is rarely documented [35]. The risk of femoral fractures increases with age, female gender and a history of fracture of the femoral neck [30, 36, 37]. In addition to these common factors shared with patients with normal kidney function, diabetes and cardiovascular diseases such as hypertension and vascular calcifications are predominant and might explain part of the bone fragility [32, 34]. Nevertheless, no specific mechanism has been shown and this might be related to an amplification of comorbidity factors in relation to uremia and mineral disorders.

Fragility fractures related to low bone strength involves a reduction of both bone quantity and quality. Quantity of bone can be easily measured by the bone mineral density (BMD) which is a predictive factor as each reduction of one standard deviation (−1 SD) doubled the risk of fractures. Bone quality includes several factors such as the geometry, bone microarchitecture, the properties of the matrix and the rate of bone remodeling. The relationship between BMD and fracture is not clear in CKD patients. At the lumbar spine, this measurement is biased by spinal osteoarthritis and by the presences of vascular calcification particularly in CKD patients on dialysis [18]. The radius and the hip are better site for the assessment of the risk of fracture as the cortical component represent up to 90 % of the site proximal bone density. Indeed, there is a negative correlation between BMD at the radius and serum PTH levels [38]. In a recent meta-analysis carried out on six of these studies, it was observed the decrease of BMD at the spine and radius, but not at the femoral neck, was significantly associated with the risk of fractures [39]. However, the number of patients included in that meta-analysis was weak and the difference in BMD between patients with and without fractures was too small to allow guidelines for clinical practice. However, adding the assessment of FRAX indices to BMD could be an useful tool for risk fracture prediction [40]. Overall, BMD measure is not as useful in patients with CKD as in the general population. One of the reason is that there is no long term prospective study in CKD in which it is possible to assess the value of BMD to predict fractures and follows the patients. Moreover, the weak predictive value can be explained by the lack of discrimination of the measure of cortical bone which is the target of PTH. This could be now addressed by micro-computerized tomography (μCT). Indeed, the 1-year follow-up of 53 patients with CKD demonstrated that bone loss affects mainly the cortical bone [41]. The thickness of cortical bone was reduced due to increased bone resorption at the endocortical surface and was correlated to the serum levels of PTH, the levels of 25(OH) vitamin D being within the normal range. These results are consistent with a higher prevalence of peripheral fracture in patients with the highest PTH levels (above 900 pg/ml) in the DOPPS cohort [37]. The attempts to reduce PTH are also associated with a reduction of fracture occurrence in the presence of risk factors. Indeed, the 12 % incidence of peripheral fractures is similar with cinacalcet than with placebo in 3,883 patients on hemodialysis, but was significantly reduced when adjusted to factors predisposing to fracture such as fracture history or tobacco [42]. Finally, abnormalities of extracellular bone matrix due to diabetes (glycation of collagen, modification of crosslinks or accumulation of cations such as aluminum, fluoride, strontium) may well have a role in the bone fragility.

A major point is to liaise the above parameters that are available in order to draw guidelines. Each one of the parameters described above such as BMD, bone histology, microarchitecture and the degree of bone remodeling contribute to bone fragility and the increase risk of fractures in CKD-MBD. However, the lack of correlation between them does not allow an accurate prediction. High bone remodeling assessed by PTH appears to be the more consistent. Indeed, in patients without CKD, high bone remodeling is associated with an increased risk of fracture while it is prevented by treatment that reduce bone turnover. This relationship is not clear-cut in CKD. Hip fractures occur in the presence of low PTH levels only in small cross-sectional studies [35, 43]. However, prospective studies demonstrated that high bone turnover assessed by PTH is the main risk factor. Undoubtedly, high PTH levels are one of the targets, but not the only one.

12.5   Impact of Low Vitamin D on Bone Metabolism in CKD

There are only a scarce number of studies looking at the impact of vitamin D insufficiency and deficiency on mineral metabolism, bone mineral density and the risk of bone fracture in CKD patients. In an Italian retrospective study carried out in 104 CKD patients undergoing chronic hemodialysis and not receiving any vitamin D compound, the bone histology showed that subjects with serum 25(OH)D lower than 15 ng/ml had decreased bone formation rate and lower trabecular mineralization surfaces than the control group, and these alterations were independent of PTH and calcitriol values [44]. A second study comprising 130 patients with CKD not yet treated by dialysis showed that patients exhibiting skeletal fractures had significantly lower serum 25(OH)D levels (15.8 ng/ml) than those without fractures (30.0 ng/ml), they were also more likely female, had longer duration of CKD and lower BMD values at the distal radius. In multivariate analyses serum 25(OH)D levels, radius BMD, and low PTH (<100 pg/ml), and history of fractures were independently associated with high risk of suffering a new skeletal fracture after initiation of dialysis therapy [45]. Another study in 69 hemodialysis patients showed a high prevalence of vitamin D deficiency (59 %), a significant negative correlation between serum 25(OH)D and PTH levels, and a positive correlation between 25(OH)D and BMD at the radius. Low vitamin D values were also independently associated with reduced BMD at the calcaneous as assessed by ultrasounds [46]. Vitamin D insufficiency has also been largely recognized to be associated with increased subperiostal bone resorption and with decreased BMD at the lumbar spine and the wrist in CKD dialysis patients [47, 48].

12.6   Treatment of Bone Fragility in Patients with CKD

The treatment of CKD-MBD should target the correction of mineral disorders, the prevention of osteoporosis and the reduction of the risk of fracture. The treatment of osteoporosis in CKD is restricted as the therapies available for the common osteoporosis are contraindicated in CKD patients with a GFR below 30 ml/min. CKD reduces the elimination of bisphosphonates and strontium ranelate, which therefore may accumulate a greater extent with the potential risk of inducing a bone mineralization defect. Unlike common osteoporosis, fractures and low BMD in CKD can be accompanied by low or high bone turnover, which raised the question of the rationale of reducing bone resorption in the first situation. Therefore, antiresorptive treatment should not be prescribed in CKD without a prior bone biopsy in order to eliminate the presence of an adynamic bone disease that could be aggravated by such a therapy. This is reasonable also in the case of therapy by bisphosphonates, which appear to further decrease bone remodeling in case of CKD [18].

Because of these reasons, there is no randomized clinical trial in CKD assessing the effect of bisphosphonates on BMD and fracture risk. However, there are very few observational reports with these treatments whose results are not convincing in terms of BMD or risk of fractures, the number of events being too small. A controlled clinical trial carried out on 50 women with CKD undergoing hemodialysis and treated by raloxifene, a molecule not cleared by the kidney, showed an increase in BMD at the lumbar spine and the absence of important side effects [49], the treatment was restricted to postmenopausal women.

If fractures or low BMD are associated with high PTH levels, reduction of PTH levels should improve bone quality and decrease the risk of fracture. Indeed, analysis of 4 placebo controlled trials with Cinacalcet, designed to reduce PTH in CKD patients undergoing dialysis and with secondary hyperparathyroidism, also significantly reduced the incidence of fracture [50]. However, the large prospective randomized clinical trial EVOLVE failed to decrease the fracture risk in the intention-to-treat analysis [42]. One of the reasons of this failure might be the number of confounding factors that could influence the occurrence of fractures in these patients. Indeed, the fracture rate was lower in patients with risk factor such as history of fracture or tobacco use. These data demonstrate that a reduction in serum PTH levels should be reinforced in dialysis patients exposed to additional risk of fracture. Finally, Denosumab, an anti-RANKL biotherapy, efficient for the treatment of osteoporosis, has not been assessed for BMD and risk of fractures in patients with CKD. Although the use of Denosumab will be limited to patients with high bone remodeling, this treatment may also induce mineral disorders that should retain attention [51].

12.7 Treatment of Bone Fragility by Vitamin D in Patients with CKD

The treatment of CKD-MBD should also target the mineral disorders in particular should refrain PTH secretion by vitamin D. In subjects with normal kidney function, administration of natural vitamin D or calcidiol is necessary to reduce secondary hyperparathyroidism related to 25-hydroxy vitamin D deficiency. A supplementation of 50,000 IU of vitamin D weekly contributes to the significantly reduction of PTH in subjects with CKD stage 3, but not with CKD stage 5 [52]. Such a treatment is however needed as calcidiol might also contribute to the mineralization of bone which is of particular interest in high remodeling states despite negative results [44] or reduce the risk of mortality [53, 54]. A recent meta-analysis, including 17 observational studies and 5 RCTs, showed that natural vitamin D supplementation, ergocalciferol or cholecalciferol, significantly increased serum 25(OH)D levels and reduced serum PTH concentration, which was more pronounced in dialysis patients. These changes were induced with a very low incidence of mild and reversible hypercalcemia (<3 %) and hyperphosphatemia (<7 %). However, in none of these studies bone related outcomes such as bone pain, BMD and bone fractures as well as cardiovascular outcomes were assessed. The studies were also of low to moderate quality [55].

Administration of calcitriol is based on the failure of 1a-hydroxylation, the supplementation of which might reduce PTH levels. Administration of calcitriol reduces serum PTH levels and improved the survival, but the impact on fractures is unknown [13, 56, 57]. The limitation is that doses of calcitriol (>3 µg/week) are associated with hypercalcemia and worse control of hyperphosphatemia. Several derivatives have been developed such as Paricalcidol, which provided similar effects [58] and can be used in association with Cinacalcet, however no clinical studies has assessed the protective effect on BMD and the risk of fracture.

In conclusion, the complexity of CKD-MBD relies on the presence of several confounding factors that include mineral metabolism and regulation of bone remodeling as well as the structure of bone. All these factors contribute to the bone fragility and the promotion of skeletal fractures, which when occurring greatly impair the quality of life of these subjects. Better understanding of the pathophysiology of CKD-MBD and the development of tools to identify patients at risk are needed to prevent skeletal fractures.

References

1. Cozzolino M, Urena-Torres P, Vervloet MG, et al. Is chronic kidney disease-mineral bone disorder (CKD-MBD) really a syndrome? Nephrol Dial Transplant 2014;29:1815–20.
2. Slatopolsky E, Brown A, Dusso A. Calcium, phosphorus and vitamin D disorders in uremia. Contrib Nephrol. 2005;149:261–71.
3. Tominaga Y. Kidney and bone update : the 5-year history and future of CKD-MBD. Parathyroidectomy for secondary hyperparathyroidism. Clin Calcium. 2012;22:1083–8.
4. Vervloet M, Massy Z, Brandenburg VM, et al. Bone: a new endocrine organ at the heart of chronic kidney disease and mineral disorders. Lancet Diabetes-Endocrinol. 2014;2:427–36.
5. Urena P, Ferreira A, Morieux C, Drueke T, de Vernejoul MC. PTH/PTHrP receptor mRNA is down-regulated in epiphyseal cartilage growth plate of uraemic rats. Nephrol Dial Transplant. 1996;11:2008–16.
6. Brandenburg VM, Vervloet MG, Marx N. The role of vitamin D in cardiovascular disease: from present evidence to future perspectives. Atherosclerosis. 2012;225:253–63.
7. Holick MF. Vitamin D, for health and in chronic kidney disease. Semin Dial. 2005;18:266–75.

8. Brandenburg VM, Kruger T. Calcifediol – more than the stepchild of CKD-MBD therapy? Curr Vasc Pharmacol. 2014;12:286–93.
9. Urena-Torres P, Metzger M, Haymann JP, et al. Association of kidney function, vitamin D deficiency, and circulating markers of mineral and bone disorders in CKD. Am J Kidney Dis. 2011;58:544–53.
10. Gal-Moscovici A, Sprague SM. Use of vitamin D in chronic kidney disease patients. Kidney Int. 2010;78:146–51.
11. Anderson PH, Lam NN, Turner AG, et al. The pleiotropic effects of vitamin D in bone. J Steroid Biochem Mol Biol. 2013;136:190–4.
12. Malluche HH, Mawad H, Monier-Faugere MC. Effects of treatment of renal osteodystrophy on bone histology. Clin J Am Soc Nephrol. 2008;3 Suppl 3:S157–63.
13. Palmer SC, McGregor DO, Craig JC, Elder G, Macaskill P, Strippoli GF. Vitamin D compounds for people with chronic kidney disease not requiring dialysis. Cochrane Database Syst Rev. 2009;(4):CD008175.
14. Moe S, Drueke T, Cunningham J, et al. Definition, evaluation, and classification of renal osteodystrophy: a position statement from Kidney Disease: Improving Global Outcomes (KDIGO). Kidney Int. 2006;69:1945–53.
15. KDIGO. KDIGO clinical practice guideline for the diagnosis, evaluation, prevention, and treatment of Chronic Kidney Disease-Mineral and Bone Disorder (CKD-MBD). Kidney Int. 2009;Suppl 113:S1–130.
16. Malluche HH, Porter DS, Monier-Faugere MC, Mawad H, Pienkowski D. Differences in bone quality in low- and high-turnover renal osteodystrophy. J Am Soc Nephrol. 2012;23:525–32.
17. Ott SM. Bone histomorphometry in renal osteodystrophy. Semin Nephrol. 2009;29:122–32.
18. Ott SM. Review article: bone density in patients with chronic kidney disease stages 4–5. Nephrology (Carlton). 2009;14:395–403.
19. Malluche HH, Mawad HW, Monier-Faugere MC. Renal osteodystrophy in the first decade of the new millennium: analysis of 630 bone biopsies in black and white patients. J Bone Miner Res. 2011;26:1368–76.
20. Urena P, Hruby M, Ferreira A, Ang KS, de Vernejoul MC. Plasma total versus bone alkaline phosphatase as markers of bone turnover in hemodialysis patients. J Am Soc Nephrol. 1996;7:506–12.
21. Barreto FC, Barreto DV, Moyses RM, et al. K/DOQI-recommended intact PTH levels do not prevent low-turnover bone disease in hemodialysis patients. Kidney Int. 2008;73:771–7.
22. Sprague SM, Bellorin-Font E, Jorgetti V, et al. Diagnostic accuracy of bone turnover markers and bone histology in patients with CKD treated by dialysis. Am J Kidney Dis. 2016;67: 559–66.
23. Urena Torres P, Friedlander G, de Vernejoul MC, Silve C, Prie D. Bone mass does not correlate with the serum fibroblast growth factor 23 in hemodialysis patients. Kidney Int. 2008;73: 102–7.
24. Wesseling-Perry K, Pereira RC, Tseng CH, et al. Early skeletal and biochemical alterations in pediatric chronic kidney disease. Clin J Am Soc Nephrol. 2012;7:146–52.
25. Cejka D, Herberth J, Branscum AJ, et al. Sclerostin and Dickkopf-1 in renal osteodystrophy. Clin J Am Soc Nephrol. 2011;6:877–82.
26. Drechsler C, Evenepoel P, Vervloet MG, et al. High levels of circulating sclerostin are associated with better cardiovascular survival in incident dialysis patients: results from the NECOSAD study. Nephrol Dial Transplant. 2015;30:288–93.
27. Viaene L, Behets GJ, Claes K, et al. Sclerostin: another bone-related protein related to all-cause mortality in haemodialysis? Nephrol Dial Transplant. 2013;28:3024–30.
28. Malluche HH, Davenport DL, Cantor T, Monier-Faugere MC. Bone mineral density and serum biochemical predictors of bone loss in patients with CKD on dialysis. Clin J Am Soc Nephrol. 2014;9:1254–62.
29. Beaubrun AC, Kilpatrick RD, Freburger JK, Bradbury BD, Wang L, Brookhart MA. Temporal trends in fracture rates and postdischarge outcomes among hemodialysis patients. J Am Soc Nephrol. 2013;24:1461–9.

30. Maravic M, Ostertag A, Torres PU, Cohen-Solal M. Incidence and risk factors for hip fractures in dialysis patients. Osteoporos Int. 2014;25:159–65.
31. Naylor KL, McArthur E, Leslie WD, et al. The three-year incidence of fracture in chronic kidney disease. Kidney Int. 2014;86:810–8.
32. Tentori F, McCullough K, Kilpatrick RD, et al. High rates of death and hospitalization follow bone fracture among hemodialysis patients. Kidney Int. 2014;85:166–73.
33. Alem AM, Sherrard DJ, Gillen DL, et al. Increased risk of hip fracture among patients with end-stage renal disease. Kidney Int. 2000;58:396–9.
34. Maravic M, Briot K, Roux C, College Francais des Medecins R. Burden of proximal humerus fractures in the French National Hospital Database. Orthop Traumatol Surg Res. 2014;100:931–4.
35. Atsumi K, Kushida K, Yamazaki K, Shimizu S, Ohmura A, Inoue T. Risk factors for vertebral fractures in renal osteodystrophy. Am J Kidney Dis. 1999;33:287–93.
36. Dooley AC, Weiss NS, Kestenbaum B. Increased risk of hip fracture among men with CKD. Am J Kidney Dis. 2008;51:38–44.
37. Jadoul M, Albert JM, Akiba T, et al. Incidence and risk factors for hip or other bone fractures among hemodialysis patients in the Dialysis Outcomes and Practice Patterns Study. Kidney Int. 2006;70:1358–66.
38. Urena P, Bernard-Poenaru O, Ostertag A, et al. Bone mineral density, biochemical markers and skeletal fractures in haemodialysis patients. Nephrol Dial Transplant. 2003;18:2325–31.
39. Jamal SA, Hayden JA, Beyene J. Low bone mineral density and fractures in long-term hemodialysis patients: a meta-analysis. Am J Kidney Dis. 2007;49:674–81.
40. Jamal SA, West SL, Nickolas TL. The clinical utility of FRAX to discriminate fracture status in men and women with chronic kidney disease. Osteoporos Int. 2014;25:71–6.
41. Nickolas TL. The utility of circulating markers to predict bone loss across the CKD spectrum. Clin J Am Soc Nephrol. 2014;9:1160–2.
42. Moe SM, Abdalla S, Chertow GM, et al. Effects of cinacalcet on fracture events in patients receiving hemodialysis: the EVOLVE trial. J Am Soc Nephrol. 2015;26:1466–75.
43. Coco M, Rush H. Increased incidence of hip fractures in dialysis patients with low serum parathyroid hormone. Am J Kidney Dis. 2000;36:1115–21.
44. Coen G, Mantella D, Manni M, et al. 25-hydroxyvitamin D levels and bone histomorphometry in hemodialysis renal osteodystrophy. Kidney Int. 2005;68:1840–8.
45. Ambrus C, Almasi C, Berta K, et al. Vitamin D insufficiency and bone fractures in patients on maintenance hemodialysis. Int Urol Nephrol. 2011;43:475–82.
46. Mucsi I, Almasi C, Deak G, et al. Serum 25(OH)-vitamin D levels and bone metabolism in patients on maintenance hemodialysis. Clin Nephrol. 2005;64:288–94.
47. Fournier A, Bordier P, Gueris J, et al. Comparison of 1 alpha-hydroxycholecalciferol and 25-hydroxycholecalciferol in the treatment of renal osteodystrophy: greater effect of 25-hydroxycholecalciferol on bone mineralization. Kidney Int. 1979;15:196–204.
48. Stanbury SW. Azotaemic renal osteodystrophy. Br Med Bull. 1957;13:57–60.
49. Hernandez E, Valera R, Alonzo E, et al. Effects of raloxifene on bone metabolism and serum lipids in postmenopausal women on chronic hemodialysis. Kidney Int. 2003;63:2269–74.
50. Cunningham J, Danese M, Olson K, Klassen P, Chertow GM. Effects of the calcimimetic cinacalcet HCl on cardiovascular disease, fracture, and health-related quality of life in secondary hyperparathyroidism. Kidney Int. 2005;68:1793–800.
51. Chen CL, Chen NC, Liang HL, et al. Effects of denosumab and calcitriol on severe secondary hyperparathyroidism in dialysis patients with low bone mass. J Clin Endocrinol Metab. 2015;100:2784–92.
52. Al-Aly Z. Vitamin D, as a novel nontraditional risk factor for mortality in hemodialysis patients: the need for randomized trials. Kidney Int. 2007;72:909–11.
53. Barreto DV, Barreto Fde C, Carvalho AB, et al. Association of changes in bone remodeling and coronary calcification in hemodialysis patients: a prospective study. Am J Kidney Dis. 2008;52:1139–50.

54. Mehrotra R, Kermah DA, Salusky IB, et al. Chronic kidney disease, hypovitaminosis D, and mortality in the United States. Kidney Int. 2009;76:977–83.
55. Kandula P, Dobre M, Schold JD, Schreiber Jr MJ, Mehrotra R, Navaneethan SD. Vitamin D supplementation in chronic kidney disease: a systematic review and meta-analysis of observational studies and randomized controlled trials. Clin J Am Soc Nephrol. 2011;6:50–62.
56. Baker LR, Abrams L, Roe CJ, et al. 1,25(OH)2D3 administration in moderate renal failure: a prospective double-blind trial. Kidney Int. 1989;35:661–9.
57. Cozzolino M, Brancaccio D, Cannella G, et al. VDRA therapy is associated with improved survival in dialysis patients with serum intact PTH </= 150 pg/mL: results of the Italian FARO Survey. Nephrol Dial Transplant. 2012;27:3588–94.
58. Sprague SM, Lerma E, McCormmick D, Abraham M, Batlle D. Suppression of parathyroid hormone secretion in hemodialysis patients: comparison of paricalcitol with calcitriol. Am J Kidney Dis. 2001;38:S51–6.

Chapter 13
Vitamin D in Children with Chronic Kidney Disease: A Focus on Longitudinal Bone Growth

Justine Bacchetta and Isidro B. Salusky

Abstract Growth retardation, decreased final height and renal osteodystrophy (ROD) are common complications of childhood chronic kidney disease (CKD), resulting from a combination of abnormalities in the growth hormone (GH) axis, vitamin D deficiency, hyperparathyroidism, hypogonadism, inadequate nutrition, cachexia and drug toxicity. The impact of CKD-associated bone and mineral disorders (CKD-MBD) may be immediate (serum phosphate/calcium disequilibrium) or delayed (poor growth, ROD, fractures, vascular calcifications, increased morbidity and mortality). Vitamin D metabolism is completely modified by CKD, and children with CKD are particularly prone to 25-D deficiency whilst beneficial effects of vitamin D on immunity, anemia, and cardiovascular outcomes have been described in pediatric CKD. Vitamin D also has a direct effect on bone biology and mineral metabolism. Native vitamin supplementation and active vitamin D analogs are currently the mainstay of therapy for children with CKD-MBD, decreasing PTH levels whilst increasing FGF23 levels. However, over-suppression of PTH levels in dialyzed children using vitamin D analogs may lead to adynamic bone disease, growth failure, cardiovascular calcifications, and growth plate inhibition. The aim of this review is therefore to focus on vitamin D effects on bone and longitudinal growth, and on the therapeutic use of the different vitamins D in pediatric CKD in 2015.

Keywords Vitamin D • Chronic kidney disease • Dialysis • Children • Paediatrics • Longitudinal growth

J. Bacchetta (✉)
Centre de Référence des Maladies Rénales Rares, Service de Néphrologie Rhumatologie Dermatologie Pédiatriques, Hôpital Femme Mère Enfant, Bron, France
e-mail: justine.bacchetta@chu-lyon.fr

I.B. Salusky
Division of Pediatric Nephrology, David Geffen School of Medicine at UCLA, University of California Los Angeles, Los Angeles, CA, USA
e-mail: isalusky@mednet.ucla.edu

© Springer International Publishing Switzerland 2016
P.A. Ureña Torres et al. (eds.), *Vitamin D in Chronic Kidney Disease*,
DOI 10.1007/978-3-319-32507-1_13

13.1 Introduction

Growth retardation, decreased final height and renal osteodystrophy (ROD) are common complications of childhood chronic kidney disease (CKD), resulting from a combination of abnormalities in the growth hormone (GH) axis, vitamin D deficiency, hyperparathyroidism, hypogonadism, inadequate nutrition, cachexia and drug toxicity [1]. The impact of CKD-associated bone and mineral disorders (CKD-MBD) may be immediate (serum phosphate/calcium disequilibrium) or delayed (poor growth, ROD, fractures, vascular calcifications, increased morbidity and mortality) [1]. Not only do these complications impact overall quality of life through their effects on both physical and mental well-being in children with CKD, but alterations in mineral metabolism and bone disease are linked to cardiovascular disease, the leading cause of death in children with CKD [1].

Vitamin D metabolism is completely modified by CKD, and children with CKD exhibit altered catabolism and concentrations of DBP (D-binding protein) and bioavailable 25-D levels, with an important impact of the underlying renal disease (glomerular diseases inducing lower 25-D levels) [2]. Indeed, such patients are particularly prone to 25 OH vitamin D (25-D) deficiency (most often defined by values below 30 ng/mL or 75 nmol/L), as described in different pediatric studies from different parts of the world: 77 % of children presented 25-D deficiency in a cohort of 57 CKD stages II-IV American children [3], 26 % in a cohort of 143 CKD British children [4], 40 % in a cohort of 227 CKD stage 1–4 French children [5], and 32 % in a cohort of 59 pediatric dialysis patients from Korea [6]. In the recent report from the CKID (Chronic Kidney Disease in Children Cohort Study) study in 506 children with CKD, Kumar described a 28 %-prevalence of 25-D deficiency; moreover, significant predictors of 25-D deficiency were the following factors: older age, non-white ethnicity, higher body mass index, assessment during winter, less often than daily milk intake, non-use of nutritional vitamin D supplement and proteinuria [7].

Moreover, in addition to reporting a 65 % prevalence of 25-D deficiency in CKD stages 2–4 children, Shroff et al. also demonstrated in a placebo-controlled randomized trial that ergocalciferol was able to prevent the development of secondary hyperparathyroidism [8].

Apart from the beneficial effects of vitamin D on immunity [9], anemia [10, 11], and cardiovascular outcomes, that are detailed in other chapters of this textbook, the aim of this review is to focus on vitamin D effects on bone and longitudinal growth, and on the therapeutic use of the different vitamins D in the global pediatric CKD-MBD picture.

13.2 Physiology of Normal Growth and Bone Formation

Linear growth is a unique feature of childhood, occurring through the modeling of new bone by skeletal accretion and longitudinal growth in the growth plate. In this process, chondrocytes play a key role, as well as growth hormone (GH) [12]. One third of the total growth occurs during the first 2 years of life, on a primarily nutrition-dependent basis [12]. Later childhood is marked by a lesser, although constant, growth velocity (5–7 cm/year), driven primarily by the actions of GH and thyroid hormone. At the onset of puberty, estrogen and testosterone induce a second increase of growth velocity. During growth, the epiphyseal cartilage goes through a process of progressive maturation, and when no additional epiphyseal cartilage remains to provide further long bone growth, bone fusion occurs between the shaft and the epiphysis, ending the linear growth process.

Bone formation in children occurs by two distinct mechanisms: the first one is similar to that observed in adults (i.e., skeletal remodeling of existing mineralized tissue that is controlled by osteoclasts and osteoblasts) whereas the second one is specific to the pediatric population (i.e., modeling of new bone by skeletal accretion and longitudinal growth from the growth plate, through the action of chondrocytes) [13]. The growth plate is an avascular tissue between the epiphyses and metaphyses of long bones; endochondral bone formation corresponds to its progressive replacement by bone. The regulation of this process is complex, with a key role for GH and the PTH/PTH related protein-receptor (PTHrP) axis [14].

1,25(OH)$_2$D has an intracrine role in endochondral ossification and chondrocyte development in vivo: indeed, the inactivation of both alleles of the *CYP27B1* gene encoding the 1-alfa hydroxylase inhibits osteoclastogenesis and increases the width of the hypertrophic zone of the growth plate at embryonic D15.5 in mice. In this model, the expression of chondrocytic differentiation markers such as Indian Hedgehog and PTH/PTHrP receptor was increased, whilst the expression of the angiogenic marker VEGF was decreased in the neonatal growth plate, suggesting a delayed vascularization. In contrast, the transgenic mice overexpressing *CYP27B1* presented with a mirror image phenotype with a reduction in the width of the hypertrophic zone of the embryonic growth plate, decreased bone volume in neonatal long bones, and inverse expression patterns of chondrocytic differentiation markers [15].

13.3 The Roles of Vitamin D in Bone Physiology

From a clinical point of view, vitamin D also has a direct effect on bone biology, independent of its effects on mineral metabolism; the role of vitamin D deficiency to explain rickets has long been known, and Priemel et al. demonstrated in a cohort of 675 deceased adults that pathologic mineralization defects could occur when serum 25-D level was below 30 ng/mL [16]. Recent data also showed abnormal growth plate histology with lower 25-D levels in an English cohort of 52 postmortem pediatric cases (aged 2 days to 10 years) [17].

From a more fundamental point of view, the role of vitamins D on bone has also been evaluated: conversion of 25-D to 1,25-D in osteoblasts, osteocytes, chondrocytes and osteoclast indeed regulate fundamental physiological processes such as cell proliferation, maturation, mineralization and resorption, with a key-role described for the vitamin D receptor VDR [18]. As such, increased vitamin D activity in mature osteoblasts improves bone mineral volume; however, results can be conflicting, some authors demonstrating a dual role for vitamin D in osteoblasts. Indeed, a treatment of pre-osteoblast cells leads to an inhibition of collagen I and alkaline phosphatase levels whilst a treatment of mature osteoblasts leads to a stimulation of these two markers [19]. The role of vitamins D has also been evaluated on osteoclast differentiation and on bone resorption activity, again with conflicting results: active 1,25-D has been shown to strongly inhibit human osteoclast formation by some authors, whereas others have rather demonstrated a positive effect, performing cultures with both vitamin D and dexamethasone [20]. In terms of resorption activity, 1,25-D appears to inhibit osteoclast activity when osteoclast differentiation and bone resorption are not studied separately; however we recently demonstrated in human osteoclasts a significant inhibitory effect of 1,25-D on osteoclast differentiation, without any significant impact on bone resorption when evaluating resorption per cell [20]. Last, Lieben highlighted a potential role of vitamin D in mineralization: indeed, in intestine-specific VDR knockout mice, maintaining normocalcemia has priority over skeletal integrity. In such a setting, to maintain normal circulating calcium levels (and therefore to minimize skeletal calcium storage), 1,25-D not only increases calcium release from bone, but also inhibits calcium incorporation in bone [21].

13.4   Vitamin D Metabolism in Pediatric CKD

In early stages of CKD, increments in FGF23 levels and decreased klotho levels are the first biochemical abnormalities associated with CKD-MBD; increased FGF23 levels play an important role on the inhibition of calcitriol synthesis; however the primary stimuli for such response remains to be determined. The progressive decline in 1,25-D levels is followed by increasing PTH levels and it is important to highlight that such hormonal changes occur while serum calcium and phosphorus levels still remain within the normal range [22]. Hypocalcemia and hyperphosphatemia develop later in the course of CKD in response to decreased intestinal calcium absorption (from critically low calcitriol concentrations) and decreased phosphate excretion (from critically low renal mass), respectively [23]. Finally, 25-D deficiency, which is prevalent worldwide, likely also contributes to the development of secondary hyperparathyroidism.

   As already detailed above, patients with CKD are particularly prone to 25-D deficiency, due to several combined factors including decreased sunlight exposure, relative scarcity of vitamin D in occidental diets, lack of supplementation in vitamin D due to the current underestimation for recommended daily intake, type of primary renal disease and increased body fat mass in populations [1].

13.5   Vitamin D and Longitudinal Growth in Pediatric CKD

In pediatric patients with CKD, growth failure develops early in the course of CKD and affects up to 35 % of this population; by the time of renal transplantation, a significant proportion of children present with severe short stature [24]. The etiology of this poor growth is multifactorial and includes both potentially modifiable factors (e.g., protein and calorie malnutrition, anemia, metabolic acidosis, hypothyroidism and salt-wasting) and less modifiable factors such as abnormalities in the GH-IGF1 axis, resistance to GH, ROD and therapies [24].

From a more basic point of view, in sub-totally nephrectomised rats presenting with mild or advanced secondary hyperparathyroidism, the assessment of epiphyseal growth plate (using quantitative histology, mRNA levels of selected markers of chondrocyte proliferation and differentiation) showed that the width of the growth plate cartilage in the proximal tibia and mRNA levels for PTH/PTHrP receptor were markedly decreased in nephrectomised rats in comparison to controls. While a treatment with growth hormone increased growth plate thickness in rats with secondary hyperparathyroidism, in contrast, the administration of calcitriol attenuated these responses, thus demonstrating that calcitriol counteracts the trophic actions of growth hormone on epiphyseal growth plate cartilage in rats, modifying chondrocyte differentiation in vivo [25].

Interestingly, in children with CKD, diminished linear growth was also observed in children undergoing chronic peritoneal dialysis during intermittent calcitriol therapy. In this study evaluating 16 pre-pubertal patients with bone biopsy-proven secondary hyperparathyroidism who completed a 12-month prospective clinical trial of intermittent calcitriol therapy (after a 12-month period of daily calcitriol therapy), Kuizon et al. showed that Z-scores for height did not change during 12 months of daily calcitriol therapy whereas they significantly decreased from -1.8 ± 0.3 to -2.0 ± 0.3, during intermittent calcitriol therapy. The largest reductions were seen in patients who developed adynamic bone lesions. Thus, these data suggested that high dose intermittent calcitriol therapy adversely affects linear growth, particularly in patients with adynamic bone disease. As such, the higher doses of calcitriol or the intermittent schedule of calcitriol administration may directly inhibit chondrocyte activity in the growth plate cartilage of children with end-stage renal disease [26]. These data were described during an era when patients were given large doses of calcium-based binders, thus questioning their validity in 2015, with lower daily doses of vitamin D analogs and the availability of calcium-free phosphate binders. Indeed, the use of such binders with high doses of active vitamin D sterols in dialysis patients was associated with skeletal improvement of the lesions of secondary hyperparathyroidism without increments in serum calcium levels in dialysis patients [27].

13.6   Vitamin D and Bone Metabolism in Pediatric CKD

The bone and growth consequences of CKD have been highlighted in a cohort of 249 young Dutch adults with onset of end-stage renal failure before the age of 14 years: in this cohort, 61 % of patients had severe growth retardation, 37 % severe bone disease (as defined by at least one of the following conditions: deforming bone abnormalities, chronic pain related to the skeletal system, disabling bone abnormalities, aseptic bone necrosis and low-traumatic fractures) and 18 %

disabilities resulting from bone impairment [28]. More recently, fracture histories were obtained at baseline as well as at years 1, 3, and 5 in the prospective CKID cohort including 537 children with CKD. At enrollment, median age was 11 years, and 16 % of patients reported a past of fracture. Over a median of 3.9 years, 43 boys and 24 girls presented with incident fractures, corresponding to 395 (95 % confidence interval [95 % CI], 293–533) and 323 (95 % CI, 216–481) fractures per 10,000 person-years, respectively. These rates were two- to threefold higher than published general pediatric rates. By multivariable analysis, advanced pubertal stage, greater height Z-score, walking difficulties, and higher PTH levels were independently associated with greater fracture risk; interestingly 25-D levels did not correlate with fracture risk. Phosphate binder treatment (predominantly calcium-based) was associated with lower fracture risk (hazard ratio, 0.37; 95 % CI, 0.15–0.91; P = 0.03). Participation in more than one team sport was associated with a higher risk of fracture [29]. In addition, evidence of vascular calcifications has been demonstrated in young adult dialysis patients with ESRD therapy initiated in childhood [30].

Bone biopsy from the anterior iliac crest (after double tetracycline labeling) remains the reference standard to evaluate bone status in CKD patients. Even though it is rarely performed in clinical practice, bone biopsy followed by histomorphometry analysis are the only available techniques leading to an accurate evaluation of renal osteodystrophy (ROD) [31]. ROD is characterized by alterations in bone turnover, mineralization and volume; these three components should be evaluated independently to characterize the different subtypes of ROD, as defined by the K-DIGO in 2006 [32].

High bone turnover (secondary hyperparathyroidism, *osteitis fibrosa cystica*) is the primary skeletal lesion of pediatric ROD, and is present in virtually all untreated incident pediatric dialysis patients. This lesion is caused by a long-term exposure to high serum PTH levels and $1,25(OH)_2D$ deficiency. By contrast, low turnover lesions (i.e., adynamic bone disease) may occur as a result of excess treatment with vitamin D analogs and calcium salts and are characterized by relative low PTH and alkaline phosphatase levels as well as high serum calcium levels. Low bone turnover has been associated with an increased risk of vascular calcifications, fractures and more severe growth retardation [26].

Defects in skeletal mineralization are also prevalent in pediatric patients with CKD—occurring in 30 % in stage 2 CKD and increasing in prevalence as CKD progresses, even though bone turnover remains normal in the earliest CKD stages and becomes apparent while GFR decreases [23, 33]. In contrast to adult patients, nearly 80 % of pediatric dialysis patients display some defect in skeletal mineralization, a problem that is not corrected by traditional therapy with vitamin D sterols and phosphate binders [23]. Although alterations in skeletal mineralization (i.e. rickets) contribute to increased fracture rates, bone deformities, and growth retardation in children with normal renal function, their exact role in these clinical symptoms in children with CKD, remains to be elucidated.

Although active vitamin D sterols are currently the mainstay of therapy for elevated PTH levels, over-suppression of PTH levels in dialyzed children may lead to adynamic bone disease which is associated with growth failure and cardiovascular calcifications [13]. Moreover, as detailed above, active vitamin D sterols, particularly calcitriol, may also inhibit the growth-plate [26]. Taken together, these data illustrate that active vitamin D sterols exert a positive role in controlling PTH levels and *osteitis fibrosa* but, with excessive use, may result in excessive PTH suppression, adynamic bone disease, growth failure, and progressive cardiovascular calcifications. However, such potential complications associated to active vitamin D sterols are minimized with the concomitant use of calcium-free phosphate binders. A randomized controlled trial in pediatric patients undergoing peritoneal dialysis was performed to evaluate the impact of recombinant human growth hormone (rhGH) therapy depending on the underlying renal osteodystrophy at baseline; rhGH increases bone formation rates in patients with low turnover renal osteodystrophy, whereas increases in bone formation rate are attenuated by calcitriol therapy in patients with high turnover renal osteodystrophy [34].

From a more basic point of view, it was recently demonstrated that doxercalciferol was able to modify the expression of osteocytic markers (notably increase of the full-length form of FGF23, decrease of the 57 kDa form of DMP1 and increase sclerostin) in 11 children with end stage renal disease, thus highlighting a potential of vitamin D analog on bone mineralization and skeletal response to PTH [35].

13.7   The Interplay Between Vitamin D and FGF23 in Pediatric CKD

FGF23 is a protein synthesized by osteocytes that has a key role in the 'bone-parathyroid-kidney' axis and the regulation of phosphate/calcium metabolism. Three main effects have been classically described: hypophosphatemia (through an inhibition of phosphate reabsorption in the proximal tubule), decreased PTH levels and decreased $1,25(OH)_2D$ levels (through an inhibition of 1α hydroxylase and an activation of 24 hydroxylase activity in the kidney) [36]. Off-target effects of FGF23 have also been demonstrated, notably on cardiomyocytes [37], monocytes [38], and osteoclasts [20]. Recently, the effects of FGF23 in the distal renal tubule have been more precisely defined: it stimulates calcium reabsorption through TRPV5 [39], whereas it also stimulates sodium handling and increases blood pressure [40]. In terms of physiology, the links between iron metabolism and FGF23 seems also of importance, although still under investigation [41].

A number of studies have focused on FGF23 during CKD, this biomarker being indeed the first to be deregulated in early CKD. In such a setting, increased FGF23 levels have been shown to be a risk factor for cardiovascular mortality, general mortality, progression of renal disease, resistance to vitamin D analogs, and more recently infections [42–45]. In healthy volunteers, oral phosphate loading stimulates FGF23 synthesis while it is the contrary for dietary phosphate restriction. FGF23 levels increase progressively as renal function declines, well before the onset of a critical reduction in the nephron number. However, the increase in FGF23 levels in blood and bone in early CKD (observed well before increased phosphate/ PTH or decreased $1,25(OH)_2D$ levels), and the exact mechanisms/triggers of this increase still remain to be elucidated: it could be secondary to a decreased renal clearance compensatory mechanism to the loss of the kidney-secreted klotho protein, and/or an increased production of FGF23 in bone cells among others [46]. Another potential important factor in the regulation of FGF23 production is iron and indeed iron deficiency is a potent stimulator of FGF23 production [41]. Iron deficiency anemia is one of the early manifestations associated to CKD, but the role of iron on FGF23 in CKD remains to be investigated.

It remains to be determined whether and how decreasing FGF23 levels could improve overall morbidity and mortality in CKD patients. Indeed, the current standard therapies affect FGF23 levels differently. Briefly, dietary phosphate restriction may decrease FGF23 levels but long-term compliance with such diets is difficult, non-calcium-based binders appear to reduce FGF23 levels, mainly sevelamer carbonate and ferric citrate whereas calcium-based binders either increase or have no effect on FGF23 levels; active vitamin D sterols increase FGF23 levels in blood and bone whilst calcimimetics decrease FGF23 levels [47]. Theorically, the use of anti-FGF23 agents in CKD could be of interest, but results from animal models have been disappointing, enabling the correction of hyperparathyroidism while increasing phosphate levels and mortality as expected because of the significant increase in phosphate levels [48]. With all these data in mind, the appropriate therapy in CKD that will minimize the rise in FGF23 and most importantly prevent cardiovascular morbidity remains to be defined.

In that setting, two clinical trials evaluating the role of the calcimimetic cinacalcet were performed in patients with CKD. The ADVANCE trial provided evidence that cinacalcet combined with low doses of vitamin D may slow the progression of coronary artery calcifications compared to therapy using larger, varying doses of vitamin D [49]. However, the EVOLVE trial, including 3,883 hemodialysis patients with moderate to severe hyperparathyroidism randomized either to cinacalcet or placebo and followed up to 64 months, did not meet its clinical primary endpoint (time to all-cause mortality, myocardial infarction, hospitalization for unstable angina, heart failure or a peripheral vascular event) using an unadjusted intention-to-treat analysis, although secondary and sensitivity analysis suggested a beneficial effect [50]. One main issue of this important clinical trial was the extensive non-adherence, thus leading the intention-to-treat analysis quite challenging [51]. Secondary analyses of the EVOLVE study were recently published. Another secondary analysis including 2,602 patients (out of the initial 3,883) with samples at both baseline and week 20 showed that a significantly larger proportion of patients randomized to cinacalcet had $\geq 30\%$ reductions in FGF23 levels. Among patients randomized to cinacalcet, a $\geq 30\%$ reduction in FGF23 between baseline and week 20 was associated with a nominally significant reduction in the primary composite end point (relative hazard, 0.82; 95% confidence interval, 0.69–0.98); results were similar for cardiovascular mortality, sudden cardiac death, and heart failure [52]. However, these results should really be interpreted cautiously due to the methodological limitations observed in this trial, and are far from pediatric questions… In the future, specific questions should be addressed before advancing to a full-scale clinical outcomes trial, as recently summarized in the review from Isakova [53]. If the secondary conclusions of the EVOLVE trial are proven to be true despite the absence of statistical difference with the intent-to-treat analysis, FGF23 levels may become an important target in the clinical management of CKD patients, and these results could therefore become of the utmost interest for pediatric patients. However, international clinical trials on cinacalcet in pediatric dialysis are ongoing, and we should stay cautious with these results from secondary analyses.

Moreover, FGF23 is not the only biomarker we could modify in CKD. The single-pass trans-membrane klotho protein, well known for its biological properties in vivo to enhance FGF23-mediated receptor activation, also has mineral effects by itself (increased calcium reabsorption due to a direct modification of the sugar chains of TRPV5 in the distal tubule and direct regulation of PTH synthesis), and cardiovascular effects [54]. Indeed, low klotho levels (isolated or secondary to high uremic toxins levels) have been shown recently to be associated with left ventricular hypertrophy in murine models of CKD [55–57]. With these data in mind, other therapeutic options such as FGF-R modulation that are currently under evaluation, or pharmacological increase of klotho levels may also become promising tools for cardiovascular outcomes and overall mortality in pediatric CKD.

13.8   Native Vitamin D Supplementation and Vitamin D Analogs in CKD Children

13.8.1   Global Management of Pediatric CKD-MBD

The clinical management of CKD-MBD in children is currently focused on three main objectives: (1) to provide an optimal growth in order to maximize the final height with an early management with recombinant GH therapy when required, (2) to equilibrate calcium/phosphate metabolism so as to obtain acceptable bone quality and cardiovascular status, and (3) to correct all metabolic and clinical abnormalities that can worsen bone disease, growth and cardiovascular disease, i.e., metabolic acidosis, anemia, malnutrition, and 25-D deficiency. All the following measures are used by pediatric nephrologists to optimize the CKD-MBD management: correction of hyperphosphatemia (dietary restriction of phosphorus, calcium-based phosphate binders, non-calcium based phosphate binders, notably sevelamer but also maybe in a next future iron-based phosphate binders), correction of 25-D deficiency, correction of hypocalcemia, and correction of hyperparathyroidism (vitamin D analog, calcimimetics, and exceptionally in 2015 parathyroidectomy) [1].

13.9 Native Vitamin D Therapy

In addition to providing a substrate for the formation of calcitriol, thus indirectly suppressing PTH levels, Ritter et al. identified that 25-D continues to directly suppress PTH synthesis even when parathyroid gland 1 alpha hydroxylase is inhibited, thus demonstrating a direct effect of 25-D on PTH synthesis, independent of 1,25-D [58]. Moreover, a recent placebo-controlled randomized trial also demonstrated that ergocalciferol was able to delay the onset of secondary hyperparathyroidism in pediatric patients with pre-dialysis CKD [8]. As such, native vitamin D supplementation appears to be a cornerstone of pediatric CKD-MBD management. Although current international guidelines suggest that increased PTH levels, in face of 25-D insufficiency/deficiency (<30 ng/ml) be first treated with native vitamin D supplementation, no 'practical' guidelines are provided concerning the dose (daily, monthly, quarterly?) and the type of vitamin D (ergocalciferol or cholecalciferol) depending on age, body weight, severity of 25-D deficiency and CKD stage. In the future, clinical trials my focus on this rather simple but critical question.

13.9.1 Vitamin D Analogs

Following 25-D repletion, if hyperparathyroidism is not controlled according to specific CKD stage, active vitamin D sterols should be initiated to help controlling serum PTH values. However, one should keep in mind that optimal PTH levels remain to be defined: indeed, the international KDIGO guidelines recommend PTH levels two to nine times the upper normal limit in CKD stage V [32], whereas European pediatric guidelines recommend PTH levels two to three times the upper normal limit in CKD stage V [59]. This threshold remains discussed, but high PTH levels are also well known to be associated with anemia, left ventricular hypertrophy and vascular calcifications; a recent 2013 report from the international pediatric peritoneal dialysis (PD) registry (IPPN) proposed a PTH target between 100 and 200 pg/ml in children undergoing chronic PD [60], keeping in mind that it can be difficult to propose guidelines for PTH levels since the assays can have a 30–50 % variability across the world

In 2010, a Cochrane review emphasized the paucity of long-term data on safety and efficacy of different active vitamin D sterols for the treatment of pediatric secondary hyperparathyroidism; however, PTH levels have been shown to decrease similarly with all preparations [61]. Although vitamin D sterols are currently the mainstay of therapy for elevated PTH levels, over-suppression of PTH levels in maintenance dialysis children may lead to adynamic bone disease, a condition associated with growth failure and cardiovascular calcifications. Active vitamin D sterols, particularly calcitriol, may also inhibit the growth plate. Taken together, these data illustrate that active vitamin D sterols exert a positive role in controlling PTH levels and *osteitis fibrosa* but, with excessive use, may result in excessive PTH suppression, adynamic bone disease, growth failure, and progressive cardiovascular calcifications but such suppression of secondary hyperparathyroidism is associated with progressive rise of FGF23 [1]. Since there are currently no data demonstrating any differences on the control of secondary hyperparathyroidism or renal osteodystrophy between the various active vitamin D sterols the choice may depend on local prescription options; and when calcitriol was compared to doxercalciferol similar control of secondary hyperparathyroidism was obtained but doxercalciferol had a greater degree of osteoclastic suppression.

13.9.2 Calcimimetics

Calcimimetics have been used in pediatric CKD, but their use remains off-label [62–64]. As discussed above, recent clinical trials in CKD adults receiving cinacalcet or placebo have shown that cinacalcet significantly decreases FGF23 levels [52]. In the meantime, international pediatric clinical trials on cinacalcet in dialysis are ongoing, and may change our daily management of pediatric ROD and CKD-MBD in a near future. Figure 13.1 summarizes the current understanding on phosphate/calcium metabolism in human physiology, while Fig. 13.2 summarizes the effects of different CKD-MBD therapies on this complex pathway.

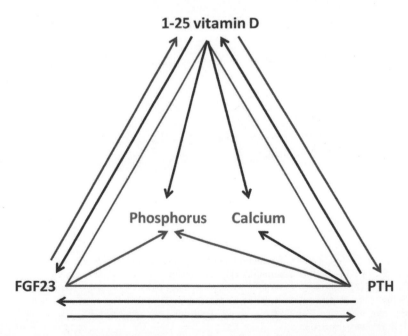

Fig. 13.1 The current understanding of calcium/phosphate metabolism regulation in human physiology. *Grey arrows* corresponding to an inhibiting effect; *Red arrows* corresponding to a stimulating effect

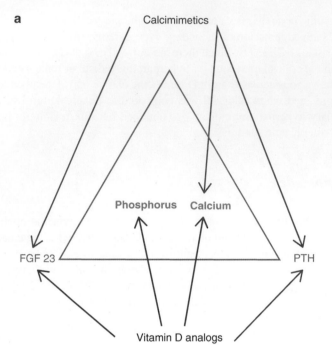

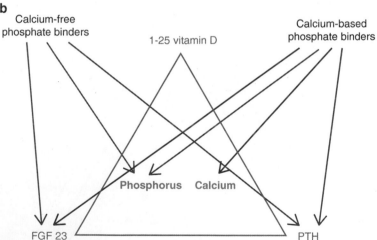

Fig. 13.2 The different effects on calcium, phosphate, FGF23 and PTH levels of the current therapies used for CKD-MBD management. (**a**) Effects of active vitamin D analogs and calcimimetics. (**b**) Effects of calcium-based and calcium-free phosphate binders. *Grey arrows* corresponding to an inhibiting effect; *Red arrows* corresponding to a stimulating effect. It is noteworthy that not all the Ca-free binders reduce FGF23; for example, lanthanum can reduce FGF23 levels mainly when used with dietary restriction

13.9.3   *Vitamin D After Pediatric Renal Transplantation*

Vitamin D deficiency remains an important problem after renal transplantation [65, 66]; in this context, regular vitamin D supplementation may serve as a potentially modifiable factor. Indeed, vitamin D plays an important role for bone quality after renal transplantation, but it also has critical roles in immunity (through a natural inhibition of the mTor signalling) [67]. In that setting, low 25D levels before transplantation have also been shown to be associated with an increased risk of cancer after transplantation whilst low 25(OH)D levels have been linked with an increased risk of delayed graft function [68, 69].

13.10   Conclusions

Recent research has confirmed that 25(OH)D has plenty of metabolic actions, including beneficial effects on bone, vessels, inflammation, defense against infection and muscle function, all being frequent conditions in pediatric CKD patients; however the impact of vitamin D therapy on each of these specific conditions remain to be defined. Recently, normal 25(OH)D levels have been shown to be associated with less proteinuria and to attenuate renal failure progression in 167 CKD children (median GFR 51 mL/min per 1.73 m^2) from the ESCAPE trial. In this study, renal survival increased by 8.2 % per 10 nmol/L increase in 25-D levels, independently of GFR, proteinuria, blood pressure and FGF23 levels; the threshold for observing such an effect was 50 nmol/L [70].

Although there are no large randomized controlled trial on the effects on nutritional vitamin D in CKD patients (and especially in children!), and since vitamin D should be considered as a hormone, it seems prudent to restore sufficient serum levels. Over dosage is quite uncommon despite extensive administration, and could be easily monitored by serum calcium and 25(OH)D levels, a routine measure in pediatric CKD. In the future, international and large clinical trials should provide not also practical guidelines for 25-D supplementation but also evidence for global beneficial effects of this non-expensive and well-tolerated drug.

Disclosure of Interest   JB: research grants from Amgen, Sandoz, Novartis and Crinex; consulting fees from Amgen, Genzyme, Otsuka and Pfizer.
   IBS: Amgen, OPKO, Abbvie and Sanofi

References

1. Bacchetta J, Harambat J, Cochat P, Salusky IB, Wesseling-Perry K. The consequences of chronic kidney disease on bone metabolism and growth in children. Nephrol Dial Transplant. 2012;27:3063–71.

2. Denburg MR, Kalkwarf HJ, de Boer IH, Hewison M, Shults J, Zemel BS, et al. Vitamin D bioavailability and catabolism in pediatric chronic kidney disease. Pediatr Nephrol. 2013;28:1843–53.
3. Menon S, Valentini RP, Hidalgo G, Peschansky L, Mattoo TK. Vitamin D insufficiency and hyperparathyroidism in children with chronic kidney disease. Pediatr Nephrol. 2008;23:1831–6.
4. Belostotsky V, Mughal MZ, Berry JL, Webb NJ. Vitamin D deficiency in children with renal disease. Arch Dis Child. 2008;93:959–62.
5. Bacchetta J, Dubourg L, Harambat J, Ranchin B, Abou-Jaoude P, Arnaud S, et al. The influence of glomerular filtration rate and age on fibroblast growth factor 23 serum levels in pediatric chronic kidney disease. J Clin Endocrinol Metab. 2010;95:1741–8.
6. Cho HY, Hyun HS, Kang HG, Ha IS, Cheong HI. Prevalence of 25(OH) vitamin D insufficiency and deficiency in pediatric patients on chronic dialysis. Perit Dial Int. 2013;33:398–404.
7. Kumar J, McDermott K, Abraham AG, Friedman LA, Johnson VL, Kaskel FJ, et al. Prevalence and correlates of 25-hydroxyvitamin D deficiency in the Chronic Kidney Disease in Children (CKiD) cohort. Pediatr Nephrol. 2016;31:121–9.
8. Shroff R, Wan M, Gullett A, Ledermann S, Shute R, Knott C, et al. Ergocalciferol supplementation in children with CKD delays the onset of secondary hyperparathyroidism: a randomized trial. Clin J Am Soc Nephrol. 2012;7:216–23.
9. Bacchetta J, Chun RF, Gales B, Zaritsky JJ, Leroy S, Wesseling-Perry K, et al. Antibacterial responses by peritoneal macrophages are enhanced following vitamin D supplementation. PLoS One. 2014;9:e116530.
10. Bacchetta J, Zaritsky JJ, Sea JL, Chun RF, Lisse TS, Zavala K, et al. Suppression of iron-regulatory hepcidin by vitamin D. J Am Soc Nephrol. 2014;25:564–72.
11. Rianthavorn P, Boonyapapong P. Ergocalciferol decreases erythropoietin resistance in children with chronic kidney disease stage 5. Pediatr Nephrol. 2013;28:1261–6.
12. Mahesh S, Kaskel F. Growth hormone axis in chronic kidney disease. Pediatr Nephrol. 2008;23:41–8.
13. Salusky IB, Goodman WG. Growth hormone and calcitriol as modifiers of bone formation in renal osteodystrophy. Kidney Int. 1995;48:657–65.
14. Kuizon BD, Salusky IB. Growth retardation in children with chronic renal failure. J Bone Miner Res. 1999;14:1680–90.
15. Naja RP, Dardenne O, Arabian A, St Arnaud R. Chondrocyte-specific modulation of Cyp27b1 expression supports a role for local synthesis of 1,25-dihydroxyvitamin D3 in growth plate development. Endocrinology. 2009;150:4024–32.
16. Priemel M, von Domarus C, Klatte TO, Kessler S, Schlie J, Meier S, et al. Bone mineralization defects and vitamin D deficiency: histomorphometric analysis of iliac crest bone biopsies and circulating 25-hydroxyvitamin D in 675 patients. J Bone Miner Res. 2010;25:305–12.
17. Scheimberg I, Perry L. Does low vitamin D have a role in pediatric morbidity and mortality? An observational study of vitamin D in a cohort of 52 postmortem examinations. Pediatr Dev Pathol. 2014;17:455–64.
18. Anderson PH, Lam NN, Turner AG, Davey RA, Kogawa M, Atkins GJ, et al. The pleiotropic effects of vitamin D in bone. J Steroid Biochem Mol Biol. 2013;136:190–4.
19. Owen TA, Aronow MS, Barone LM, Bettencourt B, Stein GS, Lian JB. Pleiotropic effects of vitamin D on osteoblast gene expression are related to the proliferative and differentiated state of the bone cell phenotype: dependency upon basal levels of gene expression, duration of exposure, and bone matrix competency in normal rat osteoblast cultures. Endocrinology. 1991;128:1496–504.
20. Allard L, Demoncheaux N, Machuca-Gayet I, Georgess D, Coury-Lucas F, Jurdic P, et al. Biphasic effects of vitamin D and FGF23 on human osteoclast biology. Calcif Tissue Int. 2015;97:69–79.
21. Lieben L, Masuyama R, Torrekens S, Van Looveren R, Schrooten J, Baatsen P, et al. Normocalcemia is maintained in mice under conditions of calcium malabsorption by vitamin D-induced inhibition of bone mineralization. J Clin Invest. 2012;122:1803–15.

22. Heidbreder E, Naujoks H, Brosa U, Schramm L. The calcium-parathyroid hormone regulation in chronic renal failure investigation of its dynamic secretion pattern. Horm Metab Res. 1997;29:70–5.
23. Wesseling-Perry K, Pereira RC, Tseng CH, Elashoff R, Zaritsky JJ, Yadin O, et al. Early skeletal and biochemical alterations in pediatric chronic kidney disease. Clin J Am Soc Nephrol. 2012;7:146–52.
24. Harambat J, Cochat P. Growth after renal transplantation. Pediatr Nephrol. 2009;24: 1297–306.
25. Sanchez CP, Salusky IB, Kuizon BD, Abdella P, Juppner H, Goodman WG. Growth of long bones in renal failure: roles of hyperparathyroidism, growth hormone and calcitriol. Kidney Int. 1998;54:1879–87.
26. Kuizon BD, Goodman WG, Juppner H, Boechat I, Nelson P, Gales B, et al. Diminished linear growth during intermittent calcitriol therapy in children undergoing CCPD. Kidney Int. 1998;53:205–11.
27. Wesseling-Perry K, Pereira RC, Sahney S, Gales B, Wang HJ, Elashoff R, et al. Calcitriol and doxercalciferol are equivalent in controlling bone turnover, suppressing parathyroid hormone, and increasing fibroblast growth factor-23 in secondary hyperparathyroidism. Kidney Int. 2011;79:112–9.
28. Groothoff JW, Offringa M, Van Eck-Smit BL, Gruppen MP, Van De Kar NJ, Wolff ED, et al. Severe bone disease and low bone mineral density after juvenile renal failure. Kidney Int. 2003;63:266–75.
29. Denburg MR, Kumar J, Jemielita T, Brooks ER, Skversky A, Portale AA, et al. Fracture burden and risk factors in childhood CKD: results from the CKiD cohort study. J Am Soc Nephrol. 2015;10:571–7.
30. Goodman WG, Goldin J, Kuizon BD, Yoon C, Gales B, Sider D, et al. Coronary-artery calcification in young adults with end-stage renal disease who are undergoing dialysis. N Engl J Med. 2000;342(20):1478–83.
31. Hernandez JD, Wesseling K, Pereira R, Gales B, Harrison R, Salusky IB. Technical approach to iliac crest biopsy. Clin J Am Soc Nephrol. 2008;3:S164–9.
32. Moe S, Drueke T, Cunningham J, Goodman W, Martin K, Olgaard K, et al. Definition, evaluation, and classification of renal osteodystrophy: a position statement from Kidney Disease: Improving Global Outcomes (KDIGO). Kidney Int. 2006;69:1945–53.
33. Bakkaloglu SA, Wesseling-Perry K, Pereira RC, Gales B, Wang HJ, Elashoff RM, et al. Value of the new bone classification system in pediatric renal osteodystrophy. Clin J Am Soc Nephrol. 2010;5:1860–6.
34. Bacchetta J, Wesseling-Perry K, Kuizon B, Pereira RC, Gales B, Wang HJ, et al. The skeletal consequences of growth hormone therapy in dialyzed children: a randomized trial. Clin J Am Soc Nephrol. 2013;8:824–32.
35. Pereira RC, Juppner H, Gales B, Salusky IB, Wesseling-Perry K. Osteocytic protein expression response to doxercalciferol therapy in pediatric dialysis patients. PLoS One. 2015;10(3):e0120856.
36. Bacchetta J, Salusky IB. Evaluation of hypophosphatemia: lessons from patients with genetic disorders. Am J Kidney Dis. 2012;59:152–9.
37. Faul C, Amaral AP, Oskouei B, Hu MC, Sloan A, Isakova T, et al. FGF23 induces left ventricular hypertrophy. J Clin Invest. 2011;121:4393–408.
38. Bacchetta J, Sea JL, Chun RF, Lisse TS, Wesseling-Perry K, Gales B, et al. Fibroblast growth factor 23 inhibits extrarenal synthesis of 1,25-dihydroxyvitamin D in human monocytes. J Bone Miner Res. 2013;28:46–55.
39. Andrukhova O, Smorodchenko A, Egerbacher M, Streicher C, Zeitz U, Goetz R, et al. FGF23 promotes renal calcium reabsorption through the TRPV5 channel. EMBO. 2014;33: 229–46.
40. Andrukhova O, Slavic S, Smorodchenko A, Zeitz U, Shalhoub V, Lanske B, et al. FGF23 regulates renal sodium handling and blood pressure. EMBO. 2014;6:744–59.

41. Farrow EG, Yu X, Summers LJ, Davis SI, Fleet JC, Allen MR, et al. Iron deficiency drives an autosomal dominant hypophosphatemic rickets (ADHR) phenotype in fibroblast growth factor-23 (Fgf23) knock-in mice. Proc Natl Acad Sci U S A. 2011;108(46):E1146–55.

42. Gutierrez OM, Mannstadt M, Isakova T, Rauh-Hain JA, Tamez H, Shah A, et al. Fibroblast growth factor 23 and mortality among patients undergoing hemodialysis. N Engl J Med. 2008;359:584–92.

43. Fliser D, Kollerits B, Neyer U, Ankerst DP, Lhotta K, Lingenhel A, et al. Fibroblast growth factor 23 (FGF23) predicts progression of chronic kidney disease: the Mild to Moderate Kidney Disease (MMKD) Study. J Am Soc Nephrol. 2007;18:2600–8.

44. Isakova T, Xie H, Yang W, Xie D, Anderson AH, Scialla J, et al. Fibroblast growth factor 23 and risks of mortality and end-stage renal disease in patients with chronic kidney disease. JAMA. 2011;305:2432–9.

45. Chonchol M, Greene T, Zhang Y, Hoofnagle AN, Cheung AK. Low vitamin D and high fibroblast growth factor 23 serum levels associate with infectious and cardiac deaths in the HEMO study. J Am Soc Nephrol. 2016;27:227–37.

46. Pereira RC, Juppner H, Azucena-Serrano CE, Yadin O, Salusky IB, Wesseling-Perry K. Patterns of FGF-23, DMP1, and MEPE expression in patients with chronic kidney disease. Bone. 2009;45:1161–8.

47. Khouzam NM, Wesseling-Perry K, Salusky IB. The role of bone in CKD-mediated mineral and vascular disease. Pediatr Nephrol. 2015;30:1379–88.

48. Shalhoub V, Shatzen EM, Ward SC, Davis J, Stevens J, Bi V, et al. FGF23 neutralization improves chronic kidney disease-associated hyperparathyroidism yet increases mortality. J Clin Invest. 2012;122:2543–53.

49. Bellasi A, Reiner M, Petavy F, Goodman W, Floege J, Raggi P. Presence of valvular calcification predicts the response to cinacalcet: data from the ADVANCE study. J Heart Valve Dis. 2013;22:391–9.

50. Investigators ET, Chertow GM, Block GA, Correa-Rotter R, Drueke TB, Floege J, et al. Effect of cinacalcet on cardiovascular disease in patients undergoing dialysis. N Engl J Med. 2012;367:2482–94.

51. Kubo Y, Sterling LR, Parfrey PS, Gill K, Mahaffey KW, Gioni I, et al. Assessing the treatment effect in a randomized controlled trial with extensive non-adherence: the EVOLVE trial. Pharm Stat. 2015;14:242–51.

52. Moe SM, Chertow GM, Parfrey PS, Kubo Y, Block GA, Correa-Rotter R, et al. Cinacalcet, fibroblast growth factor-23, and cardiovascular disease in hemodialysis: the evaluation of cinacalcet HCl therapy to lower cardiovascular events (EVOLVE) trial. Circulation. 2015;132:27–39.

53. Isakova T, Ix JH, Sprague SM, Raphael KL, Fried L, Gassman JJ, et al. Rationale and approaches to phosphate and fibroblast growth factor 23 reduction in CKD. J Am Soc Nephrol. 2015;26:2328–39.

54. Olauson H, Vervloet MG, Cozzolino M, Massy ZA, Urena Torres P, Larsson TE. New insights into the FGF23-Klotho axis. Semin Nephrol. 2014;34:586–97.

55. Fu H, Liu Y. Loss of Klotho in CKD breaks one's heart. J Am Soc Nephrol. 2015;26:2305–7.

56. Xie J, Yoon J, An SW, Kuro-o M, Huang CL. Soluble Klotho protects against uremic cardiomyopathy independently of fibroblast growth factor 23 and phosphate. J Am Soc Nephrol. 2015;26:1150–60.

57. Yang K, Wang C, Nie L, Zhao X, Gu J, Guan X, et al. Klotho protects against indoxyl sulphate-induced myocardial hypertrophy. J Am Soc Nephrol. 2015;26:2434–46.

58. Ritter CS, Brown AJ. Direct suppression of Pth gene expression by the vitamin D prohormones doxercalciferol and calcidiol requires the vitamin D receptor. J Mol Endocrinol. 2011;46:63–6.

59. Klaus G, Watson A, Edefonti A, Fischbach M, Ronnholm K, Schaefer F, et al. Prevention and treatment of renal osteodystrophy in children on chronic renal failure: European guidelines. Pediatr Nephrol. 2006;21:151–9.

60. Haffner D, Schaefer F. Searching the optimal PTH target range in children undergoing peritoneal dialysis: new insights from international cohort studies. Pediatr Nephrol. 2013;28: 537–45.
61. Geary DF, Hodson EM, Craig JC. Interventions for bone disease in children with chronic kidney disease. Cochrane. 2010;(1):CD008327.
62. Bacchetta J, Plotton I, Ranchin B, Vial T, Nicolino M, Morel Y, et al. Precocious puberty and unlicensed paediatric drugs for severe hyperparathyroidism. Nephrol Dial Transplant. 2009;24:2595–8.
63. Silverstein DM, Kher KK, Moudgil A, Khurana M, Wilcox J, Moylan K. Cinacalcet is efficacious in pediatric dialysis patients. Pediatr Nephrol. 2008;23:1817–22.
64. Platt C, Inward C, McGraw M, Dudley J, Tizard J, Burren C, et al. Middle-term use of Cinacalcet in paediatric dialysis patients. Pediatr Nephrol. 2010;25:143–8.
65. Bacchetta J, Ranchin B, Demede D, Allard L. The consequences of pediatric renal transplantation on bone metabolism and growth. Curr Opin Organ Transplant. 2013;18:555–62.
66. Ebbert K, Chow J, Krempien J, Matsuda-Abedini M, Dionne J. Vitamin D insufficiency and deficiency in pediatric renal transplant recipients. Pediatr Transplant. 2015;19:492–8.
67. Lisse TS, Liu T, Irmler M, Beckers J, Chen H, Adams JS, et al. Gene targeting by the vitamin D response element binding protein reveals a role for vitamin D in osteoblast mTOR signaling. FASEB. 2011;25:937–47.
68. Ducloux D, Courivaud C, Bamoulid J, Kazory A, Dumoulin G, Chalopin JM. Pretransplant serum vitamin D levels and risk of cancer after renal transplantation. Transplantation. 2008;85:1755–9.
69. Falkiewicz K, Boratynska M, Speichert-Bidzinska B, Magott-Procelewska M, Biecek P, Patrzalek D, et al. 1,25-dihydroxyvitamin D deficiency predicts poorer outcome after renal transplantation. Transplant Proc. 2009;41:3002–5.
70. Shroff R, Aitkenhead H, Costa N, Trivelli A, Litwin M, Picca S, et al. Normal 25-hydroxyvitamin D levels are associated with less proteinuria and attenuate renal failure progression in children with CKD. J Am Soc Nephrol. 2016;27:314–22.

Part III
Non-classical Effects of Vitamin D

Chapter 14
Vitamin D and Progression of Renal Failure

Marc De Broe

Abstract In addition to his widely recognized endocrine effects on the calcium, phosphate, PTH metabolism, vitamin D has many other pleiotropic effects on the vascular function, blood pressure, proteinuria, insulin resistance, lipid metabolism, inflammation, immunity which all may play a role in the progression of renal failure. Angiotensin-converting enzyme inhibitors (ACEi) for renin-angiotensin-aldosterone system (RAAS) blockade are routinely used to slow CKD progression. Natural vitamin D and active vitamin D analogs may further reduce proteinuria in CKD patients in addition to these current treatment regimens. The inverse correlation of blood pressure and vitamin D plasma levels as well as promising data from small intervention studies of vitamin D supplementation provide a rationale for well performed RCT addressing efficacy and safety of vitamin D in hypertension/cardiovascular diseases. Unfortunately, up to now three RCT have not been able to support this.

Determination of the optimal vitamin D analogue and its optimal dosage in case of protection or slowing down the development of vascular calcifications remains to be investigated in depth in pre-clinical and clinical conditions. Vitamin D supplementation may lead to a small but significant improvement in mortality but did not appear to prevent the development of diabetes in the largest clinical trial to date.

Effects of Vitamin D on renal fibrosis and slowing down/preventing progressive renal damage has been investigated thoroughly in vitro, in vivo and in humans but currently limited to a promising item. The increase in serum creatinine observed during several studies is not attributable to a decrease of the glomerular filtration rate but on the increased creatinine generation, an anabolic effect of vitamin D. Natural vitamin D and active vitamin D preparations are among the few reasonable and evident candidates to be tested in a multicenter, prospective RCT as a potential protector of the failing kidney in patients with CKD 3 and 4.

Keywords Chronic kidney disease • Proteinuria • Hypertension • Renin • Angiotensin • Aldosterone • Calcium • Parathyroid hormone • Phosphate • VDR • Inflammation • FGF23 • Randomized clinical trial (RCT)

M. De Broe, MD, PhD
University Antwerpen, Antwerp, Belgium
e-mail: marc.debroe@uantwerpen.be

© Springer International Publishing Switzerland 2016
P.A. Ureña Torres et al. (eds.), *Vitamin D in Chronic Kidney Disease*,
DOI 10.1007/978-3-319-32507-1_14

14.1 Introduction

Patients with progressive chronic kidney disease (CKD) develop phosphate retention becoming apparent in the serum when CKD stage 3–4 is reached. Indeed FGF23 is secreted by osteocytes at early stage of renal insufficiency and because of his potent phosphaturic effect (by decreasing the brush-border abundance of the sodium phosphate (NaPi2a co-transporter channels) is able to control this phosphate retention at least up to estimated glomerular filtration rate (eGFR) of 50 ml/min/1.73 m^2. Concomitantly FGF23 inhibit synthesis of active vitamin D (calcitriol), inducing a decrease of gastro-intestinal absorption of calcium and hence less inhibitory effect of PTH synthesis at the level of the PTH gland [1].

Klotho expression, an essential co-factor for the phosphatonin FGF23 signaling, is reduced in the failing kidney also at early stages. This reduced klotho levels results in relative FGF23 resistance/less effective elevated levels of FGF23 in promoting renal phosphate excretion The decreased synthesis of active vitamin D, the progressive phosphate retention inducing a relative decrease in ionized calcium (counter ion effect) stimulate PTH synthesis and secretion resulting in the classical secondary hyperparathyroidism (SHPT) of patients with CKD stage 5 [2].

In 1978, a study published in *The Lancet* reported 18 patients who had advanced CKD, and presence of renal osteodystrophy and were treated with either natural vitamin D3 (4,000 IU/day) or 1,25-dihydroxyvitamin D (1,25(OH)$_2$D; 1 µg/day) along with 500 mg of calcium after a 6-month observation period [3]. In the group treated with 1,25(OH)$_2$D, seven of eight patients developed hypercalcemia that necessitated a reduction in dosage. The percentage fall in creatinine clearance was greater during treatment than before treatment in all patients who were on 1,25(OH)$_2$D ($P<0.01$) and in seven of nine patients on vitamin D3 treatment. The authors concluded that deterioration of renal function was a major limitation of the clinical use of 1,25(OH)$_2$D and vitamin D3 in non-dialyzed patients with CKD. Time and things have changed. Currently vitamin D may be considered as one of the leading substances opening perspectives, never thought of, not only concerning his well established favorable effects on the bone and mineral metabolism but as having the potential to slow down the progression of CKD.

The discovery that most tissues and cells in the body have a vitamin D receptor and that several possess the enzymatic machinery to convert the primary circulating form of vitamin D, 25-hydroxyvitamin D, to the active form, 1,25-dihydroxyvitamin D, has opened the way for the currently, discovered many effects of vitamin D in almost any organ/system of the body.

The pleiotropic effects of vitamin D in CKD have been previously reviewed by several authors [4–6]. The specific vitamin D related effects on retarding CKD progression is the main issue of this review. In this context the anti-proteinuric anti-hypertensive, anti-inflammatory and anti-fibrotic effects of vitamin D will be discussed.

14.2 Anti-proteinuric Effect

Already 15 years ago evidence was provided for the functional effects of $1,25(OH)_2D_3$ on mesangial cells [7–9], demonstrating the beneficial action of $1,25(OH)_2D_3$ and 22-oxa-calcitol in regulating mesangial proliferation in vivo. In the anti-thy-1 glomerulonephritis model, both 22-oxa-calcitol and $1,25(OH)_2D_3$ not only inhibited mesangial cell proliferation, but also decreased the degree of glomerulosclerosis and albuminuria, as well as the expression of type I and type IV collagen and a-SMA.

More recent reports indicate that $1,25(OH)_2D_3$ decreases podocyte loss and inhibits podocyte hypertrophy in the subtotal nephrectomy rats [10]. Mean podocyte volume was significantly higher in the subtotal nephrectomy rats, compared with both the sham and $1,25(OH)_2D_3$-treated SNX groups. These findings indicate that hypertrophy of podocytes could be prevented by treatment with $1,25(OH)_2D_3$ and that the podocyte, the key cell in the evolution of proteinuria, is a target for renal protective action of vitamin D. A nice summary on the most important experimental studies using different animal models was written by R Agarwall [11]. The beneficial effect of active vitamin D on glomerular structures is consistent with the results of proteinuria reductions in several animal models [12, 13]. It is well known that glomerular hemodynamic changes, podocyte abnormality and mesangial activation are associated with proteinuria.

There have been several single case reports and small observational studies suggesting an anti-proteinuria benefit of vitamin D therapy [11]. Agarwal reported reduction in proteinuria detected semi-quantitatively by dipstick using an automated analysis in patients who had stages 3 and 4 CKD with secondary hyperparathyroidism and participated in three randomized, controlled trials of oral paricalcitol. In that post hoc analysis, reduction in dipstick proteinuria occurred in the face of the frequent use of agents that block the renin-angiotensin-aldosterone system (RAAS).

Alborzi et al. [14] reported a prospective pilot trial of 24 patients who had CKD2-3 and were randomly allocated in a double-blind manner to three equal groups to receive 0, 1, or 2 µg of paricalcitol, a vitamin D analog, orally for 1 month. It seems from that study that paricalcitol-induced reduction in albuminuria and inflammation may be mediated independent of its effects on hemodynamics or PTH suppression. In an uncontrolled trial, reported from Hong Kong [15], ten patients with biopsy-proven IgA nephropathy and persistent proteinuria despite angiotensin-converting enzyme inhibition and angiotensin II receptor blockade were treated with 0.5 µg calcitriol twice weekly for 12 weeks. After calcitriol treatment, there was a significant overall decrease in urine protein-creatinine during the first 6 weeks that persisted throughout the study period. No significant change in blood pressure (BP) or renal function was noted.

Lowering of albuminuria or proteinuria in these trials, occurred without changes in BP even when recorded by ambulatory BP monitoring, raising the notion that the decrease in proteinuria (improvement in kidney disease?) conferred by the use of these drugs may occur via non hemodynamic pathways.

In a large multinational, placebo-controlled, double-blind trial (VITAL) [16], patients with type 2 diabetes and albuminuria who were receiving angiotensin-converting enzyme inhibitors (ACEi) or angiotensin receptor blockers were enrolled and received during 24 weeks' treatment with placebo, 1 µg/day paricalcitol, or 2 µg/day paricalcitol. Addition of 2 µg/day of paricalcitol to RAAS inhibition safely lowered residual albuminuria in patients with diabetic nephropathy. The anti-proteinuric effect was particularly seen in patients on a high salt diet who had poor response to RAAS therapy. Persistent RAAS activity may be due to incomplete blockade or a rebound rise in renin during treatment; renin inhibition is shown to augment the anti-proteinuric effect.

In an important prospective observational [17] study it was determined whether nutritional vitamin D repletion can have additional beneficial effects in patients with type 2 diabetic nephropathy already established on RAAS inhibition. During a 7-month period, 63 patients were enrolled and those with low levels of circulating 25(OH)D were treated with oral cholecalciferol for 4 months. Baseline serum 25(OH)D and 1,25(OH)$_2$D levels showed no significant correlation with baseline urinary monocyte chimioattractant-1 (MCP-1), transforming growth factor β-1 (TGFβ1), or albuminuria measured as the urinary albumin-to-creatinine ratio. Of the 63 patients, 54 had insufficient or deficient levels of serum 25(OH)D and 49 complied with cholecalciferol therapy and follow-up. Both 25(OH)D and 1,25(OH)$_2$D were significantly increased at 2 and 4 months of treatment. Albuminuria (25 %) and urinary TGFβ1 decreased significantly at both time points compared to their baseline values, while urinary MCP-1 did not change.

Thus, in the short term, dietary vitamin D repletion with cholecalciferol had a beneficial effect in delaying the progression of diabetic nephropathy, as measured by albuminuria and pro-fibrotic urinary markers, above that due to established RAAS-inhibition [18].

MH de Borst et al. [19] performed very recently a systematic review of the literature on active treatment for reduction of residual proteinuria. All randomized controlled trials of vitamin D analogs in patients with CKD that reported an effect on proteinuria with sample size >50 were selected. From 907 citations retrieved six studies providing data for 688 patients were included in the meta-analysis. Active vitamin D analogs reduced (−16 %) proteinuria compared with controls. Active vitamin D further reduce proteinuria in CKD patients even in fully RAAS-inhibited patients. Natural, nutritional vitamin D seems to have short-term beneficial effects in diabetic patients with CKD treated with RAAS-inhibition.

14.3   Anti-hypertensive Effects of Vitamin D

Seminal discoveries by Li et al. [20] demonstrated that vitamin D is a potent negative endocrine regulator of the RAAS by suppressing of renin biosynthesis [21]. This vitamin D repression of renin expression is independent of calcium metabolism, the volume- and salt-sensing mechanisms, and the angiotensin II feedback regulation [20]. In normal mice, vitamin D deficiency stimulates renin expression, whereas injection of $1,25(OH)_2D$ reduces renin synthesis.

Mice that lack the vitamin D receptor (VDR) have elevated production of renin and angiotensin II, leading to hypertension, cardiac hypertrophy, and increased water intake [20]. Vitamin D receptor knock-out mice have increased the production of renin and angiotensin II with resultant arterial hypertension and left ventricular hypertrophy (LVH) [22]. Mice deficient in $1,25(OH)_2D$ synthesis develop hypertension, cardiac hypertrophy and reduced systolic function due to overstimulation of renal and cardiac RAAS [23] (Fig. 14.1).

The inverse correlation of blood pressure and vitamin D plasma levels as well as promising data from small intervention studies of vitamin D supplementation provide a rationale for well performed RCT addressing efficacy and safety of vitamin D in hypertension/cardiovascular diseases [24, 25].

A meta-analysis of 18 randomized controlled trials showed that there were fewer deaths in participants randomized to vitamin D supplementation as compared to those on placebo [26]. When the relative risk for incident hypertension was computed amongst participants of two large and independent prospective cohort studies, during the 4-year follow-up subjects with a 25(OH)D level <15 ng/mL were threefold more likely to develop hypertension than those with a 25(OH)D level ≥30 ng/mL [26].

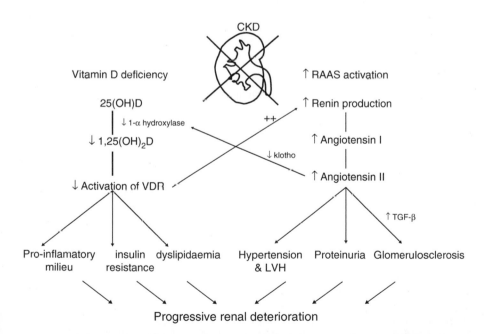

Fig. 14.1 The vit D axis and the renin-angiotensin-aldosterone system (RAAS) in chronic kidney disease (CKD) and their interactions. *VDR* Vit D receptor, *LVH* left ventricular hypertrophy, *25(OH)D* 25-hydroxyvitamin D, *1,25(OH)₂D* 1,25-dihydroxyvitamin-D, *TGF-β* transforming growth factor beta (Adapted from Shroff et al. [6])

The important role for vitamin D deficiency in the pathogenesis and maintenance of hypertension in African Americans has recently been described as a unifying hypothesis encompassing his anti-RAAS, insulin sensitivity, anti-inflammatory and vascular effects [27].

Secondary hyperparathyroidism, seen in all patients with CKD4-combined or not with vitamin D deficiency/insufficiency, could be a mechanism for hypertension. It is a well known that high PTH levels affect vascular smooth muscle cells and increase vascular stiffness and promotes atherosclerosis [28]. Two clinical trials in hemodialysis patients have shown that treatment with vitamin D analogues lead to a reduction in renin and angiotensin II levels and a significant regression of LVH [29, 30].

In patients receiving peritoneal dialysis, a lower serum 25(OH)D concentration was shown to be associated with an increased risk of cardiovascular events, those with a 25(OH)D level of $\geq$45.7 nmol/L had a significantly higher cardiovascular event-free survival probability than those with a 25(OH)D level $\leq$45.7 nmol/L [31].

Despite plenty of observation al data on the association of vitamin with decreased cardiovascular- related morbidity and mortality the Paricalcitol Capsule Benefits in Renal Failure-Induced Cardiac Morbidity (PRIMO) trial, a randomized controlled trial on a group of 227 patients with CKD with mild-to-moderate LVH and preserved left-ventricular ejection fraction, could not show the influence of 48 weeks of paricalcitol therapy on the left ventricular mass index or on Döppler measures of diastolic dysfunction [32, 33].

Paricalcitol and ENdothelial fuNction in chronic kidneY disease (PENNY trial) is a double-blinded randomized controlled trial testing the effect of an active form of vitamin D, paricalcitol (2 μg/day × 12 weeks) on endothelium-dependent and endothelium-independent vasodilatation in 88 patients with stage 3–4 CKD and serum PTH levels >65 pg/mL (paricalcitol, n=44; placebo, n=44). Baseline flow-mediated dilation was identical in patients on paricalcitol (3.6±2.9%) and placebo (3.6±2.9%) groups. After 12 weeks of treatment, flow-mediated dilation rose in the paricalcitol but not in the placebo group, and the between-group difference in flow-mediated dilation changes (the primary end point, 1.8%; 95% confidence interval, 0.3–3.1%) was significant (P=0.016), and the mean proportional change in flow-mediated dilation was 61% higher in paricalcitol-treated patients than in placebo-treated patients. Such an effect was abolished 2 weeks after stopping the treatment. No effect of paricalcitol on endothelium-independent vasodilatation was registered. Paricalcitol improves endothelium-dependent vasodilatation in patients with stage 3–4 CKD.

The recently reported effect of paricalcitol on left ventricular mass and function in CKD (the OPERA trial) did not find a left ventricular mass difference for the chronic administration of paricalcitol to patients with CKD stages 3–5 [34].

As Goldsmith wrote recently with first the Paricalcitol Capsule Benefits in Renal Failure-Induced Cardiac Morbidity (PRIMO) study the PENNY trial and now the OPERA trial, the fat lady has indeed finished singing, at least her first act [35].

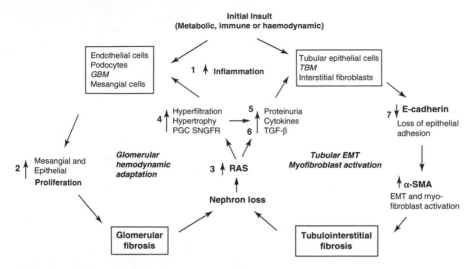

Fig. 14.2   Active vitamin D (*1*) has anti-inflammatory effects; (*2*) inhibits mesangial and podocyte proliferation; (*3*) down-regulates the renin-angiotensin system (RAS) by inhibiting renin production; (*4*) prevents glomerular hypertrophy as measured by glomerular volume in 5/6 subtotal nephrectomized rats; (*5*) decreases proteinuria in different animal models of CKD; (*6*) decreases fibrogenic cytokine production in the kidney by regulating Smad3 and TGF-b pathways; (*7*) has the potential to block the EMT and myofibroblast activation. *RAS* renin-angiotensin system, *PGC* glomerular capillary pressure, *SNGFR* single-nephron glomerular filtration rate, *a-SMA* a-smooth muscle actin, *EMT* epithelial to mesenchymal transition [9]

14.4   Non RAAS-Mediated Effects on the Cardiovascular System

CKD particularly CKD dialysis [36] population is characterized by intimal and even more medial arterial calcifications and arterial stiffness resulting in a vascular phenotype that is seen with advanced age [37] in adults [38] and in children [39]. Secondary hyperparathyroidism, seen in most of patients with CKD4-combined or not with vitamin D deficiency/insufficiency, could be a mechanism for hypertension and cardiac hypertrophy. It is well known that high circulating PTH levels affect vascular smooth muscle cells and increase vascular stiffness and promotes atherosclerosis [28, 40].

At the level of the vascular smooth muscle cell, VDR activators (VDRAs) can promote increased calcium uptake by the cells both through systemic effects and local effects mediated via the VDR and calcium channels in the vessel wall [41]. However, VDRAs also have a protective role and have been shown to suppress smooth muscle cell proliferation [42], down-regulate osteoblastic gene expression [43], decrease (Fig. 14.2) TGFβ1 expression in plaques [44] and up-regulate local production of the calcification inhibitor matrix gla-protein (MGP) [43] (Fig. 14.3

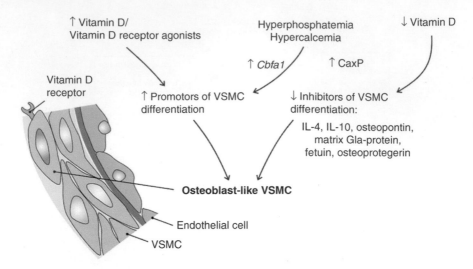

Fig. 14.3 Vascular calcification in chronic kidney disease (CKD) is induced via both passive Ca ×
P deposition and active transformation of vascular smooth muscle cells (*VSMCs*) into an osteoblast-
like phenotype. The vitamin D receptor (VDR) agonist paricalcitol is useful in the treatment of
CKD patients. Besides effectively suppressing secondary hyperthyroidism, paricalcitol seems to
be less phosphatemic and calcemic, therefore decreasing the risk for vascular calcification
(Adapted from Huybers and Bindels [45])

[45]). Determination of the optimal vitamin D analogue and its optimal dosage in
case of protection or slowing down the development of vascular calcifications
remains to be investigation in depth (Fig. 14.2).

14.5   Vitamin D and Insulin Resistance, Obesity and Lipid Metabolism

Data from observational studies and animal-experimental models suggest that vitamin D therapy holds promise for improving health outcomes in CKD. Improved
glucose metabolism is one potential mechanism through which vitamin D may exert
beneficial effects.

Data from the hemodialysis population consistently suggest that calcitriol
improves short-term insulin secretion and insulin sensitivity in ESRD. Data
addressing long-term outcomes are only available in the general population, in
which vitamin D supplementation may lead to a small but significant improvement
in mortality but did not appear to prevent the development of diabetes in the largest
clinical trial to date [46]. One potential explanation is that patients with CKD may
derive more benefit from vitamin D interventions, given their more profound defi-
ciencies in vitamin D at baseline. In particular, vitamin D therapy may be most
effective when intrinsic 1-α hydroxylase activity is most impaired [47].

Obesity-associated vitamin D insufficiency is likely due to the decreased bio-availability of vitamin D from cutaneous and dietary sources because of its sequestration in the body fat [48]. Unfortunately, weight reduction is unlikely to occur with vitamin D supplementation alone [49].

Rodriguez-Rodriguez et al. have shown that vitamin D deficiency is an independent predictor of elevated triglycerides [50]. Motiwala and Wang [51] and Zittermann [52] have shown that vitamin D modulates lipid metabolism by decreasing the level of serum triglyceride (TG) in overweight subjects. However, studies using 25(OH)D supplementation in the general population as well as in adults with CKD have not shown any lowering of HDL cholesterol [53].

14.6   Vitamin D and Inflammation and Immune Modulation

CKD has to be considered as a chronic inflammatory clinical setting. Markers of inflammation such as CRP and IL-6 predict major disease (cardiovascular diseases and infection) outcome in dialysis patients. Wolf et al. [54] found an increased mortality among incident hemodialysis patients in those with low circulating vitamin D levels. Zehnder et al. [55] described a relation between reduced vitamin D hormonal system in kidney disease with increased inflammation. Within the kidney $1,25(OH)_2D$ can attenuate TNFα induced MCP-1 expression by the proximal tubular cells and sequestration of NFkappa-beta signaling [56].

In innate immune responses, activation of Toll-like receptors (TLRs) triggers direct anti-microbial activity against intracellular bacteria, which in murine monocytes and macrophages is mediated principally by nitric oxide. TLR activation of human macrophages is up-regulating the expression of the vitamin D receptor and the vitamin D-1–hydroxylase genes, leading to induction of the anti-microbial peptide cathelicidin and killing of intracellular *Mycobacterium tuberculosis*. Sera from African-American individuals, known to have increased susceptibility to tuberculosis, had low 25-hydroxyvitamin D levels and were inefficient in supporting cathelicidin messenger RNA induction. These data demonstrate a link between TLRs and vitamin D–mediated innate immunity and suggest that differences in ability of human populations to produce vitamin D may contribute to susceptibility to microbial infection [57].

Salamon et al. [58] reported a novel, metabolic role for vitamin D in tuberculosis identified through integrated transcriptome and mechanistic studies. Transcriptome analysis revealed an association between the VDR and lipid metabolism in human tuberculosis and infected macrophages. Vitamin D treatment of infected macrophages abrogated infection-induced accumulation of lipid droplets, which are required for intracellular M. tuberculosis growth. Additional transcriptomics results showed that vitamin D down-regulates the pro-adipogenic peroxisome proliferator-activated receptor γ (PPARγ) in infected macrophages. PPARγ agonists reversed the anti-adipogenic and the anti-microbial effects of VDR, indicating a link between VDR and PPARγ signaling in regulating both vitamin D functions. These findings suggest the potential for host-based, adjunct anti-tuberculosis therapy targeting lipid metabolism [58].

How far this anti-inflammatory actions of vitamin D are able to limit the renal invasion of inflammatory cells hence fibrosis and slowing down the progression of the CKD process is unknown.

14.7   Vitamin D and Renal Fibrosis and Slowing Down or Preventing Progressive Nephropathy

This aspect of the pleiotropic gamma of activities of vitamin D is a fascinating but currently limited to be a promising item.

Active vitamin D has been shown to inhibit several of the pathogenic pathways in renal fibrosis as is depicted schematically in Fig. 14.3.

Direct evidence for vitamin D inhibition of interstitial fibrogenesis was obtained in cultured interstitial fibroblasts. It was found that $1,25(OH)_2D_3$ suppressed the myofibroblast activation from interstitial fibroblast [59], a critical event in generating a-smooth muscle actin (a-SMA)-positive, matrix-producing effector cells in diseased kidney. Myofibroblast activation was initiated by incubation with TGFβ1, and treatment of rat renal interstitial fibroblasts (NRK-49F) with $1,25(OH)_2D_3$ suppressed TGFβ1 induced a-SMA expression in a dose-dependent manner. Similarly, $1,25(OH)_2D_3$ suppressed type collagen and thrombospondin-1 expression triggered by TGFβ1. These results establish the anti-fibrotic activities of active vitamin D, through its counteraction of the pro-fibrotic TGFβ1. The mechanism underlying vitamin D's ability to inhibit myofibroblast activation was further investigated. It turns out that $1,25(OH)_2D_3$-induced anti-fibrotic hepatocyte growth factor (HGF) mRNA expression and protein secretion in renal interstitial fibroblasts [59].

The TGFβ superfamily comprises pleiotropic cytokines that regulate SMAD and non-SMAD signaling. TGFβ–SMAD signal transduction is known to be involved in tissue fibrosis, including renal fibrosis. Ito et al. [60] found that 1,25-dihydroxyvitamin D_3–bound [$1,25(OH)_2D_3$-bound] vitamin D receptor (VDR) specifically inhibits TGFβ–SMAD signal transduction through direct interaction with SMAD3. In mouse models of tissue fibrosis, $1,25(OH)_2D_3$ treatment prevented renal fibrosis through the suppression of TGFβ–SMAD signal transduction. Based on the structure of the VDR-ligand complex, 2 synthetic ligands were generated. These ligands selectively inhibited TGFβ–SMAD signal transduction without activating VDR-mediated transcription and significantly attenuated renal fibrosis in mice. These results indicate that $1,25(OH)_2D_3$-dependent suppression of TGFβ–SMAD signal transduction is independent of VDR-mediated transcriptional activity. In addition, these ligands did not cause hypercalcemia resulting from stimulation of the transcriptional activity of the VDR. This study provides a new strategy for generating chemical compounds that specifically inhibit TGF-β–SMAD signal transduction. Since TGFβ–SMAD signal transduction is reportedly involved in several disorders. This non-classical vitamin D receptor pathway suppressing renal fibrosis will aid in the development of new drugs that do not cause detectable adverse effects, such as hypercalcemia.

Zhang et al. [61] in a hallmark paper demonstrated that combined treatment of diabetic mice with losartan and paricalcitol completely prevents albuminuria, restores glomerular filtration barrier structure, and markedly reduces glomerulosclerosis blockade of intra-renal renin and angiotensin II induced by hyperglycemia and losartan is observed indicating that inhibition of RAAS combined with vitamin D is able to prevent development of diabetic nephropathy.

Other vitamin D analogues have similar effects; when subtotally nephrectomized rats were treated with calcitriol, doxercalciferol or oxacalcitriol, there was a 16–25 % reduction in proteinuria by 8 weeks, and this was accompanied by reduced mesangial cell proliferation, reduced interleukin-6 (IL-6) levels, glomerular inflammation and glomerulosclerosis [62].

Paricalcitol can suppress the progression of renal insufficiency (remnant kidney model) via mediation of the TGFβ1 signaling pathway, and this effect is amplified when BP is controlled via renin-angiotensin system (RAS) blockade [62].

Tan et al. [63] evaluated the efficacy of active vitamin D in mouse model with nephropathy induced by unilateral ureteral obstruction, a widely used, aggressive interstitial fibrosis model characterized by rapid tubular atrophy and interstitial expansion and matrix deposition. The activation of vitamin D receptor, through the use of paricalcitol, significantly reduced the fibrotic lesions in obstructed kidney in a dose-dependent fashion, as demonstrated by a reduced interstitial volume and decreased deposition of interstitial matrix components [63]. Paricalcitol substantially inhibited renal mRNA expression of fibronectin, type I and type III collagen, and fibrogenic TGFβ1, while preserved E-cadherin and VDR expression, block epithelial to mesenchymal transition and inhibit apoptosis, cell proliferation in the obstructed kidney [63].

In another study Tan et al. [64] have compared the individual renal protective efficacy of paricalcitol and trandolapril (an ACEi) in obstructive nephropathy, and examined any potential additive effects of their combination on attenuating renal fibrosis and inflammation. Mice underwent unilateral ureteral obstruction and were treated individually with paricalcitol or trandolapril or their combination. Compared to vehicle-treated controls, monotherapy with paricalcitol or trandolapril inhibited the expression and accumulation of fibronectin and type I and type III collagen, suppressed a-SMA, vimentin, and Snail-1 expression, and reduced total collagen content in the obstructed kidney. Combination therapy led to a more profound inhibition of all parameters. Monotherapy also suppressed renal RANTES (regulated on activation, normal T cell expressed and secreted) and TNFα-expression and inhibited renal infiltration of T cells and macrophages, whereas the combination had additive effects. Renin expression was induced in the fibrotic kidney and was augmented by trandolapril. Paricalcitol blocked renin induction in the absence or presence of trandolapril.

To address the role of the VDR in renal fibrogenesis, Zhang et al. [65] underwent VDR-null mice to unilateral ureteral obstruction for 7 days. Compared with wild-type mice, VDR-null mice developed more severe renal damage in the obstructed kidney, with marked tubular atrophy and interstitial fibrosis. Significant induction of extracellular matrix proteins (fibronectin and collagen I), pro-fibrogenic and pro-inflammatory factors (TGFβ, connective tissue growth factor, and monocyte che-moattractant protein 1), and epithelial-to-mesenchymal transition were present together with morphologic lesions. Because VDR ablation activates the RAS and leads to accumulation of angiotensin II in the kidney, they assessed whether ele-vated angiotensin II in the VDR-null kidney promotes injury. Treatment with the angiotensin 1 antagonist losartan eliminated the difference in obstruction-induced interstitial fibrosis between wild-type and VDR-null mice, suggesting that angiotensin II contributes to the enhanced renal fibrosis observed in obstructed VDR-null kidneys.

A recent interesting paper by R Shroff et al. [66] consisted in a retrospective analysis of the ESCAPE (Effect of Strict Blood Pressure Control and ACE Inhibition on Progression of CKD in Pediatric Patients) cohort on the effect of vitamin D on proteinuria and CKD progression in children. The annualized loss of eGFR was inversely associated with baseline 25(OH)D level (P<0.001, r=0.32).

Five-year renal survival was 75 % in patients with baseline 25(OH)D ≥50 nmol/L and 50 % in those with lower 25(OH). This retrospective study has his limitations but at least it's a solid base for its conclusion: vitamin D is an effective, easily avail-able, safe, and cheap nutritional supplement that may be a useful adjunctive treat-ment to RAAS blockade to retard progressive renal function decline.

Interestingly, a retrospective analysis of 76 renal transplant patients with chronic allograft nephropathy found that treatment with calcitriol was associated with a significant improvement of graft survival at 3 years compared with the group that was not treated with calcitriol [67]. However, there are no prospective trials that have studied the possible reno-protective effect of active vitamin D on renal out-come using appropriate hard end points [67].

14.8   Vitamin D and Estimated Glomerular Filtration Rate

In clinical studies, vitamin D receptor activation facilitates an anti-proteinuric response that is incremental to blood pressure reduction and RAS blockade, sug-gesting an explanation for the benefit of reduction of proteinuria and decreased mortality in patients with kidney disease and receiving active vitamin D. Yet the increase in serum creatinine observed during these studies raises important ques-tions about the overall long-term benefit of vitamin D receptor activation for kidney function.

The effect of vitamin D on serum creatinine was reversible after the cessation of therapy [68]. In small studies, the reduction in creatinine clearance associated with vitamin D therapy was not seen in patients who had simultaneous measurement of GFR [68].

Perez et al. [69] and older studies, have suggested that vitamin D receptor activation may alter creatinine metabolism and/or its handling by the kidney.

Recently, Agarwal et al. [70] examined the effect of VDR activation on creatinine metabolism and measured GFR. A 7-day course of paricalcitol (2 µgr daily) resulted in an increase in serum creatinine and urine creatinine, while creatinine clearance did not change. Simultaneous measurement of GFR with iothalamate was not altered by paricalcitol therapy. Moreover, within 4 days of cessation of vitamin D therapy, they observed changes in creatinine generation and serum creatinine reversed back to near the baseline. In other words short term VDR activation increases creatinine generation and serum creatinine, but it does not influence the GFR. Hence theses changes have nothing to do with a nephrotoxic effect of vitamin D on the kidney. How far this anabolic effect of vitamin D receptor activation may be improving skeletal and myocardial function and have a beneficial effect on mortality in chronic renal failure patients remains to be determined.

14.9 Conclusions

Almost 40 years after the paper by Christiansen et al. describing the deterioration of renal function during vitamin D treatment there is more than a profuse literature on the beneficial effect of active and natural vitamin D, on several important aspects of the progression of a CKD patient towards renal failure [3].

The major problem is that the vast majority of this pinpointed investigations in vitro, in vivo and also in man have not been able to answer simple but essential clinical questions.

More and better clinical work using the appropriate methodology such as randomized clinical trials (RCTs) [71] is needed to e.g. elucidate whether formal repletion at early stage of CKD, nowadays a very common practice in renal centers, using cholecalciferol or ergocalciferol can prevent the renal, cardiac, and skeletal complications associated with CKD.

Despite numerous observational data on the association of vitamin D with decreased cardiovascular related morbidity and mortality three RCT "PRIMO" "PENNY" and "OPERA" showed no differences on the left ventricular mass index and function of vitamin D analogs compared to untreated patients.

The demonstration has been made several times that in vitro experiments, experimental studies and simplistic clinical observations/trials become irrelevant when applied in a proper way to a patient group with moderate to severe renal failure [72].

It is more than time that the renal community leaves his weak reputation when evaluating the number of relevant high quality controlled studies performed by the different disciplines of internal medicine [71]. Natural vitamin D is one of the few reasonable and evident candidates to be tested in a multicenter, prospective RCT as a potential protector of the failing kidney in patients with CKD 3 and 4.

Acknowledgement Erik Snelders was a more than relevant help in the realization of this manuscript.

References

1. Levin A, Bakris GL, Molitch M, Smulders M, Tian J, Williams LA, Andress DL. Prevalence of abnormal serum vitamin D, PTH, calcium, and phosphorus in patients with chronic kidney disease: results of the study to evaluate early kidney disease. Kidney Int. 2007;71(1):31–8.
2. Shroff R, Shanahan C. Klotho: an elixir of youth for the vasculature. JASN. 2011;22:5–7.
3. Christiansen C, Rødbro P, Christensen MS, Hartnack B, Transbøl I. Deterioration of renal function during treatment of chronic renal failure with 1,25-dihydroxycholecalciferol. Lancet. 1978;2(8092 Pt 1):700–3.
4. Holick MF. Vitamin D, deficiency. N Engl J Med. 2007;357(3):266–81.
5. Shroff R, Knott C, Rees L. The virtues of vitamin D – but how much is too much? Pediatr Nephrol. 2010;25(9):1607–20.
6. Shroff R, Wan M, Rees L. Can vitamin D slow down the progression of chronic kidney disease? Pediatr Nephrol. 2012;27(12):2167–73.
7. Makibayshi K, Tatematsu M, Hirata M, et al. A vitamin D analog ameliorates glomerular injury on rat glomerulonephritis. Am J Pathol. 2001;158(5):1733–41.
8. Panichi V, Migliori M, Taccola D, et al. Effects of 1,25(OH)$_2$D$_3$ in experimental mesangial proliferative nephritis in rats. Kidney Int. 2001;60(1):87–95.
9. Tian J, Liu Y, Williams LA, de Zeeuw D. Potential role of active vitamin D in retarding the progression of chronic kidney disease. Nephrol Dial Transplant. 2007;22(2):321–8.
10. Kuhlmann A, Haas CS, Gross ML, Reulbach U, Holzinger M, Schwarz U, Ritz E, Amann K. 1,25-Dihydroxyvitamin D3 decreases podocyte loss and podocyte hypertrophy in the subtotally nephrectomized rat. Am J Physiol Renal Physiol. 2004;286(3):F526–33.
11. Agarwal R. Vitamin D, proteinuria, diabetic nephropathy, and progression of CKD. Clin J Am Soc Nephrol. 2009;4(9):1523–8.
12. Schwarz U, Amann K, Orth SR, Simonaviciene A, Wessels S, Ritz E. Effect of 1,25(OH)$_2$ vitamin D3 on glomerulosclerosis in subtotally nephrectomized rats. Kidney Int. 1998;53(6): 1696–705.
13. Hirata M, Makibayashi K, Katsumata K, Kusano K, Watanabe T, Fukushima N, Doi T. 22-Oxacalcitriol prevents progressive glomerulosclerosis without adversely affecting calcium and phosphorus metabolism in subtotally nephrectomized rats. Nephrol Dial Transplant. 2002;17(12):2132–7.
14. Alborzi P, Patel NA, Peterson C, Bills JE, Bekele DM, Bunaye Z, Light RP, Agarwal R. Paricalcitol reduces albuminuria and inflammation in chronic kidney disease: a randomized double-blind pilot trial. Hypertension. 2008;52(2):249–55.
15. Szeto CC, Chow KM, Kwan BC, Chung KY, Leung CB, Li PK. Oral calcitriol for the treatment of persistent proteinuria in immunoglobulin A nephropathy: an uncontrolled trial. Am J Kidney Dis. 2008;51(5):724–31.
16. de Zeeuw D, Agarwal R, Amdahl M, Audhya P, Coyne D, Garimella T, Parving HH, Pritchett Y, Remuzzi G, Ritz E, Andress D. Selective vitamin D receptor activation with paricalcitol for reduction of albuminuria in patients with type 2 diabetes (VITAL study): a randomised controlled trial. Lancet. 2010;376(9752):1543–51.
17. Kim MJ, Frankel AH, Donaldson M, Darch SJ, Pusey CD, Hill PD, Mayr M, Tam FW. Oral cholecalciferol decreases albuminuria and urinary TGF-β1 in patients with type 2 diabetic nephropathy on established renin-angiotensin-aldosterone system inhibition. Kidney Int. 2011;80(8):851–60.
18. Kumar R. New clinical trials with vitamin D and analogs in renal disease. Kidney Int. 2011;80(8):793–6.
19. de Borst MH, Hajhosseiny R, Tamez H, Wenger J, Thadhani R, Goldsmith DJ. Active vitamin D treatment for reduction of residual proteinuria: a systematic review. J Am Soc Nephrol. 2013;24(11):1863–71.
20. Li YC, Kong J, Wei M, Chen ZF, Liu SQ, Cao LP. 1,25-Dihydroxyvitamin D(3) is a negative endocrine regulator of the renin-angiotensin system. J Clin Invest. 2002;110(2):229–38.

21. Lindner A, Charra B, Sherrard DJ, Scribner BH. Accelerated atherosclerosis in prolonged maintenance hemodialysis. N Engl J Med. 1974;290(13):697–701.
22. Xiang W, Kong J, Chen S, Cao LP, Qiao G, Zheng W, Liu W, Li X, Gardner DG, Li YC. Cardiac hypertrophy in vitamin D receptor knockout mice: role of the systemic and cardiac renin-angiotensin systems. Am J Physiol Endocrinol Metab. 2005;288(1):E125–32.
23. Zhou C, Lu F, Cao K, Xu D, Goltzman D, Miao D. Calcium-independent and 1,25(OH)2D3-dependent regulation of the renin-angiotensin system in 1alpha-hydroxylase knockout mice. Kidney Int. 2008;74(2):170–9.
24. Forman JP, Giovannucci E, Holmes MD, Bischoff-Ferrari HA, Tworoger SS, Willett WC, Curhan GC. Plasma 25-hydroxyvitamin D levels and risk of incident hypertension. Hypertension. 2007;49(5):1063–9.
25. Feneis JF, Arora RR. Role of vitamin D in blood pressure homeostasis. Am J Ther. 2010;17(6):e221–9.
26. Wang TJ, Pencina MJ, Booth SL, Jacques PF, Ingelsson E, Lanier K, Benjamin EJ, D'Agostino RB, Wolf M, Vasan RS. Vitamin D deficiency and risk of cardiovascular disease. Circulation. 2008;117(4):503–11.
27. Rostand SG. Vitamin D, blood pressure, and African Americans: toward a unifying hypothesis. Clin J Am Soc Nephrol. 2010;5(9):1697–703.
28. Pilz S, Tomaschitz A, Ritz E, Pieber TR. Vitamin D status and arterial hypertension: a systematic review. Nat Rev Cardiol. 2009;6(10):621–30.
29. Park CW, Oh YS, Shin YS, Kim CM, Kim YS, Kim SY, Choi EJ, Chang YS, Bang BK. Intravenous calcitriol regresses myocardial hypertrophy in hemodialysis patients with secondary hyperparathyroidism. Am J Kidney Dis. 1999;33(1):73–81.
30. Kim HW, Park CW, Shin YS, Kim YS, Shin SJ, Kim YS, Choi EJ, Chang YS, Bang BK. Calcitriol regresses cardiac hypertrophy and QT dispersion in secondary hyperparathyroidism on hemodialysis. Nephron Clin Pract. 2006;102(1):c21–9.
31. Wang AY, Lam CW, Sanderson JE, Wang M, Chan IH, Lui SF, Sea MM, Woo J. Serum 25-hydroxyvitamin D status and cardiovascular outcomes in chronic peritoneal dialysis patients: a 3-y prospective cohort study. Am J Clin Nutr. 2008;87(6):1631–8.
32. Tamez H, Zoccali C, Packham D, Wenger J, Bhan I, Appelbaum E, Pritchett Y, Chang Y, Agarwal R, Wanner C, Lloyd-Jones D, Cannata J, Thompson BT, Andress D, Zhang W, Singh B, Zehnder D, Pachika A, Manning WJ, Shah A, Solomon SD, Thadhani R. Vitamin D reduces left atrial volume in patients with left ventricular hypertrophy and chronic kidney disease. Am Heart J. 2012;164(6):902–9.
33. Thadhani R, Appelbaum E, Pritchett Y, Chang Y, Wenger J, Tamez H, Bhan I, Agarwal R, Zoccali C, Wanner C, Lloyd-Jones D, Cannata J, Thompson BT, Andress D, Zhang W, Packham D, Singh B, Zehnder D, Shah A, Pachika A, Manning WJ, Solomon SD. Vitamin D therapy and cardiac structure and function in patients with chronic kidney disease: the PRIMO randomized controlled trial. JAMA. 2012;307(7):674–84.
34. Wang AY, Fang F, Chan J, Wen YY, Qing S, Chan IH, Lo G, Lai KN, Lo WK, Lam CW, Yu CM. Effect of paricalcitol on left ventricular mass and function in CKD – the OPERA trial. J Am Soc Nephrol. 2014;25(1):175–86.
35. Goldsmith DJ, Massy ZA, Brandenburg V. The uses and abuses of Vitamin D compounds in chronic kidney disease-mineral bone disease (CKD-MBD). Semin Nephrol. 2014;34(6):660–8.
36. Nakamura S, Ishibashi-Ueda H, Niizuma S, Yoshihara F, Horio T, Kawano Y. Coronary calcification in patients with chronic kidney disease and coronary artery disease. Clin J Am Soc Nephrol. 2009;4(12):1892–900.
37. Shroff RC, McNair R, Figg N, Skepper JN, Schurgers L, Gupta A, Hiorns M, Donald AE, Deanfield J, Rees L, Shanahan CM. Dialysis accelerates medial vascular calcification in part by triggering smooth muscle cell apoptosis. Circulation. 2008;118(17):1748–57.
38. London GM, Guérin AP, Verbeke FH, Pannier B, Boutouyrie P, Marchais SJ, Métivier F. Mineral metabolism and arterial functions in end-stage renal disease: potential role of 25-hydroxyvitamin D deficiency. J Am Soc Nephrol. 2007;18(2):613–20.

39. Shroff R, Egerton M, Bridel M, Shah V, Donald AE, Cole TJ, Hiorns MP, Deanfield JE, Rees L. A bimodal association of vitamin D levels and vascular disease in children on dialysis. J Am Soc Nephrol. 2008;19(6):1239–46.
40. Shroff RC, Donald AE, Hiorns MP, Watson A, Feather S, Milford D, Ellins EA, Storry C, Ridout D, Deanfield J, Rees L. Mineral metabolism and vascular damage in children on dialysis. J Am Soc Nephrol. 2007;18(11):2996–3003.
41. Shroff RC, Shanahan CM. The vascular biology of calcification. Semin Dial. 2007;20(2):103–9.
42. Carthy EP, Yamashita W, Hsu A, Ooi BS. 1,25-Dihydroxyvitamin D3 and rat vascular smooth muscle cell growth. Hypertension. 1989;13(6 Pt 2):954–9.
43. Mathew S, Lund RJ, Chaudhary LR, Geurs T, Hruska KA. Vitamin D receptor activators can protect against vascular calcification. J Am Soc Nephrol. 2008;19(8):1509–19.
44. Becker LE, Koleganova N, Piecha G, Noronha IL, Zeier M, Geldyyev A, Kökeny G, Ritz E, Gross ML. Effect of paricalcitol and calcitriol on aortic wall remodeling in uninephrectomized ApoE knockout mice. Am J Physiol Renal Physiol. 2011;300(3):F772–82.
45. Huybers S, Bindels RJ. Vascular calcification in chronic kidney disease: new developments in drug therapy. Kidney Int. 2007;72(6):663–5.
46. de Boer IH, Tinker LF, Connelly S, Curb JD, Howard BV, Kestenbaum B, Larson JC, Manson JE, Margolis KL, Siscovick DS, Weiss NS. Calcium plus vitamin D supplementation and the risk of incident diabetes in the Women's Health Initiative. Diabetes Care. 2008;31(4):701–7.
47. de Boer IH. Vitamin D and glucose metabolism in chronic kidney disease. Curr Opin Nephrol Hypertens. 2008;17(6):566–72.
48. Wortsman J, Matsuoka LY, Chen TC, Lu Z, Holick MF. Decreased bioavailability of vitamin D in obesity. Am J Clin Nutr. 2000;72(3):690–3.
49. Sneve M, Figenschau Y, Jorde R. Supplementation with cholecalciferol does not result in weight reduction in overweight and obese subjects. Eur J Endocrinol. 2008;159(6):675–84.
50. Rodríguez-Rodríguez E, Ortega RM, González-Rodríguez LG, López-Sobaler AM, UCM Research Group VALORNUT (920030). Vitamin D deficiency is an independent predictor of elevated triglycerides in Spanish school children. Eur J Nutr. 2011;50(5):373–8.
51. Motiwala SR, Wang TJ. Vitamin D and cardiovascular risk. Curr Hypertens Rep. 2012;14(3):209–18.
52. Zittermann A, Frisch S, Berthold HK, Götting C, Kuhn J, Kleesiek K, Stehle P, Koertke H, Koerfer R. Vitamin D supplementation enhances the beneficial effects of weight loss on cardiovascular disease risk markers. Am J Clin Nutr. 2009;89(5):1321–7.
53. Zittermann A, Gummert JF, Börgermann J. The role of vitamin D in dyslipidemia and cardiovascular disease. Curr Pharm Des. 2011;17(9):933–42.
54. Wolf M, Shah A, Gutierrez O, Ankers E, Monroy M, Tamez H, Steele D, Chang Y, Camargo Jr CA, Tonelli M, Thadhani R. Vitamin D levels and early mortality among incident hemodialysis patients. Kidney Int. 2007;72(8):1004–13.
55. Zehnder D, Quinkler M, Eardley KS, Bland R, Lepenies J, Hughes SV, Raymond NT, Howie AJ, Cockwell P, Stewart PM, Hewison M. Reduction of the vitamin D hormonal system in kidney disease is associated with increased renal inflammation. Kidney Int. 2008;74(10):1343–53.
56. Tan X, Wen X, Liu Y. Paricalcitol inhibits renal inflammation by promoting vitamin D receptor-mediated sequestration of NF-kappaB signaling. J Am Soc Nephrol. 2008;19(9):1741–52.
57. Liu PT, Stenger S, Li H, Wenzel L, Tan BH, Krutzik SR, Ochoa MT, Schauber J, Wu K, Meinken C, Kamen DL, Wagner M, Bals R, Steinmeyer A, Zügel U, Gallo RL, Eisenberg D, Hewison M, Hollis BW, Adams JS, Bloom BR, Modlin RL. Toll-like receptor triggering of a vitamin D-mediated human antimicrobial response. Science. 2006;311(5768):1770–3.
58. Salamon H, Bruiners N, Lakehal K, Shi L, Ravi J, Yamaguchi KD, Pine R, Gennaro ML. Cutting edge: vitamin D regulates lipid metabolism in Mycobacterium tuberculosis infection. J Immunol. 2014;193(1):30–4.

59. Li Y, Spataro BC, Yang J, Dai C, Liu Y. 1,25-dihydroxyvitamin D inhibits renal interstitial myofibroblast activation by inducing hepatocyte growth factor expression. Kidney Int. 2005;68(4):1500–10.
60. Ito I, Waku T, Aoki M, Abe R, Nagai Y, Watanabe T, Nakajima Y, Ohkido I, Yokoyama K, Miyachi H, Shimizu T, Murayama A, Kishimoto H, Nagasawa K, Yanagisawa J. A nonclassical vitamin D receptor pathway suppresses renal fibrosis. J Clin Invest. 2013;123(11):4579–94.
61. Zhang Z, Zhang Y, Ning G, Deb DK, Kong J, Li YC. Combination therapy with AT1 blocker and vitamin D analog markedly ameliorates diabetic nephropathy: blockade of compensatory renin increase. Proc Natl Acad Sci U S A. 2008;105(41):15896–901.
62. Mizobuchi M, Morrissey J, Finch JL, Martin DR, Liapis H, Akizawa T, Slatopolsky E. Combination therapy with an angiotensin-converting enzyme inhibitor and a vitamin D analog suppresses the progression of renal insufficiency in uremic rats. J Am Soc Nephrol. 2007;18(6):1796–806.
63. Tan X, Li Y, Liu Y. Paricalcitol attenuates renal interstitial fibrosis in obstructive nephropathy. J Am Soc Nephrol. 2006;17(12):3382–93.
64. Tan X, He W, Liu Y. Combination therapy with paricalcitol and trandolapril reduces renal fibrosis in obstructive nephropathy. Kidney Int. 2009;76(12):1248–57.
65. Zhang Y, Kong J, Deb DK, Chang A, Li YC. Vitamin D receptor attenuates renal fibrosis by suppressing the renin-angiotensin system. J Am Soc Nephrol. 2010;21(6):966–73.
66. Shroff R, Aitkenhead H, Costa N, Trivelli A, Litwin M, Picca S, Anarat A, Sallay P, Ozaltin F, Zurowska A, Jankauskiene A, Montini G, Charbit M, Schaefer F, Wühl E; ESCAPE Trial Group. Normal 25-hydroxyvitamin D levels are associated with less proteinuria and attenuate renal failure progression in children with CKD. J Am Soc Nephrol. 2015. pii: ASN.2014090947. [Epub ahead of print].
67. O'Herrin JK, Hullett DA, Heisey DM, Sollinger HW, Becker BN. A retrospective evaluation of 1,25-dihydroxyvitamin D(3) and its potential effects on renal allograft function. Am J Nephrol. 2002;22(5–6):515–20.
68. Bertoli M, Luisetto G, Ruffatti A, Urso M, Romagnoli G. Renal function during calcitriol therapy in chronic renal failure. Clin Nephrol. 1990;33(2):98–102.
69. Perez A, Raab R, Chen TC, Turner A, Holick MF. Safety and efficacy of oral calcitriol (1,25-dihydroxyvitamin D3) for the treatment of psoriasis. Br J Dermatol. 1996;134(6):1070–8.
70. Agarwal R, Hynson JE, Hecht TJ, Light RP, Sinha AD. Short-term vitamin D receptor activation increases serum creatinine due to increased production with no effect on the glomerular filtration rate. Kidney Int. 2011;80(10):1073–9.
71. Palmer SC, Sciancalepore M, Strippoli GF. Trial quality in nephrology: how are we measuring up? Am J Kidney Dis. 2011;58(3):335–7.
72. Novak JE, Inrig JK, Patel UD, Califf RM, Szczech LA. Negative trials in nephrology: what can we learn? Kidney Int. 2008;74(9):1121–7.

Chapter 15
Vitamin D and Diabetes in Chronic Kidney Disease

Emilio González Parra, Maria Luisa González-Casaus, and Ricardo Villa-Bellosta

Abstract The relation between the kidney and vitamin D is well known. Vitamin D has also been recognized to regulate endocrine pancreatic function; it stimulates pancreatic beta cells proliferation and insulin secretion. And several studies suggest that vitamin D status may have a significant role in glucose homeostasis in general, and on the pathophysiology and progression of metabolic syndrome and type-2 diabetes in particular. The deficiency in vitamin D is associated with a reduced insulin secretion, which might be an important factor for the susceptibility of developing diabetes. Vitamin D has been proposed also as a possible therapeutic agent in the prevention and treatment of type-1 and type-2 diabetes. In diabetic patients at various CKD stages, circulating 25(OH)D levels are negatively correlated with glycosylated hemoglobin (HbA_{1c}) values, which suggests that increasing circulating vitamin levels may have a beneficial effect of the glycemic control. Likewise, the activation of the vitamin D receptor (VDR) can reduce proteinuria and contribute to the nephroprotection. Low circulating 25(OH)D levels in CKD patients have been associated with a higher risk of all-cause mortality and faster progression of kidney disease. Unfortunately, the level of evidence to support 25(OH)D therapy for CKD or diabetes mellitus is low. Several studies of nutritional vitamin D supplementation in patients with CKD and type-2 diabetes are actually ongoing, although their results are not yet available.

Keywords Uremia • CKD • Diabetes • Proteinuria • Insulin • Insulin resistance • Pancreas • Vitamin D receptor (VDR) • VDR activators

E. González Parra, MD (✉)
Servicio de Nefrología, Universidad Autónoma, Fundación Jiménez Díaz, Madrid, Spain
e-mail: EGParra@idcsalud.es; egparra@fjd.es

M.L. González-Casaus, MD
Laboratory of Nephrology and Mineral Metabolism, Biochemistry/Biopathology,
Hospital Central de la Defensa Gomez Ulla, Madrid, Spain
e-mail: mlgcasaus@gmail.com

R. Villa-Bellosta, PhD
Department of Nephrology, IIS-Fundación Jiménez Díaz, Madrid, Spain
e-mail: ricardo.villa@fjd.es

© Springer International Publishing Switzerland 2016
P.A. Ureña Torres et al. (eds.), *Vitamin D in Chronic Kidney Disease*,
DOI 10.1007/978-3-319-32507-1_15

15.1 Basic Approach Between Diabetes and Vitamin D

Vitamin D is a forms of fat-soluble secosteroids, a type of steroid with a "broken" ring that is responsible for enhancing intestinal absorption of calcium, phosphate, magnesium, iron, and zinc. In humans, the most important compounds in this group are vitamin D_3 (also known as cholecalciferol) and vitamin D_2 or ergocalciferol (also found in fungi and plants). Humans receive vitamin D through sunlight exposure and dietary intake. Vitamin D is only found in a limited number of foods, such as fatty fish, egg yolks, mushrooms, and dietary supplements, and the primary natural source of vitamin D is UVB-radiation-dependent synthesis in the skin. Vitamin D_2 and Vitamin D_3 are synthesized through UVB irradiation of ergosterol and 7-dehydrocholesterol, respectively, during sunlight exposure.

Vitamin D_2 and D_3 are inert and are converted to 25-hydroxyvitamin D or 25(OH) D (25-hydroxyergocalciferol [25(OH)D_2] and 25-hydroxycholecalciferol [25(OH) D_3] or calcidiol, respectively) by the microsomal enzyme vitamin D 25-hydroxylase in hepatocytes (Fig. 15.1). These two specific vitamin D metabolites are measured in serum and plasma to determine a patient's vitamin D status. In the kidney, part of the calcidiol is converted to calcitriol (1-α,25-dihydroxicholecalciferol or 1,25(OH)$_2$D$_3$)—the biologically active vitamin D metabolite—by 1α-hydroxylase. The renal production of calcitriol is tightly regulated by calcium, phosphate, serum levels of both parathyroid hormone (PTH) and fibroblast growth factor 23 (FGF23), and calcitriol itself. Calcitriol has a short half-life (4–6 h) and circulates as a hormone in the blood, promoting healthy bone growth and remodeling and regulating the concentration of calcium/phosphate in the bloodstream. The 24-hydroxylase enzyme degrades both 25-hydrovitamin D and calcitriol into biologically inactivate water-soluble calcitroic acid (see Fig. 15.1).

The active vitamin D metabolite calcitriol mediates its biological effects by binding to the vitamin D receptor (VDR), which is primarily located in the core of target cells in most organs, including several white blood cells, such as monocytes and activated T and B cells. Although all vitamin D metabolites bind to the VDR, most biological effects are likely mediated by calcitriol, as it has the greatest receptor affinity.

Accumulating evidence suggests that calcitriol possesses (a) **anti-inflammatory properties** [1]: reducing pro-inflammatory cytokines (such as TNFα), increasing anti-inflammatory cytokines (such as IL-10) and suppressing NF-kB activity; (b) **anti-oxidative effects**: reducing reactive oxygen species (ROS) generation and restoring cellular ROS-scavenging enzyme activity; and (c) **anti-hypertrophic and anti-fibrotic properties** [2]: suppressing hypertrophy gene expression and regulating heart extracellular matrix metabolism. (d) Calcitriol also possesses **anti-atherosclerotic actions** by increasing fibrinolysis and inhibition of both foam cell formation and vascular smooth muscle cell proliferation and migration. (e) Moreover, calcitriol **promotes vascular calcification** [3] via hypercalcemia, hyperphosphatemia, and by inducing transformation of vascular smooth muscle cells. In vitro, calcitriol affects the synthesis of neurotrophic factors, nitric oxide synthesis, and glutathione.

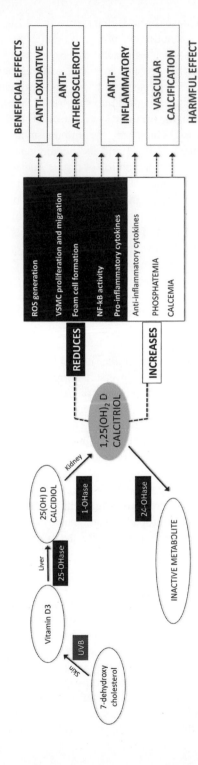

Fig. 15.1 Vitamin D biochemistry and its beneficial or harmful effects. *UVB* ultraviolet B radiation, *25 OHase* vitamin D 25-hydroxylase, *25(OH) D* 25-hydrovitamin D, *1 OHase* vitamin D 1α-hydroxylase, *1,25(OH)₂ D* 1,25-hydrovitamin D *24 OHase* vitamin D 24-hydroxylase

Diabetes mellitus (DM) is a disease characterized by hyperglycemia and is caused by absolute or relative insulin deficiency, sometimes associated with insulin resistance. Type-1 diabetes is an autoimmune disease in which the patient's own immune system reacts against islet antigens and destroys beta cells. Invarious immune cells CYP27B1 has been discovered, the 1α-hydroxylase responsible for the final activation of circulating calcidiol into calcitriol, makes it possible for calcitriol to be produced locally in the immune system itself. T- and B-lymphocytes are also direct targets of calcitriol. Therefore, the immune-modulating properties of active calcitriol suggest that vitamin D and its metabolites or analogs could be potential therapeutic agents for the prevention of type-1 diabetes.

An indirect sign of the importance of vitamin D in the pancreatic function is the presence of VDR in pancreatic cells, including beta cells. These cells possess the 1-alpha hydroxylase enzyme and can locally produce calcitriol, which is capable of exerting autocrine/paracrine action. Therefore, vitamin D has been proposed as a possible therapeutic agent in the prevention and treatment of type-1 and type-2 diabetes. Patients with vitamin D deficiency have a dysfunction of pancreatic beta cells with impaired insulin secretion and increased tissular resistance to insulin. The role of vitamin D in insulin secretion appears to be due to a direct effect of this hormone on the VDR receptor on pancreatic cells, or indirectly through the calcium-binding proteins. The increase in intracellular calcium increases the conversion of proinsulin to insulin. It also improves tissue sensitivity to insulin. For these reasons, vitamin D deficiency could be responsible for the susceptibility of developing diabetes, as studies show that vitamin D status is inversely correlated to diabetes.

Type-2 diabetes is associated with exposure of beta cells to chronically elevated levels of glucose and free fatty acids (FFA)—conditions referred to as glucotoxicity and lipotoxicity, respectively—leading to oxidative and endoplasmatic reticulum (ER) stress (see Fig. 15.2). These phenomena result in functional impairment and cell death, which are mediated through excessive generation of reactive oxygen species (ROS), mitochondrial dysfunction, and inflammation of pancreatic beta cells. As calcitriol possesses anti-inflammatory and anti-oxidative effects, this hormone could prevent detrimental effects such as these. Chronic hyperglycemia is the proximate cause of retinopathy, chronic kidney failure, neuropathies, and macrovascular disease in diabetes. In type-2 diabetes, beta cells are also adversely affected by chronic hyperglycemia and secrete less and less insulin, thereby adding to a downward spiral of loss of function.

Both types of diabetes display increased levels of ROS such as free radicals. For this reason, the onset of diabetes is closely associated with increased oxidative stress, which also causes of glomerulonephritis in grafted kidneys, rheumatoid arthritis in joints, and atherosclerosis in vessels. Moreover, the dialysis procedure contributes to the exacerbation of oxidative stress.

The precise mechanism by which oxidative stress accelerates diabetes complications is only partly understood, but protein damage protein is recognized to be one contributing factor. In physiological concentration, endogenous ROS production helps maintaining protein homeostasis. However, when ROS excessively accumulate for prolonged periods of time, it causes chronic oxidative stress and adverse effects, especially in islet cells that are vulnerable to ROS due to their low intrinsic

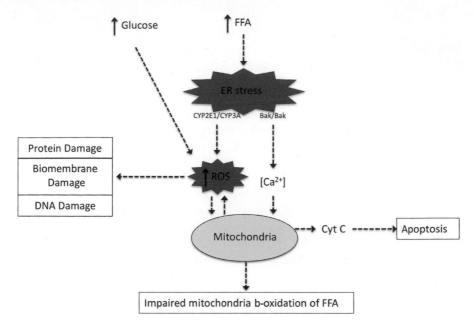

Fig. 15.2 Mechanism of action in diabetes. *ROS* reactive oxygen species, *FFA* free fatty acid, *Cyt C* cytochrome C, *ER* endoplasmic reticulum

levels of antioxidant enzymes. For example, in a model of type-2 diabetes, high glucose concentration increased intracellular peroxide levels in islet cells [4].

Multiple biochemical pathways and mechanisms of action have been implicated in the deleterious effects of chronic hyperglycemia and oxidative stress on the function of pancreatic beta cells and vascular and renal tissues. At least six pathways are emphasized in the literature as being major contributors to ROS, including (1) α-ketoaldehyde by glyceraldehyde autoxidation, (2) PKC activation, (3) glycation, (4) sorbitol metabolism, (5) hexosamine metabolism, and (6) oxidative phosphorylation. Chronic exposure of pancreatic beta cells to supra-physiologic concentration of glucose also causes abnormal insulin secretion and defective insulin gene expression and transcription. The defect in insulin gene expression is due to the loss of a least two critical proteins (PDX-1 and MafA) that activate the insulin promoter.

Clinical diabetes mellitus is often accompanied by elevated blood levels of cholesterol, triglycerides, and free fatty acid (FFA). Prolonged exposure of pancreatic beta cells to fatty acids has been reported to inhibit insulin gene expression. Simultaneous presence of hyperglycemia and elevated fatty acid levels causes accumulation of cytosolic citrate, the precursors of malonyl-CoA, which inhibits carnitine palmitoyl-transferase-1, the enzyme responsible for fatty acid transport into the mitochondria. Moreover, recent studies have revealed that palmitate inhibits insulin gene expression by inhibition of insulin promoter activity and increased levels of intracellular ceramide. However, palmitate-induced generation of ceramide has been reported to lead to apoptosis (X34), and palmitate-induced apoptosis causes generation of ROS.

Calcitriol may exert beneficial effects on altered cardiac metabolism in diabetic cardiomyopathy and improve insulin secretion and sensitivity. The imbalance of FFA and glucose utilization results in the accumulation of toxic intermediates of FFA, increased oxidative stress, mitochondrial dysfunction, abnormalities in calcium handling, and subsequently diabetic cardiomyopathy. Calcitriol restores impaired insulin secretion in vitamin D-deficient rats and activates the expression of the human insulin receptor gene. Calcitriol improves diabetic cardiomyopathy, regulating peroxisome proliferator-activated receptors and increasing glucose utilization via glucose transporter 4. Moreover, vitamin D-deficient rats activated the glycolytic pathway and reduced β-oxidation, which is also characteristic of cardiac remodeling and heart failure [5].

Finally, expression of receptors for calcitriol and 1α-hydroxylase has been described in all tissues involved in the pathogenesis of type-2 diabetes, including pancreatic beta cells, liver, kidney, fat tissue, and muscle [6]. Moreover, the formation of the bioactive metabolite of vitamin D (calcitriol) occurs mainly in the kidney; therefore, disturbance in kidney function could impair the synthesis of calcitriol and its degradation by 24-hydroxylase, also taking place in kidney.

15.2 Relationship Between Vitamin D and Diabetes in Healthy Populations

15.2.1 Epidemiology of Diabetes Mellitus

Diabetes mellitus is a common chronic disease, with an estimated global prevalence of 9 % among adults aged >18 as of 2014. In 2012, an estimated 1.5 million deaths were directly caused by diabetes, and the World Health Organization (WHO) projects that diabetes will be the seventh leading cause of death by 2030. Type-1 diabetes (juvenile or insulin-dependent diabetes mellitus) is an autoimmune disorder in which the immune system reacts against the pancreatic beta cells, leading to a deficit of insulin. This type mainly affects children and adolescents, and its susceptibility is linked to specific HLA genotypes. Moreover, type 2 diabetes (non insulin-dependent or adult-onset) results from the body's ineffective use of insulin, probably by primary dysfunction in peripheral insulin target organs (mainly liver, fat, and skeletal muscle), although beta-cell dysfunction is also present. Type-2 diabetes comprises 90 % of people with diabetes around the world, and is largely the result of excess body weight and physical inactivity.

15.2.2 Relationship Between Vitamin D and Diabetes

Taking into account the important pleiotropic role of vitamin D, suggested by the presence of VDR, the expression of CYP27B1-hydroxylase in pancreatic beta cells, and the presence of a vitamin D-responsive element in the human insulin receptor gene promoter, it is reasonable to hypothesize that a relationship exists between vitamin D and diabetes mellitus. Via its ability to regulate calcium fluxes, vitamin D may furthermore influence insulin release as well as insulin action. Moreover, by affecting cytokine production, vitamin D plays a beneficial role in pancreatic beta-cell survival and insulin sensitivity. Nevertheless, while rickets and osteomalacia are rarely diagnosed disorders, subclinical hypovitaminosis D is recognized as a common condition. Studies from all over the world clearly report that an inadequate vitamin D status is a global issue and, even more, that vitamin D deficiency is a recognized risk factor for increased risk of mortality in the general population. Due to the key role of UV-B radiation of the skin in vitamin D synthesis, sunscreen use, clothing, skin pigmentation, and the winter season reduces vitamin D production. At latitudes above 33° (i.e., all of Europe), UV-B radiation is only effective during the summer months; indeed, studies have shown that even in Mediterranean countries—often considered to receive bountiful sunlight—elevated prevalence of hypovitaminosis D has been found during the winter months. Our group reported a prevalence of vitamin D insufficiency of 84 % according to a cutoff of 50 nmol/L for calcidiol serum levels in a population of outpatient postmenopausal women from a rheumatology clinic [7]. Recently, a 57 % prevalence of vitamin D insufficiency was observed in a population of patients with coronary artery disease, with both studies being performed in Madrid (Spain) [8]. What is more, in studying a control group made up of healthy, young military personnel on active duty receiving adequate outdoor physical activity and aged 27.9 years (SD 5.2 years), we recorded mean serum calcidiol levels under the threshold of vitamin D sufficiency (75 nmol/L), showing a prevalence of insufficiency of 75 and 44 % for respective cut-offs of 75 and 50 nmol/L in circulating 25-hydroxyvitamin D.

15.2.3   Type 1 Diabetes and Vitamin D

Based on experimental models showing that vitamin D deficiency inhibits insulin secretion by the pancreas and that this beta-cell function is normalized by calcitriol and on epidemiologic studies in populations with hypovitaminosis D suggestive of pancreatic beta-cell dysfunction, vitamin D deficiency has been associated with risk of diabetes. It has been suggested that *CYP27B1* polymorphism variants that lead to a decrease in the local expression of 1α-hydroxylase would increase the risk of both diabetes type-1 and hypovitaminosis D [9]. Also, epidemiological similarities exist between diabetes type 1 and vitamin D deficiency, as incidence rates of both disorders are more elevated in the geographic areas with less ultraviolet irradiance [10]. Similarly, some studies have found an inverse correlation between vitamin D and diabetes type-1, although studies of vitamin D deficiency in these diabetic patients are limited. Another cross-sectional study reported a prevalence of inadequate levels of vitamin D in type-1 diabetic patients of 76 %, employing a cut-off of 75 nmol/L in calcidiol serum levels to define hypovitaminosis D. A later study showed that children who have multiple positive islet autoantibodies without manifest type-1 diabetes have lower levels of vitamin D in their blood than children without the autoantibodies; however, the progression of the disease remained unaffected by the vitamin D levels in the pre-diabetic group (defined as the presence of multiple islet autoantibodies) [11]. These studies mostly examined the links between vitamin D levels in pregnancy or childhood and the risk of type-1 diabetes in children, although about 60 % of type 1 diabetes cases occur after age 20. A 6-year study of 2,000 individuals by the European Association for the Study of Diabetes tested the association between vitamin D deficiency and risk of type-1 diabetes in a way that provided a dose response relationship. A comparison of serum 25(OH)D levels between healthy people who later developed type 1 diabetes and healthy controls estimated that the level of calcidiol needed to prevent half the cases of type 1 diabetes is 50 ng/mL (125 nmol/L). Another prospective case-control study of U.S. military personnel analyzed serum samples of 310 individuals diagnosed as having type-1 diabetes between 1997 and 2009 and collected before the onset of the disease, comparing the obtained values with those of 613 healthy subjects. The results of the study showed that healthy young adults with serum levels of vitamin D above 75 nmol/L had about half the risk of developing type-1 diabetes as those individuals with lower levels. Another study that evaluated vitamin D as a predictor of microvascular complications and mortality in type-1 diabetes after a 5-year follow-up concluded that severe vitamin D deficiency independently predicts all-cause mortality (hazard ratio for mortality 2.7), but not development of microvascular complication in the eye and kidney [12]. Nevertheless, most of these studies do not focus on the adverse effects of vitamin D inadequacy on beta-cell function.

15.2.4   Type 2 Diabetes and Vitamin D

Vitamin D deficiency is reported to be more common in type 2 than in type-1 diabetes. Several studies evidence the relationship between vitamin D and type 2-diabetes [13]. The National Health and Nutrition Examination Survey (NHANES) demonstrated that serum calcidiol levels were inversely correlated with the incidence of type-2 diabetes and insulin resistance. Also, in elderly subjects—a population at increased risk of vitamin D deficiency and in whom type 2 diabetes is particularly common—serum calcidiol levels <50 nmol/L doubled the risk of newly diagnosed type 2 diabetes after adjustment for confounding factors. Furthermore, low vitamin D status was associated with markers of impaired glucose metabolism, such as glycosylated hemoglobin (HbA1c). The link between vitamin D and type-2 diabetes is different than that of type-1 diabetes. Several factors may contribute to this difference. Obesity, an important determinant of type-2 diabetes, is commonly associated with hypovitaminosis D. Several polymorphisms in vitamin D binding protein (VDBP) and VDR genes could be associated with impaired glucose tolerance and obesity [14]. Absolute fat mass is inversely related to serum calcidiol levels, but at present, it is unclear whether vitamin D deficiency itself contributes to obesity. Fat-soluble vitamin D3 sequestered in the large adipose compartment may contribute to inadequate circulating levels of calcidiol and calcitriol, though at same time this vitamin D unavailability could increase intracellular calcium in adipocytes and stimulate adipogenesis and the development of obesity. In this regard, some evidence shows a role for leptin in downregulation of calcitriol synthesis, as leptin levels are positively correlated with obesity. A recent study [15] has helped clarify the connection between vitamin D, obesity, and diabetes by comparing vitamin D levels in people at a wide range of weights (from lean to morbidly obese subjects). The results of this study evidenced a decrease in calcidiol serum levels in pre-diabetic and diabetic subjects compared to normoglycemic subjects (independently of body mass index (BMI)). Also, vitamin D levels were closely related to glucose metabolism, suggesting that hypovitaminosis D is more closely associated with carbohydrate metabolism than with obesity [15]. Furthermore, the authors also analyzed VDR gene expression during pre-adipocyte differentiation and in vitro stimulation with $1,25(OH)_2D_3$ of adipose tissue from donors with different BMI values, finding that VDR gene expression was higher in tissue from obese patients. On the other hand, central obesity (using waist circumference as a surrogate marker) is related to metabolic syndrome. Some authors find a powerful association between hypovitaminosis D and metabolic syndrome in obese patients independently of body fat mass. The relationship between vitamin D with altered carbohydrate metabolism and activation of the renin-angiotensin system—mechanisms involved in the pathophysiology of metabolic syndrome—make this association plausible. Finally, current data suggest that type-2 diabetic patients with vitamin D deficiency have elevated C-reactive protein (CRP), fibrinogen, and HbA1c levels compared with healthy controls, indicating that inflammation is implicated in insulin resistance and type-2 diabetes. What is more, the exogenous administration of vitamin D ameliorates markers of systemic inflammation and possibly improves insulin sensitivity and beta-cell function by directly modulating the generation and effect of inflammatory cytokines.

15.2.5 Treatment with Vitamin D

On the basis of these links, vitamin D sufficiency may provide protection against the development of diabetes mellitus, and intervention studies are needed to elucidate whether vitamin D supplementation could prevent development of diabetes in at-risk populations or improve prognosis in diabetic patients. Several animal trials with vitamin D_3 or active vitamin D in glucose metabolism have been performed. Early intervention with calcitriol in non-obese diabetic (NOD) mice diminished the incidence of both insulitis and diabetes, and late intervention throughout childhood and puberty also reduced clinical diabetes in NOD mice [16]. In spite of this, clinical trials in humans have yielded conflicting results. The EURODIAB group suggested an association between vitamin D supplementation in infancy and a decreased risk of type-1 diabetes in a multicenter case-control study [17]. A recent study concluded that vitamin D_3 supplement improves HbA1c in pediatric patients with type-1 diabetes and vitamin D deficiency. Another intervention trial involving administration of a small dose of $1,25(OH)_2D_3$ in new-onset diabetic children showed no improvements of C-peptide levels, although insulin requirements decreased. However, there is scarce clinical data on diabetes intervention with $1,25(OH)_2D_3$ starting at the decline of beta-cell function, and they failed to induce preservation of the same, possibly due to a safety concern, as the doses of calcitriol or analogs needed to prevent or ameliorate type 1 diabetes have a hypercalcemic effect. Results of intervention studies on type-2 diabetes have also yielded unconvincing results. While some studies show that administration of vitamin D_2 or D_3 could prevent or improve the disease, other trials have found no benefits after supplementation with vitamin D. A review and meta-analysis of fifteen trials comparing vitamin D or analogs with placebo showed insufficient evidence of a beneficial effect to recommend vitamin D supplementation as a means of improving glycemic control or insulin resistance in patients with diabetes [18]. However, these contradictory results could be explained by several factors including, dose size, method of supplementation, genetics, and previous status of vitamin D. Moreover, vitamin D deficiency should be avoided in populations at risk of diabetes. Long-term intervention studies are needed to demonstrate whether vitamin D treatment decreases the risk of diabetes. At present, more than fifty clinical trials are evaluating the effects of vitamin D supplementation on different aspects of diabetes mellitus (Table 15.1).

15.3 Vitamin D and Diabetes in Chronic Kidney Disease

The kidney plays an important role in the systemic endocrine action of vitamin D. These actions, which are analyzed in depth in this chapter, are compromised in diabetic patients with chronic kidney disease.

As renal function declines, serum levels of $1,25(OH)_2D$ decrease progressively, leading to active vitamin D deficiency. Somewhat less commonly recognized is the high prevalence of nutritional vitamin D deficiency in patients with renal disorders. Serum 25(OH)D levels begin to decrease in stage 2 CKD, and 25(OH)D deficiency is prevalent in all subsequent stages of CKD, including ESRD [19]. Proteinuria may be accompanied by high urinary loss of vitamin D-binding protein, leading to increased renal loss of vitamin D metabolites.

15.3.1 Relationship Between Vitamin D and Diabetes in Patients with Chronic Kidney Disease

Several studies suggest that vitamin D status may also have a significant role in glucose homeostasis in general and on pathophysiology and progression of metabolic syndrome and type-2 diabetes in particular [20]. In diabetic patients at various CKD stages, 25(OH)D levels were negatively correlated with HbA1c values. These observations may suggest a beneficial effect of vitamin D on HbA1c levels in CKD patients.

Table 15.1 Main clinical trials about vitamin D supplementation in patients with diabetes mellitus

Code	Title	Conditions	Intervention	Recruitment	Study results
NTC 01741181	Vitamin D supplementation in patients with diabetes mellitus type 2	DM2/VD deficiency	Vitamin D vs placebo	Completed	No available
NTC 02101151	Effect of vitamin D supplementation on the metabolic control and body composition of type 2 diabetes	DM2/obesity	Cholecalciferol	Completed	No available
NTC 01412710	Effect of vitamin D supplementation on cardiovascular risk factors among Hispanic and African americans with type 2 diabetes	DM2	Cholecalciferol	Completed	No available
NTC 02112721	Can vitamin D supplementation prevent type 2 diabetes?	DM2	Vitamin D vs placebo	Recruiting	No available
NTC 00400491	Vitamin D supplementation to patients with type 2 diabetes	DM2	Cholecalciferol vs placebo	Completed	No available
NTC 01991054	The effects of vitamin D supplementation on patients with type 2 diabetes and vitamin D deficiency	DM2/VD deficiency	cholecalciferol	Recruiting	No available
NTC 00985361	Effect of vitamin D supplementation on haemoglobin A1c in patients with uncontrolled type 2 diabetes	DM2	VD3/vitamin C	Completed	No available
NTC 01854463	The effect of vitamin D supplementation in type 2 diabetes	DM2	Cholecalciferol vs placebo	Completed	No available
NTC 01942694	Vitamin D and type 2 diabetes study	Prediabetes/DM2	Cholecalciferol vs placebo	Recruiting	No available
NTC 01726777	Effect of vitamin D supplementation on glucose tolerance in subjects at risk for diabetes with low vitamin D	DM2/VD deficiency	Vitamin D vs placebo	Recruiting	No available
NTC 02513888	Prevention of type 2 diabetes with vitamin D supplementation	Prediabetes	Vitamin D + diet and lifestyle/placebo + diet and lifestyle	Recruiting	No available

(continued)

Table 15.1 (continued)

Code	Title	Conditions	Intervention	Recruitment	Study results
NTC 01585051	Effect of vitamin D supplementation on blood pressure and HbA1c levels in patients with T2D	DM2	Calcidiol vs NaCl 0.9 %	Completed	No available
NCT 02513875	Prevention of type 2 diabetes with vitamin D	Prediabetes	Vitamin D vs placebo	Recruiting	No available
NCT 01354262	Effect of vitamin D supplementation on hemoglobin A1c	DM2/VD deficiency	Vitamin D	Completed	No available
NCT 01855321	Effects of treating vitamin D deficiency in poorly controlled type 2 diabetes	DM2	Vitamin D vs placebo	Completed	No available
NCT 01500005	The effect of vitamin D supplementation on arterial stiffness on diabetic patients	Diabetes	Baby D3 drops	Completed	No available
NCT 01736865	Vitamin D for established type 2 diabetes	DM2	Cholecalciferol vs placebo	Recruiting	No available
NCT 02464462	The role of vitamin D3 and calcium supplementation in attenuating T2DM severity	DM2	Vitamin D3 vs placebo	Completed	No available
NCT 01889810	Effect of vitamin D supplementation on insulin resistance-the DIR study	Prediabetes/ suboptimal vitamin D status	Vitamin D3	Recruiting	No available
NCT 00784511	Vitamin D, glucose control and insulin sensitivity in African-Americans	DM2	Cholecalciferol vs microcrystalline cellulose	Completed	No available
NCT 01386736	Vitamin D and glucose metabolism in pediatrics	Insulin resistance/ VD deficiency	Vd drops/placebo	Recruiting	No available
NCT 01662193	Effects of vitamin D and calcium supplementation on inflammatory biomarkers and adipocytokines in diabetic patients	Metabolic disease	VD/Ca/VD+Ca/placebo	Recruiting	No available
NCT 00858247	Effect of vitamin D3 supplementation on insulin resistance and cardiovascular risk factors in obese adolescents	Obesity	Cholecalciferol	Completed	Has results

NCT 01856946	Effect of vitamin D supplementation on oral glucose tolerance among obese adolescents	Insulin resistance	4,000 UI cholecalciferol	Recruiting	No available
NCT 00436475	Vitamin D and calcium homeostasis for prevention of type 2 diabetes	Glucose intolerance/ DM2	2000UI VD3/Ca/placebo	Completed	No available
NCT 00552409	Randomized controlled trial of vitamin D3 in diabetic kidney disease	DM/ CKD	Cholecalciferol/placebo	Completed	Has results
NCT 00347542	A trial to study the effect of vitamin D supplementation on glucose and insulin metabolism in centrally obese men	DM non insulin dependent/obesity	Vitamin D	Completed	No available
NCT 00320853	A study to evaluate the effect of vitamin D supplementation on insulin sensitivity and secretion	DM non insulin dependent	Vitamin D	Completed	No available
NCT 01170442	Does vitamin D improve glycemic control in type 2 DM?	DM/VD deficiency	2,000 IU VD3/5,000 IU VD3/placebo	Terminated	No available

Evidence indicates that vitamin D is important in the pathogenesis of glucose intolerance and insulin resistance (IR) in patients with CKD. IR is present in the early stages of CKD and has an inverse association with 25(OH)D levels. Calcitriol treatment of CKD patients treated by hemodialysis (HD) and with secondary hyperparathyroidism is associated with increased insulin secretion; this is linked to decreased intracellular free calcium. It is possible that the effect of altered calcium content in beta cells on insulin secretion depends on the magnitude and duration of the change. The goal of IR treatment is traditionally aimed at etiologies including uremic toxins, protein catabolism, vitamin D deficiency, metabolic acidosis, anemia, poor physical fitness, and cachexia.

15.3.2   Vitamin D and Proteinuria in Diabetes Mellitus

Although the close relationship between vitamin D and kidney seems to have even greater importance, as it is known to activate VDR and can reduce proteinuria and contribute to nephroprotection [21]. Experimental models have shown the effect of vitamin D on the blockade of the renin-angiotensin-aldosterone system (RAAS), protection of podocytes and mesangial cells, inflammation and tubulointerstitial fibrosis [22].

Albuminuria is a typical finding in patients with diabetic nephropathy (DN). Evidence from clinical trials and associated data from the NHANES III cohort demonstrated an inverse relationship between 25(OH)D levels and degree of albuminuria. Furthermore, diabetes is closely associated with low 25(OH)D levels. Given the above findings, patients with established DN are expected to have even lower 25(OH)D levels than patients with CKD from other causes but a similar estimated glomerular filtration rate (eGFR). In fact, the prevalence of 25(OH)D insufficiency (93%) and deficiency (51.5%) was high in CKD patients with and without diabetes.

Several clinical studies in patients with proteinuric nephropathy have analyzed the activation role of VDR in relation the decrease in proteinuria, progression of renal disease, and mortality, some in diabetic nephropathy. The study that has had the most profound impact is the VITAL study in patients with type-2 diabetes and renal failure with albuminuria in stages 2–4. This was a double blind, randomized, case-control study using 2 mg of paricalcitol, a specific activator of VDR, in combination with an inhibitor of RAAS. The findings showed a greater decrease in proteinuria, better control of blood pressure, and a decrease in the progression of kidney failure. Proteinuria predicts the occurrence of cardiovascular events, mortality, and hospital admissions, though there is also a deteriorating relationship between proteinuria and glomerular filtration. Studies have shown that vitamin D has a renoprotective effect in patients with diabetes mellitus, possibly due to the reduction in proteinuria, a reduction of the activity of the renin-angiotensin system, or due to direct renal effects [22]. However, a recent meta-analysis that included 18 studies of treatment with vitamin D observed a reduction in proteinuria but without modification on renal function.

15.3.3 Vitamin D and Progression of Renal Disease

Few studies have analyzed the effect of 25(OH)D deficiency on progression of kidney disease in patients with type-2 diabetes. In studies of patients with CKD of any cause, lower 25(OH)D levels were associated with an increased risk of incident ESRD and contributed to decreased eGFR in early and advanced stages of CKD. In the study by Ravani et al. baseline 25(OH)D levels correlated directly and significantly with eGFR. The prevalence of 25(OH)D deficiency was observed in several studies, and the Cox regression analysis showed the 25(OH)D level to be an independent predictor of death and ESRD. The association between lower 25(OH)D levels and reduced eGFR was strongest in patients with diabetes.

Low 25(OH)D levels in patients with CKD have been associated with a higher risk of all-cause mortality and faster progression of kidney disease. In the NHANES III cohort, individuals with 25(OH)D levels, 15 ng/ml had a higher risk for all-cause mortality despite adjustments for CKD stage and for potential confounders. Individuals with lower 25(OH)D levels were more likely to have diabetes. 25(OH)D deficiency is independently associated with a more than 50 % increase in baseline serum creatinine, end state renal disease, or death in type II diabetic nephropathy in patients with type II diabetic nephropathy [23].

15.3.4 Vitamin D Supplement Need Among CKD Patients

Stimulation of VDR exerts protective activity through multiple mechanisms, including inhibition of the RAAS, regulation of cell proliferation and differentiation, reduction of proteinuria, anti-inflammation, and anti-fibrosis. Growing evidence indicates that vitamin D exerts anti-proteinuric and renoprotective effects in diabetic patients with CKD. Additionally, it has been shown that vitamin D_3 repletion has beneficial effects on urinary albumin and transforming growth factor-$\beta 1$ excretion in type-2 diabetic patients with CKD undergoing established RAAS inhibition therapy. Treatment with cholecalciferol led to significantly higher levels of circulating 25(OH)D and 1,25(OH)$_2$D$_3$ levels relative to baseline, and increased levels of active forms of vitamin D were correlated with a decrease in urinary albumin creatinine ratio and transforming growth factor (TGF)-$\beta 1$. These data indicate that vitamin D compounds may be useful tools for delaying the progression of diabetic CKD beyond the effects expected from established RAAS inhibition protocols.

Vitamin D supplementation in CKD has now shifted to ensure that both classic and non-classic requirements are met. In contrast to the classic endocrine function of vitamin D, the autocrine/paracrine function of vitamin D appears to remain intact as long as 25(OH)D, the necessary substrate, is available. 1α-hydrolyase activity is maintained, even in anephric patients. In patients with DM, circulating 25(OH)D level is almost universally, lower than 30 ng/ml. Therefore, supplementation should be universally considered in this population. Unfortunately, the level of evidence to support 25(OH)D therapy for CKD or DM is low [24]. Several studies of nutritional vitamin D supplementation in patients with type-2 diabetes are ongoing, although their results are not yet available. Scant data are available on combining therapy with both nutritional and active vitamin D compounds; thus, caution should be exercised in clinical practice because of the possibility of vitamin D intoxication. Further data are necessary in this area [23].

We can hypothesize that vitamin D supplementation decreases insulin resistance and reduces HbA1c levels in patients with diabetes. However, supplementation studies have not unambiguously found that vitamin D favors an improvement in glucose homeostasis parameters.

15.4 Conclusions

Vitamin D supplementation for the general population may lead to a small but significant improvement in mortality, though it did not appear to prevent the development of DM in the largest clinical trial to date [25]. Data from the HD population consistently suggest that calcitriol improves short-term insulin secretion and insulin sensitivity. In patients with end-stage renal disease, insulin resistance is an independent predictor of cardiovascular disease and is linked to protein energy wasting and malnutrition, as well as with systemic inflammation, oxidative stress, elevated serum adipokines and fetuin-A, metabolic acidosis, vitamin D deficiency, depressed serum erythropoietin, endoplasmic reticulum stress, and suppressors of cytokine signaling. All these mechanisms cause insulin resistance by suppressing insulin receptor-PI3K-Akt pathways in CKD.

References

1. Aragno M, Mastrocola R, Medana C, Catalano MG, Vercellinatto I, Danni O, Boccuzzi G. Oxidative stress-dependent impairment of cardiac-specific transcription factors in experimental diabetes. Endocrinology. 2006;147(12):5967–74.
2. Chen S, Law CS, Grigsby CL, Olsen K, Hong TT, Zhang Y, Yeghiazarians Y, Gardner DG. Cardiomyocyte-specific deletion of the vitamin D receptor gene results in cardiac hypertrophy. Circulation. 2011;124(17):1838–47.
3. Bas A, Lopez I, Perez J, Rodriguez M, Aguilera-Tejero E. Reversibility of calcitriol-induced medial artery calcification in rats with intact renal function. J Bone Miner Res. 2006;21(3):484–90.
4. Tanaka Y, Tran PO, Harmon J, Robertson RP. A role for glutathione peroxidase in protecting pancreatic beta cells against oxidative stress in a model of glucose toxicity. Proc Natl Acad Sci U S A. 2002;99(19):12363–8.
5. Assalin HB, Rafacho BP, dos Santos PP, et al. Impact of the length of vitamin D deficiency on cardiac remodeling. Circ Heart Fail. 2013;6:809–16.
6. Takiishi T, Gysemans C, Bouillon R, et al. Vitamin D and diabetes. Rheumatol Dis Clin N Am. 2012;38:179–206.
7. Aguado P, Del Campo MT, Garcés MV, González Casaús ML, Coya J, Torrijos A, Bernad M, Gijón-Baños J, Martín Mola E, Martinez ME. Low Vitamin D levels in outpatient

postmenopausal women in the Madrid area of Spain: its relationship with bone mineral density. Osteoporos Int. 2000;11:739–44.

8. Gonzalez Parra E, Aceña A, Lorenzo O, Tarín N, Gonzalez Casaus ML, Cristobal C, Huelmos A, Mahillo I, Pello AM, Carda R, Hernandez-Gonzalez I, Alonso J; Rodriguez Artalejo F, Lopez-bescos L, Ortiz A, Egido J, Tuñon J. Important abnormalities of bone and mineral metabolism are present in patients with coronary artery disease with mild decrease in stimated glomerulat filtratio rate. J Bone Miner Metab. 2015; in press.

9. Lopez ER, Regula K, Pani MA, Krause M, Usadel KH, Badenhoop K. CYP27B1 polimorphism variants are associated with type 1 diabetes mellitus n Germans. J Steroid Biochem Mol Biol. 2004;89-90:155–7.

10. Mohr SB, Garland CF, Gorham ED, Garland FC. The association between ultraviolet irradiance, vitamin D status and incidence rates of type 1 diabetes in 51 regions worldwide. Diabetologia. 2008;51:1391–8.

11. Raab J, Giannopoulou EZ, Schneider S, Warncke K, Krasmann M, Winkler C, Ziegler AG. Prevalence of vitamin D deficiency in pre-type 1 diabetes and its association with disease progression. Diabetologia. 2014. doi:10.1007/s00125-014-3181-4.

12. Joergensen C, Hovind P, Schmedes A, Parving HH, Rossing P. Vitamin D levels, microvascular complications, and mortality in type 1 diabetes. Diabetes Care. 2011;34:1081–5.

13. Mattila C, Knekt P, Mannistö S, Rissanen H, Laaksonen MA, Montonen J, et al. Serum 25-hydroxivitamin D concentration and subsequent risk of type 2 diabetes. Diabetes Care. 2007;30:2560–70.

14. Valdivielso JM, Fernandez E. Vitamin D receptor polymorphism and disease. Clin Chim ACta. 2006;37:1–12.

15. Clemente Postigo M, Muñoz Garach A, Serrano M, Garrido Sanchez L, Bernal Lopez MR, Fernandez Garcia D, Moreno Santos I, Garriga N, Castellano Castillo D, et al. Serum 25-hydroxyvitamin D and adispose tissue vitamin D receptor gene expression: relationship with obesity and type 2 diabetes. J Clin Endocrinol Metab. 2015;100(4):E 591–5.

16. Giulietti A, Gysemans C, Stoffels K, van Etten E, Decallone B, Overbergh L. Vitamin D deficiency in early life accclerates type 1 diabetes in non-obese diabetic mice. Diabetologia. 2004;47:451–62.

17. Vitamin D supplement in early childhood and risk for type 1 (insulin dependent) diabetes mellitus. The EURODIAB Su-study 2 Study group. Diabetologia. 1999;42: 51–4.

18. George PS, Pearson ER, Witham MD. Effect of vitamin D supplementation on glycaemic control and insulin resistance: a systematic review and meta-analysis. Diabet Med. 2012;29: e142–50.

19. Gonzalez-Parra E, Rojas-Rivera J, Tuñón J, Praga M, Ortiz A, Egido J. Vitamin D receptor activation and cardiovascular disease. Nephrol Dial Transplant. 2012;27 Suppl 4: iv17–21.

20. González-Parra E, Egido J. Vitamin D, metabolic syndrome and diabetes mellitus. Med Clin (Barcelona). 2014;142(11):493–6. 6.

21. Egido J, Ruiz-Ortega M, González Parra E, Rico Zalba L, Fernández Fernández B, Mallavia B, Ortiz A, Gómez Guerrero C. Tratamiento de la nefropatía diabética: más allá del bloqueo del sistema renina-angiotensina. Nefrol Sup Ext. 2011;2(5):77–84.

22. Rojas-Rivera J, de la Piedra C, Ramos A, Ortiz A, Egido J. The expanding spectrum of biological actions of vitamin D. Nephrol Dial Transplant. 2010;25:2850–65.

23. Fernández-Juárez G, Luño J, Barrio V, García de Vinuesa S, Praga M, Goicoechea M, Lahera V, Casas L, Oliva J, on behalf of the PRONEDI Study Group. 25 (OH) vitamin D levels and renal disease progression in patients with type 2 diabetic nephropathy and blockade of the renin-angiotensin system. Clin J Am Soc Nephrol. 2013;8:1870–6.

24. González-Parra E, Avila PJ, Mahillo-Fernández I, Lentisco C, Gracia C, Egido J, Ortiz A. High prevalence of winter 25-hydroxyvitamin D deficiency despite supplementation according to guidelines for hemodialysis patients. Clin Exp Nephrol. 2012;16(6):945–51.

25. De Boer IH, Tinker LF, Connelly S, et al. Calcium plus vitamin D supplementation and the risk of incident diabetes in the women's health initiative. Diabetes Care. 2008;31(4):701–7.

Chapter 16
Vitamin D and Muscle in Chronic Kidney Disease

Philippe Chauveau and Michel Aparicio

Abstract Skeletal muscle is frequently impacted in uraemic patients with both mechanical and metabolic consequences. Muscle wasting, weakness and structural changes, fundamentally as atrophy of type II muscle fibers, but also insulin resistance are common and however readily overlooked. Beyond a negative effect on physical activity and quality of life, skeletal muscle loss was reported to be also a powerful and independent predictor of survival, at least partly in relation with insulin resistance. Muscle loss in uraemic patients appears to be multifactorial. Among the different mechanisms liable to contribute to muscle wasting vitamin D deficiency, which is present in 50–80 % of incident dialysis patients, is a well-known factor of reduction of muscle mass, strength, physical performance and of increased risk of falls.

In these circumstances, vitamin D supplementation appears to be a reasonable, simple and potentially adequate therapy. Vitamin D supplementation seems to be an effective strategy to replenish vitamin D stores and to control PTH and more scarcely other biochemical endpoints. As only few observational studies have been performed, there are not enough data to draw definitive conclusions about the effects of natural vitamin D supplementation on patients' outcomes, including mortality, and a fortiori on muscle disorders and their mechanical and metabolic consequences.

Large, well-designed, randomized controlled trials are still requested to assess the possible benefits of natural vitamin D supplementation on skeletal muscle in CKD patients.

Keywords Vitamin D • Muscle • Kidney disease • Uremia • Sarcopenia

P. Chauveau, MD (✉)
Centre Hospitalier Universitaire de Bordeaux, Bordeaux, France
e-mail: Ph.chauveau@gmail.com

M. Aparicio, MD
Service de Néphrologie Transplantation Dialyse, Centre Hospitalier,
Universitaire de Bordeaux, Bordeaux, France

© Springer International Publishing Switzerland 2016   285
P.A. Ureña Torres et al. (eds.), *Vitamin D in Chronic Kidney Disease*,
DOI 10.1007/978-3-319-32507-1_16

16.1 Introduction

Muscle wasting and weakness were reported in patients with chronic kidney disease (CKD) more than 50 years ago under the term of uremic myopathy [1] similar muscle features have also been observed in several varieties of chronic diseases with normal renal function and in the elderly general population. Multiple observational studies have shown that, in these different circumstances, circulating 25(OH)D levels were also frequently reduced in parallel to the severity of muscle symptoms, but such association was neither observed with serum 1,25(OH)$_2$D nor PTH concentrations [2]. It is difficult to clearly delineate the respective role of CKD, age and vitamin D deficiency in the reduction of skeletal muscle mass and function, only scarce data have been reported in this field in the literature.

Vitamin D deficiency results in muscle wasting and weakness but there are suggestions that muscle metabolism is also altered, specifically its sensitivity to insulin resulting in an increase in cardiovascular risk and muscle protein breakdown. These latter can explain, at least partly, that skeletal muscle wasting and circulating low 25(OH)D levels are independent predictors of poor outcomes including increased all-cause and cardiovascular mortality in CKD patients as within healthy populations and in a number of clinical situations [3–6]. The resulting morbidity and mortality risk justifies a high priority for early detection of muscle wasting, prevention and treatment. Among various therapeutic possibilities, correction of vitamin D deficiency has logically raised up a growing interest [7].

In the present chapter, we will first describe muscle abnormalities in CKD, then the effects of vitamin D deficiency and of vitamin D supplementation on muscle function and their contractile and metabolic impact. Vitamin D epidemiology and relationship between vitamin D deficiency and fractures are described elsewhere in this book.

16.2 Skeletal Muscle Abnormalities in CKD Patients

16.2.1 Alteration of Muscle Mass and Function

Loss of muscle function is frequently overlooked in CKD patients, and yet muscle wasting and reduction in maximal exercise capacity have been reported at every CKD stage, their prevalence usually runs in parallel with the progression of renal failure to concern more than 50 % of patients on dialysis treatment [8].

The term of uremic sarcopenia has been recently proposed to characterize this muscle wasting which affects predominantly the proximal lower limb associated with proximal myalgia. The different physical performance testing and self-reports confirm the decline in physical activity and muscle force associated with an early weakness in response to exercise, particularly pronounced in CKD malnourished patients. Values of VO2 max and of tests of overall exercise capacity and strength do not exceed 50 % of those of age-matched controls [9]. Given the old age of most dialysis patients, age-related sarcopenia is a likely contributor to muscle wasting, however not all studies have confirmed this proposal [10].

Physical examination, electromyographical studies and muscle enzymes are usually normal. There is no evidence of defective excitation-contraction coupling, the most prominent abnormality of muscle function is slowing of relaxation likely linked to the atrophy of type II fibers which have fast-twitch contractile characteristics and a high rate of energy utilization [11]. Assessment of body composition confirms the reduction of the cross sectional area (CSA) of the contractile tissue, without a mandatory reduction in total muscle area because of a frequent increase in non-contractile tissue content (fat and collagen) negatively related with the values of the physical performance tests [12].

Muscle biopsies have shown predominance of type II muscle fibers loss and atrophy. Type II fibers are quicker to fatigue and the first to be recruited when fast reaction is needed, such as in the prevention of fall, their proportion and diameter is significantly predictor for falls. Mean muscle type II fiber cross-sectional area is 25–30 % smaller than in healthy age- and sex-matched controls [13]. In addition, scattered necrosis, enlarged intermyofibrillar spaces and infiltration with amorphous material, predominantly fat, are frequently observed, independently of BMI and visceral fat. Substantial alteration of mitochondria shape and number is common, associated with a decrease in mitochondrial enzymes activity and a slower energy production. Compared to controls muscle fiber capillarization is reduced [14]. Interestingly, similar histological abnormalities have been observed as well in non-locomotor (rectus abdominis) and semi-non-locomotor (deltoid) muscles suggesting that, these lesions are not only resulting from a potential disuse atrophy [15].

As above-mentioned for the clinical symptoms, the morphological changes which affect type II muscle fibers correlate with serum 25(OH)D levels, they are not a specific hallmark of CKD since quite similar findings have been found in adults with severe vitamin D deficiency not related to CKD and in individuals with age-related sarcopenia.

16.2.2   Pathophysiology

The loss of muscle mass observed in CKD results from persistent imbalances between reduced protein synthesis and stimulated protein degradation. Complications associated with CKD such as metabolic acidosis, inflammation, increased angiotensin II levels, "uremic toxins" and poor vitamin D status have in common to lead to defects in the insulin growth factor -1 (IGF-1)/Insulin/PI3K/Akt intracellular signaling pathway which result in the up-regulation of the main catabolic pathways involved in the development of muscle wasting: caspase-3, ATP-dependent ubiquitin proteasome (UPS) and myostatin [16–19].

Among the different factors liable to impact negatively skeletal muscle in CKD patients we will emphasize more particularly on vitamin D deficiency.

16.3   Vitamin D and Skeletal Muscle Mass and Function

16.3.1   Vitamin D and Skeletal Muscle: Mode of Action

Apart from its classic effects on bone and on the regulation of calcium and phosphate homeostasis, vitamin D has also ubiquitous non-calcemic functions, linked to the presence of receptors (VDRs) that are distributed in almost every tissue including skeletal muscle [20]. Activation of muscle VDRs accounts for the range of effects that vitamin D exerts in skeletal muscle, so the decline of muscle VDR expression with age makes the elderly more vulnerable to vitamin D deficiency.

On a cellular level, vitamin D metabolites modulate the function of skeletal muscle via three different mechanisms:

- A genomic transcriptional effect. It has been suggested that activation of the nuclear VDR resulted in a regulatory effect on calcium flux, mineral homeostasis and signaling pathways promoting muscle growth and myogenic differentiation.
- A non genomic effect mediated by a VDR translocated in the cell-membrane of muscle fibers, supporting a rapid non-transcriptional calcium transport, within seconds to minutes, into the muscle cell relevant to muscle contraction.
- VDR polymorphisms associated with variability in muscle contractile capacity.

16.3.2   Vitamin D Supplementation and Muscle Function

Vitamin D deficiency is common in the elderly and institutionalized people and most studies on the effects of vitamin D supplementation on muscle mass and function have been performed in these populations.

Numerous observational studies have linked vitamin D deficiency (serum 25(OH)D levels <20 ng/mL) with muscle wasting, mainly related to the reduction in type II muscle fibers number and size. Proximal muscle weakness, diffuse muscle pain, gait impairments and increased susceptibility to falls and fractures, these latter favored by an associated fragile skeleton, are the main clinical consequences of muscle wasting.

Positive effects of vitamin D on muscle performance are well known for a very long time. As early as the ancient Greece, sun exposure was already prescribed as a cure for weak and flabby muscles and Olympian athletes were instructed to train in sunlight to improve their physical performance. During the last 50 years, an extensive literature has widely shown that UV radiation and vitamin D compounds, nutritional or active forms, had a positive effect on serum 25(OH)D levels, bone mineral density and the associated muscle dysfunction: physical performance, weakness, decreased mobility, body sway and rate of falls and fractures, the effect on other functional outcomes such as pain and quality of life is less clear [21]. Lastly, biopsies in a handful of cases have shown that vitamin D supplementation induced a potentially increase in the relative number and cross-sectional size of type II muscle fibers [22].

It is noticeable that, there was a substantial heterogeneity in study design among the different trials concerning: type of vitamin D native or D analogs, optimal dose and timing, route of administration, duration, calcium co-administration, target 25(OH)D levels etc.... The evidence for muscle outcomes does not seem to favor one mode of treatment over the others, but positive effects of vitamin D supplementation appear to be more prominent in patients with low baseline levels, on the contrary there is no evidence to support supplementation in patients with normal baseline levels. In this last population, essentially in the elderly, some other confounding factors such as orthostatic hypotension, mental status, psychoactive drugs, cane or walker use may better account for muscle symptoms, particularly falls, than any vitamin D deficiency.

16.4 Vitamin D Supplementation in CKD Patients: Effects on Skeletal Muscle Functions

While beneficial effects of vitamin D supplementation on muscle strength and physical performance have been mostly reported in the elderly general population and more scarcely in younger adults and children, results of the few studies performed in CKD patients appear more debatable.

16.4.1 Contractile Function and Vitamin D Supplementation in CKD Patients

The most specific abnormality of the metabolic pathway of vitamin D in CKD patients is the lack of ability to convert 25(OH)D into the active $1,25(OH)_2D_3$ form of the molecule, due to the reduced activity of renal 1-alpha hydroxylase enzyme. However, vitamin D deficiency, assessed as low 25(OH)D serum level, is also frequently observed when renal function is severely lost. Over 80 % of incident hemodialysis patients suffer from both 25(OH)D deficiency and $1,25(OH)_2D$ deficiency independently of disorders of mineral metabolism [6].

Different cross sectional studies have shown that health-related quality of life, muscle strength, falls risk, physical performance and variance in muscle CSA were significantly associated with 25(OH)D serum levels and/or with $1,25(OH)_2D$ [23–25].

In most studies on vitamin D supplementation in CKD patients the primary endpoint was the mean percentage change from baseline in serum PTH levels, the effects on biochemical endpoints: 25(OH)D, PTH, calcium and phosphate homeostasis and on the risk of all-cause and cardiovascular mortality were less frequently assessed. Several meta-analyses have shown that vitamin D supplementation was an effective strategy to replenish vitamin D stores but this did not lead constantly to significant results on patient outcomes and on biochemical end points, except PTH levels [26].

In the RCTs and meta-analyses concerning vitamin D supplementation and CKD patients, skeletal muscle mass and function and risks of falls were not included among the potential targets of the different forms of active and nutritional vitamin D in systems outside of bone and mineral metabolism. Only relatively scarce observational and case-controls studies have dealt with the effects of vitamin D supplementation on skeletal muscle mass and function and the resulting quality of life, independence and ability to perform activity of daily living.

In a retrospective and cross-sectional study, hemodialysis patients supplemented with calcitriol or with its analogue paricalcitol, had larger muscle size and greater muscle strength than non-treated patients [27]. In an other study concerning stage 3-4 CKD patients and stage 5 CKD patients on peritoneal dialysis, all with vitamin D deficiency, physical performance tests, static and dynamic balance tests and isometric strength tests improved in both groups after vitamin D replacement [28]. In a recent randomized controlled trial, patients on hemodialysis with low 25(OH)D levels received oral cholecalciferol or placebo for 6 months. At the end of the follow-up period, patients allocated to cholecalciferol had higher levels of 25(OH)D and 1,25(OH)$_2$D and a greater reduction in phosphorus levels compared with the placebo group. However, there was no significant difference between the two groups in serum PTH levels, tests of functional capacity, muscle strength and health-related quality of life [29].

Given the impact of falls and fractures on morbidity and mortality of patients, it would be important to have some information on a potentially preventive effect of vitamin D supplementation on the risk of falls, to our knowledge no randomized controlled trials have been performed in this field.

16.4.2 Insulin Resistance and Vitamin D Supplementation in CKD Patients

Skeletal muscle is a highly metabolic tissue that responds to a large range of hormones, so the impact of vitamin D deficiency on skeletal muscle is not limited to the alteration of force and locomotion, it may also concern muscle metabolism pathways, specifically its sensitivity to insulin.

Insulin resistance (IR) is closely and independently associated with increased cardio-vascular risk, as part of the metabolic syndrome [30]. Insulin resistance is also associated with increased skeletal muscle protein breakdown contributing to the uremic muscle wasting, this latter could explain the accelerated loss of lean body mass observed in patients with type II diabetes compared to hemodialysis patients without diabetes [31]. The post receptor defect in the insulin-receptor signaling pathway in skeletal muscle, which is the likely primary abnormality results from a number of reversible factors, one of them is vitamin D deficiency.

Several observational studies have confirmed, in the general population, a significant association between vitamin D status and insulin sensitivity. Low circulating 25(OH)D levels are negatively associated with various measures of glucose metabolism such as homeostasis model assessment of insulin resistance (HOMA-IR), fasting glucose as well as insulin levels reflecting a state of hyperinsulinemia confirmed by clamp studies. In prospective studies, vitamin D deficiency is associated with a long-term risk of developing insulin resistance and is highly prevalent in patients with type II diabetes. The pathophysiology of type II diabetes includes a range of reversible factors, among them vitamin D deficiency could play an important role by affecting both insulin sensitivity and insulin secretory capacity independently of PTH, calcitriol and intracellular calcium.

Moreover, evidence from in vitro studies suggests that vitamin D may improve insulin sensitivity by increasing the expression of insulin receptors via effects on Akt and on early steps of insulin signaling pathway.

In the Third National Health and Nutrition Examination Survey (NHANES III) which included more than 14,000 participants, Vitamin D and kidney function had independent, inverse association with insulin resistance, as in the general population, although vitamin D was altered at a later stage than insulin sensitivity in the course of renal failure, on this different grounds, vitamin D supplementation should be a logical treatment of this dreadful complication [32]. Unfortunately, only few small studies have been performed on the effects of vitamin D supplementation on insulin resistance in CKD patients.

Mixed results of vitamin D supplementation on glucose metabolism and insulin sensitivity and insulin secretion have been reported in experimental animal models and in CKD patients [33–35]. Moreover, in these different studies, there was no assessment to compare the outcomes of muscle mass and function on the one hand with the outcome of insulin sensitivity in response to supplementation with vitamin D on the other hand, obviously larger well-designed trials devoted to this topic are needed.

16.5   Conclusions

Clinical muscular consequences of vitamin D deficit have been described some decades ago in the general population, mostly in the elderly, as well as in CKD patients, likewise molecular mechanisms by which vitamin D impacts on muscle mass and function have been elucidated. It could appear that supplementation with various forms of vitamin D should be a reasonably safe, simple and potentially effective intervention, actually, a significant improvement in muscle performance is frequently observed with this treatment in the elderly. If results of vitamin D supplementation on muscle function are rather convincing in the elderly, the results are more questionable in CKD patients.

A few years ago, a meta-analysis including 76 trials concluded to the unproven efficacy of vitamin D supplementation in CKD patients except positive effects on some biochemical indices [26]. Since then, although multiple observational studies and clinical trials have confirmed the impact of vitamin D supplementation on PTH levels, there are not enough data to draw conclusions about the effects of this therapy on patients' outcomes, including mortality, and a fortiori on muscle disorders and their mechanical and metabolic consequences. Large, well-designed, randomized controlled trials are still requested to assess the possible benefits of vitamin D supplementation on skeletal muscle in CKD patients.

References

1. Serratrice G, Toga M, Roux H, Murisasco A, de Bisschop G. Neuropathies, myopathies and neuromyopathies in chronic uremic patients. Presse Med. 1967;75(37):1835–8.
2. Boudville N, Inderjeeth C, Elder GJ, Glendenning P. Association between 25-hydroxyvitamin D, somatic muscle weakness and falls risk in end-stage renal failure. Clin Endocrinol (Oxf). 2010;73(3):299–304.
3. Stenvinkel P, Heimbürger O, Lindholm B. Wasting but not malnutrition predicts cardiovascular mortality in end-stage renal disease. Nephrol Dial Transplant. 2004;19:2181–3.
4. Sietsema KE, Amato A, Adler SG, Brass EP. Exercise capacity as a predictor of survival among ambulatory patients with end-stage renal disease. Kidney Int. 2004;65:719–24.
5. Pilz S, Tomaschitz A, Friedl C, Amrein K, Drechsler C, Ritz E, et al. Vitamin D status and mortality in chronic kidney disease. Nephrol Dial Transplant. 2011;26(11):3603–9.
6. Wolf M, Shah A, Gutierrez O, Ankers E, Monroy M, Tamez H, et al. Vitamin D levels and early mortality among incident hemodialysis patients. Kidney Int. 2007;72(8):1004–13.
7. Melamed ML, Thadani RI. Vitamin D therapy in chronic kidney disease and end-stage renal disease. Clin J Am Soc Nephrol. 2012;7(2):358–65.
8. Clyne N, Jogestrand T, Lins LE, Pehrsson SK. Progressive decline in renal function induces a gradual decrease in total hemoglobin and exercise capacity. Nephron. 1994;67:322–6.
9. Fahal IH. Uraemic sarcopenia: aetiology and implications. Nephrol Dial Transplant. 2014;29:1655–65.
10. Hall RK, Landerman LR, O'Hare AM, Anderson RA, Colón-Emeric CS. Chronic kidney disease and recurrent falls in nursing home residents: a retrospective cohort study. Geriatr Nurs. 2015;36(2):136–41.
11. Fahal IH, Bell GM, Bonc JM, Edwards RH. Physiological abnormalities of skeletal muscle in dialysis patients. Nephrol Dial Transplant. 1997;12(1):119–27.
12. Cheema B, Abas H, Smith B, et al. Investigation of skeletal muscle quality and quantity in end-stage renal disease. Nephrology. 2010;15:454–63.
13. Ceglia L. Vitamin D, and its role in skeletal muscle. Curr Opin Clin Nutr Metab Care. 2009;12(6):628–33.
14. Diesel W, Emms M, Knight BK, et al. Morphology features of the myopathy associated with chronic renal failure. Am J Kidney Dis. 1993;22:677–84.
15. Sakkas GK, Ball D, Mercer TH, Sargeant AJ, Tolfrey K, Naish PF. Atrophy of non-locomotor muscle in patients with end-stage renal failure. Nephrol Dial Transplant. 2003;18:2074–81.
16. Workenech BT, Mitch WE. Review of muscle wasting associated with chronic kidney disease. Am J Clin Nutr. 2010;91(Suppl):1128 S–32 S.
17. Du J, Wang X, Miereles C, et al. Activation of caspase-3 is an initial step triggering accelerated muscle proteolysis in catabolic conditions. J Clin Invest. 2004;113:115–23.
18. Zhang L, Wang XH, Wang H, Du J, Mitch WE. Satellite cell dysfunction and impaired IGF-1 signaling cause CKD-induced muscle atrophy. J Am Soc Nephrol. 2010;21:419–27.
19. Wang XH, Mitch WE. Mechanisms of muscle wasting in chronic kidney disease. Nat Rev Nephrol. Nature Publishing Group; 2014;10:501–16.
20. Holick MF. Vitamin D, deficiency. N Engl J Med. 2007;357(3):266–81.
21. Girgis CM, Clifton-Bligh RJ, Turner N, Lau SL, Gunton JE. Effects of vitamin D in skeletal muscle: falls, strength, athletic performance and insulin sensitivity. Clin Endocrinol (Oxf). 2014;80(2):169–81.

22. Sato Y, Iwamoto J, Kanoko T, Satoh K. Low-dose vitamin D prevents muscular atrophy and reduces falls and hip fractures in women after stroke: a randomized controlled trial. Cerebrovasc Dis. 2005;20(3):187–92.
23. Gordon PL, Doyle JW, Johansen KL. Association of 1,25-dihydroxyvitamin D levels with physical performance and thigh muscle cross-sectional area in chronic kidney disease stage 3 and 4. J Ren Nutr. 2012;22(4):423–33.
24. Beyer I, Mets T, Bautmans I. Chronic low-grade inflammation and age-related sarcopenia. Curr Opin Clin Nutr Metab Care. 2012;15:12–22.
25. Anand S, Kaysen GA, Chertow GM, Johansen KL, Grimes B, Dalrymple LS, et al. Vitamin D deficiency, self-reported physical activity and health-related quality of life: the Comprehensive Dialysis Study. Nephrol Dial Transplant. 2011;26(11):3683–8.
26. Palmer SC, McGregor DO, Macaskill P, Craig JC, Elder GJ, Strippoli GFM. Meta-analysis: vitamin D compounds in chronic kidney disease. Ann Intern Med. 2007;147(12):840–53.
27. Gordon PL, Sakkas GK, Doyle JW, Shubert T, Johansen KL. Relationship between vitamin D and muscle size and strength in patients on hemodialysis. J Ren Nutr. 2007;17:397–407.
28. Taskapan H, Bayral O, Karahan D, Durmus B, Altay Z, Ulutas O. Vitamin D and muscle strength, functional ability and balance in peritoneal dialysis patients with vitamin D deficiency. Clin Nephrol. 2011;76:110–6.
29. Hewitt NA, O'Connor AA, O'Shaughnessy DV, Elder GJ. Effects of cholecalciferol on functional, biochemical, vascular, and quality of life outcomes in hemodialysis patients. Clin J Am Soc Nephrol. 2013;8(7):1143–9.
30. Shinohara K, Shoji T, Emoto M, Tahara H, Koyama H, Ishimura E, et al. Insulin resistance as an independent predictor of cardiovascular mortality in patients with end-stage renal disease. J Am Soc Nephrol. 2002;13(7):1894–900.
31. Siew ED, Pupim LB, Majchrzak KM, Shintani A, Flakoll PJ, Ikizler TA. Insulin resistance is associated with skeletal muscle protein breakdown in non-diabetic chronic hemodialysis patients. Kidney Int. 2007;71(2):146–52.
32. Chonchol M, Scragg R. 25-Hydroxyvitamin D, insulin resistance, and kidney function in the Third National Health and Nutrition Examination Survey. Kidney Int. 2007;71(2):134–9.
33. de Boer IH, Sachs M, Hoofnagle AN, Utzschneider KM, Kahn SE, Kestenbaum B, et al. Paricalcitol does not improve glucose metabolism in patients with stage 3–4 chronic kidney disease. Kidney Int. 2013;83(2):323–30.
34. Blair D, Byham-Gray L, Lewis E, McCaffrey S. Prevalence of vitamin D [25(OH)D] deficiency and effects of supplementation with ergocalciferol (vitamin D2) in stage 5 chronic kidney disease patients. J Ren Nutr. 2008;18(4):375–82.
35. Mak RH. 1,25-Dihydroxyvitamin D3 corrects insulin and lipid abnormalities in uremia. Kidney Int. 1998;53(5):1353–7.

Chapter 17
Vitamin D Deficiency and Infection in Chronic Kidney Disease

Jean-Paul Viard

Abstract Infections are an important cause of morbidity and mortality in chronic, particularly end stage, renal disease. Uremia and dialysis are associated with immune impairment at multiple levels: decreased innate and adaptive immunity, increased inflammation. The role of vitamin D in the regulation of immune functions, particularly as an enhancer of innate immunity and as an anti-inflammatory agent, is now well recognized. Since vitamin D deficiency is frequent in patients with chronic kidney disease, several studies examined the relationships between vitamin D insufficiency and immune impairment or infectious diseases in this population. Vitamin D deficiency could contribute to decreased innate immunity and increased inflammation or immune cell activation, including through modulating the microbiome and intestinal permeability. Convincing data from epidemiological studies have associated vitamin D deficiency with inflammation, all-cause mortality, cardiovascular and infectious outcomes. However, intervention studies are still needed to validate the causality relationship and determine whether vitamin D supplementation can reduce infections in chronic kidney disease patient.

Keywords Vitamin D • Chronic kidney disease • Infection • Immune responses • Inflammation

17.1   Introduction

Vitamin D has been studied in chronic kidney disease (CKD) for many years because of the disturbances of its metabolism and their consequences on mineral and bone homeostasis. Among extra-skeletal effects of vitamin D, its role as a potential regulator of immune functions and inflammation has more recently been extensively studied. In large epidemiological studies conducted in the general

J.-P. Viard, MD
UF de Thérapeutique en Immuno-infectiologie, Hôtel-Dieu, Paris, France
e-mail: jean-paul.viard@htd.aphp.fr

© Springer International Publishing Switzerland 2016   295
P.A. Ureña Torres et al. (eds.), *Vitamin D in Chronic Kidney Disease*,
DOI 10.1007/978-3-319-32507-1_17

population, vitamin D deficiency has been associated with an increased susceptibility to infections, especially tuberculosis and respiratory tract infections) [1, 2], and, although this remains debated, vitamin D supplementation could reduce the risk of some of these infections [3].

Since patients with CKD (and other chronic conditions) have a higher morbidity and mortality burden from, in particular, infectious (and cardiovascular) diseases, the role of vitamin D deficiency in the pathogeny of these complications has been examined, and supplementation trials have been implemented. This chapter will examine whether and why vitamin D deficiency could be considered a risk factor for infection in CKD, and whether there is any evidence that vitamin D supplementation may reduce infections in CKD patients.

17.2 Chronic Kidney Disease, Infection, Immune Impairment and Inflammation

Infections are an important cause of morbidity and mortality in CKD [4]. For example, a single-center study in France showed that, over a 7-month observation period, 30 % of critical care unit admission of patients with CKD were linked to bacterial infections [5]. In particular, patients with end-stage renal disease (ESRD) accumulate factors leading to an increased risk of infection, such as malnutrition, comorbidities (such as diabetes), the presence of vascular access devices, but also immune dysfunction [4, 6]. Of note, it has been shown in the US dialysis population that, while infection-related deaths have decreased over the last years, infection-related hospitalizations have not and failed to decrease with the decline of catheter use [7]. The impairment of host response to pathogens in CKD therefore appears as a plausible underlying risk factor, while risk factors linked to dialysis procedures have been progressively reduced [6, 7].

Impaired immune functions are a feature of CKD and ESRD [6, 8], as exemplified by the lower response rate to vaccines and the accelerated decline of antibody titers in ESRD patients. Uremia reduces innate host responses to pathogens, through negative effects on the activation and function of monocytes (decreased TLR and costimulatory molecules expression, reactive oxygen species release and phagocytosis) and neutrophils (decreased phagocytosis). Adaptive immunity is also impaired through the reduction of antigen presentation (by dendritic cells, macrophages and B cells), an altered distribution of T cell subpopulations (abnormal CD4/CD8 ratio, reduction of the naive and central-memory compartments), increased T-cell apoptosis and a shift towards the production of Th2 cytokines.

It is interesting to note that many of the immune abnormalities found in CKD are reminiscent of the immune phenotype found, of course at different degrees, in other conditions such as extreme ageing [9] and HIV infection [10]. CKD, ageing and HIV infection also have in common that immune impairment is paralleled by persistent inflammation and the consequences thereof, mediated by an increased production of proinflammatory cytokines and chronic cell activation [4, 6, 9, 10].

Much attention has recently been paid to the link that could exist between immune impairment and chronic inflammation on the one hand, and the impact of dysbiosis and bacterial translocation form the gut, on the other hand [11]. Among other conditions, both CKD [6, 12] and HIV infection [13] appear as promising fields of investigation in this emerging research area. In CKD patients [6, 12], bacterial compounds (endotoxin, ribosomal DNA) have been detected in the blood stream of patients, and correlate with the intensity of systemic inflammation assessed through the levels of soluble biomarkers such as C-reactive protein, interleukin-6 and monocyte activation markers. Interestingly, the levels of endotoxin/lipopolysaccharide increase with the progression of CKD, reaching the highest levels in patients on dialysis, being then an independent predictor of mortality. Several studies have also documented disorders in the gut microbiome of CKD patients, with a dominance of bacteria with urease, uricase and p-cresol-producing activities and a decrease of species with butyrate-producing activities, resulting in an increased production in gut-derived uremic toxins (e.g. indoxyl sulfate and p-cresyl sulfate), which in turn activate leucocytes and inflammatory cytokine production.

17.3 Possible Role of Vitamin D Deficiency in the Immune Dysfunction of CKD

17.3.1 Vitamin D and Immunity

Vitamin D is increasingly recognized as an important factor of immune regulation because virtually all immune cells are equipped with the vitamin D receptor and are able to activate 25-hydroxy vitamin D [14–16].

17.3.1.1 Vitamin D and Innate Immunity

Epithelial cells and monocytes/macrophages express both toll-like receptors (TLR), recognizing ligands originating from pathogens, CYP27B1, a cytochrome component that activates 25-hydroxyvitamin D [25(OH)D] through 1α-hydroxylation, and the vitamin D receptor (VDR) [14–16]. This makes an intracrine system that plays an important role in the production de of bactericidal peptides, such as cathelicidin, with largely proven activity against *Mycobacterium tuberculosis*, and β-defensin 4A. Activation of TLRs induces the synthesis of bactericidal peptides via CYP27B1 transcription, binding of 1,25-dihydroxyvitamin D [1,25(OH)$_2$D] to the VDR, and formation of a heterodimer with the retinoid X receptor (RXR), that regulates the expression of vitamin D-responsive genes.

Vitamin D induces proliferation and cytokine production in natural killer (NK) cells. Vitamin D also induces autophagy in macrophages. Autophagy is a finely regulated phenomenon that is important in the defence against pathogens, particularly intracellular pathogens such as viruses and mycobacteria. In a dose-dependent manner, $1,25(OH)_2D$ induces autophagy in monocyte-derived macrophages, and this has been shown to reduce the intracelluar replication of HIV and *Mycobacterium tuberculosis*. In human macrophages, TLR8 activation induces the expression of cathelicidin, VDR and CYP27B1. Experiments using interfering RNAs, inhibitory chemicals and vitamin D-depleted culture media have shown that it is through vitamin D and cathelicidin-dependent autophagy that TLR8 agonistes inhibit HIV cell infection in this model [17].

Altogether, these results suggest that vitamin D could play an important role in the first line of defence against pathogens.

17.3.1.2 Vitamin D in Adaptive Immunity

The literature on vitamin D and T cell function supports the assumption that vitamin D deficiency is a risk factor for the onset and a poorer evolution of autoimmune diseases, the strongest example being multiple sclerosis. It is widely admitted that vitamin D decreases the differentiation and proliferation of dendritic cells, favors the production of Th2, rather than Th1 cytokines, decreases the CD4/CD8 ratio, and induces the differentiation of regulatory T cells (Treg), while it prevents the differentiation of Th17 cells and inhibits differentiation and antibody production in B cells [14, 18].

At first sight, all these actions of vitamin D appear contrary to mounting a good response against pathogens, but this should probably be nuanced for two reasons. First, it has been shown, in CKD patients, that vitamin D deficiency is associated with a low T-cell proliferation ability, corrected by the addition $1,25(OH)_2D$, and furthermore that the vitamin D-VDR system is active in the signal transduction through the T cell receptor in naïve T cells [19]. This suggests that vitamin D plays a role in primary T cell activation, upstream to cytokine orientation. Second, it has been shown in a mouse model [20] that Tregs play an important role in T CD8 cell priming. While Tregs are widely known for suppressing autoimmune responses, their depletion induces activation and expansion of CD8+ cells with low avidity for the antigen, due to an overproduction of the CCL-3/4/5 chemokines, which stabilize the interactions between dendritic cells and low avidity T cells. In the absence of Tregs, antigen avidity of the primary immune response remained low, resulting in an impaired memory response to *Listeria monocytogenes*. These results suggest that Tregs are important regulatory agents of T CD8 cell homeostasis and priming, conditioning high avidity primary response and strong memory response.

17.3.1.3 Vitamin D and Inflammation

Vitamin D deficiency has been associated with inflammation. In patients having performed a coronary angiography, vitamin D deficiency was associated with higher mortality, but also with higher levels of cell adhesion molecules, of oxidative stress markers and of inflammatory markers such as C-reactive protein (CRP) and interleukin 6 (IL-6) [21]. In a placebo-controlled study in patients with heart failure, vitamin D supplementation induced a decrease of TNF-α levels and an increase in the level of the anti-inflammatory cytokine interleukin 10 (IL-10) [22]. In a large general population cohort, low 25(OH)D levels were associated with higher levels of coagulation activation markers, plasminogen tissue activator and D-dimers [23]. Higher concentrations of these markers of inflammation and coagulation activation have been associated with mortality in persons living with HIV showing good control of viral replication on treatment [24]. Vitamin D deficiency has been associated with poorer clinical outcomes in persons with treated or untreated HIV infection [25, 26], with ongoing inflammation [27], with an increase over time of inflammatory markers and a poorer CD4 cell count restoration [28]. Finally, in a small trial in virologically controlled HIV-infected persons, vitamin D supplementation allowed to obtain a decrease of CD8 cell activation markers [29]. In the setting of tuberculosis, vitamin D supplementation, added to anti-tuberculous drugs, was associated with a much faster correction of immune/inflammation parameters than anti-tuberculous drugs alone [30].

A reasonable conclusion is that vitamin D could not only favour a stronger innate immune response (and possibly a stronger adaptive cell responses) to pathogens, but could also reduce inflammation and cell activation linked to the presence of pathogens, particularly in subacute or chronic infections. It can be hypothesized that this would also apply to other conditions, such as CKD/ESRD, where chronic inflammation, which is not triggered by a specific pathogen, has also been associated with higher mortality [31].

However, interestingly, a recent study in a mouse model of systemic *Candida* infection showed that animals receiving low doses of $1,25(OH)_2D_3$ had a lower fungic load and a longer survival than controls, while animals receiving high doses of $1,25(OH)_2D_3$ had poorer outcomes: these surprising results suggest that low vitamin D doses favors beneficial inflammatory response (e.g. by targeting the IFN-γ gene), while high doses would reduce the inflammatory response to the point of being detrimental [32]. This indication of a bimodal influence of vitamin D on host responses adds complexity but might help interpreting apparently conflicting results of supplementation trials.

Recent studies indicate that vitamin D could also play a role in the interplay between the microbiome and immune dysregulation and inflammation, by modulating the microbiome and intestinal permeability [33, 34].

17.3.2 Contribution of Low Vitamin D in Immune Impairment in CKD

As summarized above, immune dysfunction in CKD concerns both innate and adaptive immunity, and persistent inflammation. From the description of the immunological effects of vitamin D, it is reasonable to speculate that vitamin D deficiency may be involved in the immune impairment of CKD and that supplementation could reinforce innate immunity and decrease inflammation in CKD patients, while it would certainly be much more difficult to anticipate its effects on adaptive immunity.

As a matter of fact, it has been recently shown that treating peritoneal macrophages from patients on peritoneal dialysis with vitamin D ex vivo increased mRNA expression of cathelicidin, and that supplementing patients with vitamin D had the same effect (after adjustment for cell population number) [35]. Interestingly, the same study showed that vitamin D (ex vivo treatment and administration to patients) decreased the synthesis of hepcidin, which normally inhibits ferroportin, the only known exporter of intracellular iron to date. Since many bacteria use iron for growth, depletion of intracellular iron could be another, indirect, vitamin-D induced antibacterial effect.

Another factor of immune dysregulation has been proposed in CKD patients, in relation with vitamin D metabolism and phosphocalcic homeostasis. Bone-derived fibroblast growth factor 23 (FGF23) is a phosphaturic hormone that inhibits CYP27B1 and induces $1,25(OH)_2D$ inactivation, and serum levels of FGF23 are increased in CKD. Recent studies indicate that FGF23 could also have immune regulatory functions. Treatment of monocytes (from blood of healthy donors or from peritoneal dialysis effluents of uremic patients) with FGF23 decreased CYP27B1 mRNA expression in these cells [36]. This could interfere negatively with the intracrine system responsible for the production of bactericidal peptides and contribute to an increased susceptibility to infections.

17.4   Observational Studies in CKD

One recent large study from the HEMO cohort of hemodialysis patients [37] examined the association between yearly serum levels of $25(OH)D$, $1,25(OH)_2D$ and FGF23 and clinical cardiovascular and infectious outcomes using time-dependent Cox regression models, after controlling for important covariates.

Correlations between vitamin D, FGF23 and inflammation markers were also examined. $25(OH)D$ levels correlated positively with serum calcium, $1,25(OH)_2D$, FGF23, and inversely with PTH, hsCRP and IL-6. FGF23 levels also correlated positively with serum phosphorus, PTH, and $1,25(OH)_2D$, but there was no correlation with hsCRP or IL-6.

After a median follow-up of 3 years, 582 deaths were reported in 1,340 participants, and 499 participants were hospitalized or died because of an infection. Patients with $25(OH)D$ levels in the highest quartile had the lowest risk of infectious events (hazard ratio [HR]: 0.66 vs lowest quartile, 95 % CI: 0.49–0.89), cardiovascular events (HR: 0.71, 95 % CI: 0.53–0,96) and all-cause mortality (HR: 0 0.46, 95 % CI: 0.34–0.62). No significant association of $1,25(OH)_2D$ with clinical outcomes was observed. In contrast, patients with FGF23 in the highest quartile had the highest risk of infection (HR: 1.57, vs lowest quartile, 95 % CI: 1.13–2.18), cardiovascular events (HR: 1.49, 95 % CI: 1.06–2.08) and all-cause death (HR: 1.50, 95 %

CI: 1.07–2.12). Interestingly, the addition of inflammation markers (including also TNF-α and IFN-Y) in the models did not attenuate the associations.

This important study underlines that high 25(OH)D levels, as a time-dependent variable had a graded relationship with the decreased risk of events, in particular infections, and that this was independent of systemic inflammation. As frequently debated, this can generate two series of hypotheses: the first one would evoke the direct immunological effects of vitamin D, the second one would view high 25(OH)D levels only as a marker of better general health. Of particular interest, however, is the finding that higher FGF23 levels were predictive of infections, and this was also independent of inflammation. The inhibitory effect of FGF23 on 1,25(OH)$_2$D synthesis in monocytes, resulting in decreased bactericidal abilities, is a plausible explanation.

17.5 Intervention Trials in CKD

To our knowledge, there is no convincing data from large cohorts or randomized controlled trials assessing whether vitamin D supplementation could reduce infectious diseases morbidity or mortality in CKD. However, meta-analyses have been produced examining its effects on all-cause mortality or cardiovascular deaths, and we can hypothesize that infectious events would follow the same trends (as in ref [37]). One meta-analysis of observational cohorts [38] concluded that vitamin D supplementation and a protective effect on all-cause mortality (HR: 0.71, 95 % CI: 0.57–0.89, in a time-dependent Cox model). A meta-analysis of randomized, placebo-controlled trials found no significant effect [39]. The heterogeneity of trials, particularly in terms of vitamin D dosing and duration of supplementation, is a recurrent difficulty for analysis. In addition, another meta-analysis examined whether the effect of drugs (vitamin D compounds, phosphate binders, cinacalcet, biphosphonates, calcitonin) on PTH, calcemia and phosphoremia were associated with all-cause and cardiovascular deaths: only PTH levels were significantly, but loosely, negatively associated with mortality [40]. This is important to keep in mind, because there is probably no direct relationship between bone/mineral-related endpoints and other, extra-skeletal (e.g. immunoregulatory, anti-infectious) effects of vitamin D.

17.6 Conclusions

In CKD, as in other chronic conditions, vitamin D deficiency could act as an aggravating factor of immune dysregulation and inflammation. Since vitamin D supplementation is easy, unexpensive and well tolerated, it is of great interest to determine whether it can translate into the correction of immunological abnormalities and ultimately into clinical benefit, e.g. the prevention of infections. Controlled trials are needed but one should not underestimate the difficulties pertaining due to the selection of adequate at-risk populations, the definition of relevant and realistic outcomes, the numbers of participants necessary to reach a valid conclusion, and the definition of the dosing and timing of vitamin D supplementation. The latter issue should not be overlooked, because, there is no agreement on desirable target vitamin D levels when examining non-skeletal outcomes, and some effects of vitamin D, particularly in the field of inflammation, might follow a "U" curve.

Studying the effects of vitamin D supplementation on especially relevant biological markers, in carefully designed trials, may still represent an unavoidable intermediate step on the basis of current knowledge.

References

1. Ralph AR, Lucas RM, Norval M. Vitamin D and solar ultraviolet radiation in the risk and treatment of tuberculosis. Lancet Infect Dis. 2013;13:77–88.
2. Ginde AA, Mansbach JM, Camargo Jr CA. Association between serum 25-hydroxyvitamin D level and upper respiratory tract infection in the Third National Health and Nutrition Examination Survey. Arch Intern Med. 2009;169:384–90.
3. Bergman P, Lindh ÅU, Björkhem-Bergman L, Lindh JD. Vitamin D and respiratory tract infections: a systematic review and meta-analysis of randomized controlled trials. PLoS One. 2013;8(6):e65835. doi:10.1371/journal.pone.0065835.
4. Dalrymple LS, Go AS. Epidemiology of acute infections among patients with chronic kidney disease. Clin J Am Soc Nephrol. 2008;3:1487–93. doi:10.2215/CJN.01290308.
5. Contu D, d'Ythurbide G, Messka J, et al. J Infect. 2014;68(2):105–15. doi:10.1016/j.jinf.2013.10.003.
6. Anders HJ, Andersen K, Stecher B. The intestinal microbiota, a leaky gut, and abnormal immunity in kidney disease. Kidney Int. 2013;83:1010–6. doi:10.1038/ki.2012.440.
7. Collins AJ, Foley RN, Gilbertson DT, et al. United States Renal Data System public health surveillance of chronic kidney disease and end-stage renal disease. Kidney Int Suppl. 2015;5:2–7. doi:10.1038/kisup.2015.2.
8. Lang CL, Wang MH, Chiang CK, et al. Vitamin D and the immune system from the nephrologist's point of view. IRSN Endocrinol. 2014. doi:10.1155/2014/10546.
9. Wikby A, Ferguson F, Forsey R, et al. An immune risk phenotype, cognitive impairment, and survival in very late life: impact of allostatic load in Swedish octogenarian and nonagenarian humans. J Gerontol. 2005;60A(5):556–65.
10. Paiardini M, Müller-Trutwin M. HIV-associated chronic immune activation. Immunol Rev. 2013;254:78–101.
11. West CE, Jenmalm MC, Kozyrskyi AL, et al. The gut microbiota and inflammatory non communicable diseases : associations and potentials for gut microbiota therapies. J Allergy Clin Immunol. 2015;135(1):3–13. doi:10.1016/jaci.2014.11.012.
12. Lau WL, Kalantar-zadeh K, Vaziri ND. The gut as a source of inflammation in chronic kidney disease. Nephron. 2015;130:92–8. doi:10.1159/000381990.
13. Novati S, Sacchi P, Cima S, et al. General issues on microbial translocation in HIV-infected patients. Eur Rev Med Pharmacol Sci. 2015;19(5):866–78.
14. Mora JR, Iwata M, von Andrian UH. Vitamin effects on the immune system : vitamins A and D take centre stage. Nat Rev Immunol. 2008;8:685–97. doi:10.103/nri2378.
15. Peelen E, Knioppenberg S, Muris AH, Thewissen M, Smolders J, Tervaert C, Hupperts R, Damoiseaux J. Effects of vitamin D on the peripheral adaptive immune system: a review. Autoimmun Rev. 2011;10:733–43.

16. Hewison M. Antibacterial effects of vitamin D. Nat Rev Endocrinol. 2011;7:337–45.
17. Campbell GR, Spector SA. Toll-like receptor 8 ligands activate a vitamin D mediated autophagic response that inhibits human immunodeficiency virus type 1. PLoS Pathog. 2012;8(11): e1003017.
18. Cantorna M, Waddell A. The vitamin D receptor turns off chronically activated T cells. Ann N Y Acad Sci. 2014;1317:70–5.
19. Von Essen MR, Kongsbak M, Schjerling P, Olgaard K, Odum N, Geisler C. Vitamin D controls T cell antigen receptor signaling and activation of human T cells. Nat Immunol. 2010;11: 344–9.
20. Pace L, Tempez A, Arnold-Schrauf C, Lemaitre F, Bousso P, Felter L, et al. Regulatory T cells increase the avidity of primary CD8+ T cell responses and promote memory. Science. 2012;338:532–6.
21. Dobnig H, Pilz S, Scharnagl H, Renner W, Seelhorst U, Wellnitz B, et al. Independent association of low serum 25-hydroxyvitamin D and 1,25-dihydroxyvitamin D levels with all-cause and cardiovascular mortality. Arch Intern Med. 2008;168:1340–9.
22. Schleithoff SS, Zittermann A, Tenderich G, Berthold HK, Stehle P, Koerfer R. Vitamin D supplementation improves cytokine profiles in patients with congestive heart failure: a double-blind, randomized, placebo-controlled study. Am J Clin Nutr. 2006;83:754–9.
23. Hyppönen E, Berry D, Cortina-Borja M, Power C. 25-Hydroxyvitamin D and pre-clinical alterations in inflammatory and hemostatic markers : a cross sectional analysis in the 1958 British birth cohort. PLoS One. 2010;5(5):e10801.
24. Kuller LH, Tracy R, Belloso W, De Witt S, Dumond F, Lane HC, et al. Inflammatory and coagulation biomarkers and mortality in patients with HIV infection. PLoS Med. 2008; 5(10):e203.
25. Mehta S, Hunter DJ, Mugusi FM, Spiegelman D, Manji KP, Giovanucci EL, et al. Perinatal outcomes, including mother-to-child transmission of HIV, and child mortality and their association with maternal vitamin D status in Tanzania. J Infect Dis. 2009;200:1022–30.
26. Viard JP, Souberbielle JC, Kirk O, Knysz B, Losso M, Gatell J, et al. Vitamin D and clinical disease progression in HIV infection: results from the EuroSIDA study. AIDS. 2011;25: 1305–15.
27. Legeai C, Vigouroux C, Souberbielle JC, Bouchaud O, Boufassa F, Bastard JP, et al. Associations between 25-hydroxyvitamin D andimmunologic, metabolic, inflammatory markers in treatment-naive HIV-infected persons : the ANRS CO09 "COPANA" cohort study. PLoS One. 2013;8(9):e74868. doi:10.1371/journal.pone.0074868.
28. Shepherd L, Souberbielle JC, Bastard JP, Fellahi S, Capeau J, Reekie J, et al. Prognostic value of vitamin D level for all-cause mortality, and association with inflammatory markers, in HIV-infected persons. J Infect Dis. 2014;210:234–43.
29. Fabre-Mersseman V, Tubiana R, Papagno L, Bayard C, Briceno O, Fastenackels S, et al. Vitamin D supplementation is associated with reduced immune activation levels in HIV-1-infected patients on suppressive antiretroviral therapy. AIDS. 2014;28:2677–82.
30. Coussens AK, Wilkinson RJ, Hanifa Y, et al. Vitamin D accelerates resolution of inflammatory responses during tuberculosis. Proc Natl Acad Sci U S A. 2012;109:15449–54.
31. van Tellingen A, Grooteman MP, Schoorl M, et al. Intercurrent clinical events are predictive of plasma C-reactive protein levels in hemodialysis patients. Kidney Int. 2002;62:632–8.
32. Lim JH, Ravikumar S, Wang YM, Thamboo TP, Ong L, Chen J, et al. Bimodal influence of vitamin D in host response to systemic candida infection-vitamin D dose matters. J Infect Dis. 2015;212:635–44. pii: jiv033. [Epub ahead of print].
33. Lucas RM, Gorman S, Geldenhuys S, et al. Vitamin D and immunity. F1000Prime Rep. 2014;6:118. doi:10.12703/P6-118.
34. Assa A, Vong L, Pinnell LJ, et al. Vitamin D deficiency promotes epithelial barrier dysfunction and intestinal inflammation. J Infect Dis. 2014;210:12961305. doi:10.1093/infdis/jiu235.
35. Bacchetta J, Chun RF, Gales B, et al. Antibacterial responses by peritoneal macrophages are enhanced following vitamin D supplementation. PLoS One. 2014;9(12):e116530. doi:10.137/journal.pone.0116530.

36. Bacchetta J, Sea JL, Chun RF, et al. FGF 23 inhibits extra-renal synthesis of 1,25-dihydroxyvitamin D in human monocytes. J Bone Miner Res. 2013;28(1):46–55. doi:10.1002/jbmr.1740.
37. Chonchol M, Greene T, Zhang Y, et al. Low vitamin D and high fibroblast growth factor 23 serum levels associate with infectious and cardiac deaths in the HEMO study. J Am Soc Nephrol. 2015. doi:10.1681/ASN.2014101009.
38. Zheng Z, Shi H, Jia J, et al. Vitamin D supplementation and mortality risk in chronic kidney disease: a meta-analysis of 20 observational studies. BMC Nephrol. 2013;14:199. doi:10.1186/1471-2369-14-199.
39. Mann MC, Hobbs AJ, Hemmelgarn BR, et al. Effect of oral vitamin D analogs on mortality and cardiovascular outcomes among adults with chronic kidney disease: a meta-analysis. Clin Kidney J. 2015;8:41–8. doi:10.1093/ckj/sfu122.
40. Palmer SC, Teixeira-Pinto A, Saglimbene V, et al. Association of drug effects on serum parathyroid hormone, phosphorus, and calcium levels with mortality in CKD: a meta-analysis. Am J Kidney Dis. 2015. doi:10.1053/j.ajkd.2015.03.36.

Chapter 18
Vitamin D and Inflammation in Chronic Kidney Disease

Javier Donate-Correa, Ernesto Martín-Núñez, and Juan F. Navarro-González

Abstract Vitamin D deficiency, defined by low serum levels of 25-hydroxyvitamin D, is prevalent in patients with chronic kidney disease, a disorder characterized by a state of chronic low-grade inflammation. This inflammatory state is especially marked in end-stage renal disease and it has been disclosed as an important factor contributing to the progression of renal disease and the high cardiovascular morbidity and mortality found in these patients. This chapter highlights clinical and experimental studies that could potentially explain the link between vitamin D and inflammation. Whether correction of vitamin D deficiency and the associated improvement of inflammatory markers has beneficial effects on cardiovascular outcomes should be investigated in controlled clinical trials.

Keywords Chronic kidney disease • Vitamin D • Inflammation • Vitamin D receptor • Cardiovascular disease • Inflammatory cytokines • RAAS • Vitamin D receptor activators • Paricalcitol • Immunomodulation

18.1 Introduction

Inflammation is recognized as an important factor contributing to the progression of chronic kidney disease (CKD) as well as a hallmark of the high cardiovascular (CV) morbidity and mortality present in these patients. Vitamin D deficiency, defined by low serum levels of 25-hydroxyvitamin D, is especially prevalent in CKD patients who present a dysregulation of vitamin D and mineral metabolism [1].

J. Donate-Correa, PhD (✉) • E. Martín-Núñez
Research Unit, University Hospital Nuestra Señora de Candelaria,
Santa Cruz de Tenerife, Spain
e-mail: jdonate@ull.es

J.F. Navarro-González, MD, PhD, FASN
Research Unit and Nephrology Service, University Hospital Nuestra Señora de Candelaria,
Santa Cruz de Tenerife, Spain
e-mail: jnavgon@gobiernodecanarias.org

© Springer International Publishing Switzerland 2016   305
P.A. Ureña Torres et al. (eds.), *Vitamin D in Chronic Kidney Disease*,
DOI 10.1007/978-3-319-32507-1_18

Vitamin D has important roles in many physiological processes although is primarily involved in calcium and phosphorus homeostasis and bone metabolism. However, beyond these regulatory capabilities, experimental and clinical data suggest beneficial effects of vitamin D on proteinuria, blood pressure, inflammation, and cardiovascular outcomes. Different epidemiological studies have shown an association between vitamin D deficiency with inflammatory disorders such as rheumatoid arthritis, inflammatory bowel disease, systemic lupus erythematous, while has been also considered as a risk factor for developing cancer, cardiovascular disease, hypertension, and diabetes [2]. Importantly, in animal models for some of these diseases, vitamin D supplementation has showed therapeutic effects [3].

The active form of vitamin D, also called calcitriol or 1-alpha,25-dihydroxyvitamin D_3 ($1,25(OH)_2D_3$) is primarily synthesized in the kidneys from $25(OH)D$ (calcidiol) by the action of the enzyme 1α-hydroxylase. This active form binds posteriorly to the vitamin D receptor (VDR) to exert its functions. However, there is increasing evidence that the kidneys are not unique in its ability to generate calcitriol. Many tissues possess 1α-hydroxylase activity, suggesting a paracrine role for $1,25(OH)_2D_3$, which is not well understood. However, in vitro experiments indicate that $1,25(OH)_2D_3$ may be involved in diverse physiological functions, including regulation of cytokines, inflammatory and/or fibrotic pathways, the renin-angiotensin-aldosterone system (RAAS), vascular and cardiac cell function, modulation of immune response, cell growth and differentiation, and others [4–12].

The existence of this wide range of physiological actions is enhanced by the ubiquitous distribution of the VDR in the human body (intestine, kidney, bone, parathyroid glands, immune system, smooth muscle, and myocardium),which is responsible for the pleiotropic effects of VDR activation [4].

Therefore, despite its classical actions in mineral metabolism homeostasis, vitamin D may play important roles on the cardiovascular system, systemic inflammation, oxidative stress, and immune regulation [13]. Importantly, epidemiological studies suggest an inverse association between vitamin D levels and inflammatory markers [14–16]. This chapter highlights clinical and experimental studies that could potentially explain the link between vitamin D and inflammation in the renal patient.

18.2 Inflammation in CKD Patients

Among the many complications of CKD that contribute to the high morbidity and mortality observed in these patients, systemic low-grade inflammation has a prominent role as one of the most typical features and major contributors to the uremic phenotype in advanced stages of CKD. This chronic low-grade inflammation is almost universally present in CKD patients and is fuelled by several independent mechanisms, including accumulation of advanced glycation end products and advanced oxidative protein products, enhanced lipid oxidation, elevation of pro-inflammatory cytokine levels, and stimulated T-cells [17, 18]. Although the prevalence of inflammation is variable and depends of multiple factors like residual renal function, geographic and genetic differences, and dialysis therapy [19], is particularly elevated in end stage renal disease (ESRD) patients, where inflammatory cytokines are associated with higher all-cause and CV mortality [19–21].

Systemic inflammation in these patients is intrinsically linked not only to renal dysfunction but also to other factors, including a state of acquired immune dysfunction, metabolic and nutritional derangements, and protein-energy wasting [22]. Inflammation is an underlying phenomenon in atherosclerosis and vascular disease, and the inflammatory status strongly correlates with increased CV morbidity and mortality. Recent evidence suggests that persistent inflammation is also a major cause of premature general and vascular aging [23]. In addition, inflammation is thought to play a major role in the pathophysiology and progression of renal dysfunction [24].

In these patients, C-reactive protein (CRP) and pro-inflammatory cytokines such as tumor necrosis factor (TNF)-α, interleukin (IL)-1, and IL-6 are elevated [19–21]. In a prospective study involving patients on hemodialysis (HD), Jung et al. [25] used computed tomography imaging to demonstrate that elevated CRP was a strong and independent predictor of progression of coronary artery calcification, even after adjusting for baseline calcification. Likewise, Zocalli et al. demonstrated in this population that IL-6 captures almost entirely the prediction power of the overall inflammation burden, and therefore, IL-6 seems to be an almost ideal indicator of the severity of inflammation [26]. Since inflammatory parameters are sensitive predictors of the outcomes, inflammation appears to be a logical target for preventive and therapeutic interventions in patients with CKD [27, 28].

Many therapeutic strategies can be addressed for treating inflammation in renal patients by targeting inflammatory pathways at different levels, including treating the source of inflammation, changing lifestyle and nutritional habits, and implementing therapeutic strategies commonly used in these patients, which may induce pleiotropic beneficial effects. From this point of view, therapy with vitamin D may be considered as a common therapeutic approach in patients with CKD with additional positive impact on systemic inflammation.

18.3   Vitamin D in Cardiovascular Disease

There is increased recognition that vitamin D deficiency plays a role in the development of CV disease. In addition to regulating mineral metabolism homeostasis and skeletal health, vitamin D plays important metabolic roles which are important for renal and CV protection [29]. Observational studies in general population showed that vitamin D deficiency is associated with classical CV risk factors [30] as well as with clinical events such as congestive heart failure, coronary artery disease, peripheral artery disease, and stroke [31–33], an association that persists in prospective studies [34–36]. Importantly, in one of this observational studies [37] it was shown that low levels of circulating 25(OH)D were significantly correlated with two markers of inflammation (CRP and IL-6), suggesting a link between low vitamin D levels and inflammation. Posteriorly, a study conducted in middle-aged and older healthy volunteers [38] revealed that vascular endothelial cells from subjects with 25(OH)D deficiency showed increased expression levels of the inflammatory cytokine IL-6 and the pro-inflammatory transcription nuclear factor kappa B (NF-kB). More recently, an inverse correlation between 25(OH)D and CRP and IL-6 levels was described in 182 patients (ages 5–21) with CKD stages 2–5, an association that remained significant after adjusting for the severity of CKD [39].

Animal studies point to vitamin D as an important regulator of the RAAS. In a very interesting study, Xiang et al. [40] showed that VDR knockout mice shared hypertension with cardiac hypertrophy and, importantly, up-regulation of the cardiac RAAS. In this model, $1,25(OH)_2D_3$ acted as an endocrine suppressor of renin biosynthesis. Conversely, treatment with VDR activators (VDRAs) like paricalcitol attenuated the development of left ventricular hypertrophy (LVH) in Dahl salt-sensitive [41] and uremic rats [42]. Likewise, amelioration of cardiac hypertrophy and, cardiac remodeling, and an improvement of left ventricular diastolic measures have been observed in uremic rats and in rats with spontaneous hypertension treated with vitamin D analogs [43].

Clinical studies also point to the cardio-protective effects of vitamin D. HD patients treated with intravenous calcitriol [44] or with oral cholecalciferol [45, 46] shared reduced cardiac hypertrophy accompanied by a decrease in the levels of inflammatory markers [45, 46]. Administration of cholecalciferol to ESRD patients was found to reduce circulating IL-8, IL-6, and TNF-α levels by approximately 55 %, 30 %, and 60 %, respectively [47]. Similarly, one study showed that vitamin D deficiency in HD patients who did not received therapy with vitamin D receptor agonists was associated with an increased risk of all-cause mortality [48]. However, in the recent multicenter double-blinded, randomized, placebo-controlled PRIMO study, treatment with paricalcitol did not alter left ventricular mass index or improve measures of diastolic dysfunction in patients with CKD [49]. Therefore, the impact of vitamin D therapy on long-term outcomes in patients with CKD, and its potential relationship with modulation of inflammation, needs to be evaluated in prospective adequately designed and powered studies.

18.4   Mechanisms Linking Vitamin D and Inflammation

As discussed above, inflammation has been associated with vitamin D deficiency in CKD patients. Several mechanisms have been recently proposed to explain this link.

The active form of the vitamin D generates biological responses both by regulating gene transcription (genomic responses) and by rapidly activating a variety of signal transduction pathways (rapid responses). Vitamin D regulates the expression of diverse genes in a variety of tissues. These genomic actions are mediated by the VDR, a kind of nuclear receptor which, after heterodimerization with the retinoid X receptor (RXR) to form the VDR/RXR/co-factor complex, interacts with specific

DNA sequences called vitamin D response elements (VDRE) located in the promoter regions of the target genes [50]. Although the majority of activities associated with vitamin D appear to be initiated through this nuclear VDR, there is evidence that calcitriol may also act in a "nongenomic" manner generating rapid responses. This suggests the existence of a membrane associated VDR, which probably has the ability to bind different ligands than the nuclear VDR [51, 52].

It is estimated that about 3 % of the human genome is regulated by $1,25(OH)_2D_3$ with actions on a wide variety of physiological processes which can be summarized in: regulation of the functioning of B and T lymphocytes (the adaptative immune system); control of the innate immune system; secretion of insulin by pancreatic cells; the functioning of the heart and blood pressure regulation; and the brain activity [53–55]. Specifically, the mechanisms by which vitamin D exert these physiological effects include the regulation of the synthesis and production of cytokines, inflammation, fibrogenesis, RAAS, immune response and cell growth and differentiation.

Macrophage and monocyte activation is a key element in the inflammatory response, leading to the generation of a number of pro-inflammatory factors, such as TNF-α, interferons (IFNs), IL-1, IL-2, IL-6, IL-8, and IL-12, leptin and adiponectin, as well as the anti-inflammatory cytokine IL-10. The synthesis of these proteins may be modulated by vitamin D either as a result of direct interaction with monocytes or indirectly through its effects on calcium, phosphorus, and parathyroid hormone (PTH) metabolism (Fig. 18.1). In addition, these cytokines modulate the hepatic production of acute-phase proteins, such as the CRP [56]. The majority of HD patients present high serum levels of CRP, which have been associated with accelerated atherosclerosis and increased CV morbidity and mortality [56]. Vitamin D supplementation has been related to a decrease in CRP levels in healthy subjects [57] and in CKD patients [58].

The effects of vitamin D on the inflammatory status can be partially explained by the presence of the VDR in a group of immune cells that includes monocytes, antigen-presenting cells (macrophages and dendritic cells) and T and B cells (Fig. 18.1) [59–66]. Hence, vitamin D could exert a regulatory function on the immune system unrelated to mineral metabolism homeostasis. A number of studies support this hypothesis, confirming the capacity of vitamin D to act as a modulator of the immune response and cell differentiation [66–68]. These effects include a decline in the synthesis of pro-inflammatory cytokines (such as IL-6, IL-12, IFN-γ, and TNF-α), the increase of IL-10, and a VDR-mediated sequestration of NF-kB signaling, all of which favor a less inflamed state [69, 70].

Is remarkable that intracrine conversion from 25(OH)D to calcitriol in these cells (Fig. 18.1), which present 1α-hydroxylase activity, has potent anti-inflammatory effects through the reduction in the production of the T helper type 1 cytokines IL-2, interferon-γ, and TNF-α, and the suppression of the inflammatory macrophage response [70]. Such improvement of the inflammation status occurs even in moderate stages of CKD [71].

Vitamin D is able to inhibit the activation the TNF-α converting enzyme (TACE), also called ADAM17, which plays an important role in the generation of renal

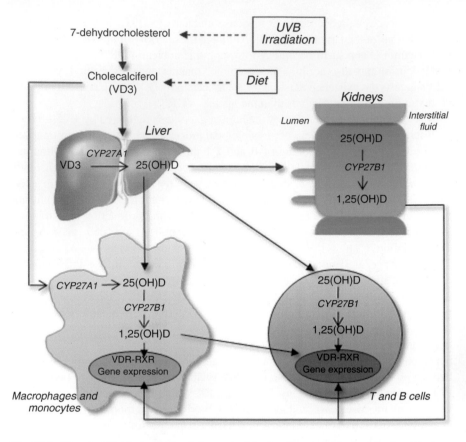

Fig. 18.1 Vitamin D3 (cholecalciferol) is acquired in the diet or synthesized in the skin from cholesterol and hydroxylated in the liver to 25(OH)D, the main circulating form of the vitamin D. Later, is hydroxylated in the kidneys by the 25-hydroxyvitamin D-1 α-hydroxylase, also known as protein CYP27B1, to become 1,25(OH)D, the physiologically most active form. Cells of the immune system, including macrophages, dendritic cells, T and B cells also express this enzyme, and therefore can generate 1,25(OH)D. Importantly, 1,25(OH)D acts on immune cells in an autocrine or paracrine manner by binding to the VDR. *VDRE* VD response element

fibrosis, glomerulosclerosis, and proteinuria [4]. Studies in patients on HD have demonstrated that expression of TACE in peripheral monocytes, and serum levels of TNF-α, ICAM-1, and VCAM-1, are increased compared to normal controls, and that the combination of vitamin D supplementation and paricalcitol reduced TACE expression and activity. Moreover, TACE activation is usually secondary to activation of the renal RAAS system, which, as discussed below, is also directly inhibited by the VDR activation [4, 72]. Thus, vitamin D suppresses TACE activation and subsequent inflammation at multiple levels. Moreover, TACE activation in renal cells also leads to subsequent release of TNF-α, ICAM-1, and VCAM-1 into the circulation, promoting systemic inflammation. Importantly, the activation of renal TACE can be also blocked by administration of vitamin D analogs [73].

Another mechanism for the control of the inflammatory status could be associated with proteinuria. Vitamin D deficiency is associated with an increased risk for developing proteinuria [74]. Specifically, albuminuria is a major risk factor for the progression of renal and CV disease and is linked to all-cause and CV mortality [75], which is associated with increased levels of IL-6 in CKD patients [76]. Importantly, treatment with active vitamin D compounds seems to have a beneficial effect on proteinuria in patients with CKD [77, 78].

Vitamin D could also control inflammation through regulation of the transcription factor NF-kB. In a study using a mouse model of obstructed nephropathy, paricalcitol reduced the infiltration of inflammatory T-cells and renal expression of the RANTES (regulated and normal T-cell expressed and secreted) protein [79]. In this work, Tan et al. [79] demonstrated that induction of the pro-inflammatory RANTES protein, which is dependent on NF-kB signaling, is prevented by repressing the NF-kB-mediated gene transcription through the nuclear VDR.

Finally, vitamin D is now considered as a negative regulator of the activation of the RAAS, which exerts hemodynamic and pro-inflammatory actions and plays an important role in the progression of CKD. Renin is synthesized in the kidney by juxtaglomerular cells stimulating the formation of angiotensin I, which is metabolized to angiotensin II. Angiotensin II is a very active vasoconstrictor molecule and stimulates aldosterone secretion by adrenal cells [36]. *In vitro* studies using a juxtaglomerular cell model have shown that $1,25(OH)_2D_3$, as well as other vitamin D analogs, directly suppress renin gene expression via a VDRE present in the renin gene [80]. In fact, VDR knockdown mice have higher expression of renin and angiotensin II synthesis, and develop sodium retention, elevated arterial blood pressure, and LVH [81] due to the absence of the normal suppression of RAAS activation by vitamin D [82]. In humans, low concentrations of serum calcidiol are accompanied by higher levels of circulating angiotensin, concluding that in patients with arterial hypertension, vitamin D supplementation helps to reduce the concentrations of renin and angiotensin II in the serum [83].

18.5 Anti-inflammatory Effects of Vitamin D Receptor Activators in CKD Patients

Treatment with VDRAs is considered a mainstay strategy for preventing the onset and delaying the progression of secondary hyperparathyroidism (SHPT), and also with potential benefits on long term outcomes in patients with CKD. Going beyond the primary therapeutic goal of PTH suppression, the results of several large observational studies in HD patients have demonstrated improved survival in the patients that received VDRA therapy compared those with no VDRA treatment [84–87]. One of the proposed additional benefits of VDRA-based therapy in CKD patients resides in its potential anti-inflammatory activity since VDR activation presents anti-inflammatory, immunologic and nephroprotective actions [88]. Preclinical data also suggests the existence of modulatory effects on inflammation by decreasing inflammatory biomarkers after treatment with VDRAs [79, 89].

Currently, several VDRAs are used for the treatment or prevention of SHPT in patients with CKD and include calcitriol (that was the first compound commercially available), doxercalciferol and alfacalcidol (both of them require 25-hydroxylation in the liver to produce the active moieties), and maxacalcitol and paricalcitol (which do not require the additional step of enzymatic activation) [90, 91].

Importantly, these VDRAs differ in their functional selectivity at the VDR [92]. The survival benefits and the differential effects of selective VDRAs have been linked to nonclassical effects of VDRAs, which are distinct from their effects on the parathyroid gland, gut and bone, and include anti-inflammatory actions. The immunomodulatory effects of the selective VDRA paricalcitol have been analyzed *in vitro* in human peripheral blood mononuclear cells (PBMC), revealing a significant reduction of the pro-inflammatory cytokines IL-8 and TNF-α and an increase in anti-inflammatory factors [93, 94]. These effects were also observed in an experimental rat model of obstructive nephropathy, where paricalcitol was able to inhibit local, renal inflammatory infiltration of T cells and macrophages, accompanied by decreased gene expression of TNF-α [79].

In vitro studies in PBMCs obtained from HD patients [95] and in cultures of rat osteoblasts [96] have made evident the effect of VDRAs on the inhibition of the production of cytokines involved in atheroma formation and calcification. This inhibitory effect extends to proteins implicated in arterial calcification in human osteoblasts *in vitro* [97] and on preventing thrombosis in mice [98].

As mentioned above, vitamin D suppresses renin production. In As4.1 cells transiently transfected with the human VDR complementary DNA, both calcitriol and paricalcitol suppressed renin mRNA expression in similar dose-dependent fashions [99]. These data suggest that paricalcitol may have a greater therapeutic window for providing beneficial effects on the RAAS with less risk of hypercalcemic effects, just as it does for PTH suppression. Experimental studies with VDRAs have demonstrated strong suppressive effects on inflammatory mechanisms and oxidative stress. Treatment with the VDRA paricalcitol significantly decreased cardiac oxidative stress in uremic rats, and especially when it was administered in combination with enalapril, prevented inflammation and oxidative injury in uremic rats and in apoE deficient, atherosclerosis-prone mice [100].

From the above-mentioned findings, it appears that selective VDRA therapy should improve the chronic inflammation status of CKD patients at least in a similar way as non-selective activators. However, only a few studies have focused on the potential immunomodulatory effect of selective VDRAs in CKD patients. In a randomized, placebo-controlled study by Moe et al. [101], intravenous injection of paricalcitol in HD patients did not significantly affected cytokine release from the isolated monocytes. However, this study has two drawbacks: only patients with low PTH levels were included, and the blood for the monocyte study was collected after dialysis sessions, when serum concentrations of paricalcitol were lowest. In another double blind, randomized, placebo-controlled pilot trial with CKD patients stage 2 and 3, Alborzi et al. [58] observed a paricalcitol-induced decline in albuminuria and inflammation (revealed by a sharp fall in CRP levels) after only 1 month of treatment. Results were independent of the effects on hemodynamics or PTH suppression. Sochorová et al. [102] demonstrated *in vitro* that both calcitriol and paricalcitol exert potent immunomodulatory effects, with a reduction of bioactive IL-2 and a decrease in the induction of antigen-specific T cells, by inhibiting the maturation of dendritic cells despite potent Toll-like receptor mediated stimulation. In accordance with previous studies, a decrease in CRP, IL-6, IL-8, and TNF-α, and a rise in IL-10 were detected after treatment. Recently, Izquierdo et al. [103] demonstrated an improvement in the inflammation status of HD patients after only 3 months of treatment with paricalcitol. Also in HD patients, a significant decline in CRP and TNF-α and increased ratio values for TNF-α/IL-10 and IL-6/IL-10 has been found after treatment with paricalcitol, which reflects an immunomodulatory activity of this selective VDRA [104]. These results were replicated in a small group of CKD patients in stage 3b and 4. After 5 months of paricalcitol administration, significant reductions were also detected in serum CRP and in serum and PBMCs cell gene expression of TNF-α and IL-6 [105]. Taken together, these works indicate that treatment with the selective VDRA paricalcitol may shift the balance toward an improved inflammation status, which in turn, could reduce the risk of atherosclerosis in CKD patients.

There is a lack of studies on the immunomodulatory effects of selective vs. non-selective VDRAs in CKD. Although an influence on the chronic inflammation status has been suggested to explain some of the differential characteristics of paricalcitol in the improvement of renal patients' outcomes, this possibility has not been clarified yet. In a recent work, Guerrero et al. [106] evaluated the effects of calcitriol and paricalcitol in experimentally inflamed rats, rat aortic rings, and human VSMCs treated with phosphate and TNF-α. The data indicated that treatment with paricalcitol resulted in a more pronounced anti-inflammatory effect than treatment with calcitriol and, as opposed to calcitriol; paricalcitol was able to prevent vascular calcification.

18.6 Conclusions

In patients with CKD, inflammation appears to be a logical target for preventive and therapeutic interventions. There is emerging evidence linking inflammation to vitamin D deficiency and suggesting that sufficient levels of 25(OH)D and sufficient local production of $1,25(OH)_2D_3$ and/or treatment with VDRAs might be beneficial in the control of systemic inflammation in patients with CKD. The whole spectrum of interrelated beneficial effects and potential mechanisms by which vitamin D homeostasis may lower cardiovascular risk evidences the need of randomized controlled studies examining the effect of vitamin D administration on inflammatory markers and cardiovascular outcomes.

References

1. Lo W-K. Serum parameters, inflammation, renal function and patient outcome. Contrib Nephrol. 2006;150:152–5.
2. Gouni-Berthold I, Krone W, Berthold HK. Vitamin D and cardiovascular disease. Curr Vasc Pharmacol. 2009;7(3):414–22.
3. Guillot X, Semerano L, Saidenberg-Kermanac'h N, Falgarone G, Boissier M-C. Vitamin D and inflammation. Joint Bone Spine. 2010;77(6):552–7.
4. Dusso AS, Brown AJ, Slatopolsky E. Vitamin D. Am J Physiol Renal Physiol. 2005;289(1): F8–28.
5. Al-Badr W, Martin KJ. Vitamin D and kidney disease. Clin J Am Soc Nephrol. 2008;3(5): 1555–60.
6. Liu PT, Stenger S, Li H, Wenzel L, Tan BH, Krutzik SR, et al. Toll-like receptor triggering of a vitamin D-mediated human antimicrobial response. Science. 2006;311(5768):1770–3.
7. Saggese G, Federico G, Balestri M, Toniolo A. Calcitriol inhibits the PHA-induced production of IL-2 and IFN-gamma and the proliferation of human peripheral blood leukocytes while enhancing the surface expression of HLA class II molecules. J Endocrinol Invest. 1989;12(5):329–35.
8. Tan X, Li Y, Liu Y. Paricalcitol attenuates renal interstitial fibrosis in obstructive nephropathy. J Am Soc Nephrol. 2006;17(12):3382–93.
9. Wu-Wong JR, Nakane M, Ma J. Effects of vitamin D analogs on the expression of plasminogen activator inhibitor-1 in human vascular cells. Thromb Res. 2006;118(6):709–14.
10. Zhang Z, Sun L, Wang Y, Ning G, Minto AW, Kong J, et al. Renoprotective role of the vitamin D receptor in diabetic nephropathy. Kidney Int US. 2008;73(2):163–71.
11. Li YC, Kong J, Wei M, Chen Z-F, Liu SQ, Cao L-P. 1,25-Dihydroxyvitamin D(3) is a negative endocrine regulator of the renin-angiotensin system. J Clin Invest US. 2002;110(2): 229–38.
12. Artaza JN, Norris KC. Vitamin D reduces the expression of collagen and key profibrotic factors by inducing an antifibrotic phenotype in mesenchymal multipotent cells. J Endocrinol Engl. 2009;200(2):207–21.
13. Grant WB, Holick MF. Benefits and requirements of vitamin D for optimal health: a review. Altern Med Rev. 2005;10(2):94–111.
14. Liu LC, Voors AA, van Veldhuisen DJ, van der Veer E, Belonje AM, Szymanski MK, et al. Vitamin D status and outcomes in heart failure patients. Eur J Heart Fail. 2011;13(6): 619–25.
15. Björkhem-Bergman L, Nylén H, Norlin AC, Lindh JD, Ekström L, Eliasson E, et al. Serum levels of 25-hydroxyvitamin D and the CYP3A biomarker 4β-hydroxycholesterol in a high-dose vitamin D supplementation study. Drug Metab Dispos. 2013;41(4):704–8.
16. Hopkins MH, Owen J, Ahearn T, Fedirko V, Flanders WD, Jones DP, et al. Effects of supplemental vitamin D and calcium on biomarkers of inflammation in colorectal adenoma patients: a randomized, controlled clinical trial. Cancer Prev Res (Phila). 2011;4(10):1645–54.
17. Petchey WG, Johnson DW, Isbel NM. Shining D' light on chronic kidney disease: mechanisms that may underpin the cardiovascular benefit of vitamin D. Nephrology (Carlton). 2011;16(4):351–67.
18. Silverstein DM. Inflammation in chronic kidney disease: role in the progression of renal and cardiovascular disease. Pediatr Nephrol. 2009;24(8):1445–52.
19. Wanner C, Metzger T. C-reactive protein a marker for all-cause and cardiovascular mortality in haemodialysis patients. Nephrol Dial Transplant Engl. 2002;17 Suppl 8:29–40.
20. Zimmermann J, Herrlinger S, Pruy A, Metzger T, Wanner C. Inflammation enhances cardiovascular risk and mortality in hemodialysis patients. Kidney Int. 1999;55(2):648–58.
21. Stenvinkel P, Wanner C, Metzger T, Heimbürger O, Mallamaci F, Tripepi G, et al. Inflammation and outcome in end-stage renal failure: does female gender constitute a survival advantage? Kidney Int. 2002;62(5):1791–8.

22. Machowska A, Carrero JJ, Lindholm B, Stenvinkel P. Therapeutics targeting persistent inflammation in chronic kidney disease. Transl Res. 2015. doi:10.1016/j.trsl.2015.06.012. pii: S1931-5244(15)00217-0, [Epub ahead of print].
23. Stenvinkel P, Larsson TE. Chronic kidney disease: a clinical model of premature aging. Am J Kidney Dis. 2013;62(2):339–51.
24. Hiramoto JS, Katz R, Peralta CA, Ix JH, Fried L, Cushman M, et al. Inflammation and coagulation markers and kidney function decline: the Multi-Ethnic Study of Atherosclerosis (MESA). Am J Kidney Dis. 2012;60(2):225–32.
25. Jung HH, Kim SW, Han H. Inflammation, mineral metabolism and progressive coronary artery calcification in patients on haemodialysis. Nephrol Dial Transplant. 2006;21(7):1915–20. Epub 2006 Mar 22.
26. Zoccali C, Tripepi G, Mallamaci F. Dissecting inflammation in ESRD: do cytokines and C-reactive protein have a complementary prognostic value for mortality in dialysis patients? J Am Soc Nephrol. 2006;17(12 Suppl 3):S169–73.
27. Meuwese CL, Stenvinkel P, Dekker FW, Carrero JJ. Monitoring of inflammation in patients on dialysis: forewarned is forearmed. Nat Rev Nephrol. 2011;7(3):166–76.
28. Meuwese CL, Snaedal S, Halbesma N, Stenvinkel P, Dekker FW, Qureshi AR, et al. Trimestral variations of C-reactive protein, interleukin-6 and tumour necrosis factor-alpha are similarly associated with survival in haemodialysis patients. Nephrol Dial Transplant. 2011;26(4):1313–8.
29. Tentori F, Blayney MJ, Albert JM, Gillespie BW, Kerr PG, Bommer J, et al. Mortality risk for dialysis patients with different levels of serum calcium, phosphorus, and PTH: the Dialysis Outcomes and Practice Patterns Study (DOPPS). Am J Kidney Dis. 2008;52(3):519–30.
30. Querfeld U, Mak RH. Vitamin D deficiency and toxicity in chronic kidney disease: in search of the therapeutic window. Pediatr Nephrol. 2010;25(12):2413–30.
31. Martins D, Wolf M, Pan D, Zadshir A, Tareen N, Thadhani R, et al. Prevalence of cardiovascular risk factors and the serum levels of 25-hydroxyvitamin D in the United States: data from the Third National Health and Nutrition Examination Survey. Arch Intern Med. 2007;167(11):1159–65.
32. Kim DH, Sabour S, Sagar UN, Adams S, Whellan DJ. Prevalence of hypovitaminosis D in cardiovascular diseases (from the National Health and Nutrition Examination Survey 2001 to 2004). Am J Cardiol. 2008;102(11):1540–4.
33. Scragg R, Jackson R, Holdaway IM, Lim T, Beaglehole R. Myocardial infarction is inversely associated with plasma 25-hydroxyvitamin D3 levels: a community-based study. Int J Epidemiol. 1990;19(3):559–63.
34. Kojima G, Bell C, Abbott RD, Launer L, Chen R, Motonaga H, et al. Low dietary vitamin D predicts 34-year incident stroke: the Honolulu Heart Program. Stroke. 2012;43(8):2163–7.
35. Giovannucci E, Liu Y, Hollis BW, Rimm EB. 25-hydroxyvitamin D and risk of myocardial infarction in men: a prospective study. Arch Intern Med. 2008;168(11):1174–80.
36. Wang TJ, Pencina MJ, Booth SL, Jacques PF, Ingelsson E, Lanier K, et al. Vitamin D deficiency and risk of cardiovascular disease. Circulation. 2008;117(4):503–11.
37. Dobnig H, Pilz S, Scharnagl H, Renner W, Seelhorst U, Wellnitz B, et al. Independent association of low serum 25-hydroxyvitamin d and 1,25-dihydroxyvitamin d levels with all-cause and cardiovascular mortality. Arch Intern Med. 2008;168(12):1340–9.
38. Jablonski KL, Chonchol M, Pierce GL, Walker AE, Seals DR. 25-Hydroxyvitamin D deficiency is associated with inflammation-linked vascular endothelial dysfunction in middle-aged and older adults. Hypertension. 2011;57(1):63–9.
39. Kalkwarf HJ, Denburg MR, Strife CF, Zemel BS, Foerster DL, Wetzsteon RJ, et al. Vitamin D deficiency is common in children and adolescents with chronic kidney disease. Kidney Int. 2012;81(7):690–7.
40. Xiang W, Kong J, Chen S, Cao LP, Qiao G, Zheng W, et al. Cardiac hypertrophy in vitamin D receptor knockout mice: role of the systemic and cardiac renin-angiotensin systems. Am J Physiol Endocrinol Metab. 2005;288(1):E125–32.
41. Bodyak N, Ayus JC, Achinger S, Shivalingappa V, Ke Q, Chen YS, et al. Activated vitamin D attenuates left ventricular abnormalities induced by dietary sodium in Dahl salt-sensitive animals. Proc Natl Acad Sci U S A. 2007;104(43):16810–5.

42. Mizobuchi M, Nakamura H, Tokumoto M, Finch J, Morrissey J, Liapis H, et al. Myocardial effects of VDR activators in renal failure. J Steroid Biochem Mol Biol. 2010;121(1–2):188–92.
43. Koleganova N, Piecha G, Ritz E, Gross ML. Calcitriol ameliorates capillary deficit and fibrosis of the heart in subtotally nephrectomized rats. Nephrol Dial Transplant. 2009;24(3):778–87.
44. Kim HW, Park CW, Shin YS, Kim YS, Shin SJ, Kim YS, et al. Calcitriol regresses cardiac hypertrophy and QT dispersion in secondary hyperparathyroidism on hemodialysis. Nephron Clin Pract. 2006;102(1):c21–9.
45. Matias PJ, Jorge C, Ferreira C, Borges M, Aires I, Amaral T, et al. Cholecalciferol supplementation in hemodialysis patients: effects on mineral metabolism, inflammation, and cardiac dimension parameters. Clin J Am Soc Nephrol. 2010;5(5):905–11.
46. Bucharles S, Barberato SH, Stinghen AE, Gruber B, Piekala L, Dambiski AC, et al. Impact of cholecalciferol treatment on biomarkers of inflammation and myocardial structure in hemodialysis patients without hyperparathyroidism. J Ren Nutr. 2012;22(2):284–91.
47. Stubbs JR, Idiculla A, Slusser J, Menard R, Quarles LD. Cholecalciferol supplementation alters calcitriol-responsive monocyte proteins and decreases inflammatory cytokines in ESRD. J Am Soc Nephrol. 2010;21:353–61.
48. Ogawa T, Kyono A, Sato M, Sugimoto H, Otsuka K, Nitta K. Vitamin D receptor agonist supplementation and suppression of inflammation may have advantage for all-cause mortality in hemodialysis patients. Clin Exp Nephrol. 2012;16(5):779–85.
49. Thadhani R, Appelbaum E, Pritchett Y, Chang Y, Wenger J, Tamez H, et al. Vitamin D therapy and cardiac structure and function in patients with chronic kidney disease: the PRIMO randomized controlled trial. JAMA. 2012;307(7):674–84.
50. Wu-Wong JR. Vitamin D, receptor: a highly versatile nuclear receptor. Kidney Int. 2007;72(3):237–9.
51. Nemere I, Schwartz Z, Pedrozo H, Sylvia VL, Dean DD, Boyan BD. Identification of a membrane receptor for 1,25-dihydroxyvitamin D3 which mediates rapid activation of protein kinase C. J Bone Miner Res. 1998;13(9):1353–9.
52. Marcinkowska E. A run for a membrane vitamin D receptor. Biol Signals Recept. 2001;10(6):341–9.
53. Carlberg C. Current understanding of the function of the nuclear vitamin D receptor in response to its natural and synthetic ligands. Recent Results Cancer Res. 2003;164:29–42.
54. Bouillon R, Carmeliet G, Verlinden L, van Etten E, Verstuyf A, Luderer HF, et al. Vitamin D and human health: lessons from vitamin D receptor null mice. Endocr Rev. 2008;29(6):726–76.
55. Norman AW. From vitamin D to hormone D: fundamentals of the vitamin D endocrine system essential for good health. Am J Clin Nutr. 2008;88(2):491S–9.
56. Wanner C, Zimmermann J, Schwedler S, Metzger T. Inflammation and cardiovascular risk in dialysis patients. Kidney Int Suppl. 2002;80:99–102.
57. Timms PM, Mannan N, Hitman GA, Noonan K, Mills PG, Syndercombe-Court D, et al. Circulating MMP9, vitamin D and variation in the TIMP-1 response with VDR genotype: mechanisms for inflammatory damage in chronic disorders? QJM England. 2002;95(12):787–96.
58. Alborzi P, Patel NA, Peterson C, Bills JE, Bekele DM, Bunaye Z, et al. Paricalcitol reduces albuminuria and inflammation in chronic kidney disease: a randomized double-blind pilot trial. Hypertension. 2008;52(2):249–55.
59. Provvedini DM, Manolagas SC. 1 Alpha,25-dihydroxyvitamin D3 receptor distribution and effects in subpopulations of normal human T lymphocytes. J Clin Endocrinol Metab. 1989;68(4):774–9.
60. Tsoukas CD, Provvedini DM, Manolagas SC. 1,25-dihydroxyvitamin D3: a novel immunoregulatory hormone. Science. 1984;224(4656):1438–40.
61. Norman PE, Powell JT. Vitamin D and cardiovascular disease. Circ Res. 2014;114(2):379–93.
62. Veldman CM, Cantorna MT, DeLuca HF. Expression of 1,25-dihydroxyvitamin D(3) receptor in the immune system. Arch Biochem Biophys. 2000;374(2):334–8.
63. Penna G, Adorini L. 1 Alpha,25-dihydroxyvitamin D3 inhibits differentiation, maturation, activation, and survival of dendritic cells leading to impaired alloreactive T cell activation. J Immunol. 2000;164(5):2405–11.

64. Yu XP, Mocharla H, Hustmyer FG, Manolagas SC. Vitamin D receptor expression in human lymphocytes. Signal requirements and characterization by western blots and DNA sequencing. J Biol Chem. 1991;266(12):7588–95.
65. Hewison M, Freeman L, Hughes SV, Evans KN, Bland R, Eliopoulos AG, et al. Differential regulation of vitamin D receptor and its ligand in human monocyte-derived dendritic cells. J Immunol. 2003;170(11):5382–90.
66. Kizaki M, Norman AW, Bishop JE, Lin CW, Karmakar A, Koeffler HP. 1,25-Dihydroxyvitamin D3 receptor RNA: expression in hematopoietic cells. Blood. 1991;77(6):1238–47.
67. Seibert E, Levin NW, Kuhlmann MK. Immunomodulating effects of vitamin D analogs in hemodialysis patients. Hemodial Int. 2005;9 Suppl 1:S25–9.
68. van Etten E, Mathieu C. Immunoregulation by 1,25-dihydroxyvitamin D3: basic concepts. J Steroid Biochem Mol Biol. 2005;97(1–2):93–101.
69. Mathieu C, Adorini L. The coming of age of 1,25-dihydroxyvitamin D(3) analogs as immunomodulatory agents. Trends Mol Med. 2002;8(4):174–9.
70. Helming L, Bose J, Ehrchen J, Schiebe S, Frahm T, Geffers R, et al. 1alpha,25-Dihydroxyvitamin D3 is a potent suppressor of interferon gamma-mediated macrophage activation. Blood. 2005;106(13):4351–8.
71. Navarro-Gonzalez JF, Mora-Fernandez C, Muros M, Herrera H, Garcia J. Mineral metabolism and inflammation in chronic kidney disease patients: a cross-sectional study. Clin J Am Soc Nephrol. 2009;4(10):1646–54.
72. Freundlich M, Quiroz Y, Zhang Z, Zhang Y, Bravo Y, Weisinger JR, et al. Suppression of renin-angiotensin gene expression in the kidney by paricalcitol. Kidney Int. 2008;74(11): 1394–402.
73. Dusso A, Arcidiacono MV, Yang J, Tokumoto M. Vitamin D inhibition of TACE and prevention of renal osteodystrophy and cardiovascular mortality. J Steroid Biochem Mol Biol. 2010;121(1–2):193–8.
74. de Boer IH, Ioannou GN, Kestenbaum B, Brunzell JD, Weiss NS. 25-Hydroxyvitamin D levels and albuminuria in the Third National Health and Nutrition Examination Survey (NHANES III). Am J Kidney Dis. 2007;50(1):69–77.
75. Levey AS, de Jong PE, Coresh J, El Nahas M, Astor BC, Matsushita K, et al. The definition, classification, and prognosis of chronic kidney disease: a KDIGO Controversies Conference report. Kidney Int. 2011;80:17–28.
76. Isakova T, Gutierrez OM, Patel NM, Andress DL, Wolf M, Levin A. Vitamin D deficiency, inflammation, and albuminuria in chronic kidney disease: complex interactions. J Ren Nutr. 2011;21(4):295–302.
77. de Zeeuw D, Agarwal R, Amdahl M, Audhya P, Coyne D, Garimella T, et al. Selective vitamin D receptor activation with paricalcitol for reduction of albuminuria in patients with type 2 diabetes (VITAL study): a randomised controlled trial. Lancet (Lond Engl). 2010;376(9752): 1543–51.
78. Liu L-J, Lv J-C, Shi S-F, Chen Y-Q, Zhang H, Wang H-Y. Oral calcitriol for reduction of proteinuria in patients with IgA nephropathy: a randomized controlled trial. Am J Kidney Dis. 2012;59(1):67–74.
79. Tan X, Wen X, Liu Y. Paricalcitol inhibits renal inflammation by promoting vitamin D receptor-mediated sequestration of NF-kappaB signaling. J Am Soc Nephrol. 2008;19(9):1741–52.
80. Li YC, Kong J, Wei M, Chen Z-F, Liu SQ, Cao L-P. 1,25-Dihydroxyvitamin D(3) is a negative endocrine regulator of the renin-angiotensin system. J Clin Invest. 2002;110(2):229–38.
81. Heaney RP, Holick MF. Why the IOM recommendations for vitamin D are deficient. J Bone Miner Res. 2011;26(3):455–7.
82. K/DOQI Workgroup. K/DOQI clinical practice guidelines for cardiovascular disease in dialysis patients. Am J Kidney Dis US; 2005;45(4 Suppl 3):S1–153.
83. Pilz S, Tomaschitz A, Ritz E, Pieber TR. Vitamin D status and arterial hypertension: a systematic review. Nat Rev Cardiol. 2009;6(10):621–30.
84. Teng M, Wolf M, Ofsthun MN, Lazarus JM, Hernan MA, Camargo CAJ, et al. Activated injectable vitamin D and hemodialysis survival: a historical cohort study. J Am Soc Nephrol. 2005;16(4):1115–25.

85. Kalantar-Zadeh K, Kuwae N, Regidor DL, Kovesdy CP, Kilpatrick RD, Shinaberger CS, et al. Survival predictability of time-varying indicators of bone disease in maintenance hemodialysis patients. Kidney Int. 2006;70(4):771–80.
86. Young EW, Albert JM, Akiba T, et al. Vitamin D therapy and mortality in the Dialysis Outcomes and Practice Patterns Study (DOPPS). J Am Soc Nephrol. 2005;16:278A.
87. Teng M, Wolf M, Lowrie E, Ofsthun N, Lazarus JM, Thadhani R. Survival of patients undergoing hemodialysis with paricalcitol or calcitriol therapy. N Engl J Med. 2003;349(5): 446–56.
88. Perez-Gomez MV, Ortiz-Arduan A, Lorenzo-Sellares V. Vitamin D and proteinuria: a critical review of molecular bases and clinical experience. Nefrologia. 2013;33(5):716–26.
89. Tan X, He W, Liu Y. Combination therapy with paricalcitol and trandolapril reduces renal fibrosis in obstructive nephropathy. Kidney Int. 2009;76(12):1248–57.
90. Andress DL. Vitamin D, treatment in chronic kidney disease. Semin Dial. 2005;18(4): 315–21.
91. Hudson JQ. Secondary hyperparathyroidism in chronic kidney disease: focus on clinical consequences and vitamin D therapies. Ann Pharmacother. 2006;40(9):1584–93.
92. Brancaccio D, Bommer J, Coyne D. Vitamin D receptor activator selectivity in the treatment of secondary hyperparathyroidism: understanding the differences among therapies. Drugs NZ. 2007;67(14):1981–98.
93. Eleftheriadis T, Antoniadi G, Liakopoulos V, Stefanidis I, Galaktidou G. Inverse association of serum 25-hydroxyvitamin D with markers of inflammation and suppression of osteoclastic activity in hemodialysis patients. Iran J Kidney Dis. 2012;6(2):129–35.
94. Muller K, Haahr PM, Diamant M, Rieneck K, Kharazmi A, Bendtzen K. 1,25-Dihydroxyvitamin D3 inhibits cytokine production by human blood monocytes at the post-transcriptional level. Cytokine. 1992;4(6):506–12.
95. Panichi V, De Pietro S, Andreini B, Bianchi AM, Migliori M, Taccola D, et al. Calcitriol modulates in vivo and in vitro cytokine production: a role for intracellular calcium. Kidney Int. 1998;54(5):1463–9.
96. Bellows CG, Reimers SM, Heersche JN. Expression of mRNAs for type-I collagen, bone sialoprotein, osteocalcin, and osteopontin at different stages of osteoblastic differentiation and their regulation by 1,25 dihydroxyvitamin D3. Cell Tissue Res. 1999;297(2):249–59.
97. Drissi H, Pouliot A, Koolloos C, Stein JL, Lian JB, Stein GS, et al. 1,25-(OH)2-vitamin D3 suppresses the bone-related Runx2/Cbfa1 gene promoter. Exp Cell Res. 2002;274(2): 323–33.
98. Aihara K, Azuma H, Akaike M, Ikeda Y, Yamashita M, Sudo T, et al. Disruption of nuclear vitamin D receptor gene causes enhanced thrombogenicity in mice. J Biol Chem. 2004;279(34):35798–802.
99. Wu-Wong JR, Nakane M, Traylor L, Ruan X, Kroeger PE, Tian J. Cardiovascular disease in chronic kidney failure: is there a role for vitamin D analogs? Curr Opin Investig Drugs. 2005;6(3):245–54.
100. Husain K, Suarez E, Isidro A, Hernandez W, Ferder L. Effect of paricalcitol and enalapril on renal inflammation/oxidative stress in atherosclerosis. World J Biol Chem. 2015;6(3):240–8.
101. Moe SM, Zekonis M, Harezlak J, Ambrosius WT, Gassensmith CM, Murphy CL, et al. A placebo-controlled trial to evaluate immunomodulatory effects of paricalcitol. Am J Kidney Dis. 2001;38(4):792–802.
102. Sochorova K, Budinsky V, Rozkova D, Tobiasova Z, Dusilova-Sulkova S, Spisek R, et al. Paricalcitol (19-nor-1,25-dihydroxyvitamin D2) and calcitriol (1,25-dihydroxyvitamin D3) exert potent immunomodulatory effects on dendritic cells and inhibit induction of antigen-specific T cells. Clin Immunol. 2009;133(1):69–77.
103. Izquierdo MJ, Cavia M, Muniz P, de Francisco ALM, Arias M, Santos J, et al. Paricalcitol reduces oxidative stress and inflammation in hemodialysis patients. BMC Nephrol. 2012;13:159.
104. Navarro-Gonzalez JF, Donate-Correa J, Mendez ML, de Fuentes MM, Garcia-Perez J, Mora-Fernandez C. Anti-inflammatory profile of paricalcitol in hemodialysis patients: a prospective, open-label, pilot study. J Clin Pharmacol. 2013;53(4):421–6.

105. Donate-Correa J, Dominguez-Pimentel V, Mendez-Perez ML, Muros-de-Fuentes M, Mora-Fernandez C, Martin-Nunez E, et al. Selective vitamin D receptor activation as anti-inflammatory target in chronic kidney disease. Mediators Inflamm. 2014;2014:670475.
106. Guerrero F, Montes de Oca A, Aguilera-Tejero E, Zafra R, Rodriguez M, Lopez I. The effect of vitamin D derivatives on vascular calcification associated with inflammation. Nephrol Dial Transplant. 2012;27(6):2206–12.

Chapter 19
Vitamin D and Heart Structure and Function in Chronic Kidney Disease

Stefan Pilz, Vincent Brandenburg, and Pablo A. Ureña Torres

Abstract The relationship between vitamin D and heart structure and function is of crucial importance in chronic kidney disease (CKD) because cardiovascular events including sudden cardiac death are, beside cancer, the major cause of premature mortality in these patients. The vitamin D receptor (VDR) is expressed in the heart and the vessels, and experimental studies have documented various molecular effects of vitamin D that may protect against heart diseases. Epidemiological studies in CKD patients identified vitamin D deficiency as a risk marker for adverse cardiovascular outcomes. Randomized controlled trials (RCT) have shown that vitamin D treatment exerts beneficial effects on some cardiovascular risk factors such as parathyroid hormone and proteinuria, but there was no effect on myocardial hypertrophy. Whether vitamin D treatment can significantly reduce cardiovascular events in CKD patients is still unclear because available data are based on very few and relatively small RCTs. It should, however, be noted that some RCTs including one meta-analysis suggest that patients on active vitamin D treatment experience fewer cardiovascular events. Regarding clinical use of vitamin D in CKD patients, it must therefore be stressed that although patients on active vitamin D treatment are at increased risk of hypercalcemia, there is no clear indication that this potential adverse effect translates into higher cardiovascular risk. These safety considerations

S. Pilz, MD, PhD (✉)
Department of Endocrinology and Metabolism, Medical University of Graz,
Graz, Styria, Austria
e-mail: stefan.pilz@chello.at

V. Brandenburg, MD
Department of Cardiology and Center for Rare Diseases (ZSEA), RWTH University Hospital,
Aachen, Germany
e-mail: Vincent.Brandenburg@post.rwth-aachen.de

P.A. Ureña Torres, MD, PhD
Ramsay-Générale de Santé, Service de Néphrologie et Dialyse, Clinique du Landy,
Saint Ouen, France

Department of Renal Physiology, Necker Hospital, University of Paris V, René Descartes,
Paris, France
e-mail: urena.pablo@wanadoo.fr

© Springer International Publishing Switzerland 2016   321
P.A. Ureña Torres et al. (eds.), *Vitamin D in Chronic Kidney Disease*,
DOI 10.1007/978-3-319-32507-1_19

are of great importance when considering the clinical use of active vitamin D treatment, but further large RCTs are urgently needed to better characterize the cardiovascular effects of vitamin D treatment in CKD.

Keywords Vitamin D • Calcitriol • Paricalcitol • Heart • Myocardium • Cardiovascular • Mortality • RCT • Meta-analysis • 25(OH)D

19.1   Introduction

Cardiovascular events including sudden cardiac death are, beside cancer, the major causes of mortality in chronic kidney disease (CKD) patients [1–3]. There exists a complex interplay between cardiovascular diseases and CKD–mineral and bone disorders (CKD–MBD) which are of great importance for monitoring, treatment, and outcome of CKD patients [4]. In this context, it is classically known that vitamin D effects are crucial for the regulation of calcium and phosphate homeostasis, but accumulating evidence from experimental studies indicates that vitamin D may also participate in the pathogenesis of cardiovascular diseases. In line with this, vitamin D deficiency has also been identified as a risk marker for an adverse cardiovascular risk profile and for increased cardiovascular events and mortality [5, 6]. In this book chapter, we will give an overview on the existing knowledge on vitamin D and cardiovascular disease in CKD with a particular focus on heart structure and function. In addition, we will also briefly summarize data on the relationship between vitamin D and vessel diseases as well as cardiovascular risk factors because heart diseases are frequently the final consequence of these pathologies. Our work is based on a Pubmed literature search until October 2015 using the search terms "vitamin D AND kidney AND cardiovascular" and "vitamin D AND kidney AND heart". We also checked the reference lists from the identified articles for further relevant literature. We aimed to restrict our work to data in the setting of CKD because general data on vitamin D and cardiovascular diseases have already been well reviewed elsewhere, and vitamin D metabolism in CKD differs significantly from individuals with normal kidney function [7–13]. We refer to the existing literature and to other chapters of this book with regard to basic vitamin D knowledge in CKD patients.

19.2   Experimental Studies

19.2.1   VDR Activation and Heart Structure and Function

Expression of the vitamin D receptor (VDR) as well as of 1α-hydroxylase has been identified in the heart and the vessels, i.e. in cardiomyocytes, endothelial cells and vascular smooth muscle cells (VSMC) [14–17]. Main mechanisms for direct

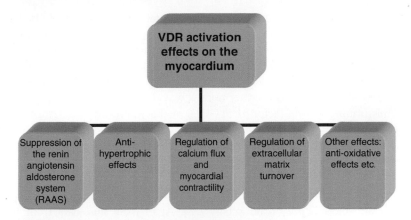

Fig. 19.1 Main mechanisms for direct vitamin D effects on the myocardium

vitamin D effects on the myocardium are shown in Fig. 19.1. Knock-out mice for either VDR or 1α-hydroxylase are hypertensive with cardiac hypertrophy that is at least partially induced by overexpression of renin with increased activity of the renin angiotensin aldosterone system (RAAS). Even mice with a cardiomyocyte-specific VDR-knockout yield myocardial hypertrophy [18]. It is well documented in experimental studies that VDR activation suppresses cardiomyocyte hypertrophy, and reduces cell proliferation and atrial natriuretic peptide (ANP) gene expression [19–21]. Consistent with this, it has also been shown that rats on a low vitamin D diet develop myocardial hypertrophy and that treatment with VDR agonists exerts antihypertrophic effects [15, 22]. Interestingly, it has also been reported that calcitriol increases the expression and the activity of the type a natriuretic peptide receptor and may thus exert beneficial effects on cardiovascular health by e.g. increasing the excretion of sodium [23, 24].

VDR activation modulates myocardial contractility probably by regulating calcium flux in the myocardium [5, 25]. Regarding the vitamin D effects on myocardial function, it has been observed that 1α-hydroxylase knockout mice suffer from reduced systolic function that can be restored by calcitriol treatment [26]. Interestingly, VDR knockout mice showed accelerated rates of myocardial contraction and relaxation [27]. The effects of VDR activation on myocardial contractility are thus still puzzling but considering that calcitriol was also able to induce accelerated relaxation of cardiomyocytes, it is conceivable that VDR activation may be important for diastolic function [27]. This is supported by data in 5/6 nephrectomized rats showing that the VDR agonist VS-105 improves, beside ejection fraction and fractional shortening, also the E/A ratio, a routine echocardiographic parameter that is used to classify diastolic function [28].

VDR activation has also been shown to regulate myocardial extracellular matrix (ECM) turnover by effects on the expression of matrix metalloproteinases (MMPs) and tissue inhibitors of metalloproteinases (TIMPs) [29]. Whether vitamin D induced regulation of ECM turnover may protect against myocardial fibrosis is, however, still not entirely clear because experimental studies were not fully consistent. While studies in nephrectomized and uremic rats reported on antifibrotic effects of calcitriol and paricalcitol, the opposite, i.e. aggravated fibrosis, has been observed in rats with renal insufficiency that were treated with paricalcitol [30–32]. In murine models of cardiac steatosis, an increase in interstitial fibrosis is, however, observed in VDR knockout mice [33]. Furthermore, it was demonstrated that calcitriol prevents transforming growth factor β1 (TGFβ1) mediated pro-fibrotic changes in primary cardiac fibroblasts [34]. In diabetic rats, calcitriol reduced fibrosis and exerted beneficial effects on cardiac function [35, 36]. Survival rate and cardiac function after experimental myocardial infarction were also reduced in VDR knockout compared to wild-type mice [37]. Moreover, VDR activation protected against myocardial reperfusion injury in mice by reducing oxidative stress, and by inhibition of apoptosis and modulation of autophagy [38]. Apart from this, data from stress-exposed mice suggest that vitamin D signaling may protect against stress-induced deteriorating effects on the heart [39]. We can therefore conclude from these experimental data that VDR signaling is indeed important for the maintenance of a physiologic heart structure and function, but we must be aware that cell culture and animal studies may not adequately reflect the pathophysiology in CKD patients.

19.3   VDR Activation and Vessels

Excess as well as deficiency of vitamin D can lead to vascular calcification. Historically, it is well known for almost a century that vitamin D intoxication induces hypercalcemia with vascular calcification [7, 40]. High dose calcitriol treatment in subtotally nephrectomized rats leads to an increased aortic calcium and phosphate content and induces an osteoblastic phenotype in VSMC with an up-regulation of proteins regulating mineralization and calcium transport, and of osteogenic transcription factors [7, 41]. VDR activation induced vascular calcification may be induced by rather a systemic than a local effect because calcitriol induced aortic calcification in uremic rats did not differ between VDR knockout and VDR wild-type aortic allografts [42]. It is also important to note that calcitriol induced vascular calcification in rats is reversible after withdrawal of calcitriol [43, 44]. High serum phosphate levels seem to be critical for calcitriol induced vascular calcification because lowering phosphate levels can prevent vascular calcification in klotho knock-out mice, which are characterized by both high calcium and high calcitriol levels [43, 44]. In contrast to calcitriol induced vascular calcification it has also been reported that mice treated with a low vitamin D diet had more aortic calcification and higher expressions of osteogenic key factors than mice fed with recommended amounts of vitamin D [45, 46]. In a mouse model of CKD, calcitriol and paricalcitol protected against aortic calcification at dosages sufficient to correct secondary hyperparathyroidism, whereas higher dosages induced aortic calcification [47]. A molecular effect of VDR activation that may protect against vascular calcification is an increased expression of the anticalcification factor osteopontin as shown in aortic medial cells [48]. The osteogenic process of VSMC mineralisation induced by phosphate and tumor necrosis factor-α (TNF- α) could also be abrogated by VDR agonists [49].

Several experimental studies have, by the majority, shown that vitamin D may protect against endothelial dysfunction and atherosclerosis. VDR agonists improved endothelial function in 5/6 nephrectomized rats and in diabetic rats with early-stage nephropathy [50–52]. Mechanistically, it has been demonstrated that VDR signaling increases NO synthesis and reduces expression of cyclooxygenase-2 (COX-2) and thromboxane-prostanoid receptors [53, 54]. Expression of endothelial adhesion molecules, e.g. ICAM-1 (intercellular adhesion molecule 1) and VCAM-1 (vascular cell adhesion molecule 1), is suppressed by VDR activation, and knock-down of the VDR in endothelial cells was associated with endothelial activation characterized by increased leukocyte-endothelial cell interactions [55]. VSMC are also target cells for vitamin D and it has been reported that VDR knockout mice have an increased production of angiotensin-II and superoxide anions leading to premature senescence of VSMC [56]. VDR agonists may also suppress VSMC proliferation, but this has not been consistently reported in all studies [57, 58]. Moreover, calcitriol has been shown to inhibit foam cell formation and cholesterol uptake in macrophages of patients with type 2 diabetes mellitus [59]. Another anti-atherosclerotic effect of VDR activation is mediated by regulation of cholesterol efflux and macrophage polarization as shown in hypercholesterolemic swine [60]. Experimental data also indicate that VDR activation may promote vascular repair [61]

19.4 VDR Activation and Cardiovascular Risk Factors

Numerous experimental studies have shown that vitamin D may protect against a variety of classic and emerging risk factors. In this context, it must be stressed that the suppression of parathyroid hormone (PTH) is an important cardiovascular-protective effect of VDR activation when considering that PTH itself exerts several harmful effects on the heart and the vessels [62, 63]. Suppression of renin expression and the RAAS by vitamin D has been shown to prevent hypertension, atherosclerosis and heart diseases in experimental studies [14, 64–66]. Several other effects of VDR activation on cardiovascular risk factors such as inflammation, diabetes mellitus, arterial hypertension, blood lipids, coagulation, and renal diseases have been extensively reviewed elsewhere [7–11, 67].

19.5 Observational Studies

19.5.1 25-Hydroxyvitamin D and Cardiovascular Disease

Most, albeit not all, epidemiological studies in CKD patients showed that low levels of 25-hydroxyvitamin D (25[OH]D) are associated with an increased risk of cardiovascular disease and mortality including sudden cardiac death [68–80]. In small clinical studies, low serum 25(OH)D concentrations were partially associated with myocardial hypertrophy in CKD patients [81, 82]. Low serum 25(OH)D concentrations were associated with vascular calcification in some but not all studies in CKD patients [83–86]. Several studied in CKD patients showed, however, a significant association between vitamin D deficiency and endothelial dysfunction as well as clinical measures of atherosclerosis [85, 87–89]. It has been largely, but not consistently, observed that low serum 25(OH)D concentrations are associated with albuminuria, and decline of glomerular filtration rate (GFR) including progression to end-stage renal disease [77, 90–95].

19.6   Calcitriol and Cardiovascular Disease

Epidemiological studies in CKD patients have largely shown that low serum concentrations of calcitriol are associated with an increased risk of mortality and cardiovascular events [61, 66, 70, 88]. In CKD patients with and without dialysis, serum calcitriol levels were either inversely or not associated with vascular calcification and atherosclerosis [76, 78, 89, 90]. Moreover, in patients with advanced kidney disease, low serum calcitriol levels were predictive for initiation of long-term dialysis treatment [78].

19.7   Vitamin D Genetics and Cardiovascular Disease

In 182 dialysis patients there was a significant association between the Bsml VDR polymorphism and left ventricular mass index [99]. Similar associations have been confirmed in non-dialysis patients [100]. There was, however, no significant association between VDR polymorphisms and end-stage renal disease in a meta-analysis including 1510 patients and 1812 controls [101].

19.8   Vitamin D Treatment and Cardiovascular Diseases

19.8.1   Natural Vitamin D Treatment: Observational and Uncontrolled Studies

Some observational studies report on use of natural vitamin D supplements and cardiovascular diseases in CKD [102–113]. It has been observed that ergocalciferol treatment was associated with reduced cardiovascular events in 126 older men with CKD stages 3 and 4 [104]. An observational study in hemodialysis patients reported on significant improvement in left ventricular function (i.e. decreased end-diastolic and end-systolic diameters) in five patients treated with 100 µg 25(OH)D for 8 months when compared to five patients without vitamin D supplementation [105]. A 1-year prospective study in hemodialysis patients showed that oral cholecalciferol supplementation was associated with significantly reduced brain natriuretic peptide (BNP) levels and left ventricular mass index [106]. Another observational study in 30 hemodialysis patients confirmed that oral cholecalciferol supplementation over 6 months was associated with significantly decreased left ventricular mass index, and similar results were also obtained in a further observational study in dialysis patients [107, 108]. Moreover, it has been observed in 15 patients with IgA nephropathy, that parameters of cardiac autonomic tone were significantly improved when comparing values at baseline and 28 days after daily vitamin D supplementation with 10,000 International Units (IU) [109]. In 26 patients with CKD stage 3 and 4 it was reported that after cholecalciferol supplementation of 300,000 IU at baseline and after 8 weeks there was a significant decrease in E-Selectin, ICAM-1, and VCAM-1 at week 16 [110]. A study in 213 hemodialysis patients reported that ergocalciferol treatment is associated with significantly reduced frequency of vascular access dysfunction [111]. Natural vitamin D supplementation was also associated with reductions in inflammatory parameters in several, but not all, observational studies [106–108, 110, 112, 113].

19.8.2   Natural Vitamin D Treatment: Randomized Controlled Trials

Some randomized controlled trials (RCTs) have already been performed to study cardiovascular effects of natural vitamin D supplementation in CKD patients. A RCT in 84 dialysis patients receiving either 50,000 IU vitamin D per week for 8–12 weeks or placebo failed to show a significant effect on circulating pro-B-type natriuretic peptide (pro-BNP) concentration [114]. In 38 vitamin D deficient patients with CKD stage 3 and 4 who were randomized to either 50,000 IU vitamin D weekly for the first month and then monthly or placebo for an overall study period of 6 months, there were significant improvements in endothelium dependent microcirculatory vasodilatation and pulse pressure, and a reduction in tissue advanced glycation end products in the vitamin D compared to the placebo group [115]. Another RCT was performed in 60 hemodialysis patients who were randomly allocated to 50,000 IU vitamin D or placebo, once weekly for 8 weeks and then monthly for 4 months [116]. There was, however, no significant effect on pulse wave velocity (PWV) in that study [116]. There was also no significant vitamin D effect on left ventricular systolic function, left ventricular diastolic function, BNP, PWV, central blood pressure, 24-h blood pressure, and augmentation index in a RCT in 50 dialysis patients randomized to 3000 IU cholecalciferol daily or placebo for 6 months [117]. A further RCT was performed in 105 hemodialysis patients who received either ergocalciferol 50,000 IU weekly, 50,000 IU monthly or placebo for 1 year

[118]. There were, apart from an increase in 25(OH)D, no significant effects on parameters of mineral metabolism or hospitalizations, but there was a non-significant trend towards reduced mortality in patients allocated to ergocalciferol with a hazard ratio (95 % confidence interval) of 0.28 (0.07–1.19). Moreover, there was no effect on arterio-vein access maturation in a cholecalciferol RCT in 52 hemodialysis patients [119]. In 96 hemodialysis patients awaiting transplantation it was evaluated in a RCT whether 50,000 IU cholecalciferol weekly for 1 year prevents alloreactive T-cell memory formation, but there were was no significant effect [120]. Another RCT in 38 hemodialysis patients did also not report on any vitamin D effect on cytokines (CRP and TNF-α), Th1 and Th2 lymphocyte frequencies and monocyte subset cell counts [121]. Regarding effects of vitamin D on vascular calcification in RCTs in CKD patients, it can be summarized that there were no relevant adverse effects but also no significant benefits, and the overall conclusion is that natural vitamin D supplementation is relatively safe in these patients [122, 123]. While it is logical that vitamin D supplementation is effective in increasing serum 25(OH)D levels across all stages of CKD, it has also been shown that PTH can also be suppressed by natural vitamin D treatment, albeit this has not been consistently confirmed in all RCTs [122–128]. Vitamin D RCT data in CKD patients on other cardiovascular risk factors such as e.g. glucose metabolism or blood pressure are sparse and did largely show no consistent and significant effect [102, 103]. Most studies performed in study cohorts without CKD did also fail to prove a significant blood pressure reduction by natural vitamin D supplementation [129, 130].

19.9   Active Vitamin D Treatment: Observational and Uncontrolled Studies

Since there are several RCTs published on active vitamin D treatment and cardiovascular diseases and its risk factors we just briefly mention some of the epidemiological studies on this topic. In this context, several observational studies have, by the majority, reported that the use of active vitamin D and its analogues is associated with significantly reduced risk of cardiovascular events and mortality [68, 96, 98, 131–150]. Some, albeit not all, observational or uncontrolled studies in CKD patients revealed that active vitamin D treatment is associated with improved left ventricular function, regression of myocardial hypertrophy, and reduction of QTc interval and dispersion [141–148]. Data on active vitamin D treatment and vascular calcification are sparse, but one study in 36 dialysis patients comparing low-dose versus high-dose calcitriol treatment for 1 year did not find any significant difference in vascular calcification [149]. Other studies, however, showed that prescription of active vitamin D treatment is associated with increased vascular calcification and vascular stiffness [150–152]. In contrast, active vitamin D treatment was associated with beneficial effects on parameters related to calcification and may thereby possibly protect against vascular damage [153–155]. Regarding observational studies on cardiovascular risk factors, it should be noted that active vitamin D treatment is, beyond its suppressive effects on PTH, associated with reduced pro-teinuria and anti-inflammatory effects in some, but not all, investigations [156–158]. It is also important to note that active vitamin D treatment causes an increase in creatinine generation without affecting glomerular filtration rate (GFR) [159].

19.9.1 Active Vitamin D Treatment: Randomized Controlled Trials

Two meta-analyses of RCTs have already addressed the research question on whether active vitamin D treatment has an effect on cardiovascular outcomes [160, 161]. Li et al. investigated the question whether active vitamin D analogues in predialysis CKD patients have an effect on cardiovascular events [161]. Five RCTs in 715 patients who experienced 35 cardiovascular events during a follow-up time of 16 weeks to 52 weeks were included into the meta-analysis [161]. As the main outcome, active vitamin D treatment was associated with a significantly reduced relative risk (RR) of 0.27 (95 % confidence interval [CI]: 0.13–0.59; p = 0.001) for cardiovascular events. In the same meta-analysis, active vitamin D treatment was also associated with reduced proteinuria, but there was no effect on left ventricular mass index, left ventricular systolic function, and systolic and dia-stolic blood pressure. There was, however, a significantly increased risk of hyper-calcemia (i.e. serum calcium concentrations above 11.0 mg/dL [2.75 mmol/L]) associated with paricalcitol treatment with a RR (95 % CI) of 7.85 (2.92–21.1; p < 0.001). While the main outcome of this meta-analysis, i.e. the significant reduction of cardiovascular events, suggests cardiovascular benefits of active vita-min D analogues, it must be acknowledged that this study is clearly limited by the relatively low number of events [161]. Another meta-analysis of RCTs by Mann et al. addressed the question whether vitamin D treatment (with either active or natural vitamin D) in patients with CKD has an effect on all-cause mortality, car-diovascular mortality, and serious adverse cardiovascular events [160]. For the main outcome all-cause mortality, 13 trials in 1469 patients with 41 fatal events and a follow-up of 3–104 weeks were included, with the vast majority of patients in RCTs on active vitamin D treatment. There was no significant effect of vitamin D treatment on all-cause mortality with a RR (95 % CI) of 0.84 (0.47–1.52). Data on cardiovascular mortality were identified in 6 RCTs in 937 patients with 8 events and a RR (95 % CI) of 0.79 (0.26–2.28). Data on serious adverse cardiovascular events were identified in 8 RCTs in 1217 patients with 15 events and a RR (95 % CI) of 1.20 (0.49–2.99). The meta-analysis by Mann et al. was thus based on fewer cardiovascular events compared to the more recent meta-analysis by Li et al. Regarding the conclusions drawn from these meta-analyses it should be noted that the RCTs included were, in general, not a priori designed to evaluate cardiovascu-lar events and that the low event rate is a clear limitation. It was thus concluded by Mann et al. that "the current state of the literature is unfit to systematically quan-tify any effect of vitamin D therapy on mortality and cardiovascular events" [160].

Specific effects of paricalcitol on myocardial structure and function have been evaluated in the PRIMO (Paricalcitol Capsule Benefits in Renal Failure-induced cardiac Morbidity) trial [162, 163]. In that RCT, 227 patients with CKD (GFR: 15–60 mL/min/1.73 m^2) and preserved left ventricular ejection fraction with mild to moderate left ventricular hypertrophy, were randomly assigned to receive paricalcitol 2 µg daily (n = 115) or placebo (n = 112). The primary end point was change in left ventricular mass index at 48 weeks and secondary end points included measures of left ventricular diastolic and systolic function, cardiac volume indexes, cardiovascular events and cardiac biomarkers. The main outcome of the PRIMO trial was that paricalcitol did not reduce left ventricular mass index. Considering that the CI was narrow and that there was a marked decrease in PTH, suggesting a strong physiologic effect of paricalcitol, the authors concluded that even a larger sample size would have yielded similar results. While there were also no meaningful effects on most secondary outcomes, there was a significantly reduced risk of cardiovascular hospitalizations in the paricalcitol (n = 1) versus the placebo group (n = 8) (p = 0.04). In a post-hoc analysis of the PRIMO trial restricted to 196 patients with available echocardiographic data, it has been shown that left atrial volume index, a measure of diastolic dysfunction severity that indicates a higher cardiovascular risk, was significantly reduced after 48 weeks in the paricalcitol group (−2.97 mL/m^2, 95 % CI: −4.00 to −1.59 mL/m^2) compared to the placebo group (−0.70 mL/m^2; 95 % CI: −1.93 to 0.53 mL/m^2; p = 0.002) [163]. The rise in BNP throughout the PRIMO trial was also significantly attenuated in the paricalcitol (+8.4 pg/mL) versus placebo group (+18.5 pg/mL; p = 0.02). These effects of paricalcitol on left atrial volume index and BNP are remarkable when considering that there was a similar blood pressure control in both groups and that RAAS inhibitor use was 80 %. It should also be noted that the effect of paricalcitol was homogeneous across all subgroups and that the changes in left atrial volume index paralleled the attenuation in BNP. Another RCT, the OPERA trial, on paricalcitol and left ventricular mass index as the primary outcome has been performed in 60 patients with CKD stage 3–5 and left ventricular hypertrophy [164]. Thirty patients were randomized to paricalcitol 1 µg daily and 30 patients to placebo. After 52 weeks, there was no significant difference in left ventricular mass index in the paricalcitol compared to the placebo group. Secondary outcome measures of left ventricular systolic and diastolic function did also not differ between the groups. Therefore, the results of the RCT by Wang et al. confirm the findings from the PRIMO trial by showing no effect of active vitamin D treatment on myocardial hypertrophy in a cohort with more severe CKD and secondary hyperparathyroidism when compared to the PRIMO study cohort. Interestingly, Wang et al. recorded two patients with hosptialization in the paricalcitol, and ten patients who were hospitalized in the placebo group (p = 0.02). Notably, no patient in the paricalcitol group had a cardiovascular-related hospitalization, whereas there were five patients with such an event in the placebo group.

Two further RCTs showed some beneficial effects of paricalcitol treatment on endothelial function [165, 166]. Zoccali et al. evaluated in a RCT in 88 patients with CKD stage 3–4 and a PTH greater than 65 pg/mL, the effect of paricalcitol 2 µg daily for 12 weeks on endothelium-dependent and endothelium-independent vaso-dilatation [166]. After 12 weeks, flow-mediated dilatation was significantly better in the paricalcitol compared to the placebo group, but there was no significant differ-ence for endothelium-independent vasodilatation. A further RCT was conducted in 36 non-diabetic patients with CKD stage 3–4 who were randomly allocated to pari-calcitol 2 µg daily (n=12), paricalcitol 1 µg daily (n=12), or placebo (n=12) for 3 months [165]. Outcome measures were parameters of sympathetic activation, macro- and microvascular functions. While most outcome measures were not affected by treatment, there was a significant decline in endothelial function in all groups, except the 2 µg paricalcitol group.

Several trials evaluated the effects of active vitamin D treatment on proteinuria [167–173]. The meta-analyses in this field found that active vitamin D treatment decreases proteinuria significantly. These findings have been well reviewed else-where [168–173].

Some other studies have also investigated the impact of active vitamin D therapy on glucose metabolism but the results were mixed. Regarding other cardiovascular risk factors it should be noted that there were e.g. no consistent and relevant effects on blood pressure [174].

The beneficial effects of active vitamin D treatment on PTH and some parame-ters of bone and mineral metabolism have also been evaluated in RCTs, and it has been clearly shown that active vitamin D treatment suppresses PTH and some bone markers such as bone alkaline phosphatase [171, 175, 176]. The clinical relevance of the interaction between vitamin D and fibroblast growth factor 23 (FGF23) as well as the significance of FGF23 in the pathogenesis of cardiovascular diseases still need to be further studies [13].

Several studies, on active as well as on natural vitamin D supplementation, are still ongoing in CKD patients and will hopefully help to clarify the role of vitamin D treatment for heart structure and function [176–181].

19.10   Conclusions

While there is compelling evidence from experimental and observational studies indicating that vitamin D may exert beneficial effects on myocardial structure and function, there are only very few and limited data addressing these issues in RCTs in CKD patients. Based on the available evidence it is thus premature to draw firm and definite conclusions on the effects of vitamin D treatment on heart structure and function in CKD. In particular, RCT data on natural vitamin D treatment in CKD are sparse, whereas there are already some RCT data available on active vitamin D treatment. Results derived from the PRIMO study on improvements in left atrial volume index and serum BNP levels by paricalcitol treatment are promising regard-ing potential beneficial effects of active vitamin D treatment on heart structure and function, but these findings need further confirmation in future RCTs. It should, however, be noted that although data on hard cardiovascular endpoints are sparse and limited by low event rates, some RCTs including one meta-analysis of RCTs suggest that patients on active vitamin D treatment experience fewer cardiovascular events. Further large RCTs are therefore needed to address the question whether vitamin D treatment is clinically indicated to prevent and treat cardiovascular diseases in CKD patients. The currently available data suggesting reduced cardiovascular events in CKD patients on active vitamin D treatment (i.e. paricalcitol) are a scientifically sound rationale for further RCTs addressing the impact of active vitamin D treatment on cardiovascular events as a primary outcome. Regarding the current relatively widespread use of vitamin D in CKD patients, it must also be stressed that although patients on active vitamin D treatment are at increased risk of hypercalcemia, there is no clear indication from RCTs that this adverse effect of active vitamin D treatment translates into higher cardiovascular risk since the available literature suggests that cardiovascular events and mortality are rather reduced than increased with active vitamin D treatment. Therefore, while proposed beneficial effects of active vitamin D treatment on heart structure and function still need to be further evaluated, the evidence from RCTs is quite convincing that active vitamin D treatment, at doses commonly used in clinical practice, is not harmful for the heart. These safety considerations are of great importance when considering the use of active vitamin D treatment in CKD patients.

References

1. Navaneethan SD, Schold JD, Arrigain S, Jolly SE, Nally Jr JV. Cause-specific deaths in non-dialysis-dependent CKD. J Am Soc Nephrol. 2015;26:2512–20.
2. Charytan DM, Lewis EF, Desai AS, Weinrauch LA, Ivanovich P, Toto RD, et al. Cause of death in patients with diabetic CKD enrolled in the trial to reduce cardiovascular events with aranesp therapy (TREAT). Am J Kidney Dis. 2015;66:429–40.
3. Di Lullo L, House A, Gorini A, Santoboni A, Russo D, Ronco C. Chronic kidney disease and cardiovascular complications. Heart Fail Rev. 2015;20:259–72.
4. Kidney-Disease: Improving Global Outcomes (KDIGO) CKD–MBD Work Group. KDIGO clinical practice guideline for the diagnosis, evaluation, prevention, and treatment of chronic kidney disease–mineral and bone disorder (CKD–MBD). Kidney Int Suppl. 2009;113: S1–130.
5. Pilz S, Tomaschitz A, Drechsler C, Dekker JM, März W. Vitamin D deficiency and myocardial diseases. Mol Nutr Food Res. 2010;54:1103–13.
6. Pilz S, Tomaschitz A, Drechsler C, de Boer RA. Vitamin D deficiency and heart disease. Kideny Int Suppl. 2011;1:111–5.
7. Zittermann A. Vitamin D, and cardiovascular disease. Anticancer Res. 2014;34:4641–8.
8. Pilz S, Gaksch M, O'Hartaigh B, Tomaschitz A, März W. The role of vitamin D deficiency in cardiovascular disease: where do we stand in 2013? Arch Toxicol. 2013;87:2083–103.
9. Beveridge LA, Witham MD. Vitamin D and the cardiovascular system. Osteoporos Int. 2013;24:2167–80.
10. Ford JA, MacLennan GS, Avenell A, Bolland M, Grey A, Witham M, RECORD Trial Group. Cardiovascular disease and vitamin D supplementation: trial analysis, systematic review, and meta-analysis. Am J Clin Nutr. 2014;100:746–55.
11. Carvalho LS, Sposito AC. Vitamin D for the prevention of cardiovascular disease: are we ready for that? Atherosclerosis. 2015;241:729–40.

12. Negri AL, Brandenburg VM. Calcitriol resistance in hemodialysis patients with secondary hyperparathyroidism. Int Urol Nephrol. 2014;46:1145–51.
13. Negri AL. Fibroblast growth factor 23: associations with cardiovascular disease and mortality in chronic kidney disease. Int Urol Nephrol. 2014;46:9–17.
14. Bouillon R, Carmeliet G, Verlinden L, van Etten E, Verstuyf A, Luderer HF, et al. Vitamin D and human health: lessons from vitamin D receptor null mice. Endocr Rev. 2008;29: 726–76.
15. Gardner DG, Chen S, Glenn DJ. Vitamin D and the heart. Am J Physiol Regul Integr Comp Physiol. 2013;305:R969–77.
16. Schnatz PF, Nudy M, O'Sullivan DM, Jiang X, Cline JM, Kaplan JR, et al. The quantification of vitamin D receptors in coronary arteries and their association with atherosclerosis. Maturitas. 2012;73:143–7.
17. Chen S, Glenn DJ, Ni W, Grigsby CL, Olsen K, Nishimoto M, et al. Expression of the vitamin d receptor is increased in the hypertrophic heart. Hypertension. 2008;52:1106–12.
18. Chen S, Law CS, Grigsby CL, Olsen K, Hong TT, Zhang Y, et al. Cardiomyocyte-specific deletion of the vitamin D receptor gene results in cardiac hypertrophy. Circulation. 2011;124: 1838–47.
19. Nibbelink KA, Tishkoff DX, Hershey SD, Rahman A, Simpson RU. 1,25(OH)2-vitamin D3 actions on cell proliferation, size, gene expression, and receptor localization, in the HL-1 cardiac myocyte. J Steroid Biochem Mol Biol. 2007;103:533–7.
20. Wu J, Garami M, Cheng T, Gardner DG. 1,25(OH)2 vitamin D3, and retinoic acid antagonize endothelin-stimulated hypertrophy of neonatal rat cardiac myocytes. J Clin Invest. 1996;97: 1577–88.
21. Panizo S, Barrio-Vázquez S, Naves-Díaz M, Carrillo-López N, Rodríguez I, Fernández-Vázquez A, et al. Vitamin D receptor activation, left ventricular hypertrophy and myocardial fibrosis. Nephrol Dial Transplant. 2013;28:2735–44.
22. Weishaar RE, Kim SN, Saunders DE, Simpson RU. Involvement of vitamin D3 with cardiovascular function. III. Effects on physical and morphological properties. Am J Physiol. 1990;258:E134–42.
23. Chen S, Ni XP, Humphreys MH, Gardner DG. 1,25 dihydroxyvitamin d amplifies type a natriuretic peptide receptor expression and activity in target cells. J Am Soc Nephrol. 2005;16:329–39.
24. Chen S, Olsen K, Grigsby C, Gardner DG. Vitamin D activates type A natriuretic peptide receptor gene transcription in inner medullary collecting duct cells. Kidney Int. 2007;72: 300–6.
25. Choudhury S, Bae S, Ke Q, Lee JY, Singh SS, St-Arnaud R, et al. Abnormal calcium handling and exaggerated cardiac dysfunction in mice with defective vitamin d signaling. PLoS One. 2014;9:e108382.
26. Zhou C, Lu F, Cao K, Xu D, Goltzman D, Miao D. Calcium-independent and 1,25(OH)2D3-dependent regulation of the renin-angiotensin system in 1alpha-hydroxylase knockout mice. Kidney Int. 2008;74:170–9.
27. Tishkoff DX, Nibbelink KA, Holmberg KH, Dandu L, Simpson RU. Functional vitamin D receptor (VDR) in the t-tubules of cardiac myocytes: VDR knockout cardiomyocyte contractility. Endocrinology. 2008;149:558–64.
28. Wu-Wong JR, Chen YW, Wessale JL. Vitamin D receptor agonist VS-105 improves cardiac function in the presence of enalapril in 5/6 nephrectomized rats. Am J Physiol Renal Physiol. 2015;308:F309–19.
29. Weber KT, Weglicki WB, Simpson RU. Macro- and micronutrient dyshomeostasis in the adverse structural remodelling of myocardium. Cardiovasc Res. 2009;81:500–8.
30. Koleganova N, Piecha G, Ritz E, Gross ML. Calcitriol ameliorates capillary deficit and fibrosis of the heart in subtotally nephrectomized rats. Nephrol Dial Transplant. 2009;24: 778–87.
31. Mizobuchi M, Nakamura H, Tokumoto M, Finch J, Morrissey J, Liapis H, et al. Myocardial effects of VDR activators in renal failure. J Steroid Biochem Mol Biol. 2010;121:188–92.

32. Repo JM, Rantala IS, Honkanen TT, Mustonen JT, Kööbi P, Tahvanainen AM, et al. Paricalcitol aggravates perivascular fibrosis in rats with renal insufficiency and low calcitriol. Kidney Int. 2007;72:977–84.
33. Glenn DJ, Cardema MC, Gardner DG. Amplification of lipotoxic cardiomyopathy in the VDR gene knockout mouse. J Steroid Biochem Mol Biol. 2015. doi:10.1016/j. jsbmb.2015.09.034. pii: S0960-0760(15)30092-3.
34. Meredith A, Boroomand S, Carthy J, Luo Z, McManus B. 1,25 dihydroxyvitamin D3 inhibits TGFβ1-mediated primary human cardiac myofibroblast activation. PLoS One. 2015;10(6): e0128655.
35. Lee TW, Kao YH, Lee TI, Chang CJ, Lien GS, Chen YJ. Calcitriol modulates receptor for advanced glycation end products (RAGE) in diabetic hearts. Int J Cardiol. 2014;173: 236–41.
36. Lee TI, Kao YH, Chen YC, Tsai WC, Chung CC, Chen YJ. Cardiac metabolism, inflammation, and peroxisome proliferator-activated receptors modulated by 1,25-dihydroxyvitamin D3 in diabetic rats. Int J Cardiol. 2014;176:151–7.
37. Bae S, Singh SS, Yu H, Lee JY, Cho BR, Kang PM. Vitamin D signaling pathway plays an important role in the development of heart failure after myocardial infarction. J Appl Physiol (1985). 2013;114:979–87.
38. Yao T, Ying X, Zhao Y, Yuan A, He Q, Tong H, et al. Vitamin D receptor activation protects against myocardial reperfusion injury through inhibition of apoptosis and modulation of autophagy. Antioxid Redox Signal. 2015;22:633–50.
39. Jiang P, Zhang WY, Li HD, Cai HL, Liu YP, Chen LY. Stress and vitamin D: altered vitamin D metabolism in both the hippocampus and myocardium of chronic unpredictable mild stress exposed rats. Psychoneuroendocrinology. 2013;38:2091–8.
40. Mallick NP, Berlyne GM. Arterial calcification after vitamin-D therapy in hyperphosphatemic renal failure. Lancet. 1968;2:1316–20.
41. Zebger-Gong H, Müller D, Diercke M, Haffner D, Hocher B, Verberckmoes S, et al. 1,25-Dihydroxyvitamin D3-induced aortic calcifications in experimental uremia: upregulation of osteoblast markers, calcium-transporting proteins and osterix. J Hypertens. 2011;29:339–48.
42. Lomashvili KA, Wang X, O'Neill WC. Role of local versus systemic vitamin D receptors in vascular calcification. Arterioscler Thromb Vasc Biol. 2014;34:146–51.
43. Bas A, Lopez I, Perez J, Rodriguez M, Aguilera-Tejero E. Reversibility of calcitriol-induced medial artery calcification in rats with intact renal function. J Bone Miner Res. 2006;21: 484–90.
44. Razzaque MS. The dualistic role of vitamin D in vascular calcifications. Kidney Int. 2011;79: 708–14.
45. Schmidt N, Brandsch C, Kühne H, Thiele A, Hirche F, Stangl GI. Vitamin D receptor deficiency and low vitamin D diet stimulate aortic calcification and osteogenic key factor expression in mice. PLoS One. 2012;7:e35316.
46. Schmidt N, Brandsch C, Schutkowski A, Hirche F, Stangl GI. Dietary vitamin D inadequacy accelerates calcification and osteoblast-like cell formation in the vascular system of LDL receptor knockout and wild-type mice. J Nutr. 2014;144:638–46.
47. Mathew S, Lund RJ, Chaudhary LR, Geurs T, Hruska KA. Vitamin D receptor activators can protect against vascular calcification. J Am Soc Nephrol. 2008;19:1509–19.
48. Lau WL, Leaf EM, Hu MC, Takeno MM, Kuro-o M, Moe OW, et al. Vitamin D receptor agonists increase klotho and osteopontin while decreasing aortic calcification in mice with chronic kidney disease fed a high phosphate diet. Kidney Int. 2012;82:1261–70.
49. Aoshima Y, Mizobuchi M, Ogata H, Kumata C, Nakazawa A, Kondo F, et al. Vitamin D receptor activators inhibit vascular smooth muscle cell mineralization induced by phosphate and TNF-α. Nephrol Dial Transplant. 2012;27:1800–6.
50. Hirata M, Serizawa K, Aizawa K, Yogo K, Tashiro Y, Takeda S, et al. 22-Oxacalcitriol prevents progression of endothelial dysfunction through antioxidative effects in rats with type 2 diabetes and early-stage nephropathy. Nephrol Dial Transplant. 2013;28:1166–74.

51. Wu-Wong JR, Li X, Chen YW. Different vitamin D receptor agonists exhibit differential effects on endothelial function and aortic gene expression in 5/6 nephrectomized rats. J Steroid Biochem Mol Biol. 2015;148:202–9.
52. Wu-Wong JR, Noonan W, Nakane M, Brooks KA, Segreti JA, Polakowski JS, et al. Vitamin d receptor activation mitigates the impact of uremia on endothelial function in the 5/6 nephrectomized rats. Int J Endocrinol. 2010;2010:625852.
53. Dong J, Wong SL, Lau CW, Liu J, Wang YX, Dan He Z, et al. Calcitriol restores renovascular function in estrogen-deficient rats through downregulation of cyclooxygenase-2 and the thromboxane-prostanoid receptor. Kidney Int. 2013;84:54–63.
54. Andrukhova O, Slavic S, Zeitz U, Riesen SC, Heppelmann MS, Ambrisko TD, et al. Vitamin D is a regulator of endothelial nitric oxide synthase and arterial stiffness in mice. Mol Endocrinol. 2014;28:53–64.
55. Bozic M, Álvarez Á, de Pablo C, Sanchez-Niño MD, Ortiz A, Dolcet X, et al. Impaired vitamin D signaling in endothelial cell leads to an enhanced leukocyte-endothelium interplay: implications for atherosclerosis development. PLoS One. 2015;10:e0136863.
56. Valcheva P, Cardus A, Panizo S, Parisi E, Bozic M, Lopez Novoa JM, et al. Lack of vitamin D receptor causes stress-induced premature senescence in vascular smooth muscle cells through enhanced local angiotensin-II signals. Atherosclerosis. 2014;235:247–55.
57. Chen S, Law CS, Gardner DG. Vitamin D-dependent suppression of endothelin-induced vascular smooth muscle cell proliferation through inhibition of CDK2 activity. J Steroid Biochem Mol Biol. 2010;118:135–41.
58. Cardús A, Parisi E, Gallego C, Aldea M, Fernández E, Valdivielso JM. 1,25-Dihydroxyvitamin D3 stimulates vascular smooth muscle cell proliferation through a VEGF-mediated pathway. Kidney Int. 2006;69:1377–84.
59. Oh J, Weng S, Felton SK, Bhandare S, Riek A, Butler B, et al. 1,25(OH)2 vitamin d inhibits foam cell formation and suppresses macrophage cholesterol uptake in patients with type 2 diabetes mellitus. Circulation. 2009;120:687–98.
60. Yin K, You Y, Swier V, Tang L, Radwan MM, Pandya AN, et al. Vitamin D protects against atherosclerosis via regulation of cholesterol efflux and macrophage polarization in hypercholesterolemic swine. Arterioscler Thromb Vasc Biol. 2015. pii: ATVBAHA.115.306132.
61. Wong MS, Leisegang MS, Kruse C, Vogel J, Schürmann C, Dehne N, et al. Vitamin D promotes vascular regeneration. Circulation. 2014;130:976–86.
62. Fitzpatrick LA, Bilezikian JP, Silverberg SJ. Parathyroid hormone and the cardiovascular system. Curr Osteoporos Rep. 2008;6:77–83.
63. Tomaschitz A, Ritz E, Pieske B, Rus-Machan J, Kienreich K, Verheyen N, et al. Aldosterone and parathyroid hormone interactions as mediators of metabolic and cardiovascular disease. Metabolism. 2014;63:20–31.
64. Li YC. Vitamin D: roles in renal and cardiovascular protection. Curr Opin Nephrol Hypertens. 2012;21:72–9.
65. Szeto FL, Reardon CA, Yoon D, Wang Y, Wong KE, Chen Y, et al. Vitamin D receptor signaling inhibits atherosclerosis in mice. Mol Endocrinol. 2012;26:1091–101.
66. Vaidya A, Williams JS. The relationship between vitamin D and the renin-angiotensin system in the pathophysiology of hypertension, kidney disease, and diabetes. Metabolism. 2012;61:450–8.
67. Pilz S, Kienreich K, Rutters F, de Jongh R, van Ballegooijen AJ, Grübler M, et al. Role of vitamin D in the development of insulin resistance and type 2 diabetes. Curr Diab Rep. 2013;13:261–70.
68. Wolf M, Shah A, Gutierrez O, Ankers E, Monroy M, Tamez H, et al. Vitamin D levels and early mortality among incident hemodialysis patients. Kidney Int. 2007;72:1004–13.
69. Wang AY, Lam CW, Sanderson JE, Wang M, Chan IH, Lui SF, et al. Serum 25-hydroxyvitamin D status and cardiovascular outcomes in chronic peritoneal dialysis patients: a 3-y prospective cohort study. Am J Clin Nutr. 2008;87:1631–8.
70. Chonchol M, Cigolini M, Targher G. Association between 25-hydroxyvitamin D deficiency and cardiovascular disease in type 2 diabetic patients with mild kidney dysfunction. Nephrol Dial Transplant. 2008;23:269–74.

71. Drechsler C, Verduijn M, Pilz S, Dekker FW, Krediet RT, Ritz E, et al. Vitamin D status and clinical outcomes in incident dialysis patients: results from the NECOSAD study. Nephrol Dial Transplant. 2011;26:1024–32.

72. Drechsler C, Pilz S, Obermayer-Pietsch B, Verduijn M, Tomaschitz A, Krane V, et al. Vitamin D deficiency is associated with sudden cardiac death, combined cardiovascular events, and mortality in haemodialysis patients. Eur Heart J. 2010;31:2253–61.

73. Pilz S, Tomaschitz A, Friedl C, Amrein K, Drechsler C, Ritz E, et al. Vitamin D status and mortality in chronic kidney disease. Nephrol Dial Transplant. 2011;26:3603–9.

74. Kramer H, Sempos C, Cao G, Luke A, Shoham D, Cooper R, et al. Mortality rates across 25-hydroxyvitamin D (25[OH]D) levels among adults with and without estimated glomerular filtration rate <60 ml/min/1.73 m2: the third national health and nutrition examination survey. PLoS One. 2012;7:e47458.

75. Ravani P, Malberti F, Tripepi G, Pecchini P, Cutrupi S, Pizzini P, et al. Vitamin D levels and patient outcome in chronic kidney disease. Kidney Int. 2009;75:88–95.

76. Barreto DV, Barreto FC, Liabeuf S, Temmar M, Boitte F, Choukroun G, et al. Vitamin D affects survival independently of vascular calcification in chronic kidney disease. Clin J Am Soc Nephrol. 2009;4:1128–35.

77. Kendrick J, Cheung AK, Kaufman JS, Greene T, Roberts WL, Smits G, et al. Associations of plasma 25-hydroxyvitamin D and 1,25-dihydroxyvitamin D concentrations with death and progression to maintenance dialysis in patients with advanced kidney disease. Am J Kidney Dis. 2012;60:567–75.

78. Marcén R, Jimenez S, Fernández-Rodriguez A, Galeano C, Villafruela JJ, Gomis A, et al. Are low levels of 25-hydroxyvitamin D a risk factor for cardiovascular diseases or malignancies in renal transplantation? Nephrol Dial Transplant. 2012;27 Suppl 4:iv47–52.

79. Mehrotra R, Kermah DA, Salusky IB, Wolf MS, Thadhani RI, Chiu YW, et al. Chronic kidney disease, hypovitaminosis D, and mortality in the United States. Kidney Int. 2009;76:977–83.

80. Pilz S, Iodice S, Zittermann A, Grant WB, Gandini S. Vitamin D status and mortality risk in CKD: a meta-analysis of prospective studies. Am J Kidney Dis. 2011;58:374–82.

81. Patange AR, Valentini RP, Gothe MP, Du W, Pettersen MD. Vitamin D deficiency is associated with increased left ventricular mass and diastolic dysfunction in children with chronic kidney disease. Pediatr Cardiol. 2013;34:536–42.

82. Lai S, Coppola B, Dimko M, Galani A, Innico G, Frassetti N, et al. Vitamin D deficiency, insulin resistance, and ventricular hypertrophy in the early stages of chronic kidney disease. Ren Fail. 2014;36:58–64.

83. de Boer IH, Kestenbaum B, Shoben AB, Michos ED, Sarnak MJ, Siscovick DS. 25-hydroxyvitamin D levels inversely associate with risk for developing coronary artery calcification. J Am Soc Nephrol. 2009;20:1805–12.

84. García-Canton C, Bosch E, Ramírez A, Gonzalez Y, Auyanet I, Guerra R, et al. Vascular calcification and 25-hydroxyvitamin D levels in non-dialysis patients with chronic kidney disease stages 4 and 5. Nephrol Dial Transplant. 2011;26:2250–6.

85. London GM, Guérin AP, Verbeke FH, Pannier B, Boutouyrie P, Marchais SJ, et al. Mineral metabolism and arterial functions in end-stage renal disease: potential role of 25-hydroxyvitamin D deficiency. J Am Soc Nephrol. 2007;18:613–20.

86. Fusaro M, Gallieni M, Rebora P, Rizzo MA, Luise MC, Riva H, et al. Atrial fibrillation and low vitamin D levels are associated with severe vascular calcifications in hemodialysis patients. J Nephrol. 2016;29:419–26.

87. Yadav AK, Banerjee D, Lal A, Jha V. Vitamin D deficiency, CD4+CD28null cells and accelerated atherosclerosis in chronic kidney disease. Nephrology (Carlton). 2012;17:575–81.

88. Zhang QY, Jiang CM, Sun C, Tang TF, Jin B, Cao DW, et al. Hypovitaminosis D is associated with endothelial dysfunction in patients with non-dialysis chronic kidney disease. J Nephrol. 2015;28:471–6.

89. Chitalia N, Recio-Mayoral A, Kaski JC, Banerjee D. Vitamin D deficiency and endothelial dysfunction in non-dialysis chronic kidney disease patients. Atherosclerosis. 2012;220:265–8.

90. Shroff R, Aitkenhead H, Costa N, Trivelli A, Litwin M, Picca S, et al. Normal 25-hydroxyvitamin D levels are associated with less proteinuria and attenuate renal failure progression in children with CKD. J Am Soc Nephrol. 2015. pii: ASN.2014090947.
91. Fernández-Juárez G, Luño J, Barrio V, de Vinuesa SG, Praga M, Goicoechea M, et al. 25 (OH) vitamin D levels and renal disease progression in patients with type 2 diabetic nephropathy and blockade of the renin-angiotensin system. Clin J Am Soc Nephrol. 2013;8:1870–6.
92. de Boer IH, Katz R, Chonchol M, Ix JH, Sarnak MJ, Shlipak MG, et al. Serum 25-hydroxyvitamin D and change in estimated glomerular filtration rate. Clin J Am Soc Nephrol. 2011;6:2141–9.
93. Sahin I, Gungor B, Can MM, Avci II, Guler GB, Okuyan E, et al. Lower blood vitamin D levels are associated with an increased incidence of contrast-induced nephropathy in patients undergoing coronary angiography. Can J Cardiol. 2014;30:428–33.
94. Lee DR, Kong JM, Cho KI, Chan L. Impact of vitamin D on proteinuria, insulin resistance, and cardiovascular parameters in kidney transplant recipients. Transplant Proc. 2011;43:3723–9.
95. de Boer IH, Ioannou GN, Kestenbaum B, Brunzell JD, Weiss NS. 25-Hydroxyvitamin D levels and albuminuria in the Third National Health and Nutrition Examination Survey (NHANES III). Am J Kidney Dis. 2007;50:69–77.
96. Inaguma D, Nagaya H, Hara K, Tatematsu M, Shinjo H, Suzuki S, et al. Relationship between serum 1,25-dihydroxyvitamin D and mortality in patients with pre-dialysis chronic kidney disease. Clin Exp Nephrol. 2008;12:126–31.
97. Andrade J, Er L, Ignaszewski A, Levin A. Exploration of association of 1,25-OH2D3 with augmentation index, a composite measure of arterial stiffness. Clin J Am Soc Nephrol. 2008;3:1800–6.
98. Ogawa T, Ishida H, Akamatsu M, Matsuda N, Fujiu A, Ito K, et al. Relation of oral 1alpha-hydroxy vitamin D3 to the progression of aortic arch calcification in hemodialysis patients. Heart Vessels. 2010;25:1–6.
99. Testa A, Mallamaci F, Benedetto FA, Pisano A, Tripepi G, Malatino L, et al. Vitamin D receptor (VDR) gene polymorphism is associated with left ventricular (LV) mass and predicts left ventricular hypertrophy (LVH) progression in end-stage renal disease (ESRD) patients. J Bone Miner Res. 2010;25:313–9.
100. Santoro D, Gagliostro G, Alibrandi A, Ientile R, Bellinghieri G, Savica V, et al. Vitamin D receptor gene polymorphism and left ventricular hypertrophy in chronic kidney disease. Nutrients. 2014;6:1029–37.
101. Yang L, Wu L, Fan Y, Ma J. Associations among four polymorphisms (BsmI, FokI, TaqI and ApaI) of vitamin D receptor gene and end-stage renal disease: a meta-analysis. Arch Med Res. 2015;746:1–7.
102. Kandula P, Dobre M, Schold JD, Schreiber Jr MJ, Mehrotra R, Navaneethan SD. Vitamin D supplementation in chronic kidney disease: a systematic review and meta-analysis of observational studies and randomized controlled trials. Clin J Am Soc Nephrol. 2011;6:50–62.
103. Alvarez J, Wasse H, Tangpricha V. Vitamin D supplementation in pre-dialysis chronic kidney disease: a systematic review. Dermatoendocrinol. 2012;4:118–27.
104. Lishmanov A, Dorairajan S, Pak Y, Chaudhary K, Chockalingam A. Treatment of 25-OH vitamin D deficiency in older men with chronic kidney disease stages 3 and 4 is associated with reduction in cardiovascular events. Am J Ther. 2013;20:480–6.
105. Coratelli P, Petrarulo F, Buongiorno E, Giannattasio M, Antonelli G, Amerio A. Improvement in left ventricular function during treatment of hemodialysis patients with 25-OHD3. Contrib Nephrol. 1984;41:433–7.
106. Matias PJ, Jorge C, Ferreira C, Borges M, Aires I, Amaral T, et al. Cholecalciferol supplementation in hemodialysis patients: effects on mineral metabolism, inflammation, and cardiac dimension parameters. Clin J Am Soc Nephrol. 2010;5:905–11.
107. Bucharles S, Barberato SH, Stinghen AE, Gruber B, Piekala L, Dambiski AC, et al. Impact of cholecalciferol treatment on biomarkers of inflammation and myocardial structure in hemodialysis patients without hyperparathyroidism. J Ren Nutr. 2012;22:284–91.

108. Kidir V, Ersoy I, Altuntas A, Gultekin F, Inal S, Dagdeviren BH, et al. Effect of cholecalciferol replacement on vascular calcification and left ventricular mass index in dialysis patients. Ren Fail. 2015;37:635–9.
109. Mann MC, Hemmelgarn BR, Exner DV, Hanley DA, Turin TC, Wheeler DC, et al. Vitamin D supplementation is associated with stabilization of cardiac autonomic tone in IgA nephropathy. Hypertension. 2015;66:e4–6.
110. Chitalia N, Ismail T, Tooth L, Boa F, Hampson G, Goldsmith D, et al. Impact of vitamin D supplementation on arterial vasomotion, stiffness and endothelial biomarkers in chronic kidney disease patients. PLoS One. 2014;9:e91363.
111. Agarwal G, Vasquez K, Penagaluru N, Gelfond J, Qunibi WY. Treatment of vitamin D deficiency/insufficiency with ergocalciferol is associated with reduced vascular access dysfunction in chronic hemodialysis patients. Hemodial Int. 2015;19:499–508.
112. Stubbs JR, Idiculla A, Slusser J, Menard R, Quarles LD. Cholecalciferol supplementation alters calcitriol-responsive monocyte proteins and decreases inflammatory cytokines in ESRD. J Am Soc Nephrol. 2010;21:353–61.
113. Jean G, Souberbielle JC, Chazot C. Monthly cholecalciferol administration in haemodialysis patients: a simple and efficient strategy for vitamin D supplementation. Nephrol Dial Transplant. 2009;24:3799–805.
114. Seirafian S, Haghdarsaheli Y, Mortazavi M, Hosseini M, Moeinzadeh F. The effect of oral vitamin D on serum level of N-terminal pro-B-type natriuretic peptide. Adv Biomed Res. 2014;3:261.
115. Dreyer G, Tucker AT, Harwood SM, Pearse RM, Raftery MJ, Yaqoob MM. Ergocalciferol and microcirculatory function in chronic kidney disease and concomitant vitamin d deficiency: an exploratory, double blind, randomised controlled trial. PLoS One. 2014;9:e99461.
116. Hewitt NA, O'Connor AA, O'Shaughnessy DV, Elder GJ. Effects of cholecalciferol on functional, biochemical, vascular, and quality of life outcomes in hemodialysis patients. Clin J Am Soc Nephrol. 2013;8:1143–9.
117. Mose FH, Vase H, Larsen T, Kancir AS, Kosierkiewic R, Jonczy B, et al. Cardiovascular effects of cholecalciferol treatment in dialysis patients – a randomized controlled trial. BMC Nephrol. 2014;15:50.
118. Bhan I, Dobens D, Tamez H, Deferio JJ, Li YC, Warren HS, et al. Nutritional vitamin D supplementation in dialysis: a randomized trial. Clin J Am Soc Nephrol. 2015;10:611–9.
119. Wasse H, Huang R, Long Q, Zhao Y, Singapuri S, McKinnon W, et al. Very high-dose cholecalciferol and arteriovenous fistula maturation in ESRD: a randomized, double-blind, placebo-controlled pilot study. J Vasc Access. 2014;15(2):88–94.
120. Li L, Lin M, Krassilnikova M, Ostrow K, Bader A, Radbill B, et al. Effect of cholecalciferol supplementation on inflammation and cellular alloimmunity in hemodialysis patients: data from a randomized controlled pilot trial. PLoS One. 2014;9:e109998.
121. Seibert E, Heine GH, Ulrich C, Seiler S, Köhler H, Girndt M. Influence of cholecalciferol supplementation in hemodialysis patients on monocyte subsets: a randomized, double-blind, placebo-controlled clinical trial. Nephron Clin Pract. 2013;123:209–19.
122. Delanaye P, Weekers L, Warling X, Moonen M, Smelten N, Médart L, et al. Cholecalciferol in haemodialysis patients: a randomized, double-blind, proof-of-concept and safety study. Nephrol Dial Transplant. 2013;28:1779–86.
123. Massart A, Debelle FD, Racapé J, Gervy C, Husson C, Dhaene M, et al. Biochemical parameters after cholecalciferol repletion in hemodialysis: results from the VitaDial randomized trial. Am J Kidney Dis. 2014;64:696–705.
124. Marckmann P, Agerskov H, Thineshkumar S, Bladbjerg EM, Sidelmann JJ, Jespersen J, et al. Randomized controlled trial of cholecalciferol supplementation in chronic kidney disease patients with hypovitaminosis D. Nephrol Dial Transplant. 2012;27:3523–31.
125. Sprague SM, Silva AL, Al-Saghir F, Damle R, Tabash SP, Petkovich M, et al. Modified-release calcifediol effectively controls secondary hyperparathyroidism associated with vitamin D insufficiency in chronic kidney disease. Am J Nephrol. 2014;40:535–45.

126. Kooienga L, Fried L, Scragg R, Kendrick J, Smits G, Chonchol M. The effect of combined calcium and vitamin D3 supplementation on serum intact parathyroid hormone in moderate CKD. Am J Kidney Dis. 2009;53:408–16.
127. Armas LA, Andukuri R, Barger-Lux J, Heaney RP, Lund R. 25-Hydroxyvitamin D response to cholecalciferol supplementation in hemodialysis. Clin J Am Soc Nephrol. 2012;7: 1428–34.
128. Wasse H, Huang R, Long Q, Singapuri S, Raggi P, Tangpricha V. Efficacy and safety of a short course of very-high-dose cholecalciferol in hemodialysis. Am J Clin Nutr. 2012;95: 522–8.
129. Beveridge LA, Struthers AD, Khan F, Jorde R, Scragg R, Macdonald HM, et al. Effect of vitamin D supplementation on blood pressure: a systematic review and meta-analysis incorporating individual patient data. JAMA Intern Med. 2015;175:745–54.
130. Pilz S, Gaksch M, Kienreich K, Grübler M, Verheyen N, Fahrleitner-Pammer A, et al. Effects of vitamin D on blood pressure and cardiovascular risk factors: a randomized controlled trial. Hypertension. 2015;65:1195–201.
131. Zheng Z, Shi H, Jia J, Li D, Lin S. Vitamin D supplementation and mortality risk in chronic kidney disease: a meta-analysis of 20 observational studies. BMC Nephrol. 2013;14:199.
132. Duranton F, Rodriguez-Ortiz ME, Duny Y, Rodriguez M, Daurès JP, Argilés A. Vitamin D treatment and mortality in chronic kidney disease: a systematic review and meta-analysis. Am J Nephrol. 2013;37:239–48.
133. Naves-Díaz M, Alvarez-Hernández D, Passlick-Deetjen J, Guinsburg A, Marelli C, Rodriguez-Puyol D, et al. Oral active vitamin D is associated with improved survival in hemodialysis patients. Kidney Int. 2008;74:1070–8.
134. Sugiura S, Inaguma D, Kitagawa A, Murata M, Kamimura Y, Sendo S, et al. Administration of alfacalcidol for patients with predialysis chronic kidney disease may reduce cardiovascular disease events. Clin Exp Nephrol. 2010;14:43–50.
135. Shoji T, Shinohara K, Kimoto E, Emoto M, Tahara H, Koyama H, et al. Lower risk for cardiovascular mortality in oral 1alpha-hydroxy vitamin D3 users in a haemodialysis population. Nephrol Dial Transplant. 2004;19:179–84.
136. Shoji T, Marubayashi S, Shigematsu T, Iseki K, Tsubakihara Y, Committee of Renal Data Registry, Japanese Society for Dialysis Therapy. Use of vitamin d receptor activator, incident cardiovascular disease and death in a cohort of hemodialysis patients. Ther Apher Dial. 2015;19:235–44.
137. Miller JE, Molnar MZ, Kovesdy CP, Zaritsky JJ, Streja E, Salusky I, et al. Administered paricalcitol dose and survival in hemodialysis patients: a marginal structural model analysis. Pharmacoepidemiol Drug Saf. 2012;21:1232–9.
138. Cozzolino M, Brancaccio D, Cannella G, Messa P, Gesualdo L, Marangella M, et al. VDRA therapy is associated with improved survival in dialysis patients with serum intact PTH ≤ 150 pg/mL: results of the Italian FARO Survey. Nephrol Dial Transplant. 2012;27:3588–94.
139. Teng M, Wolf M, Lowrie E, Ofsthun N, Lazarus JM, Thadhani R. Survival of patients undergoing hemodialysis with paricalcitol or calcitriol therapy. N Engl J Med. 2003;349:446–56.
140. Bover J, Dasilva I, Furlano M, Lloret MJ, Diaz-Encarnacion MM, Ballarin J, et al. Clinical uses of 1,25-dihydroxy-19-nor-vitamin D(2) (paricalcitol). Curr Vasc Pharmacol. 2014;12: 313–23.
141. Lemmilä S, Saha H, Virtanen V, Ala-Houhala I, Pasternack A. Effect of intravenous calcitriol on cardiac systolic and diastolic function in patients on hemodialysis. Am J Nephrol. 1998;18:404–10.
142. Park CW, Oh YS, Shin YS, Kim CM, Kim YS, Kim SY, et al. Intravenous calcitriol regresses myocardial hypertrophy in hemodialysis patients with secondary hyperparathyroidism. Am J Kidney Dis. 1999;33:73–81.
143. Ivarsen P, Povlsen JV, Christensen KL. Effect of alfacalcidol on cardiac function in patients with chronic kidney disease stage 4 and secondary hyperparathyroidism: a pilot study. Scand J Urol Nephrol. 2012;46:381–8.

144. McGonigle RJ, Timmis AD, Keenan J, Jewitt DE, Weston MJ, Parsons V. The influence of 1 alpha-hydroxycholecalciferol on left ventricular function in end-stage renal failure. Proc Eur Dial Transplant Assoc. 1981;18:579–85.
145. McGonigle RJ, Fowler MB, Timmis AB, Weston MJ, Parsons V. Uremic cardiomyopathy: potential role of vitamin D and parathyroid hormone. Nephron. 1984;36:94–100.
146. Singh NP, Sahni V, Garg D, Nair M. Effect of pharmacological suppression of secondary hyperparathyroidism on cardiovascular hemodynamics in predialysis CKD patients: a preliminary observation. Hemodial Int. 2007;11:417–23.
147. Kim HW, Park CW, Shin YS, Kim YS, Shin SJ, Kim YS, et al. Calcitriol regresses cardiac hypertrophy and QT dispersion in secondary hyperparathyroidism on hemodialysis. Nephron Clin Pract. 2006;102:c21–9.
148. Bodyak N, Ayus JC, Achinger S, Shivalingappa V, Ke Q, Chen YS, et al. Activated vitamin D attenuates left ventricular abnormalities induced by dietary sodium in Dahl salt-sensitive animals. Proc Natl Acad Sci U S A. 2007;104:16810–5.
149. Morosetti M, Jankovic L, Palombo G, Cipriani S, Dominijanni S, Balducci A, et al. High-dose calcitriol therapy and progression of cardiac vascular calcifications. J Nephrol. 2008;21: 603–8.
150. Charitaki E, Davenport A. Aortic pulse wave velocity in haemodialysis patients is associated with the prescription of active vitamin D analogues. J Nephrol. 2014;27:431–7.
151. Briese S, Wiesner S, Will JC, Lembcke A, Opgen-Rhein B, Nissel R, et al. Arterial and cardiac disease in young adults with childhood-onset end-stage renal disease-impact of calcium and vitamin D therapy. Nephrol Dial Transplant. 2006;21:1906–14.
152. Drüeke TB, Massy ZA. Role of vitamin D in vascular calcification: bad guy or good guy? Nephrol Dial Transplant. 2012;27:1704–7.
153. Hansen D, Rasmussen K, Rasmussen LM, Bruunsgaard H, Brandi L. The influence of vitamin D analogs on calcification modulators. N-terminal pro-B-type natriuretic peptide and inflammatory markers in hemodialysis patients: a randomized crossover study. MC Nephrol. 2014;15:130.
154. Cianciolo G, La Manna G, Della Bella E, Cappuccilli ML, Angelini ML, Dormi A, et al. Effect of vitamin D receptor activator therapy on vitamin D receptor and osteocalcin expression in circulating endothelial progenitor cells of hemodialysis patients. Blood Purif. 2013;35:187–95.
155. Hansen D, Rasmussen K, Rasmussen LM, Bruunsgaard H, Brandi L. The influence of vitamin D analogs on calcification modulators. N-terminal pro-B-type natriuretic peptide and inflammatory markers in hemodialysis patients: a randomized crossover study. BMC Nephrol. 2014;15:130.
156. Trillini M, Cortinovis M, Ruggenenti P, Reyes Loaeza J, Courville K, Ferrer-Siles C, et al. Paricalcitol for secondary hyperparathyroidism in renal transplantation. J Am Soc Nephrol. 2015;26:1205–14.
157. De Nicola L, Conte G, Russo D, Gorini A, Minutolo R. Antiproteinuric effect of add-on paricalcitol in CKD patients under maximal tolerated inhibition of renin-angiotensin system: a prospective observational study. BMC Nephrol. 2012;13:150.
158. Lucisano S, Arena A, Stassi G, Iannello D, Montalto G, Romeo A, et al. Role of paricalcitol in modulating the immune response in patients with renal disease. Int J Endocrinol. 2015; 2015:765364.
159. Agarwal R, Hynson JE, Hecht TJ, Light RP, Sinha AD. Short-term vitamin D receptor activation increases serum creatinine due to increased production with no effect on the glomerular filtration rate. Kidney Int. 2011;80:1073–9.
160. Mann MC, Hobbs AJ, Hemmelgarn BR, Roberts DJ, Ahmed SB, Rabi DM. Effect of oral vitamin D analogs on mortality and cardiovascular outcomes among adults with chronic kidney disease: a meta-analysis. Clin Kidney J. 2015;8:41–8.
161. Li XH, Feng L, Yang ZH, Liao YH. The effect of active vitamin D on cardiovascular outcomes in predialysis chronic kidney diseases: a systematic review and meta-analysis. Nephrology (Carlton). 2015. doi:10.1111/nep.12505.

162. Thadhani R, Appelbaum E, Pritchett Y, Chang Y, Wenger J, Tamez H, et al. Vitamin D therapy and cardiac structure and function in patients with chronic kidney disease: the PRIMO randomized controlled trial. JAMA. 2012;307:674–84.
163. Tamez H, Zoccali C, Packham D, Wenger J, Bhan I, Appelbaum E, et al. Vitamin D reduces left atrial volume in patients with left ventricular hypertrophy and chronic kidney disease. Am Heart J. 2012;164:902–9.
164. Wang AY, Fang F, Chan J, Wen YY, Qing S, Chan IH, et al. Effect of paricalcitol on left ventricular mass and function in CKD – the OPERA trial. J Am Soc Nephrol. 2014;25:175–86.
165. Lundwall K, Jörneskog G, Jacobson SH, Spaak J. Paricalcitol, microvascular and endothelial function in non-diabetic chronic kidney disease: a randomized trial. Am J Nephrol. 2015;42: 265–73.
166. Zoccali C, Curatola G, Panuccio V, Tripepi R, Pizzini P, Versace M, et al. Paricalcitol and endothelial function in chronic kidney disease trial. Hypertension. 2014;64:1005–11.
167. de Zeeuw D, Agarwal R, Amdahl M, Audhya P, Coyne D, Garimella T, et al. Selective vitamin D receptor activation with paricalcitol for reduction of albuminuria in patients with type 2 diabetes (VITAL study): a randomised controlled trial. Lancet. 2010;376:1543–51.
168. Cheng J, Zhang W, Zhang X, Li X, Chen J. Efficacy and safety of paricalcitol therapy for chronic kidney disease: a meta-analysis. Clin J Am Soc Nephrol. 2012;7:391–400.
169. de Borst MH, Hajhosseiny R, Tamez H, Wenger J, Thadhani R, Goldsmith DJ. Active vitamin D treatment for reduction of residual proteinuria: a systematic review. J Am Soc Nephrol. 2013;24:1863–71.
170. Xu L, Wan X, Huang Z, Zeng F, Wei G, Fang D, et al. Impact of vitamin D on chronic kidney diseases in non-dialysis patients: a meta-analysis of randomized controlled trials. PLoS Onc. 2013;8:e61387.
171. Han T, Rong G, Quan D, Shu Y, Liang Z, She N, et al. Meta-analysis: the efficacy and safety of paricalcitol for the treatment of secondary hyperparathyroidism and proteinuria in chronic kidney disease. Biomed Res Int. 2013;2013:320560.
172. Agarwal R, Acharya M, Tian J, Hippensteel RL, Melnick JZ, Qiu P, et al. Antiproteinuric effect of oral paricalcitol in chronic kidney disease. Kidney Int. 2005;68:2823–8.
173. Zhao J, Dong J, Wang H, Shang H, Zhang D, Liao L. Efficacy and safety of vitamin D3 in patients with diabetic nephropathy: a meta-analysis of randomized controlled trials. Chin Med J (Engl). 2014;127:2837–43.
174. de Boer IH, Sachs M, Hoofnagle AN, Utzschneider KM, Kahn SE, Kestenbaum B, et al. Paricalcitol does not improve glucose metabolism in patients with stage 3–4 chronic kidney disease. Kidney Int. 2013;83:323–30.
175. Coyne DW, Goldberg S, Faber M, Ghossein C, Sprague SM. A randomized multicenter trial of paricalcitol versus calcitriol for secondary hyperparathyroidism in stages 3–4 CKD. Clin J Am Soc Nephrol. 2014;9:1620–6.
176. Coyne DW, Andress DL, Amdahl MJ, Ritz E, de Zeeuw D. Effects of paricalcitol on calcium and phosphate metabolism and markers of bone health in patients with diabetic nephropathy: results of the VITAL study. Nephrol Dial Transplant. 2013;28:2260–8.
177. Courbebaisse M, Alberti C, Colas S, Prié D, Souberbielle JC, Treluyer JM, et al. VITamin D supplementation in renAL transplant recipients (VITALE): a prospective, multicentre, double-blind, randomized trial of vitamin D estimating the benefit and safety of vitamin D3 treatment at a dose of 100,000 UI compared with a dose of 12,000 UI in renal transplant recipients: study protocol for a double-blind, randomized, controlled trial. Trials. 2014; 15:430.
178. Levin A, Perry T, De Zoysa P, Sigrist MK, Humphries K, Tang M, et al. A randomized control trial to assess the impact of vitamin D supplementation compared to placebo on vascular stiffness in chronic kidney disease patients. BMC Cardiovasc Disord. 2014;14:156.
179. Mann MC, Exner DV, Hemmelgarn BR, Hanley DA, Turin TC, MacRae JM, et al. The VITAH trial VITamin D supplementation and cardiac Autonomic tone in Hemodialysis: a blinded, randomized controlled trial. BMC Nephrol. 2014;15:129.

180. Keyzer CA, de Jong MA, Fenna van Breda G, Vervloet MG, Laverman GD, Hemmelder M, et al. Vitamin D receptor activator and dietary sodium restriction to reduce residual urinary albumin excretion in chronic kidney disease (ViRTUE study): rationale and study protocol. Nephrol Dial Transplant. 2015. pii: gfv033. [Epub ahead of print] Review.

181. Mehrotra A, Leung WY, Joson T. Nutritional vitamin D supplementation and health-related outcomes in hemodialysis patients: a protocol for a systematic review and meta-analysis. Syst Rev. 2015;4:13.

Chapter 20
Vitamin D and Endothelial Function in Chronic Kidney Disease

Mugurel Apetrii and Adrian Covic

Abstract The endothelium is a highly active organ with numerous functions regarding endothelium-dependent vasodilation, balance of inflammation and hemostasis and finally endothelial cell repair and angiogenesis. Vitamin D deficit has been linked to endothelial dysfunction, two conditions encountered early in chronic kidney disease (CKD). Vitamin D has direct effects on the endothelium: endothelial cells are capable of activating 25(OH)D to $1,25(OH)_2D_3$, which acts locally to regulate the vascular tone, to prevent vascular inflammation and oxidative stress and to promote cell repair and survival. Vitamin D also indirectly regulates endothelial function: various conditions alter the normal functioning of the endothelium in CKD, and most of them are also aggravated by the abnormal vitamin D metabolism. In this regard, vitamin D deficit in CKD favors the development and/or perpetuation of metabolic abnormalities (hyperglycemia, dyslipidemia), secondary hyperparathyroidism, chronic inflammation and also the activation of the renin-angiotensin system, conditions that trigger endothelial dysfunction. Also, CKD-associated perturbations of the vitamin D-FGF-23-klotho axis additionally promote endothelial dysfunction. Therefore, vitamin D therapy in CKD is requisite for ameliorating endothelial dysfunction, the major initiator of CVD.

Keywords Vitamin D • Endothelial dysfunction • Endothelium-dependent vasodilation • Chronic kidney disease • Cardiovascular diseases • Atherosclerosis • Inflammation • Oxidative stress • Nitric oxide • Renin-angiotensin system

M. Apetrii, MD, PhD (✉)
Nephrology Unit, Dr CI Parhon University Hospital, Iasi, Romania
e-mail: mugurelu_1980@yahoo.com

A. Covic, MD, PhD, FRCP (London), FERA
University "Grigore T. Popa", Iasi, Romania

© Springer International Publishing Switzerland 2016
P.A. Ureña Torres et al. (eds.), *Vitamin D in Chronic Kidney Disease*,
DOI 10.1007/978-3-319-32507-1_20

20.1 Introduction

Chronic kidney disease (CKD) patients are most prone to develop cardiovascular diseases (CVD). The decline in the estimate glomerular filtration rate (eGFR) independently increases the incidence of CVD, making CKD a cardiovascular (CV) risk condition per se. Endothelial function is markedly impaired in CKD due to the presence of traditional cardiovascular risk factors such as hypertension and diabetes mellitus but also due to the presence of an unnatural milieu characterized by mineral, hormonal, inflammatory and metabolic disturbances [1, 2]. Endothelial dysfunction (ED) favors atherogenesis and arteriosclerosis which further contribute to CVD development, progression and complications [3]. Furthermore, it can be detected at early stages of CKD and contributes to a high cardiovascular mortality rate in this population [4].

Vitamin D was long time regarded simply as an anti-rachitic compound that fixes calcium to bone. However, as the number of publications on vitamin D is constantly increasing, we are acknowledging that vitamin D has numerous extra-skeletal effects not being just a simple "vitamin" but a hormone and a component of a sophisticated mechanism which includes the calcitriol, specific enzymes and receptor, a dedicated plasma transport protein and many other hormones regulating vitamin D metabolism [5].

One of the modifications that characterizes CKD is represented by the decline in circulating $1,25(OH)_2D_3$ (calcitriol) levels due to inhibitory effect of FGF23 and the decreased level of 1α-hydroxylase once the glomerular filtration rate (GFR) has declined to less than 30 mL/min/1.73 m^2 [6]. In fact, several small studies suggest that vitamin D deficiency is common in patients with CKD, reaching 70–80 % in patients with stage 3–5 disease [7]. Until recently, it was thought that 1α-hydroxylase it is mainly secreted by the kidney. However, several cell types such as vascular smooth muscle cells, osteoblasts, and endothelial cells also express 1α-hydroxylase to form $1,25(OH)_2D_3$ locally [6]. This finding opens new ways for understanding the pathogenesis of vascular calcification, left ventricular hypertrophy and even arterial hypertension. Furthermore, the activation of the vitamin D receptor (VDR) in those tissues has been implicated in suppression of the renin-angiotensin-aldosterone system (RAAS), in regulation of apoptosis, and in regulation of an inflammatory response [6].

20.2 Endothelial Function and Dysfunction

Vascular endothelium is not only the delimitating barrier between the vessels wall and blood stream, but also an active organ having endocrine, autocrine and paracrine actions upon the vasculature [8–10]. Thus the endothelium has numerous functions: firstly, it regulates vascular tone through the secretion of both vasodilator (nitric oxide, endothelium-derived hyperpolarizing factor-EDHF, prostacyclin, bradykinin, adrenomedulin) and vasoconstrictor substances (endothelins, thromboxane

A2, angiotensin II, prostaglandin H2). Secondly, the endothelium regulates vascular inflammation and leukocyte adhesion through the secretion of intercellular adhesion molecule-1 (ICAM-1), vascular adhesion molecule-1 (VCAM-1), E-selectin, P-selectin, and nuclear factor k-B (NFkB). Thirdly, the endothelium modulates hemostasis and thrombosis by releasing both prothrombotic (endothelin-1, plasminogen activator inhibitor-1, tissue factor, thromboxane A2, fibrinogen) and antithrombotic (nitric oxide, plasminogen activator, von Willebrand factor, tissue factor inhibitor) agents. Finally, the endothelium regulates smooth muscle cell proliferation and also produces vascular endothelium growth factor (VEGF) that promotes angiogenesis [8, 10, 11].

Endothelial dysfunction was initially referred to vasorelaxation impairment [3]. However, it is currently accepted that endothelial function may refer to the loss of any of the endothelial functions resulting in altered vascular homeostasis [11]. The action of various CV risk factors finally results in ED: ED is encountered in hypertension, diabetes mellitus, hypercholesterolemia, obesity, and kidney disease and even in menopause and aging [8–10]. Thus, ED is a common trigger of CV disease and also a potent surrogate for CV risk [10, 12].

20.3 Vitamin D and the Endothelium in General Population and Experimental Studies

The role and the mechanism of vitamin D in endothelial dysfunction are extremely complex. As noted above, endothelial cells express the VDR and also 1α-hydroxylase, thus being one of the extra renal sites of $1,25(OH)_2D_3$ production. Locally produced vitamin D mediates many of the endothelium functions through intracrine, autocrine, and paracrine actions (Table 20.1). However, the vitamin D effects on endothelial function are contrasting, both very low and very high levels of vitamin D being associated with negative consequences in a biphasic dose-response fashion.

Active vitamin D analogs upregulate endothelial nitric oxide synthase 3 (eNOS) expression in endothelial cells of aortic rings of wild-type mice, thus enhancing nitric oxide (NO) production. This effect is dependent of VDR signaling, as it does not occur in VDR-defective mice. The activated form of vitamin D increases eNOS expression through direct transcriptional regulation [13]. $1,25(OH)_2D_3$ also increases NO production in human umbilical vein endothelial cells [14]. Further on, chronic in vivo treatment of spontaneously hypertensive rats with $1,25(OH)_2D_3$ reduced ex vivo endothelium-dependent contractions in response to acetylcholine and calcium ionophore. This effect was rather shown to be mediated by cyclooxygenase 1 (COX1) decrease than by NO, as COX1 is known to be responsible for the increased expression of endothelium-dependent contracting factors [15].

Chronic vitamin D deficiency also seems to lead to arterial stiffness in mice: long-term VDR-defective mice have increased aortic impedance and also increased

Table 20.1 CKD-associated conditions that trigger endothelial dysfunction (ED) and vitamin D beneficial effects upon the endothelium

Conditions associated with ED in CKD	Vitamin D actions upon endothelial functions
Increased RAAS activity and hypertension	1. Improves/recovers eNOS activity
Angiotensin II	2. Mitigates AGE-induced downregulation of eNOS
Aldosterone	3. Antioxidative:
Diabetes	Downregulates NADPH oxydase
Dyslipidaemia	Upregulates SOD-1/2
Inflammation	4. Anti-inflamamtory: downregulates vascular expression of IL-6 and NF-kB
Secondary hyperparathyroidism	5. Inhibits endothelial cell apoptosis and promotes survival
Klotho- FGF23 axis	6. Promotes endothelial cell migration and proliferation
Uremic toxins	7. Angiogenesis through the induction of VEGF
ADMA	
p-cresylsulphate	
Adipocytokines	
Leptin	
Resistin	
Visfatin	

ED endothelial dysfunction, *CKD* chronic kidney disease, *RAAS* renin angiotensin aldosterone system, *FGF23* fibroblast growth factor 23, *ADMA* asymmetric dimethylarginine, *eNOS* endothelial nitric oxide synthase, *AGE* advanced glycation end-products, *NADPH* nicotinamide adenine dinucleotide phosphate oxidase, *SOD* superoxide dismutase, *IL-6* interleukin-6, *NF-kB* nuclear factor-kappa B, *VEGF* vascular endothelium growth factor

collagen and decreased elastin fibers in the ascending aorta [13]. Vitamin D also has antioxidant effects on the endothelium: in human endothelial cells, reduction of cell viability and reactive oxygen species (ROS) production due to oxidative stress is prevented by pretreatment of endothelial cells with $1,25(OH)_2D_3$ [14]. Vitamin D increases expression of the antioxidant enzyme CuZn superoxide dismutase in endothelial cells also [16]. The prevention of cell death is mediated by vitamin D through reduction of apoptotic proteins and promotion of autophagy, resulting in cell "recycling" [14].

In general population, data from a case-control study performed by Tarcin et al. [17], pointed out that vitamin D-deficient (below 25 nmol/l) subjects had a significantly lower flow mediated dilatation (FMD) as a marker of impaired endothelial function compared to the vitamin D-sufficient control group (mean level of 25(OH)D = 75 nmol/l). Also, FMD significantly increased after vitamin D supplementation in the vitamin D deficiency group [17, 18]. Vitamin D deficit also contributes to the development of arterial stiffness: suboptimal serum 25(OH)D levels are independently associated with measures of endothelial function (increased carotid-femoral pulse wave velocity (PWV) and augmentation index obtained through applanation tonometry) in asymptomatic subjects, both with and without traditional CV risk factors. ED induced by vitamin D deficiency is also mediated by vascular inflammation:

vitamin D levels are inversely correlated with proinflammatory cytokine interleukin-6 (IL-6) expression in endothelial cells and vitamin D deficiency subjects have increased expression of the proinflammatory NFkB transcription factor [18].

However, contrary to expectations, vitamin D supplementation in deficient patients with coronary artery disease failed to show any improvement in endothelial function. It seems that in high-risk patients that are already on medication that targets potential triggers of endothelial dysfunction (angiotensin converting enzyme, angiotensin receptor blockers, statins), vitamin D correction/supplementation does not bring any incremental benefit [19, 20].

Other negative effects associated with vitamin D excess include hyperphosphataemia, hypercalcaemia, medial calcification, arterial stiffness and left ventricular hypertrophy. High levels of vitamin D increases matrix metallo-proteinase-2 expression, which degrades the extracellular matrix, opening the way for endothelial cell migration [21]. Angiogenesis is also promoted by vitamin D through induction of VEGF expression in endothelial cells [16].

20.4 Vitamin D and the Endothelium in CKD

Impaired endothelium function is seen across the whole span of CKD, from predialysis patients to ESRD patients on dialysis to renal transplant recipients [22]. Endothelial cell dysfunction is a well-known culprit of cardiovascular morbidity and it develops in CKD with remarkable frequency. In fact, CV risk rises with the decline in the eGFR and the key mediator of this inverse relationship seems to be represented by ED [3]. Altered endothelial function was initially described in end-stage renal disease (ESRD) patients on dialysis. Subsequently, studies have shown that ED is actually present from the early stages of CKD. However, assessing endothelial function is challenging in renal patients since two of the main conditions that cause renal impairment – hypertension and diabetes – are also associated with ED. Therefore, it is difficult to establish whether abnormal endothelial function in CKD is due to renal impairment or it is predominantly a reflection of pre-existing vascular disease aggravated by CKD [3, 23].

In CKD patients, endothelial function is altered through various mechanisms (Table 20.1); Traditional risk factors for cardiovascular disease like hypertension or diabetes are joined by nontraditional risk factors, such as asymmetric dimethylarginine (ADMA), advanced glycation end-products (AGEs), pro-oxidants, all accumulating in CKD, to induce ED via eNOS uncoupling, which results not only in the down-regulation of NO production, but also generates oxygen free radicals [12]. Mineral bone disorders may play an important role in endothelial function, since correction of vitamin D, phosphate and FGF23 after renal transplantation correlates with improved endothelium-dependent vasodilatation [24]. Cross-sectional studies correlated serum 25(OH)D, 1,25(OH)$_2$D levels with endothelium-dependent vasodilation in patients with stage 3–4 CKD and in patients with end-stage kidney disease on dialysis, suggesting that vitamin D may have an active effect on the vascular system [25].

The effect of vitamin D analogues on the improvement of endothelial function is mediated by the recovery of NO activity [26]. In a CKD-like environment in vitro, calcitriol directly normalizes eNOS activity and also decreases the number of receptors for AGEs on the endothelial cell. Lack of coupling of AGE to their receptors blunts AGE-mediated down-regulation of eNOS [27]. Also, calcitriol reverses the function of endothelial cells exposed to a CKD-like environment: calcitriol down-regulates the expression of IL-6 and the activity of NFkB, thus having vascular anti-inflammatory properties [27]. These in vitro results are further confirmed by animal models of CKD studies (sub-total nephrectomized rats) with impaired ED defined as impaired endothelium-dependent vasorelaxation response to acethylcholine [23, 26].

The uremic environment modifies the vascular expression of a wide-range of genes that regulate oxidative stress, hormone and immune functions, inflammation and lipid and glucose metabolism (genes that encode apolipoprotein A-IV, fatty acid binding protein-2, hydroxysteroid dehydrogenase, heat shock protein 1b, etc.) finally leading to ED. VDR activators ameliorate endothelial functions also by reversing these changes at the vascular level [23].

In non-dialysis patients, endothelial function deteriorates with eGFR decrease [22, 28]. However, there are differences regarding the extent of ED between different CKD stages: ESRD patients have the worse endothelial function assessed by brachial artery FMD compared to pre-dialysis or kidney transplantation patients. At the same time, it seems that after renal transplantation, endothelial function is reversed to the pre-dialysis grade of impairment, as FMD does not differ significantly between pre-dialysis CKD and post-transplantation CKD. This is probably due to remnant kidney function impairment, preceding CV damage and immunosuppression undesirable secondary effects [28].

In observational studies, vitamin D is a significant positive independent predictor of endothelial function (FMD) in non-diabetic non-dialysis CKD patients as well in ESRD patients [28–30]. The lowest FMD is seen in vitamin D deficient patients compared to vitamin D insufficient and vitamin D sufficient patients [31]. Furthermore, vitamin D deficiency is independently associated with markers of endothelial activation such as vascular cell adhesion molecule-1 (VCAM-1) and E-selectin in non-dialysis patients [28].

These results coming from cross-sectional studies were further confirmed by clinical trials. Thus, in non-diabetic CKD patients stage 3–4 with vitamin D deficiency, 6 months supplementation with ergocalciferol significantly improved endothelium-dependent microcirculatory function assessed at the forearm level, proving the causal relationship between vitamin D deficiency and ED [32]. Moreover, ergocalciferol supplementation of CKD patients reduces oxidative stress and tissue AGE formation, the latter being predictors of CVD in CKD [32]. Also, cholecalciferol administration to non-diabetic, non-dialysis, vitamin D deficient CKD patients significantly improves FMD and decreases markers of endothelial activation including inter-cellular adhesion molecule-1 (ICAM-1), VCAM-1 and E-selectin [33]. Paricalcitol administration (2 μg/day for 12 weeks) in patients with CKD stages 3–4 resulted in a significant change in FMD compared to the placebo group [34]. However, reported results regarding the endothelial benefits of vitamin D or vitamin D analogues administration differ between trials. This may be due to differences in time of exposure, as paricalcitol administration for only 1 month does not have any effect over endothelial function, irrespective of dosage (1 μg/day or 2 μg/day) [35]. Also, endothelial function in patients with diabetes mellitus type 2 and CKD did not improve after paricalcitol administration (1 μg/day for 3 months). This may be due to low dosage or it can be explained by the confounding effects of medication that targets endothelial function (anti-hypertensive or anti-diabetic medication) [36].

20.5   Vitamin D and CKD-Associated Conditions That Predispose to Endothelial Dysfunction

Vitamin D deficiency also predisposes to a wide range of conditions that cause ED in CKD, thus having indirect effects upon the endothelium (Fig. 20.1).

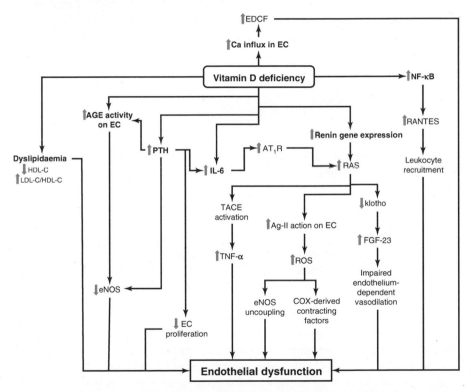

Fig. 20.1 Various pathological conditions that link vitamin D deficiency and endothelial dysfunction in chronic kidney disease. Abbreviations: *Ag-II* angiotensin II, *AGE* advanced glycation end products, *AT₁R* Angiotensin II type 1 receptor, *Ca* calcium, *COX* cyclooxygenase, *EC* endothelial cells, *EDCF* endothelial-dependent contracting factors, *eNOS* endothelial nitric oxide synthase, *FGF-23* fibroblast growth factor 23, *HDL-C* High density lipoprotein cholesterol, *IL-6* interleukin-6, *LDL-C* low-density lipoprotein cholesterol, *NF-kB* nuclear factor k-B, *PTH* parathormone, *RANTES* regulated on activation, normal T cell expressed and secreted chemokine, *RAAS* renin-angiotensin system, *ROS* reactive oxygen species, *TACE* tumor necrosis factor-α converting enzyme, *TNF-α* tumor necrosis factor

20.5.1 Diabetes

In type 2 diabetes, low circulating vitamin D levels favor poor glycemic control, and the reduction of immature endothelial progenitor cells that are involved in endothelial repair and angiogenesis, thus promoting endothelial function impairment [37]. Vitamin D protects against the negative effects of AGE on eNOS activity [38] and also has antiatherogenic effects by inhibiting foam cell formation [39]. Despite this, randomized controlled trials (RCT) of diabetic patients with suboptimal serum vitamin D levels (<30 ng/ml) did not show any significant changes induced by vitamin D repletion regarding circulating endothelial progenitor cells, FMD or blood pressure. However, FMD was significantly ameliorated by vitamin D repletion in a post-hoc analysis of diabetic patients that specifically had baseline endothelial dysfunction [40]. Clinical studies assessed only the circulating 25(OH)D form, while the active intracellular form is represented by $1,25(OH)_2D_3$. Therefore, vitamin D activation by 1α-hydroxylase may alter the relationship between 25(OH)D and markers of arterial function [41]. As mentioned before, it is also possible that in diabetic patients that are on vasoactive medication, vitamin D supplementation may not further induce any significant change.

20.5.2 Hypertension

One of the main mechanisms that is excessively activated in both hypertension and CKD having deleterious effects on vasculature is the RAAS [42]. Vitamin D regulates vascular tone through both genomic and non-genomic mechanisms [42, 43]. Through genomic mechanisms, calcitriol negatively regulates renin gene transcription: VDR-bound calcitriol inhibits the interaction between cyclic adenosine monophosphate (cAMP) response element binding and cAMP response element in the renin gene promoter, thus inhibiting the transcription of renin gene [44]. Further on, calcitriol down-regulates angiotensin II receptor 1 (AT_1R) expression in renal arteries, thus blunting the deleterious effects induced by angiotensin II binding to its receptor: in both renal and systemic arteries, vitamin D is responsible for a reduction in angiotensin II-induced ROS excessive generation [43]. ROS promote endothelium dysfunction and finally hypertension: [1] ROS alter eNOS activity, being responsible for eNOS uncoupling and thus for impaired NO-dependent endothelial function, ROS promote the expression of cyclooxygenases-derived contracting factors in the endothelium [3, 45, 46]. Also by genomic regulation, calcitriol down-regulates the expression of oxidative-stress associated enzyme, NADPH oxidase in renal arteries. The vascular anti-oxidative action of calcitriol also comprises up-regulation of SOD-1 and SOD-2 enzymes in renal arteries. The effects of calcitriol on NADPH oxidase and SOD expression may partially be mediated by the down-regulation of AT_1R, as AT_1R activation is responsible for ROS production. Thus, by regulating RAAS and ROS production, vitamin D protects both kidney and systemic vessels from ED in hypertension [43].

Through non-genomic mechanisms, calcitriol regulates calcium influx in endothelial cells. The increased production of endothelium-derived contracting factors (EDCF) depends on a high concentration of free intracellular calcium. In endothelial cells, calcitriol prevents the high calcium influx that is needed for the production of EDCF and therefore attenuates endothelium-dependent contractions [47].

Studies on animal models showed that vitamin D supplementation may improve blood pressure values, but most interventional trials failed to confirm these results in humans. Despite this, there is still convincing evidence from animal studies and in vitro studies that vitamin D contributes to endothelial function regulation in hypertension and CKD by diminishing the deleterious impact of RAAS activation and not only [42, 43].

20.5.3 Dyslipidemia

CKD is associated with major alterations of lipid metabolism resulting in dyslipidemia. Firstly, CKD patients have hypertriglyceridemia and also a high concentration of serum triglyceride-transporting lipoproteins, such as very-low-density lipoproteins (VLDLs). This is due to decreased activity of lipoprotein lipase and to CKD-associated insulin resistance which enhances VLDL production. Secondly, in CKD there is an increase in the concentration of highly atherogenic small dense low-density lipoproteins (LDL). Thirdly, CKD is associated with low levels of circulating high-density lipoprotein (HDL) particles, which also have their anti-oxidant and anti-inflammatory actions impaired [48].

Dyslipidemia in CKD promotes ED, increases CV risk and also promotes CKD progression [48, 49]. It has been suggested that vitamin D regulates endothelial function also by interfering with lipid metabolism. Vitamin D levels positively associate with HDL-cholesterol and negatively associate with triglycerides in observational studies. Unexpectedly, in some studies, vitamin D levels positively correlate with LDL-cholesterol also. Despite this, vitamin D remains negatively associated with LDL-cholesterol/HDL-cholesterol ratio, suggesting that the most significant effect of vitamin D does not regard cholesterol fractions taken individually, but implies the favorable modulation of lipid balance. However, results from interventional studies that evaluated the effects of vitamin D supplementation on lipid profile are conflicting: some did not reveal any influence; other reported significantly increased levels of LDL-cholesterol or of both LDL-cholesterol and triglycerides [50]. In a meta-analysis performed by Wang et al. [51] that included RCTs, contrary to expectations, vitamin D supplementation was shown only to increase LDL-cholesterol, without any significant effect on the other lipid fractions.

Statin therapy moderately improves vitamin D status by significantly increasing 25(OH)D levels in vitamin D-deficient, hyperlipidemic patients. Furthermore, they improves renal endothelial function by increasing basal NO activity in the renal endothelium also. The mechanisms by which statins interfere with vitamin D levels are not known. It has been speculated that the inhibition of hydroxyl-methyl-glutaryl-CoA reductase (HMG-CoA reductase) by statins favors high levels of vitamin D precursor in the skin [31]. However, contradictory results been reported by other groups; thus, patients treated by statins exhibit lower $25(OH)D_3$ values have by an unclear mechanism [52]. It is also known that statins have pleiotropic effects. Besides having anti-inflammatory and direct anti-atherogenic effects, statins also protect the endothelium: statins blunt eNOS down-regulation induced by oxidized LDL and increase eNOS expression at the post-translational level [53]. Statins also increase the number of circulating endothelial progenitor cells, which are known to promote endothelial repair and thus conserve endothelial function [10, 53].

In CKD, the triangle vitamin D-lipids-endothelial function seems to be affected at all levels. Vitamin D deficiency and dyslipidemia may have additive negative effects on endothelial function, although evidence suggests that vitamin D deficiency and lipid abnormalities may actually potentiate one another.

20.5.4 Inflammation

The pleiotropic effects of vitamin D also include immunomodulatory properties: vitamin D deficiency contributes to CKD-associated inflammatory state and also promotes cardiovascular inflammation and by this, ED [54]. Vitamin D deficiency is associated with increased expression of proinflammatory NF-kB and IL-6 in endothelial cells [55] and with high circulating levels of CRP and IL-6 [56]. Paricalcitol administration in CKD down-regulates circulating high-sensitivity CRP and both serum and mononuclear cells expression of TNF-α and IL-6 [57]. High levels of CRP activate the endothelium by promoting increased expression of adhesion molecules and lead to ED by triggering endothelin-1 release and down-regulating eNOS [49]. IL-6 triggers oxidative stress generation via up-regulation of AT_1R and RAAS activation in the vessels, leading to impaired endothelium-dependent vasodilation and, finally, atherosclerosis [58]. At the same time, inflammatory markers are predictors of CVD and mortality in the CKD population: CRP predicts CVD in CKD non-dialysis patients, CRP and IL-6 are predictors of CV and all-cause mortality in ESRD, TNF-α predicts all-cause mortality in ESRD [59].

The mechanisms through which vitamin D regulates proinflammatory cytokines expression are various. Firstly, vitamin D inhibits the activation of TNF-α converting enzyme (TACE), which causes renal and systemic inflammation by releasing TNF-α and soluble adhesion molecules. Also vitamin D suppresses RAAS activation, also a trigger of TACE activation. Secondly, vitamin D is negatively correlated with albuminuria which is per se a proinflammatory condition in CKD, where it is associated with high IL-6 concentration. Thirdly, vitamin D down-regulates NF-kB activation and subsequently the overexpression of regulated on activation, normal T cell expressed and secreted RANTES (regulated on activation, normal T cell expressed and secreted chemokine) protein, a chemokine responsible with leukocyte recruitment and promotion of chronic inflammation [54, 60].

Therefore, vitamin D deficiency triggers and maintains the low-grade inflammation in CKD, in addition to other factors (e.g. uremia, AGEs, oxidative stress, atherosclerosis, obesity, etc.). This leads to endothelial dysfunction and CV injury, thus partially explaining why CVD is the main cause of death in ESRD patients [54, 59].

20.5.5   Secondary Hyperparathyroidism

Secondary hyperparathyroidism (SHPT) due to vitamin D deficiency in CKD may also have deleterious effects on the vasculature. Increased PTH has been linked to a higher mortality and to a significant decrease in median life expectancy in elderly subjects [61]. Serum PTH levels above 250 pg/ml significantly increases the risk for coronary artery disease in chronic hemodialysis patients with SHPT [62]. In patients with primary hyperparathyroidism, high PTH independently predicts a lower FMD [63]. Even in mild primary hyperparathyroidism, parathyroidectomy improves endothelial function (FMD) in patients having endothelial dysfunction prior to the intervention [64].

In animal models of CKD, parathyroidectomy increases eNOS expression and activity, which are down-regulated in chronic renal failure rats without parathyroidectomy. Similar effects are obtained by administrating calcium channel blockers instead of performing parathyroidectomy, suggesting that NOS impairment in CKD is due to CKD-associated calcium disequilibrium [65]. However, there are studies that showed a direct effect exerted by PTH on endothelial cells. Thus, Chen at al. demonstrated that serum from SHPT patients inhibited human endothelial cell proliferation in vitro [66]. Also, PTH increases the gene and protein expression of AGE receptors, and also of IL-6 gene expression, in endothelial cells. Hence, PTH can trigger endothelium cells activation which is the first step towards the installment of ED [10, 67].

Therefore, vitamin D deficiency alters endothelial function in CKD also by triggering SHPT and subsequent calcium disturbances. SHPT promotes ED directly, and also by SHPT-induced hypercalcemia.

20.5.6   Klotho-Fibroblast Growth Factor-23 (FGF-23) Axis

FGF23 has emerged as a new biomarker for CKD progression and also for CV and bone metabolism complications associated to CKD. This is due to the fact that FGF23 rises early in CKD to enhance renal phosphate excretion and thus to maintain phosphorus homeostasis. Despite being the main phosphaturic hormone, FGF23 in high concentrations also has numerous off-target effects, especially on the cardiovascular system. This explains why FGF23 in ESRD patients is associated with vascular calcifications, left ventricular calcifications and increased mortality risk [68].

Phosphorus is the main stimulus for FGF23 production and release from the bone. High serum levels of FGF23 contribute to vitamin D deficiency in CKD by inhibiting the activity of renal 1α-hydroxylase. Experimental studies showed that calcitriol is also a potent inducer of circulating FGF23, independently of phosphate and PTH [69]. This raises the question whether calcitriol administration in CKD increases serum FGF23 levels and thus indirectly has deleterious CV effects. However, the increased serum FGF23 levels depends on vitamin D cumulative dose and may be prevented by associating cinacalcet to low-dose therapy with calcitriol or vitamin D analogs in ESRD that actually results in serum FGF23 decrease [70, 71]. The reported vitamin D effects on circulating FGF23 are inconsistent: cholecalciferol treatment did not modify serum FGF23 levels in CKD stage 3–4 patients in the study performed by Chitalia et al. [33]. In addition, escalating doses of calcitriol analogs failed to significantly increase FGF23 in ESRD patients from the ACHIEVE trial [71].

Although the effect of vitamin D supplementation on serum FGF23 levels in CKD is not yet clarified, high serum FGF23 concentration encountered in CKD triggers vitamin D deficiency and SHPT, two conditions associated with ED [72, 73]. FGF23 is associated with impaired endothelial vasodilator response to acetylcholine in elderly subjects with normal kidney function and with arterial stiffness in elderly subjects with impaired renal function [74]. It seems that high serum FGF23 levels predict not only ED, but also its progression to arterial stiffness as kidney function declines. In this direction, FGF23 is an independent positive predictor of carotid IMT, a marker of subclinical atherosclerosis, in ESRD patients [75, 76].

FGF23 signaling pathway activation requires klotho, a transmembrane protein that functions as a critical co-factor by increasing the affinity of FGF receptors for FGF23 in the kidney [77]. Klotho has pleiotropic effects: the extracellular domain is secreted into the circulation and partly mediates klotho anti-aging actions. In this regard, klotho also protects endothelial cells against senescence and apoptosis, two processes that are known to promote ED and atherosclerosis [78]. Klotho is down-regulated in CKD by increased RAAS activity [79]. This contributes to ED, as klotho deficit is associated with low NO and impaired endothelium-dependent vasodilator response to acetylcholine in mice. The mechanism by which klotho regulates NO still needs clarifying [80].

Nevertheless, CKD is associated with important imbalances of the vitamin D-FGF23-klotho axis, with all elements disturbed and contributing to ED. Vitamin D deficiency is acquired in CKD due to limited availability of 1α-hydroxylase and decreased activity but also due to increased serum FGF23 levels [72, 79]. Further on, vitamin D deficit allows renin gene to be up-regulated (see above) [44]. Activation of RAAS and overexpression of angiotensin II down-regulates klotho renal expression and thus impairs FGF23 signaling and leads to FGF23 resistance. Subsequently, hyperphosphatemia aggravates and this stimulates even a greater release of FGF23, which closes the loop by further inhibiting 1α-hydroxylase activity. Low serum vitamin D levels, high circulating FGF23 and low klotho levels and RAAS overactivation all lead to ED [79].

20.6 Conclusions

Endothelial dysfunction is the major common pathway through which CV risk factors lead to CVD in CKD. In fact, it represents the initial arterial lesion that eventually leads to atherosclerosis and arteriosclerosis. Abnormal vitamin D metabolism is a sine qua non condition of CKD that has also been related to ED. Vitamin D deficiency promotes ED in even in the early stages of CKD through both direct and indirect mechanisms. Locally activated $1,25(OH)_2D_3$ is an important regulator of endothelial functions: it promotes NO synthesis and thus endothelium-dependent vasodilation and also endothelial cell proliferation and survival. $1,25(OH)_2D_3$ also has anti-inflammatory and anti-oxidative effects in the endothelium. Moreover, in diabetic patients with CKD, vitamin D deficit favors poor glycemic control and atherogenesis. In addition, vitamin D deficit triggers overactivation of RAAS, increased generation of oxidative stress, abnormal lipid metabolism, increased systemic and renal inflammation and SHPT, all with deleterious effects on the endothelium. Further on, SHPT leads to increased FGF23 synthesis and release while RAAS downregulates klotho, two actions which bring additional injury to the vessels. Therefore, vitamin D deficiency activates a wide cascade of events that potentiate one another, finally leading to a closed loop where each element is responsible for the altering of endothelium function in CKD. Although interventional studies have proven the benefits of administering both vitamin D and vitamin D analogues in rickets/osteomalacia and osteoporotic fractures treatment, they are however limited for the improvement of endothelial function in CKD. There is much less evidence for beneficial effects on inflammation, autoimmune or cardiovascular diseases, although this could be due to the existence of different therapeutic target levels for each disease. Therefore, vitamin D supplementation for targeting ED in CKD remains an open chapter, where much remains to be written.

References

1. Hajhosseiny R, Khavandi K, Goldsmith DJ. Cardiovascular disease in chronic kidney disease: untying the Gordian knot. Int J Clin Pract. 2013;67:14–31.
2. McCullough PA, Steigerwalt S, Tolia K, Chen SC, Li S, Norris KC, Whaley-Connell A. Cardiovascular disease in chronic kidney disease: data from the Kidney Early Evaluation Program (KEEP). Curr Diab Rep. 2011;11:47–55.
3. Moody WE, Edwards N, Madhani M, Chue CD, Steeds RP, Ferro CJ, Townend JN. Endothelial dysfunction and cardiovascular disease in early-stage chronic kidney disease: cause or association? Atherosclerosis. 2012;223:86–94.
4. Stam F, et al. Endothelial dysfunction contributes to renal function-associated cardiovascular mortality in a population with mild renal insufficiency: the Hoorn study. J Am Soc Nephrol. 2006;17(2):537–45.
5. Norman AW. From vitamin D to hormone D: fundamentals of the vitamin D endocrine system essential for good health. Am J Clin Nutr. 2008;88(2):491s–9.
6. Chonchol M, Kendrick J, Targher G. Extra-skeletal effects of vitamin D deficiency in chronic kidney disease. Ann Med. 2011;43(4):273–82.

7. Holick MF. Vitamin D deficiency. N Engl J Med. 2007;357(3):266–81.
8. Malyszko J. Mechanism of endothelial dysfunction in chronic kidney disease. Clin Chim Acta. 2010;411:1412–20.
9. Seals DR, Jablonski K, Donato AJ. Aging and vascular endothelial function in humans. Clin Sci. 2011;120:357–75.
10. Dalan R, Liew H, Tan WKA, Chew DEK, Leow MKS. Vitamin D and the endothelium: basic, translational and clinical research updates. IJC Metab Endocr. 2014;4:4–17.
11. Verma S, Anderson T. Fundamentals of endothelial function for the clinical cardiologist. Circulation. 2002;105:546–9.
12. Goligorsky MS. Pathogenesis of endothelial cell dysfunction in chronic kidney disease: a retrospective and what the future may hold. Kidney Res Clin Pract. 2015;34:76–82.
13. Andrukhova O, et al. Vitamin D is a regulator of endothelial nitric oxide synthase and arterial stiffness in mice. Mol Endocrinol. 2014;28(1):53–64.
14. Uberti F, et al. Vitamin D protects human endothelial cells from oxidative stress through the autophagic and survival pathways. J Clin Endocrinol Metab. 2014;99(4):1367–74.
15. Wong MS, et al. Chronic treatment with vitamin D lowers arterial blood pressure and reduces endothelium-dependent contractions in the aorta of the spontaneously hypertensive rat. Am J Physiol Heart Circ Physiol. 2010;299(4):H1226–34.
16. Zhong W, et al. Activation of vitamin D receptor promotes VEGF and CuZn-SOD expression in endothelial cells. J Steroid Biochem Mol Biol. 2014;140:56–62.
17. Tarcin O, et al. Effect of vitamin D deficiency and replacement on endothelial function in asymptomatic subjects. J Clin Endocrinol Metab. 2009;94(10):4023–30.
18. Jablonski KL, et al. 25-Hydroxyvitamin D deficiency is associated with inflammation-linked vascular endothelial dysfunction in middle-aged and older adults. Hypertension. 2011;57(1):63–9.
19. Sokol SI, et al. The effects of vitamin D repletion on endothelial function and inflammation in patients with coronary artery disease. Vasc Med. 2012;17(6):394–404.
20. Witham MD, et al. Effect of short-term vitamin D supplementation on markers of vascular health in South Asian women living in the UK – a randomised controlled trial. Atherosclerosis. 2013;230(2):293–9.
21. Pittarella P, et al. NO-dependent proliferation and migration induced by Vitamin D in HUVEC. J Steroid Biochem Mol Biol. 2015;149:35–42.
22. Recio-Mayoral A, Banerjee D, Streather C, Kaski JC. Endothelial dysfunction, inflammation and atherosclerosis in chronic kidney disease – a cross-sectional study of predialysis, dialysis and kidney-transplantation patients. Atherosclerosis. 2011;216:446–51.
23. Wu-Wong JR, Li X, Chen YW. Different vitamin D receptor agonists exhibit differential effects on endothelial function and aortic gene expression in 5/6 nephrectomized rats. J Steroid Biochem Mol Biol. 2015;148:202–9.
24. Yilmaz MI, et al. Longitudinal analysis of vascular function and biomarkers of metabolic bone disorders before and after renal transplantation. Am J Nephrol. 2013;37(2):126–34.
25. London GM, et al. Mineral metabolism and arterial functions in end-stage renal disease: potential role of 25-hydroxyvitamin D deficiency. J Am Soc Nephrol. 2007;18(2):613–20.
26. Wu-Wong JR, Noonan W, Nakane M, Brooks KA, Segreti JA, Polakowski JS, Cox B. Vitamin d receptor activation mitigates the impact of uremia on endothelial function in the 5/6 nephrectomized rats. Int J Endocrinol. 2010;2010:625852.
27. Talmor-Barkan Y, Bernheim J, Green J, Benchetrit S, Rashid G. Calcitriol counteracts endothelial cell pro-inflammatory processes in a chronic kidney disease-like environment. J Steroid Biochem Mol Biol. 2011;124:19–24.
28. Zhang QY, Jiang C, Sun C, Tang TF, Jin B, Cao DW, He JS, Zhang M. Hypovitaminosis D is associated with endothelial dysfunction in patients with non-dialysis chronic kidney disease. J Nephrol. 2015;28:471–6.
29. Chitalia N, Recio-Mayoral A, Kaski JC, Banerjee D. Vitamin D deficiency and endothelial dysfunction in non-dialysis chronic kidney disease patients. Atherosclerosis. 2012;220:265–8.

30. London GM, Guérin A, Verbeke FH, Pannier B, Boutouyrie P, Marchais SJ, Metivier F. Mineral metabolism and arterial functions in end-stage renal disease: potential role of 25-hydroxyvitamin D deficiency. J Am Soc Nephrol. 2007;18:613–20.
31. Ott C, Raff U, Schneider MP, Titze SI, Schmieder RE. 25-hydroxyvitamin D insufficiency is associated with impaired renal endothelial function and both are improved with rosuvastatin treatment. Clin Res Cardiol. 2013;102:299–304.
32. Dreyer G, Tucker A, Dreyer G, Harwood SM, Pearse RM, Raftery MJ, Yaqoob MM. Ergocalciferol and microcirculatory function in chronic kidney disease and concomitant vitamin d deficiency: an exploratory, double blind, randomised controlled trial. PLoS One. 2014;9:e99461.
33. Chitalia N, Ismail T, Tooth L, Boa F, Hampson G, Goldsmith D, Kaski JC, Banerjee D. Impact of vitamin D supplementation on arterial vasomotion, stiffness and endothelial biomarkers in chronic kidney disease patients. PLoS One. 2014;9:e91363.
34. Zoccali C, Curatola G, Panuccio V, Tripepi R, Pizzini P, Versace M, Bolignano D, Cutrupi S, Politi R, Tripepi G, Ghiadoni L, Thadhani R, Mallamaci F. Paricalcitol and endothelial function in chronic kidney disease trial. Hypertension. 2014;64:1005–11.
35. Alborzi P, Patel N, Peterson C, Bills JE, Bekele DM, Bunaye Z, Light RP, Agarwal R. Paricalcitol reduces albuminuria and inflammation in chronic kidney disease: a randomized double-blind pilot trial. Hypertension. 2008;64:1005–11.
36. Thethi TK, Bajwa M, Ghanim H, Jo C, Weir M, Goldfine AB, Umpierrez G, Desouza C, Dandona P, Fang-Hollingsworth Y, Raghavan V, Fonseca VA. Effect of paricalcitol on endothelial function and inflammation in type 2 diabetes and chronic kidney disease. J Diabetes Complications. 2015;29:433–7.
37. Yiu Y, Chan Y, Yiu KH, Siu CW, Li SW, Wong LY, Lee SW, Tam S, Wong EW, Cheung BM, Tse HF. Vitamin D deficiency is associated with depletion of circulating endothelial progenitor cells and endothelial dysfunction in patients with type 2 diabetes. J Clin Endocrinol Metab. 2011;96:E830–5.
38. Talmor Y, Golan E, Benchetrit S, Bernheim J, Klein O, Green J, Rashid G. Calcitriol blunts the deleterious impact of advanced glycation end products on endothelial cells. Am J Physiol Renal Physiol. 2008;294:F1059–64.
39. Oh J, Weng S, Felton SK, Bhandare S, Riek A, Butler B, Proctor BM, Petty M, Chen Z, Schechtman KB, Bernal-Mizrachi L, Bernal-Mizrachi C. 1,25(OH)2 vitamin d inhibits foam cell formation and suppresses macrophage cholesterol uptake in patients with type 2 diabetes mellitus. Circulation. 2009;120:687–98.
40. Yiu YF, Yiu K, Siu CW, Chan YH, Li SW, Wong LY, Lee SW, Tam S, Wong EW, Lau CP, Cheung BM, Tse HF. Randomized controlled trial of vitamin D supplement on endothelial function in patients with type 2 diabetes. Atherosclerosis. 2013;227:140–6.
41. Andrukhova O, Slavic S, Zeitz U, Riesen SC, Heppelmann MS, Ambrisko TD, Markovic M, Kuebler WM, Erben RG. Vitamin D is a regulator of endothelial nitric oxide synthase and arterial stiffness in mice. Mol Endocrinol. 2014;28:53–64.
42. Vaidya A, Forman J. Vitamin D and vascular disease: the current and future status of vitamin D therapy in hypertension and kidney disease. Curr Hypertens Rep. 2012;14:111–9.
43. Dong J, Wong S, Lau CW, Lee HK, Ng CF, Zhang L, Yao X, Chen ZY, Vanhoutte PM, Huang Y. Calcitriol protects renovascular function in hypertension by down-regulating angiotensin II type 1 receptors and reducing oxidative stress. Eur Heart J. 2012;33:2980–90.
44. Yuan W, Pan W, Kong J, Zheng W, Szeto FL, Wong KE, Cohen R, Klopot A, Zhang Z, Li YC. 1,25-dihydroxyvitamin D3 suppresses renin gene transcription by blocking the activity of the cyclic AMP response element in the renin gene promoter. J Biol Chem. 2007;282:29821–30.
45. Yang YM, Huang A, Kaley G, Sun D. eNOS uncoupling and endothelial dysfunction in aged vessels. Am J Physiol Heart Circ Physiol. 2009;297:H1829–36.
46. Feletou M, Huang Y, Vanhoutte PM. Endothelium-mediated control of vascular tone: COX-1 and COX-2 products. Br J Pharmacol. 2011;164:894–912.
47. Wong MS, Delansorne R, Man RY, Vanhoutte PM. Vitamin D derivatives acutely reduce endothelium-dependent contractions in the aorta of the spontaneously hypertensive rat. Am J Physiol Heart Circ Physiol. 2008;295:H289–96.

48. Nitta K. Clinical assessment and management of dyslipidemia in patients with chronic kidney disease. Clin Exp Nephrol. 2012;16:522–9.
49. Husain K, Hernandez W, Ansari RA, Ferder L. Inflammation, oxidative stress and renin angiotensin system in atherosclerosis. World J Biol Chem. 2015;6:209–17.
50. Jorde R, Grimnes G. Vitamin D and metabolic health with special reference to the effect of vitamin D on serum lipids. Prog Lipid Res. 2011;50:303–12.
51. Wang H, Xia N, Peng D. Influence of vitamin D supplementation on plasma lipid profiles: a meta-analysis of randomized controlled trials. Lipids Health Dis. 2012;11:42.
52. Yuste C, et al. The effect of some medications given to CKD patients on vitamin D levels. Nefrologia. 2015;35(2):150–6.
53. Blum A, Shamburek R. The pleiotropic effects of statins on endothelial function, vascular inflammation, immunomodulation and thrombogenesis. Atherosclerosis. 2009;203:325–30.
54. Querfeld U. Vitamin D and inflammation. Pediatr Nephrol. 2013;28:605–10.
55. Jablonski KL, Chonchol M, Pierce GL, Walker AE, Seals DR. 25-Hydroxyvitamin D deficiency is associated with inflammation-linked vascular endothelial dysfunction in middle-aged and older adults. Hypertension. 2011;57:63–9.
56. Kalkwarf HJ, Denburg M, Strife CF, Zemel BS, Foerster DL, Wetzsteon RJ, Leonard MB. Vitamin D deficiency is common in children and adolescents with chronic kidney disease. Kidney Int. 2012;81:690–7.
57. Donate-Correa J, Domínguez-Pimentel V, Méndez-Pérez ML, Muros-de-Fuentes M, Mora-Fernández C, Martín-Núñez E, Cazaña-Pérez V, Navarro-González JF. Selective vitamin D receptor activation as anti-inflammatory target in chronic kidney disease. Mediators Inflamm. 2014;2014:670475.
58. Wassmann S, Stumpf M, Strehlow K, Schmid A, Schieffer B, Böhm M, Nickenig G. Interleukin-6 induces oxidative stress and endothelial dysfunction by overexpression of the angiotensin II type 1 receptor. Circ Res. 2004;94:534–41.
59. Elewa U, Sanchez-Niño NM, Martin-Cleary C, Fernandez-Fernandez B, Egido J, Ortiz A. Cardiovascular risk biomarkers in CKD: the inflammation link and the road less traveled. Int Urol Nephrol. 2012;44:1731–44.
60. Ajuebor MN, Hogaboam C, Kunkel SL, Proudfoot AE, Wallace JL. The chemokine RANTES is a crucial mediator of the progression from acute to chronic colitis in the rat. J Immunol. 2001;166:552–8.
61. Björkman MP, Sorva A, Tilvis RS. Elevated serum parathyroid hormone predicts impaired survival prognosis in a general aged population. Eur J Endocrinol. 2008;158:749–53.
62. Soubassi LP, Chiras T, Papadakis ED, Poulos GD, Chaniotis DI, Tsapakidis IP, Soubassi SP, Zerefos SN, Zerefos NS, Valis DA. Incidence and risk factors of coronary heart disease in elderly patients on chronic hemodialysis. Int Urol Nephrol. 2006;38:795–800.
63. Ekmekci A, Abaci N, Colak Ozbey N, Agayev A, Aksakal N, Oflaz H, Erginel-Unaltuna N, Erbil Y. Endothelial function and endothelial nitric oxide synthase intron 4a/b polymorphism in primary hyperparathyroidism. J Endocrinol Invest. 2009;32:611–6.
64. Carrelli AL, Walker M, Di Tullio MR, Homma S, Zhang C, McMahon DJ, Silverberg SJ. Endothelial function in mild primary hyperparathyroidism. Clin Endocrinol (Oxf). 2013;78:204–9.
65. Vaziri ND, Ni Z, Wang XQ, Oveisi F, Zhou XJ. Downregulation of nitric oxide synthase in chronic renal insufficiency: role of excess PTH. Am J Physiol. 1998;274:F642–9.
66. Chen C, Mao H, Yu X, Sun B, Zeng M, Zhao X, Qian J, Liu J, Xing C. (Abstract) Effect of secondary hyperparathyroidism serum on endothelial cells and intervention with Klotho. Mol Med Rep. 2015;12:1983–90.
67. Rashid G, Bernheim J, Green J, Benchetrit S. Parathyroid hormone stimulates endothelial expression of atherosclerotic parameters through protein kinase pathways. Am J Physiol Renal Physiol. 2007;292:F1215–8.
68. Juppner H, Wolf M, Salusky I. FGF-23: more than a regulator of renal phosphate handling? J Bone Miner Res. 2010;25:2091–7.

69. Saito H, Maeda A, Ohtomo S, Hirata M, Kusano K, Kato S, Ogata E, Segawa H, Miyamoto K, Fukushima N. Circulating FGF-23 is regulated by 1alpha,25-dihydroxyvitamin D3 and phosphorus in vivo. J Biol Chem. 2005;280:2543–9.
70. Nishi H, Nii-Kono T, Nakanishi S, Yamazaki Y, Yamashita T, Fukumoto S, Ikeda K, Fujimori A, Fukagawa M. Intravenous calcitriol therapy increases serum concentrations of fibroblast growth factor-23 in dialysis patients with secondary hyperparathyroidism. Nephron Clin Pract. 2005;101:c94–9.
71. Wetmore JB, Liu S, Krebill R, Menard R, Quarles LD. Effects of cinacalcet and concurrent low-dose vitamin D on FGF23 levels in ESRD. Clin J Am Soc Nephrol. 2010;5:110–6.
72. Dusso A, González E, Martin KJ. Vitamin D in chronic kidney disease. Best Pract Res Clin Endocrinol Metab. 2011;25:647–55.
73. Hu P, Xuan Q, Hu B, Lu L, Wang J, Qin YH. Fibroblast growth factor-23 helps explain the biphasic cardiovascular effects of vitamin D in chronic kidney disease. Int J Biol Sci. 2012;8:663–71.
74. Mirza MA, Larsson A, Lind L, Larsson TE. Circulating fibroblast growth factor-23 is associated with vascular dysfunction in the community. Atherosclerosis. 2009;205:385–90.
75. Balci M, Kirkpantur A, Gulbay M, Gurbuz OA. Plasma fibroblast growth factor-23 levels are independently associated with carotid artery atherosclerosis in maintenance hemodialysis patients. Hemodial Int. 2010;14:425–32.
76. De Backer GG. New risk markers for cardiovascular prevention. Curr Atheroscler Rep. 2014;16:427.
77. Kurosu H, Kuro-o M. The Klotho gene family as a regulator of endocrine fibroblast growth factors. Mol Cell Endocrinol. 2009;299:72–8.
78. Ikushima M, Rakugi H, Ishikawa K, Maekawa Y, Yamamoto K, Ohta J, Chihara Y, Kida I, Ogihara T. Anti-apoptotic and anti-senescence effects of Klotho on vascular endothelial cells. Biochem Biophys Res Commun. 2006;339:827–32.
79. de Borst MH, Vervloet M, ter Wee PM, Navis G. Cross talk between the renin-angiotensin-aldosterone system and vitamin D-FGF-23-klotho in chronic kidney disease. J Am Soc Nephrol. 2011;22:1603–9.
80. Saito Y, Yamagishi T, Nakamura T, Ohyama Y, Aizawa H, Suga T, Matsumura Y, Masuda H, Kurabayashi M, Kuro-o M, Nabeshima Y, Nagai R. Klotho protein protects against endothelial dysfunction. Biochem Biophys Res Commun. 1998;248:324–9.

Chapter 21
Vitamin D and Cardiovascular Calcification in Chronic Kidney Disease

Lucie Hénaut, Aurélien Mary, Said Kamel, and Ziad A. Massy

Abstract Cardiovascular calcification is a common problem among chronic kidney disease (CKD) patients. Altered vitamin D status (another key feature of CKD) has a major impact on mineral and bone disorders, including cardiovascular calcification. Preclinical and clinical studies have shown that both abnormally low and abnormally high vitamin D levels have local and systemic effects on cardiovascular calcification in CKD patients. This complex situation has major repercussions on the choice and monitoring of the dose of vitamin D prescribed to prevent and/or treat cardiovascular calcification in CKD.

Keywords Chronic kidney disease • Dialysis • Cardiovascular calcification • Vitamin D

21.1 Introduction

Chronic kidney disease (CKD) is characterized by the appearance of proteinuria and/or a progressive reduction in the glomerular filtration rate. Subsequently, blood levels of organic waste compounds called uraemic toxins rise progressively. Over the last few decades, the harmful effects of a large number of uraemic toxins on

L. Hénaut, PhD
INSERM Unit 1088 and Department of Biochemistry, University Hospital,
University of Picardie Jules Vernes and CHU d'amiens, Picardie, France

A. Mary, PharmD, PhD
INSERM Unit 1088, University of Picardie Jules Vernes, Amiens, France

S. Kamel, PharmD, PhD
INSERM Unit 1088 and Department of Biochemistry, University Hospital,
University of Picardie Jules Vernes and CHU d'amiens,
Centre Universitaire de Recherche en Santé (CURS),
Chemin du Thil, Amiens, Picardie, France

Z.A. Massy, MD, PhD, FERA (✉)
Division of Nephrology, Ambroise Paré University Hospital, Boulogne, France
e-mail: ziad.massy@aphp.fr

© Springer International Publishing Switzerland 2016   361
P.A. Ureña Torres et al. (eds.), *Vitamin D in Chronic Kidney Disease*,
DOI 10.1007/978-3-319-32507-1_21

organs and tissues (and especially the cardiovascular system) have been demonstrated.

Cardiovascular calcification is a common problem among CKD patients. The prevalence of this condition increases as kidney function fails. Cardiovascular calcification is a complex process that involves not only simple mineral precipitation (due to supersaturated phosphate and calcium concentrations in the extracellular milieu, i.e. a mineral step) but also a tightly regulated, cell-mediated process including apoptosis, osteochondrogenic differentiation, and elastin degradation (cellular step). The time course and order of appearance of these two steps in vivo have yet to be well characterized. The genesis and progression of cardiovascular calcification are controlled by inhibitory proteins and non-peptide factors (such as carboxylated matrix Gla protein, pyrophosphate (PPi), magnesium, osteopontin and calcium-sensing receptors (CaSRs)) and stimulatory proteins and non-peptide factors (such as phosphate, indoxyl sulphate, receptor activator of nuclear factor kappa-B ligand (RANKL), inflammation and the products of oxidative stress). Elevated levels of inorganic phosphate (Pi) or extracellular calcium [Ca^{2+}], inflammation and/or vascular injury lead to the conversion of vascular smooth muscle cells (VSMCs), resident fibroblasts or quiescent valve interstitial cells (VICs) into osteochondrogenic cells that start to express runx2, osterix, alkaline phosphatase (ALP), and type I collagen. This phenomenon is associated with the production and release of calcifying matrix vesicles and with extracellular matrix remodelling (type I collagen synthesis and elastin degradation). Furthermore, this calcifying environment promotes vascular cell apoptosis and consumes antioxidants, which favours the release of apoptotic bodies capable of nucleating hydroxyapatite [1]. In the medial part of the vessel, some calcifying agents (such as P_i) promote the expression of matrix metalloproteases (MMP)-2 and -9 and cathepsin S. By degrading the elastic fibers these enzymes release osteogenic products with a high affinity for calcium [2, 3].

Cardiovascular calcification is part of mineral and bone disorders, which are very common in CKD and now collectively are referred to as CKD–MBD. Altered vitamin D status (an ubiquitous feature of CKD) is a key feature of CKD–MBD and has major clinical implications. Given that the metabolism and physiopathology of vitamin D are described in detail in other chapters of this book, we shall focus here on the role of vitamin D in cardiovascular calcification. In summary, declining renal function leads to a general deficiency of vitamin D as a result of (i) a decrease in renal 1α-hydroxylase activity in response to elevated levels of phosphate, FGF-23 (a direct inhibitor of 1α-hydroxylase activity) and uraemic toxins [4, 5], (ii) a possible decrease in hepatic 25(OH)D synthesis [6], and (iii) an increase in levels of renal 24 hydroxylase (the enzyme involved in 25(OH)D and 1,25(OH)$_2$D degradation) in response to elevated FGF-23 levels [4]. Hypovitaminosis D may also be due to an insufficient dietary vitamin D intake or low photosynthetic activity. Along with the altered production and metabolism of calcitriol, renal failure is associated with calcitriol resistance as a result of (i) altered expression of the vitamin D receptor (VDR) and (ii) altered binding properties between VDR and the vitamin D response element (VDRE) [7, 8]. Thus, both native vitamin D and active vitamin D sterols (also referred to as vitamin D receptor activators or agonists (VDRAs)) may be useful treatments for secondary hyperparathyroidism (SHPT) – a condition associated with cardiovascular calcification and CKD-MBD. However, pharmacological doses of VDRAs can result in adverse effects, such as the development of adynamic bone disease, hypercalcemia and/or hyperphosphatemia – all of which favour the development of cardiovascular calcification. The more recently developed VDRAs (such as paricalcitol) are reportedly more selective in suppressing PTH secretion and are less hypercalcaemic and hyperphosphataemic. However, the relationship between native vitamin D/VDRAs on one hand and cardiovascular calcification on the other is very complex, since both high and low serum levels of native and active vitamin D have been linked to cardiovascular calcification in CKD patients. In 2008, Shroff et al. reported that paediatric dialysis patients with either low or high $1,25(OH)_2D$ serum levels had a significantly greater carotid intima-media thickness ($p<0.0001$) and significantly greater cardiovascular calcification ($p=0.0002$) than those with normal $1,25(OH)_2D$ levels [9]. These data suggest the existence of a U-shaped relationship between cardiovascular calcification and outcomes on one hand and $1,25(OH)_2D$ levels on the other. Since then, several in vitro, animal and clinical studies have sought to establish how both abnormally low and abnormally high levels of native vitamin D or VDRAs are involved in cardiovascular calcification. However, mechanistic conclusions are difficult to draw since native vitamin D or VDRAs may modulate cardiovascular calcification either through systemic effects or by local direct effects on target vascular cells.

Through an in-depth analysis of the available preclinical and clinical evidence, this chapter reviews the contrasting local and systemic effects of abnormally low and abnormally high vitamin D levels on cardiovascular calcification in CKD patients.

21.2   Vitamin D and Cardiovascular Calcification in CKD Patients

Disturbances in mineral homeostasis (such as hyperphosphatemia and SHPT as a result of calcitriol deficiency) are key factors for cardiovascular calcification in CKD patients [10]. In the first retrospective study to be published, autopsy data from children (aged 10–13) with end-stage renal disease (ESRD) suggested that VDRAs in general (and calcitriol in particular) may contribute significantly to vascular and tissue calcification [11]. A second retrospective study showed a positive correlation between circulating 25(OH)D levels and the calcification score in 38 patients undergoing long-term dialysis [12]. These observations were later confirmed in young adults with childhood-onset ESRD, in whom VDRAs intake was associated with coronary artery calcification [13].

Nevertheless, doubt persisted with regard to this adverse event, since other retrospective studies in larger cohorts of patients undergoing dialysis did not find any correlation between vitamin D intake and coronary artery calcification [14, 15]. Moreover, several epidemiological studies of CKD patients undergoing (or not) dialysis did not show a positive correlation between low 25(OH)D or 1,25(OH)D serum concentrations and coronary artery calcification [16–18]. In fact, some studies even reported a negative correlation between low levels of 25(OH)D and the calcification score in end-stage CKD patients [19, 20] and in dialysis patients [20, 21]. Furthermore, a large study (of 1,370 participants, including 394 with CKD) found an association (after adjustment) between 25(OH)D and the risk of developing incident coronary artery calcification but not the prevalence of calcification [22]. Even though these studies in CKD patients failed to observe a correlation between 1,25(OH)D and cardiovascular calcification (suggesting a possible physiological effect that was independent of renal 1α-hydroxylase), 1,25(OH)D levels were shown to be inversely correlated with coronary calcification in non-CKD patients with a moderate-to-high risk of coronary heart disease [23]. More puzzlingly, an observational study by Ogawa et al. reported that the prescription of higher dose of a VDRA (1α-hydroxy vitamin D3) appeared to protect haemodialysis patients from developing calcification of the aortic arch [24]. Accordingly, a recent meta-analysis of observational studies showed that treatment with VDRAs (but not with non-active oral medications) was associated with a decreased risk of both all-cause and cardiovascular mortality in patients with CKD not requiring dialysis and in patients with ESRD requiring dialysis [25].

To date, discrepancies between the findings of observational or retrospective studies have prevented researchers from drawing firm conclusions as to the effect of vitamin D supplementation on the development of cardiovascular calcification. All the meta-analyses in this field have been limited by the lack of adequately powered randomized controlled trials (RCTs) with cardiovascular calcification as a primary endpoint. The meta-analyses concluded that vitamin D derivatives (whatever the administration route or type of compound – non-active, active or new) effectively reduce PTH levels at all stages of CKD, although the RCTs lacked the statistical power to answer questions about any effects on mortality and cardiovascular calcification [25–28]. Accordingly, treatment with cholecalciferol was shown to be an effective, safe and manageable way of increasing 25(OH)D and 1,25(OH)$_2$D levels in haemodialysis patients without negatively affecting circulating calcium and phosphorus levels; however, cholecalciferol did not significantly impact vascular calcification in safety studies [29, 30]. As discussed below, the apparent discordance between these findings could be explained by the existence of a U-shaped relationship between cardiovascular calcification and the dose of vitamin D (as a result of a variety of complex cellular processes). This hypothesis is supported by clinical findings from Shroff et al. who reported that both carotid calcification scores and intima-media thickness were significantly higher in paediatric dialysis patients with either low or high circulating 1,25(OH)$_2$D [9], and by the Third National Health and Nutrition Examination Survey, which revealed an association between adequate concentrations of 25(OH)D (around 30–50 ng/mL) and a lower incidence of global mortality [31]. Thus, the existence of a U-shaped relationship between vitamin D status and cardiovascular outcomes could have major repercussions on the choice and monitoring of the prescribed dose of vitamin D.

21.3   Vitamin D and Cardiovascular Calcification in Animal Models of CKD

In view of early observations that the administration of toxic doses of vitamin D_2 (ergocalciferol) or D_3 (cholecalciferol) (>300,000 IU/kg every 3 days) induces massive calcification in rats [32, 33], various models of calcification have been developed with vitamin D derivatives. In male New Zealand White rabbits, vitamin D supplementation is extensively combined with cholesterol as an atherogenic diet, in order to rapidly induce atherosclerosis and arterial calcification [34, 35]. In this model, pronounced supplementation with vitamin D_2 (>100,000 IU/week) was shown to lead to the development of aortic valve stenosis, with (as in the human disease) fibrosis, calcification, inflammatory activation and atheromatous changes [36]. A similar pathophysiological process was observed in Rhesus monkeys, in which preclinical arteriosclerosis was generated by the administration of vitamin D_2, nicotine and high dietary cholesterol [37]. In non-uraemic rats, only toxic doses of calcitriol (1 µg/kg/d) induced aortic calcification [38, 39]. In uraemic rats, pharmacological doses of calcitriol (>120 ng/kg/week) were shown to efficiently promote vascular calcification [39–45]. In these models, calcitriol-induced calcification was not necessarily accompanied by the significant elevation of serum calcium levels.

The hypothesis whereby calcitriol is a powerful inductor of cardiovascular calcification became controversial when the consequences of hypovitaminosis D were studied. At lower doses (<100 ng/kg/week), administration of calcitriol protected against CKD-induced calcification of the aortic intima in a murine model of adynamic bone disorder (LDLR–/– mice fed on a fatty diet) [46]. This protective effect was confirmed in wild-type CKD mice in which medial calcification had been induced by a high-phosphate diet [47]. VDR-knockout mice showed significantly greater valvular calcification than wild-type mice when fed with a high-phosphate diet – confirming that a minimal amount of vitamin D is required to avoid cardiovascular calcification [48]. It is noteworthy that an insufficient dietary intake of cholecalciferol induced reversible, time-dependent valvular calcification of both wild type and LDLR–/– mice [48–50]. However, apart from the study of paricalcitol [46], none of the in vivo studies performed to date was well designed to demonstrate a U-shaped dose-response relationship between calcitriol or cholecalciferol and cardiovascular calcification.

The evidence from clinical and animal studies in favour of a U-shape relationship between vitamin D status and the development of vascular calcification is summarized in Fig. 21.1a.

21.4   Direct Effects of Vitamin D on Vascular Calcification: Lessons from In Vitro Models

Vitamin D has several actions, and a variety of phenomena might explain the dual, opposing effects on vascular calcification in vivo (as summarized diagrammatically in Figs. 21.1b and 21.2). Levels of vitamin D hormone are tightly regulated by

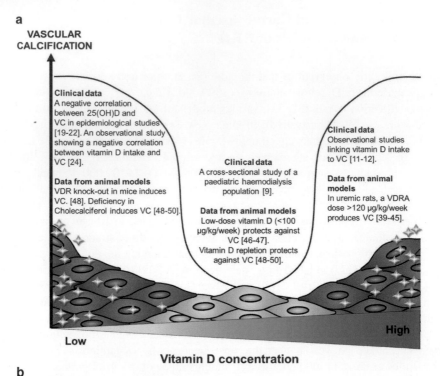

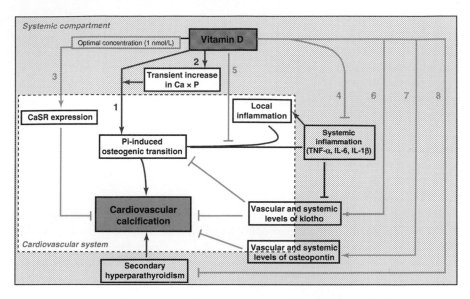

Fig. 21.2 The complexity of vitamin D's effects on vascular calcification. *Red lines* illustrate effects of vitamin D that promote vascular calcification, whereas *green lines* represent anti-calcifying effects. Vitamin D directly favors Pi-induced vascular smooth muscle cells (VSMC) calcification (*1*) and indirectly promotes elevation of the circulating Ca x Pi product concentration by enhancing absorption of the two from the intestinal tract (*2*). Vitamin D receptor activators (VDRAs) possess anti-calcific properties because they favor calcium-sensing receptor (CaSR) expression (*3*), decrease systemic inflammation (*4*) and protect against the latter's direct, pro-calcific effects (*5*). VDRAs supplementation also favors both vascular and systemic expression of klotho (*6*) and osteopontin (*7*), which are known to have anti-calcific properties. Lastly, VDRA-mediated reduction of circulating PTH levels (*8*) is involved in the regulation control of secondary hyperparathyroidism (SHPT), preventing the further development of vascular calcification

enzymes such as 25-hydroxylase, 1-alpha-hydroxylase and 24-hydroxylase. Given that (i) 1α-hydroxylase's low affinity for 25(OH)D is compensated for by higher circulating concentrations and (ii) 1α-hydroxylase is found in many tissues (other than the kidneys), both 25(OH)D and 1,25(OH)D have a significant effect on VDR activation despite CKD-related vitamin D deficiency. Interestingly, both the VDR and 1α-hydroxylase are expressed in cells found in the vasculature (e.g. VSMCs, endothelial cells and monocytes) – suggesting that calcitriol may have an autocrine role within the vascular wall in general and with regard to vascular calcification in particular (as suggested by in vitro studies).

Fig. 21.1 A schematic representation of vitamin D's varying effects on vascular calcification. Increasing vascular concentrations of calcitriol are shown on the x-axis and increasing vascular calcification (VC) is shown on the y-axis. Vascular calcification develops in the presence of abnormally low or abnormally high concentrations of calcitriol, resulting in a U-shaped correlation. (**a**) Evidence from clinical studies and in vivo animal studies of a U-shaped correlation between vitamin D status and the development of vascular calcification. (**b**) The U-shaped curve for vitamin D results from a number of complex local and systemic processes

In vitro, exposure of VSMCs to calcitriol does not induce calcification in the absence of a calcifying agent such as calcium or phosphate. The first study of this subject found that high calcitriol concentrations (>10 nmol/L) increased β-glycerophosphate-induced VSMCs calcification in vitro in a concentration-dependent manner. This effect was associated with (i) an increase in osteopontin expression and ALP activity, and (ii) a decrease in the secretion of PTH-related protein (an endogenous inhibitor of vascular calcification) [51]. Accordingly, high calcitriol concentrations also favoured the phosphate-induced overexpression of osteogenic markers such as bone morphogenetic protein 2 (BMP2), runx2, msx2, osteocalcin and osterix [52, 53]. Under high calcitriol concentrations, VDR was also found to bind to the transcription factor runx2 and thereby induce the osteogenic transformation of VSMCs [54]. In VSMCs cultured in vitro, high doses of calcitriol increase the expression of RANK-L [41], which is known to directly regulate VSMCs calcification by inducing BMP-4 expression through the alternative NF-kB pathway [55]. Furthermore, calcitriol increases VDR expression in VSMCs, which could amplify local effects. Even though most studies to date have linked high calcitriol concentrations to calcification, other studies have not observed any additive effects on phosphate-induced mineralization [56]. It is noteworthy that the addition of paricalcitol to high-phosphate medium not only reduced calcification but also downregulated the expression of BMP2 and other osteoblastic phenotype markers, which was not found with high calcitriol concentrations [41, 53]. This finding suggests that in addition to a dose effect, other factors are involved (depending on the type of vitamin D derivative).

The CaSR is a G-protein-coupled receptor expressed by parathyroid gland cells in particular. Activation of the CaSR by allosteric modulators (such as cinacalcet HCl) reduces serum PTH, Ca^{2+}_0 and P_i concentrations in dialyzed CKD patients and enables better control of SHPT [57], which may reduce the development of vascular calcification [58, 59]. Given that we and Molostvov et al. reported that the CaSR is expressed and functionally active in the vasculature [60], it is possible that calcimimetics have a direct effect on the vascular CaSR. We and others have demonstrated that an increase in CaSR expression protects against VSMCs calcification [61–63]. The mechanism has not yet been fully characterized but may involve a reduction in collagen type I secretion and BMP2 expression and an increase in MGP production. The low vascular expression of CaSR in CKD constitutes an additional calcifying factor. Studies of parathyroid, thyroid, and kidney cells have mapped VDR binding sites within two CaSR promoters [64]. In a recent study, we demonstrated that local exposure of human VSMCs to calcitriol at an optimal concentration (1 nmol/L) upregulates CaSR biosynthesis through VDR activation [65]. In turn, this increases the CaSR's availability at the cell surface and thereby its local protective effect against high-Ca^{2+}_0-induced calcification. These protective effects were centred on nanomolar concentrations, and any change in either direction by a factor of 10 or more caused a loss of calcitriol's beneficial effect. The U-shaped dose-dependent response observed in this study might explain (at least in part) the apparently paradoxical associations between cardiovascular calcification and both abnormally high and abnormally low serum $1,25(OH)_2D$ or $25(OH)D$ concentrations.

Systemic inflammation is a common feature of CKD [66] and accelerates the progression of cardiovascular calcification [67]. The inflammation marker C-reactive protein has been identified as an independent risk factor for cardiovascular morbidity and mortality in ESRD patients [68]. The circulating level of tumour necrosis factor (TNF) receptor 1 is also a strong prognostic factor for all-cause mortality in type II diabetes with renal dysfunction [69]. Interaction between members of the TNF superfamily and their receptors elicits several biological effects involved in the development of cardiovascular calcification. In vitro, TNF-α promotes P_i-induced VSMCs mineralization and osteogenic transformation [70, 71], apoptosis [72], endoplasmic reticulum stress, and Pi entry into VSMCs [73], whereas it decreases the availability of the vascular calcification inhibitor PPi [74]. TNF-α also favours the onset of calcification in valve myofibroblasts [75]. Both calcitriol and maxacalcitol were shown to abrogate the acceleration of the osteogenic process induced by phosphate and TNF-α in VSMCs in a concentration-dependent manner, through a decrease in runx2 and MMP2 expression [76]. In another study, paricalcitol was more potent than calcitriol in reducing the mineralization induced by Pi and TNF-α [77].

Taken as a whole, these data suggest that vitamin D compounds could directly and dose-dependently regulate the osteogenic transition of VSMCs. Despite all the evidence from in vitro studies, the presence of the VDR in VSMCs in vivo is still subject to debate [78].

21.5   Systemic and Indirect Effects of Vitamin D on Vascular Calcification

In addition to their direct vascular effects, VDRAs regulate more than 300 genes in all cell types. Accordingly, supplementation with VDRAs impacts the function of the main organs involved in Ca/P homeostasis (i.e. the intestine, kidney, bones and parathyroid gland) and thus affects cardiovascular calcification. It is particularly important to note that VDRAs stimulate calcium and phosphate absorption by the intestines if dietary content is low diet [79]. VDRAs also decrease calcium and phosphate reabsorption in the kidneys and can thus trigger transient or even chronic episodes of hypercalcemia or hyperphosphatemia [80]; in turn, this promotes mineral deposition in the vasculature. Lastly, VDRAs indirectly prevent cardiovascular calcification by lowering high PTH levels, which are often associated with high calcification scores [81] as a consequence of SHPT.

VDRAs supplementation also impacts inflammation, which is indirectly involved in the formation of cardiovascular calcification. High circulating levels of inflammation markers (such as CRP, TNF-α and interleukin-6 (IL-6)) are known to be associated with (i) higher levels of the bone mineral metabolism markers FGF23 and ALP, and (ii) increased prevalence, severity and progression of vascular calcification [82, 83]. Elevated serum levels of CRP, TNF-α, IL-1β and IL-6 have been reported in haemodialysis patients [84], and serum IL-6 levels are elevated in haemodialysis patients with aortic intimal and medial calcification [85] and are predictive of death [86]. Recently, the upregulation of mitogen-activated protein kinase phosphatase-1 by vitamin D was identified as a novel pathway by which vitamin D inhibits lipopolysaccharide (LPS)-induced p38 activation and cytokine production by monocytes and macrophages [87]. In accordance with this observation, treatment with vitamin D and its analogues was shown to lower serum levels of CRP, TNF-α, IL-1β and IL-6 in haemodialysis patients [88–91]. As discussed above, TNF-α is a strong inducer of Pi-induced VSMCs calcification and is also involved in the onset of valve myofibroblast calcification. In addition to the direct protective effect of calcitriol on the TNF-α-induced osteogenic transition in VSMCs, VDRAs are known to act in a paracrine manner to promote a pro-calcific to anti-calcific phenotypic transition in macrophages. The latter phenotype is characterized by low production of TNF-α and elevated levels of osteopontin (an inhibitor of calcification), which strongly reduces the VSMC calcification induced by co-culture with macrophages [92]. IL-1β was shown to promote MMP expression in calcific aortic valve stenosis [93]. Furthermore, mice lacking the IL-1β inhibitor IL-1Ra were shown to develop aortic stenosis and proximalis calcification [94]. IL-6 is a strong inducer of RANKL, and vice versa [95]. Neutralization of IL-6 reversed the RANKL-dependent regulation of osteopontin, runx2 and BMP2 in cultured VSMCs isolated from ApoE$^{-/-}$ OPG$^{-/-}$ mice [95]. In cultured human VICs, high Pi was associated with greater IL-6 secretion [96]. Pi-induced mineralization was strongly dependent on IL-6 expression in the latter study, since IL-6 blockade by siRNA decreased VICs calcification. Indeed, IL-6 increased the expression of osteoblastic genes (including runx2 and osteopontin) in cultured human VICs. Thus, by modulating the vascular response to inflammation, vitamin D sterols might interfere with vascular calcification. To address this question, Guerrero et al. evaluated the impact of vitamin D supplementation on systemic inflammation and the resulting vascular calcification in uraemic rats fed with high-phosphorus diet. Treatment with LPS increased plasma levels of TNF-α, monocyte chemotactic protein-1 and interleukin-1α, and induced calcification. Concomitant treatment with paricalcitol resulted in more marked anti-inflammatory effects than treatment with calcitriol. In contrast to calcitriol, paricalcitol prevented vascular calcification [77]. These results demonstrate that the potential anti-inflammatory effects associated with vitamin D supplementation might interfere with the process of cardiovascular calcification and therefore should not be neglected. Furthermore, they demonstrate that supplementation with various vitamin D analogues may affect vascular calcification to differing extents.

The phosphaturic hormone FGF23 and its co-factor klotho have an essential role in the control of phosphate and vitamin D metabolism. The klotho/FGF receptor-1 complex forms a specific receptor for FGF-23 signalling and mediates (in part) FGF-23's action [97]. In CKD, circulating levels of FGF23 increase dramatically as renal function decreases, whereas tissue levels of klotho decline. Since klotho-deficient mice and FGF23-null mice were shown to exhibit soft tissue calcification, some researchers have suggested that dysregulation of the FGF23–klotho axis may impact the progression of vascular calcification [98]. FGF23's putative direct effect on VSMCs calcification is still subject to debate, since the hormone was shown to induce or, in contrast, inhibit VSMCs calcification in different models [99, 100]. Uraemic, transgenic mice overexpressing klotho had greater phosphaturia, better renal function and much less calcification than wild-type mice with CKD. This klotho – associated reduction in vascular calcification might result from (i) a better control of renal function and serum phosphate and also (ii) a local protective effect, since klotho has been shown to suppress high-Pi-induced VSMCs mineralization and the osteogenic transition in vitro [101]. VDRAs were shown to stimulate FGF-23 and klotho production through the action of 1,25D-VDR/RXR on VDREs. In VDR knock-out mice, circulating levels of FGF-23 decreased more than klotho levels – suggesting that the production of FGF23 depends more tightly than klotho production on VDR activation [102]. Under calcifying conditions, VDR activation was shown to raise klotho levels and restore the VSMCs' responsiveness to FGF-23's inhibitory effects on calcification [99]. Intraperitoneal injection of VDRAs in CKD mice fed with a high-Pi diet was shown to increase serum and urinary levels of klotho. These effects were associated with an increase in vascular osteopontin expression and a decrease in aortic calcification [47].

Chronic stress factors (including pro-inflammatory TNF-α, dysregulated mineral levels, and uraemia) drive arterial klotho deficiency, which in turn is associated with the osteogenic transition of VSMCs [99]. Given that (i) pro-inflammatory factors were shown to be partly responsible for CKD-driven klotho deficiency and (ii) calcitriol reduces inflammation [90, 91], we cannot rule out the possibility that the calcitriol-driven restoration of serum and vascular klotho levels is also due to calcitriol's anti-inflammatory effects.

To distinguish between local and systemic effects of calcitriol, Lomashvili et al. grafted wild type mice with aorta from VDR knock-out mice or other wild-type mice, and then induced uraemia by feeding the animals on a high-adenine diet [103]. The researchers did not observe any intergroup differences in aorta calcification – suggesting that indirect effects of VDRAs are essential for modulating vascular calcification. However, the respective involvements of direct and indirect effects of VDRAs have not been established.

21.6 Conclusions

The link between vitamin D status and cardiovascular calcification is complex, in view of (i) the dual local and systemic effects of vitamin D products (Fig. 21.1) and (ii) the U-shaped relationship between the dose of vitamin D and cardiovascular calcification (Fig. 21.1). This complexity has major repercussions on the choice and monitoring of the dose of vitamin D prescribed to prevent and/or treat cardiovascular calcification in CKD. Future research into the role of vitamin D in cardiovascular calcification must take account of local vs. systemic effects and the U-shaped response curve.

References

1. Shanahan CM, Crouthamel MH, Kapustin A, Giachelli CM. Arterial calcification in chronic kidney disease: key roles for calcium and phosphate. Circ Res. 2011;109:697–711.
2. Pai A, Leaf EM, El-Abbadi M, Giachelli CM. Elastin degradation and vascular smooth muscle cell phenotype change precede cell loss and arterial medial calcification in a uremic mouse model of chronic kidney disease. Am J Pathol. 2011;178:764–73.
3. Bouvet C, Moreau S, Blanchette J, de Blois D, Moreau P. Sequential activation of matrix metalloproteinase 9 and transforming growth factor beta in arterial elastocalcinosis. Arterioscler Thromb Vasc Biol. 2008;28:856–62.
4. Perwad F, Zhang MYH, Tenenhouse HS, Portale AA. Fibroblast growth factor 23 impairs phosphorus and vitamin D metabolism in vivo and suppresses 25-hydroxyvitamin D-1alpha-hydroxylase expression in vitro. Am J Physiol Renal Physiol. 2007;293:F1577–83.
5. Hsu CH, Patel S. Uremic plasma contains factors inhibiting 1 alpha-hydroxylase activity. J Am Soc Nephrol. 1992;3:947–52.
6. Michaud J, Naud J, Ouimet D, Demers C, Petit J-L, Leblond FA, Bonnardeaux A, Gascon-Barré M, Pichette V. Reduced hepatic synthesis of calcidiol in uremia. J Am Soc Nephrol. 2010;21:1488–97.
7. Glorieux G, Vanholder R. Blunted response to vitamin D in uremia. Kidney Int Suppl. 2001;78:S182–5.
8. Patel SR, Ke HQ, Vanholder R, Koenig RJ, Hsu CH. Inhibition of calcitriol receptor binding to vitamin D response elements by uremic toxins. J Clin Invest. 1995;96:50–9.
9. Shroff R, Egerton M, Bridel M, Shah V, Donald AE, Cole TJ, Hiorns MP, Deanfield JE, Rees L. A bimodal association of vitamin D levels and vascular disease in children on dialysis. J Am Soc Nephrol. 2008;19:1239–46.
10. Wu-Wong JR, Melnick J. Vascular calcification in chronic kidney failure: role of vitamin D receptor. Curr Opin Investig Drugs Lond Engl 2000. 2007;8:237–47.
11. Milliner DS, Zinsmeister AR, Lieberman E, Landing B. Soft tissue calcification in pediatric patients with end-stage renal disease. Kidney Int. 1990;38:931–6.
12. Goldsmith DJ, Covic A, Sambrook PA, Ackrill P. Vascular calcification in long-term haemodialysis patients in a single unit: a retrospective analysis. Nephron. 1997;77:37–43.
13. Briese S, Wiesner S, Will JC, Lembcke A, Opgen-Rhein B, Nissel R, Wernecke K-D, Andreae J, Haffner D, Querfeld U. Arterial and cardiac disease in young adults with childhood-onset end-stage renal disease-impact of calcium and vitamin D therapy. Nephrol Dial Transplant. 2006;21:1906–14.
14. Braun J, Oldendorf M, Moshage W, Heidler R, Zeitler E, Luft FC. Electron beam computed tomography in the evaluation of cardiac calcification in chronic dialysis patients. Am J Kidney Dis. 1996;27:394–401.
15. Goodman WG, Goldin J, Kuizon BD, et al. Coronary-artery calcification in young adults with end-stage renal disease who are undergoing dialysis. N Engl J Med. 2000;342:1478–83.
16. London GM, Guérin AP, Verbeke FH, Pannier B, Boutouyrie P, Marchais SJ, Métivier F. Mineral metabolism and arterial functions in end-stage renal disease: potential role of 25-hydroxyvitamin D deficiency. J Am Soc Nephrol. 2007;18:613–20.
17. Barreto DV, Barreto FC, Liabeuf S, Temmar M, Boitte F, Choukroun G, Fournier A, Massy ZA. Vitamin D affects survival independently of vascular calcification in chronic kidney disease. Clin J Am Soc Nephrol C. 2009;4:1128–35.
18. Pillar R, G Lopes MG, Rocha LA, Cuppari L, Carvalho AB, Draibe SA, Canziani MEF. Severe hypovitaminosis D in chronic kidney disease: association with blood pressure and coronary artery calcification. Hypertens Res. 2013;36:428–32.
19. García-Canton C, Bosch E, Ramírez A, et al. Vascular calcification and 25-hydroxyvitamin D levels in non-dialysis patients with chronic kidney disease stages 4 and 5. Nephrol Dial Transplant. 2011;26:2250–6.

20. Lee S-Y, Kim H-Y, Gu SW, Kim H-J, Yang DH. 25-hydroxyvitamin D levels and vascular calcification in predialysis and dialysis patients with chronic kidney disease. Kidney Blood Press Res. 2012;35:349–54.
21. Matias PJ, Ferreira C, Jorge C, Borges M, Aires I, Amaral T, Gil C, Cortez J, Ferreira A. 25-Hydroxyvitamin D3, arterial calcifications and cardiovascular risk markers in haemodialysis patients. Nephrol Dial Transplant. 2009;24:611–8.
22. de Boer IH, Kestenbaum B, Shoben AB, Michos ED, Sarnak MJ, Siscovick DS. 25-hydroxyvitamin D levels inversely associate with risk for developing coronary artery calcification. J Am Soc Nephrol. 2009;20:1805–12.
23. Watson KE, Abrolat ML, Malone LL, Hoeg JM, Doherty T, Detrano R, Demer LL. Active serum vitamin D levels are inversely correlated with coronary calcification. Circulation. 1997;96:1755–60.
24. Ogawa T, Ishida H, Akamatsu M, Matsuda N, Fujiu A, Ito K, Ando Y, Nitta K. Relation of oral 1alpha-hydroxy vitamin D3 to the progression of aortic arch calcification in hemodialysis patients. Heart Vessels. 2010;25:1–6.
25. Zheng Z, Shi H, Jia J, Li D, Lin S. Vitamin D supplementation and mortality risk in chronic kidney disease: a meta-analysis of 20 observational studies. BMC Nephrol. 2013;14:199.
26. Wang L, Manson JE, Song Y, Sesso HD. Systematic review: vitamin D and calcium supplementation in prevention of cardiovascular events. Ann Intern Med. 2010;152:315–23.
27. Kandula P, Dobre M, Schold JD, Schreiber MJ, Mehrotra R, Navaneethan SD. Vitamin D supplementation in chronic kidney disease: a systematic review and meta-analysis of observational studies and randomized controlled trials. Clin J Am Soc Nephrol C. 2011;6:50–62.
28. Mann MC, Hobbs AJ, Hemmelgarn BR, Roberts DJ, Ahmed SB, Rabi DM. Effect of oral vitamin D analogs on mortality and cardiovascular outcomes among adults with chronic kidney disease: a meta-analysis. Clin Kidney J. 2015;8:41–8.
29. Delanaye P, Weekers L, Warling X, Moonen M, Smelten N, Médart L, Krzesinski J-M, Cavalier E. Cholecalciferol in haemodialysis patients: a randomized, double-blind, proof-of-concept and safety study. Nephrol Dial Transplant. 2013;28:1779–86.
30. Massart A, Debelle FD, Racapé J, Gervy C, Husson C, Dhaene M, Wissing KM, Nortier JL. Biochemical parameters after cholecalciferol repletion in hemodialysis: results From the VitaDial randomized trial. Am J Kidney Dis. 2014;64:696–705.
31. Melamed ML, Michos ED, Post W, Astor B. 25-hydroxyvitamin D levels and the risk of mortality in the general population. Arch Intern Med. 2008;168:1629–37.
32. Eisenstein R, Zeruolis L. Vitamin D-induced aortic calcification. Arch Pathol. 1964;77:27–35.
33. Takeo S, Anan M, Fujioka K, Kajihara T, Hiraga S, Miyake K, Tanonaka K, Minematsu R, Mori H, Taniguchi Y. Functional changes of aorta with massive accumulation of calcium. Atherosclerosis. 1989;77:175–81.
34. Hass GM, Landerholm W, Hemmens A. Production of calcific athero-arteriosclerosis and thromboarteritis with nicotine, vitamin D and dietary cholesterol. Am J Pathol. 1966;49:739–71.
35. Synetos A, Toutouzas K, Benetos G, et al. Catheter based inhibition of arterial calcification by bisphosphonates in an experimental atherosclerotic rabbit animal model. Int J Cardiol. 2014;176:177–81.
36. Ngo DTM, Stafford I, Kelly DJ, et al. Vitamin D(2) supplementation induces the development of aortic stenosis in rabbits: interactions with endothelial function and thioredoxin-interacting protein. Eur J Pharmacol. 2008;590:290–6.
37. Liu LB, Taylor CB, Peng SK, Mikkelson B. Experimental arteriosclerosis in Rhesus monkeys induced by multiple risk factors: cholesterol, vitamin D, and nictotine. Paroi Arterielle. 1979;5:25–37.
38. Bas A, Lopez I, Perez J, Rodriguez M, Aguilera-Tejero E. Reversibility of calcitriol-induced medial artery calcification in rats with intact renal function. J Bone Miner Res. 2006;21:484–90.

39. Haffner D, Hocher B, Müller D, et al. Systemic cardiovascular disease in uremic rats induced by 1,25(OH)2D3. J Hypertens. 2005;23:1067–75.
40. Henley C, Colloton M, Cattley RC, Shatzen E, Towler DA, Lacey D, Martin D. 1,25-Dihydroxyvitamin D3 but not cinacalcet HCl (Sensipar/Mimpara) treatment mediates aortic calcification in a rat model of secondary hyperparathyroidism. Nephrol Dial Transplant. 2005;20:1370–7.
41. Cardús A, Panizo S, Parisi E, Fernandez E, Valdivielso JM. Differential effects of vitamin D analogs on vascular calcification. J Bone Miner Res. 2007;22:860–6.
42. Lopez I, Mendoza FJ, Aguilera-Tejero E, Perez J, Guerrero F, Martin D, Rodriguez M. The effect of calcitriol, paricalcitol, and a calcimimetic on extraosseous calcifications in uremic rats. Kidney Int. 2008;73:300–7.
43. Koleganova N, Piecha G, Ritz E, Schmitt CP, Gross M-L. A calcimimetic (R-568), but not calcitriol, prevents vascular remodeling in uremia. Kidney Int. 2009;75:60–71.
44. Ivanovski O, Nikolov IG, Joki N, et al. The calcimimetic R-568 retards uremia-enhanced vascular calcification and atherosclerosis in apolipoprotein E deficient (apoE–/–) mice. Atherosclerosis. 2009;205:55–62.
45. Becker LE, Koleganova N, Piecha G, Noronha IL, Zeier M, Geldyyev A, Kökeny G, Ritz E, Gross M-L. Effect of paricalcitol and calcitriol on aortic wall remodeling in uninephrecto-mized ApoE knockout mice. Am J Physiol Renal Physiol. 2011;300:F772–82.
46. Mathew S, Lund RJ, Chaudhary LR, Geurs T, Hruska KA. Vitamin D receptor activators can protect against vascular calcification. J Am Soc Nephrol. 2008;19:1509–19.
47. Lau WL, Leaf EM, Hu MC, Takeno MM, Kuro-o M, Moe OW, Giachelli CM. Vitamin D receptor agonists increase klotho and osteopontin while decreasing aortic calcification in mice with chronic kidney disease fed a high phosphate diet. Kidney Int. 2012;82:1261–70.
48. Schmidt N, Brandsch C, Kühne H, Thiele A, Hirche F, Stangl GI. Vitamin D receptor defi-ciency and low vitamin D diet stimulate aortic calcification and osteogenic key factor expres-sion in mice. PLoS One. 2012;7:e35316.
49. Schmidt N, Brandsch C, Schutkowski A, Hirche F, Stangl GI. Dietary vitamin D inadequacy accelerates calcification and osteoblast-like cell formation in the vascular system of LDL receptor knockout and wild-type mice. J Nutr. 2014;144:638–46.
50. Ellam T, Hameed A, ul Haque R, Muthana M, Wilkie M, Francis SE, Chico TJA. Vitamin D deficiency and exogenous vitamin D excess similarly increase diffuse atherosclerotic calcifi-cation in apolipoprotein E knockout mice. PLoS One. 2014;9:e88767.
51. Jono S, Nishizawa Y, Shioi A, Morii H. 1,25-Dihydroxyvitamin D3 increases in vitro vascular calcification by modulating secretion of endogenous parathyroid hormone-related peptide. Circulation. 1998;98:1302–6.
52. Zebger-Gong H, Müller D, Diercke M, Haffner D, Hocher B, Verberckmoes S, Schmidt S, D'Haese PC, Querfeld U. 1,25-Dihydroxyvitamin D3-induced aortic calcifications in experi-mental uremia: up-regulation of osteoblast markers, calcium-transporting proteins and osterix. J Hypertens. 2011;29:339–48.
53. Martínez-Moreno JM, Muñoz-Castañeda JR, Herencia C, et al. In vascular smooth muscle cells paricalcitol prevents phosphate-induced Wnt/β-catenin activation. Am J Physiol Renal Physiol. 2012;303:F1136–44.
54. Han M-S, Che X, Cho G, et al. Functional cooperation between vitamin D receptor and Runx2 in vitamin D-induced vascular calcification. PLoS One. 2013;8:e83584.
55. Panizo S, Cardus A, Encinas M, Parisi E, Valcheva P, López-Ongil S, Coll B, Fernandez E, Valdivielso JM. RANKL increases vascular smooth muscle cell calcification through a RANK-BMP4-dependent pathway. Circ Res. 2009;104:1041–8.
56. Wu-Wong JR, Noonan W, Ma J, Dixon D, Nakane M, Bolin AL, Koch KA, Postl S, Morgan SJ, Reinhart GA. Role of phosphorus and vitamin D analogs in the pathogenesis of vascular calcification. J Pharmacol Exp Ther. 2006;318:90–8.
57. Block GA, Martin KJ, de Francisco ALM, et al. Cinacalcet for secondary hyperparathyroid-ism in patients receiving hemodialysis. N Engl J Med. 2004;350:1516–25.

58. Kawata T, Nagano N, Obi M, Miyata S, Koyama C, Kobayashi N, Wakita S, Wada M. Cinacalcet suppresses calcification of the aorta and heart in uremic rats. Kidney Int. 2008;74:1270–7.

59. Raggi P, Chertow GM, Torres PU, et al. The ADVANCE study: a randomized study to evaluate the effects of cinacalcet plus low-dose vitamin D on vascular calcification in patients on hemodialysis. Nephrol Dial Transplant. 2011;26:1327–39.

60. Molostvov G, James S, Fletcher S, Bennett J, Lehnert H, Bland R, Zehnder D. Extracellular calcium-sensing receptor is functionally expressed in human artery. Am J Physiol Renal Physiol. 2007;293:F946–55.

61. Alam M, Kirton JP, Wilkinson FL, et al. Calcification is associated with loss of functional calcium-sensing receptor in vascular smooth muscle cells. Cardiovasc Res. 2009;81:260–8.

62. Mendoza FJ, Martinez-Moreno J, Almaden Y, Rodriguez-Ortiz ME, Lopez I, Estepa JC, Henley C, Rodriguez M, Aguilera-Tejero E. Effect of calcium and the calcimimetic AMG 641 on matrix-Gla protein in vascular smooth muscle cells. Calcif Tissue Int. 2011;88:169–78.

63. Hénaut L, Boudot C, Massy ZA, Lopez-Fernandez I, Dupont S, Mary A, Drüeke TB, Kamel S, Brazier M, Mentaverri R. Calcimimetics increase CaSR expression and reduce mineralization in vascular smooth muscle cells: mechanisms of action. Cardiovasc Res. 2014;101: 256–65.

64. Canaff L, Hendy GN. Human calcium-sensing receptor gene. Vitamin D response elements in promoters P1 and P2 confer transcriptional responsiveness to 1,25-dihydroxyvitamin D. J Biol Chem. 2002;277:30337–50.

65. Mary A, Hénaut L, Boudot C, Six I, Brazier M, Massy ZA, Drüeke TB, Kamel S, Mentaverri R. Calcitriol prevents in vitro vascular smooth muscle cell mineralization by regulating calcium-sensing receptor expression. Endocrinology. 2015;156:1965–74.

66. Kaysen GA. The microinflammatory state in uremia: causes and potential consequences. J Am Soc Nephrol. 2001;12:1549–57.

67. Moe SM, Chen NX. Inflammation and vascular calcification. Blood Purif. 2005;23:64–71.

68. Zimmermann J, Herrlinger S, Pruy A, Metzger T, Wanner C. Inflammation enhances cardiovascular risk and mortality in hemodialysis patients. Kidney Int. 1999;55:648–58.

69. Saulnier P-J, Gand E, Ragot S, et al. Association of serum concentration of TNFR1 with all-cause mortality in patients with type 2 diabetes and chronic kidney disease: follow-up of the SURDIAGENE Cohort. Diabetes Care. 2014;37:1425–31.

70. Tintut Y, Patel J, Parhami F, Demer LL. Tumor necrosis factor-alpha promotes in vitro calcification of vascular cells via the cAMP pathway. Circulation. 2000;102:2636–42.

71. Lee H-L, Woo KM, Ryoo H-M, Baek J-H. Tumor necrosis factor-alpha increases alkaline phosphatase expression in vascular smooth muscle cells via MSX2 induction. Biochem Biophys Res Commun. 2010;391:1087–92.

72. Son B-K, Akishita M, Iijima K, Kozaki K, Maemura K, Eto M, Ouchi Y. Adiponectin antagonizes stimulatory effect of tumor necrosis factor-alpha on vascular smooth muscle cell calcification: regulation of growth arrest-specific gene 6-mediated survival pathway by adenosine 5′-monophosphate-activated protein kinase. Endocrinology. 2008;149:1646–53.

73. Masuda M, Miyazaki-Anzai S, Levi M, Ting TC, Miyazaki M. PERK-eIF2α-ATF4-CHOP signaling contributes to TNFα-induced vascular calcification. J Am Heart Assoc. 2013;2: e000238.

74. Zhao G, Xu M-J, Zhao M-M, Dai X-Y, Kong W, Wilson GM, Guan Y, Wang C-Y, Wang X. Activation of nuclear factor-kappa B accelerates vascular calcification by inhibiting ankylosis protein homolog expression. Kidney Int. 2012;82:34–44.

75. Kaden JJ, Kiliç R, Sarikoç A, Hagl S, Lang S, Hoffmann U, Brueckmann M, Borggrefe M. Tumor necrosis factor alpha promotes an osteoblast-like phenotype in human aortic valve myofibroblasts: a potential regulatory mechanism of valvular calcification. Int J Mol Med. 2005;16:869–72.

76. Aoshima Y, Mizobuchi M, Ogata H, Kumata C, Nakazawa A, Kondo F, Ono N, Koiwa F, Kinugasa E, Akizawa T. Vitamin D receptor activators inhibit vascular smooth muscle cell

mineralization induced by phosphate and TNF-α. Nephrol Dial Transplant. 2012;27: 1800–6.

77. Guerrero F, Montes de Oca A, Aguilera-Tejero E, Zafra R, Rodríguez M, López I. The effect of vitamin D derivatives on vascular calcification associated with inflammation. Nephrol Dial Transplant. 2012;27:2206–12.

78. Wang Y, DeLuca HF. Is the vitamin d receptor found in muscle? Endocrinology. 2011;152: 354–63.

79. Christakos S, Lieben L, Masuyama R, Carmeliet G. Vitamin D endocrine system and the intestine. BoneKEy Rep. 2014;3:496.

80. Mizobuchi M, Finch JL, Martin DR, Slatopolsky E. Differential effects of vitamin D receptor activators on vascular calcification in uremic rats. Kidney Int. 2007;72:709–15.

81. Coen G, Ballanti P, Mantella D, et al. Bone turnover, osteopenia and vascular calcifications in hemodialysis patients. A histomorphometric and multislice CT study. Am J Nephrol. 2009;29:145–52.

82. Stenvinkel P, Ketteler M, Johnson RJ, Lindholm B, Pecoits-Filho R, Riella M, Heimbürger O, Cederholm T, Girndt M. IL-10, IL-6, and TNF-alpha: central factors in the altered cytokine network of uremia – the good, the bad, and the ugly. Kidney Int. 2005;67:1216–33.

83. Jean G, Bresson E, Terrat J-C, Vanel T, Hurot J-M, Lorriaux C, Mayor B, Chazot C. Peripheral vascular calcification in long-haemodialysis patients: associated factors and survival consequences. Nephrol Dial Transplant. 2009;24:948–55.

84. Rysz J, Banach M, Cialkowska-Rysz A, Stolarek R, Barylski M, Drozdz J, Okonski P. Blood serum levels of IL-2, IL-6, IL-8, TNF-alpha and IL-1beta in patients on maintenance hemodialysis. Cell Mol Immunol. 2006;3:151–4.

85. Lee C-T, Chua S, Hsu C-Y, Tsai Y-C, Ng H-Y, Kuo C-C, Wu C-H, Chen T-C, Chiu TT-Y, Lee Y-T. Biomarkers associated with vascular and valvular calcification in chronic hemodialysis patients. Dis Markers. 2013;34:229–35.

86. Pecoits-Filho R, Bárány P, Lindholm B, Heimbürger O, Stenvinkel P. Interleukin-6 is an independent predictor of mortality in patients starting dialysis treatment. Nephrol Dial Transplant. 2002;17:1684–8.

87. Zhang Y, Leung DYM, Richers BN, Liu Y, Remigio LK, Riches DW, Goleva E. Vitamin D inhibits monocyte/macrophage proinflammatory cytokine production by targeting MAPK phosphatase-1. J Immunol Baltim Md 1950. 2012;188:2127–35.

88. Panichi V, De Pietro S, Andreini B, Bianchi AM, Migliori M, Taccola D, Giovannini L, Tetta C, Palla R. Calcitriol modulates in vivo and in vitro cytokine production: a role for intracellular calcium. Kidney Int. 1998;54:1463–9.

89. Matias PJ, Jorge C, Ferreira C, Borges M, Aires I, Amaral T, Gil C, Cortez J, Ferreira A. Cholecalciferol supplementation in hemodialysis patients: effects on mineral metabolism, inflammation, and cardiac dimension parameters. Clin J Am Soc Nephrol C. 2010;5:905–11.

90. Stubbs JR, Idiculla A, Slusser J, Menard R, Quarles LD. Cholecalciferol supplementation alters calcitriol-responsive monocyte proteins and decreases inflammatory cytokines in ESRD. J Am Soc Nephrol. 2010;21:353–61.

91. Verouti SN, Tsoupras AB, Alevizopoulou F, Demopoulos CA, Iatrou C. Paricalcitol effects on activities and metabolism of platelet activating factor and on inflammatory cytokines in hemodialysis patients. Int J Artif Organs. 2013;36:87–96.

92. Li X, Speer MY, Yang H, Bergen J, Giachelli CM. Vitamin D receptor activators induce an anticalcific paracrine program in macrophages: requirement of osteopontin. Arterioscler Thromb Vasc Biol. 2010;30:321–6.

93. Kaden JJ, Dempfle C-E, Grobholz R, et al. Interleukin-1 beta promotes matrix metalloproteinase expression and cell proliferation in calcific aortic valve stenosis. Atherosclerosis. 2003;170:205–11.

94. Isoda K, Matsuki T, Kondo H, Iwakura Y, Ohsuzu F. Deficiency of interleukin-1 receptor antagonist induces aortic valve disease in BALB/c mice. Arterioscler Thromb Vasc Biol. 2010;30:708–15.

95. Callegari A, Coons ML, Ricks JL, Rosenfeld ME, Scatena M. Increased calcification in osteoprotegerin deficient smooth muscle cells: dependence on receptor activator of NF-kB ligand and interleukin-6. J Vasc Res. 2014;51:118–31.
96. El Husseini D, Boulanger M-C, Mahmut A, Bouchareb R, Laflamme M-H, Fournier D, Pibarot P, Bossé Y, Mathieu P. P2Y2 receptor represses IL-6 expression by valve interstitial cells through Akt: implication for calcific aortic valve disease. J Mol Cell Cardiol. 2014;72: 146–56.
97. Shimada T, Kakitani M, Yamazaki Y, Hasegawa H, Takeuchi Y, Fujita T, Fukumoto S, Tomizuka K, Yamashita T. Targeted ablation of Fgf23 demonstrates an essential physiological role of FGF23 in phosphate and vitamin D metabolism. J Clin Invest. 2004;113:561–8.
98. Kuro-o M, Matsumura Y, Aizawa H, et al. Mutation of the mouse klotho gene leads to a syndrome resembling ageing. Nature. 1997;390:45–51.
99. Lim K, Lu T-S, Molostvov G, Lee C, Lam FT, Zehnder D, Hsiao L-L. Vascular Klotho deficiency potentiates the development of human artery calcification and mediates resistance to fibroblast growth factor 23. Circulation. 2012;125:2243–55.
100. Jimbo R, Kawakami-Mori F, Mu S, Hirohama D, Majtan B, Shimizu Y, Yatomi Y, Fukumoto S, Fujita T, Shimosawa T. Fibroblast growth factor 23 accelerates phosphate-induced vascular calcification in the absence of Klotho deficiency. Kidney Int. 2014;85:1103–11.
101. Hu MC, Shi M, Zhang J, Quiñones H, Griffith C, Kuro-o M, Moe OW. Klotho deficiency causes vascular calcification in chronic kidney disease. J Am Soc Nephrol. 2011;22:124–36.
102. Haussler MR, Whitfield GK, Kaneko I, Forster R, Saini R, Hsieh J-C, Haussler CA, Jurutka PW. The role of vitamin D in the FGF23, klotho, and phosphate bone kidney endocrine axis. Rev Endocr Metab Disord. 2012;13:57–69.
103. Lomashvili KA, Wang X, O'Neill WC. Role of local versus systemic vitamin D receptors in vascular calcification. Arterioscler Thromb Vasc Biol. 2014;34:146–51.

Chapter 22
Calciphylaxis and Vitamin D

Vincent M. Brandenburg and Pablo A. Ureña Torres

Abstract Calciphylaxis (calcific uremic arteriolopathy, CUA) is a rare disease that typically occurs in chronic dialysis patients. Clinically CUA is characterized by the stepwise development of superficial painful sensations and cutaneous lesions similar to livedo reticularis. Skin necrosis and ulceration represent the full-blown, "late" clinical picture. The aetiology of CUA is incompletely understood. Disturbances in bone and mineral metabolism as frequently seen in dialysis patients presumably play a role. Previous treatment with vitamin K antagonists for oral anticoagulation therapy is considered as a triggering and risk factor. Unfortunately, evidence-based therapeutic options are absent, since controlled treatment trials have not been conducted yet. Treatment strategies should aim at pain relief, wound care, and minimizing pro-calcifying factors. In the absence of controlled prospective trials registry studies such as the German CUA registry (www.calciphylaxis.net) are valuable tools in order to increase our understanding of the disease.

Keywords Calciphylaxis • Dialysis • Mortality • Calcitriol • Hyperparathyroidism • Sodium thiosulfate • Vitamin K antagonist

22.1 Introduction

Calciphylaxis (Calcific uremic arteriolopathy) is a rare disease primarily affecting patients on chronic hemodialysis. Exceptionally, patients without severe kidney disease are affected. Only rough estimates can be made upon the true incidence and prevalence of CUA in nephrology patient cohorts and no reliable statement can be

V.M. Brandenburg (✉)
Department of Cardiology and Center for Rare Diseases (ZSEA),
RWTH University Hospital Aachen, Aachen, Germany
e-mail: vmbrandenburg@aol.com; Vincent.Brandenburg@post.rwth-aachen.de

P.A. Ureña Torres, MD, PhD
Ramsay-Générale de Santé, Service de Néphrologie et Dialyse, Clinique du Landy,
Saint Ouen, France

Department of Renal Physiology, Necker Hospital, University of Paris V, René Descartes,
Paris, France

© Springer International Publishing Switzerland 2016   379
P.A. Ureña Torres et al. (eds.), *Vitamin D in Chronic Kidney Disease*,
DOI 10.1007/978-3-319-32507-1_22

made if these figures are changing over time. The diagnosis of CUA might be over-looked in patients with mild or abortive disease. Recent data from the US point towards an increase in incidence [1]. However, such speculations need to take into account the phenomenon of a potential pseudo-increase in incidence based on better awareness of the disease or changes in medical coding systems. Based on our experience from the German calciphylaxis registry we cannot confirm changes in incidence over time since our registry records a stable rate of 25–35 de novo CUA patients per year in Germany (2007–2014). This translates into low incidence figures clearly below those previously reported which exceeded one percent in dialysis patients [2]. Overall, calciphylaxis qualifies as a truly rare disease and is officially acknowledged (Orphanet number ORPHA280062).

22.2   Historical Perspective

Based on Hans Selye's (1907–1982) early work in the 1960s he coined the term calciphylaxis which then first appeared in human medicine. Selye's basal concept about the pathophysiology of calciphylaxis is not without obvious discrepancies to what we consider typical in CUA development nowadays. Selye's rodent experiments did not induce small-artery or arteriolar calcifications, although extensive soft-tissue calcifications were present. Nevertheless, Selye's theory is still very useful to concisely summarize our growing understanding about CUA [3]: CUA development obviously requires chronically disturbed background conditions, i.e. the breeding ground in the sense of Selye's "sensitization" factors. Chronic disturbances in mineral metabolism homeostasis (e.g. hyperparathyroidism) qualify as such latent sensitization factors. These factors need to be present for a certain latency or critical period, but CUA requires the occurrence of a final trigger or a second hit – according to Selye a "challenging" factor. Based on this theory, only the coincidence of sensitization plus challenging factor can provoke the outbreak of the full blown disease. Chronic kidney disease (CKD) or end-stage renal disease (ESRD) apparently qualify as a sensitization factor: CKD/ESRD is present in more than 90 % of all cases of calciphylaxis, both go along with disturbances in bone and mineral metabolism as well as with a chronic inflammatory state thus preparing the field for the second hit. But what exactly is the "second hit"? This issue is still unsolved and a matter of ongoing research.

CUA is not just part of the extra-osseous calcification continuum which characterizes patients with CKD/ESRD. It is noteworthy that virtually all long-term ESRD patients present with some degree of arterial calcification (both arteriosclerotic and atherosclerotic), calcific valvular disease and/or other forms of soft tissue calcifications. In sharp contrast, CUA, however, is not such a highly prevalent, creeping, slowly evolving condition – it is a more dichotomic event (i.e. present or absent). This aspect also indirectly supports the two-hit theory with some kind of acute injury as necessary additional trigger.

Severely impaired prognosis for CUA patients in terms of survival [4] plus a dramatically reduced quality of life [5] together with a high expenditure for the health system (e.g. due to long-term hospitalizations) clearly deserve our attention as caregivers and scientists in charge. Mortality rates among calciphylaxis patients were noted to be 2.5–3 times higher than average mortality rates for chronic hemo-dialysis patients [1].

22.3 The Clinical Picture of Calciphylaxis

The clinical picture of calciphylaxis exhibits some unique features. In many cases CUA presents with a mixture of large retiform ulceration with thick eschar surrounded by violaceous, indurated, tender, retiform plaques (Fig. 22.1). Some early or minor forms present like livedo reticularis (Fig. 22.2) or even as single indurated plaque. The latter may also occur as milder forms of CUA especially at the extremities (Fig. 22.3). Large, deep fat tissue ulcerations typical for the proximal form are associated with a particularly poor prognosis. Septicemia is a formidable consequence of ulcerative calciphylaxis. However, such ulcerations may also occur in the distal form of CUA. Superficial, often burning pain is virtually always part of the initial clinical picture with zoster neuralgia being a typical differential diagnosis. Therefore, pain management constitutes an integral part of adjunctive therapy in CUA patients [6]. On palpation, skin and soft tissue surrounding the necrotic areas often have a characteristic plaque-like hardening not seen in other forms of gangrene. There is a central form of calciphylaxis seen mainly at the trunk and the upper legs in obese patients which can be separated clinically from a more distal form, predominantly at the lower legs [5]. It remains unclear if these two forms are distinct but, local factors in adipose tissue such as inflammation or tissue hypoxia most likely contribute, particularly to the central form. The distal form appears to have a milder course with lower mortality rates [6].

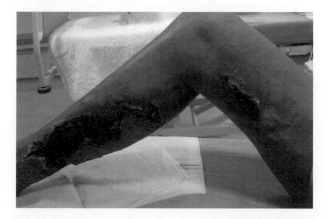

Fig. 22.1 *Right leg*: large retiform ulceration with thick eschar surrounded by violaceous, indurated, tender, retiform plaques

Fig. 22.2 Livedo-like appearance of calciphylaxis on the abdominal wall

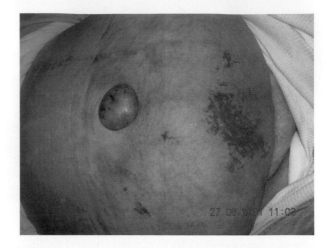

Fig. 22.3 Mild, often initial form of calciphylaxis presentation as a single indurated plaque

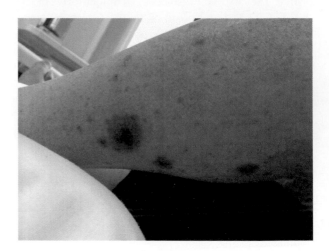

22.4 Risk Factors for Calciphylaxis

It is crucial to focus upon identification of risk factors for CUA, since once CUA has developed treatment is difficult with unsatisfactory results. Case control series might help establishing risk factors and avoid to some extent the confusion between pure associations and true causality [7]. A risk factor of outstanding importance is apparently severe CKD and ESRD. Although from time to time singular case reports emerge about CUA patients without relevant underlying kidney disease [8] these are exceptional cases and do not contradict fact that more than 90 % of all CUA cases have been reported in patients with ESRD (dialysis patients). It is still mysterious, which particular uremic factor(s) exactly predispose(s) dialysis patients to develop calciphylaxis and why the occurrence of CUA is so rare compared to the common

Table 22.1 Case-control studies elaborated the following parameters and clinical conditions as risk factors for calciphylaxis [7]

Obesity, liver disease and systemic corticosteroid usage (dose-effect association unknown) [4];
Low albumin levels and previous warfarin application [9];
High serum phosphate, high calcium-phosphate-product, previous calcium and vitamin D therapy [10];
Female gender, low albumin levels, high alkaline phosphatase, and high serum phosphorus [11];
Low albumin, previous calcitriol therapy, not using statins, high serum calcium, and previous warfarin usage [12]

forms of soft-tissue calcification such as arterial wall calcification. Most presumably a dance of uremic factors is the prerequisite for calciphylaxis development (imbalance between pro-calcifying and anti-calcifying factors). Quantifying this assumed imbalance is currently impossible. Aside from almost omnipresent uremia, several case-control studies elaborated the following list of potential additional risk factors for CUA (Table 22.1):

22.5 Vitamin D and Calciphylaxis

The particular impact of disturbances in vitamin D metabolism and/or vitamin D treatment upon CUA development is not known. High dosages of vitamin D are well established inducers of ectopic calcification – partly mediated by hypercalcemia and hyperphosphatemia [13]. Indeed, vitamin D application (dihydrotachysterol) was one of the calcification inducers used by Hans Selye in his early calciphylaxis experiments [14, 15]. Theoretically, all vitamin D compounds (active vitamin D stronger than native vitamin D) have the potency to increase calcium-phosphate product and thus promote ectopic mineral deposition. However, this association between vitamin D and calcification is not linear and depends on many influencing factors such as background vitamin D storage pools, degree of CKD and hyperparathyroidism and also upon external calcium and phosphate supply. Hence, the association between vitamin D and endpoints including vascular calcification is more appropriately described as a U-curve [16]. Such a U-curve association appreciates a potentially optimal target range for vitamin D (treatment). However, it is currently unknown if and how either optimal vitamin D treatment (whatever "optimal" vitamin D treatment looks like in a specific context), vitamin D overtreatment or undertreatment, respectively, might influence the risk for CUA. Some of the above-mentioned case-control studies have reported previous (active) vitamin D treatment as risk factor for calciphylaxis, another small case-study has shown a partially even total regression of calciphylaxis lesions in three out of nine hemodialysis patients after reducing vitamin D therapy [17], but the evidence coming out of these limited data is too weak to establish any causality. Particularly the parallel presence of several risk factor candidates such as vitamin D therapy plus additional calcium supply precludes any firm conclusions. In the German CUA registry we measured 25-hydroxyvitamin D levels in 91 unselected individuals at the time of registration. The levels indicated a highly prevalent vitamin D insufficiency: median 18.7 μg/L [IQR 9.3–33.5 μg/L] (V. Brandenburg, unpublished data).

In terms of vitamin D treatment there is general consensus among experts that calciphylaxis development is an indication for reducing the treatment regime with active compounds such as calcitriol [7, 15]. Native vitamin D supplementation might be a useful tool to stimulate wound healing and to restore mineral homeostasis in CUA patients [personal, uncontrolled experience]. Alternatively to active D, anti-PTH options should be preferred which have less potential impact upon increases of the calcium-phosphate product.

22.6   What the EVOLVE Study Adds to the Topic

Uncontrolled hyperparathyroidism (HPT) is missing among the risk factors in Table 22.1 indicating that previous case-control studies failed to establish a clear link between high PTH and CUA development. The EVOLVE trial [18] gives valuable input into the field of CUA, since EVOLVE is the largest, randomized prospective interventional trial recording CUA development among other potential adverse events. The EVOLVE study [18] stimulates the discussion about potential positive effects of calcimimetics upon CUA development with significantly less reported cases in the cinacalcet arm compared to the control arm. In EVOLVE 3,883 hemodialysis patients with moderate-to-severe hyperparathyroidism were randomly assigned to cinacalcet or placebo. Mean baseline PTH level was about 700 pg/mL and median duration of study drug exposure was 21 months. There were 6 (0.3 %) reported cases of CUA in cinacalcet-treated and 18 (0.9 %) reported cases of CUA in placebo-treated patients, corresponding to exposure-adjusted rates of 0.1 and 0.5 per 100 patient-years (p=0.009). Floege and coworkers analyzed risk factors for CUA development in this trial [19]. They found that treatment with cinacalcet and male gender are protective factors, while higher body mass index, higher diastolic blood pressure, history of dyslipidemia, smoking, and history of parathyroidectomy increase the risk for CUA in the EVOLVE cohort. It is of particular interest that on the one hand parathyroidectomy in the past increases the risk while on the other hand cinacalcet associates with reduced risk. So we might speculate about an optimal PTH range (in-between too low and too high) achievable via cinacalcet-driven PTH titration. Continuous data analysis from the CUA German registry indicate that at the time of CUA diagnosis only a minority of dialysis CUA patients had uncontrolled HPT with PTH levels exceeding 300 pg/mL (V. Brandenburg, unpublished data). Overall, the issue of how HPT influences CUA development needs further studies including data how PTH levels developed over time prior to CUA ("delta PTH" in the past) and what exactly the status of bone metabolism is. Currently, the overall very low number of CUA cases in EVOLVE, the selection bias based on inclusion criteria for this HPT trial and ambiguous diagnostic criteria prevent definite conclusions.

22.7   Vitamin K: A Key Factor in CUA?

Two of the case-control studies listed in Table 22.1 reported previous vitamin K antagonist (VKA, coumadin) usage as potential risk factor for CUA development [9, 12]. These findings are in line with data from the German calciphylaxis registry. Within our patient cohort, the prevalence of previous vitamin K antagonist usage was about 50%. This potentially causative association deserves our particular attention: CUA development might have iatrogenic aspects or in other words might be a severe adverse event from VKA prescription. Moreover, the potential association between vitamin K antagonists and CUA in chronic HD patients support Selye's two-hit theory by providing a convincing candidate for a "challenging factor". In other words, VKA application might be the straw that breaks the camel's back. The aggravation of calcification by VKA is pathophysiologically plausible. VKA interfere with the posttranslational activation of Matrix-Gla protein (MGP). MGP is of outstanding importance in inhibiting vascular calcification. Absence of MGP causes premature death in rodents due to fracture-like lesions in the aorta [20]. Moreover, VKA interfere with beta-catenin signalling via transglutaminase A, which may also contribute to vascular calcification [21]. There is substantiated evidence pointing to an accelerating effect of vitamin K antagonist application upon vascular calcification processes in humans [22–24]. Based on these findings a prospective randomized trial will test vitamin K replenishment as a therapeutic approach against uremic vascular calcification in dialysis patients (the VitaVasK trial, NCT01742273). It is unknown whether stopping therapy with VKA, application of an alternative anticoagulant, and /or vitamin K substitution is really a successful therapeutic intervention in CUA patients. However, such an approach is widely applied by treating physicians based on interim analyses from the German registry. Such a coumadin-avoiding approach is also reported from other countries [6]. We acknowledge that stopping VKA is not without risk and might create complex situations in those patients in whom anticoagulation alternatives are absent and the need for oral anticoagulation therapy is obvious (e.g. patients with prosthetic heart valves) [25]. The most common indication for VKA treatment in ESRD patients is for stroke prevention in patients with atrial fibrillation. The evidence for the efficacy of VKA treatment for stroke prevention in end-stage renal disease patients is, however, weak and coupled with potential side effects such as bleeding and vascular calcification. Therefore, we generally recommend reservation and individualized approaches in terms of VKA treatment in ESRD [25].

A pilot clinical trial to investigate the role of vitamin K supplementation in calciphylaxis is currently underway (NCT02278692), which investigates the modification of MGP levels and the reduction in pain sensation in CUA patients treated with vitamin K. Patients will be randomized to Vitamin K (phylloquinone) 10 mg orally three times a week after dialysis for 12 weeks or to placebo.

22.8   CUA Treatment: What Can We Do?

Does absence of evidence for therapeutic success justify therapeutic nihilism? No. Unassertive passivity is not an option. Many aspects of CUA treatment deal with "making dialysis patient care better" (Table 22.2). Whatever obscure nephrological expectations regarding "optimal" dialysis patient care may be these interventions can be shortly summarized as more intense and longer dialysis aiming at better CKD-MBD control. Reducing calcium supply via lowering oral calcium intake, lowering dialysis bath calcium and reducing active vitamin D treatment is another mainstay of therapy. Additionally important aspects of therapy are personalized pain relief according to WHO standards, individualized wound management and infection control.

More specifically, more purposive are three additional therapeutic interventions (Table 22.3).

Table 22.2 Current general treatment strategies in CUA based upon recordings in the German calciphylaxis registry

Intensification of dialysis therapy by
Increasing dialysis length, frequency (weekly dialysis dosage)
Switch from hemodialysis to hemodiafiltration
Switch from peritoneal dialysis to hemodialysis / hemodiafiltration
Reduction of calcium supply and calcium intake
Switch to calcium-free or calcium-reduced phosphate binders (such as sevelamer or lanthanum, magnesium- or iron-based binders)
Reduction of active vitamin D dosage
Stop vitamin K antagonist treatment and start vitamin K supplementation instead
Use alternative long-term anticoagulation therapy such as intravenous heparin or low-molecular weight heparin in reduced dosage
Therapy of hyperparathyroidism, but avoid "over-treatment" and development of adynamic bone disease
Application of cinacalcet
Parathyroidectomy
Optimal CKD-MBD therapy including native vitamin D supplementation (ergocalciferol, cholecalciferol)
Reduction of calcification pressure (please refer to Table 22.3)
Improve oxygen supply e.g. via hyperbaric O2-therapy
Supportive therapy
Wound management
Treat local and systemic infection, regular wound swabs
Pain management according to WHO standards
Limb amputation in uncontrolled clinical settings
Psychological care for patients and family

Table 22.3 Specific interventions in
CUA patients aiming at a new balance
between pro-calcifying and anti-
calcifying factors:

Sodium-thiosulfate (STS),
Bisphosphonates, and
Parathyroidectomy/cinacalcet

22.9 Myth or Reality: Sodium Thiosulfate for Patients with Calciphylaxis?

The most intensively discussed therapeutic options for CUA is currently sodium-thiosulfate (STS), which holds some promise due to reports about potential effectiveness and acceptable tolerability in CUA patients. The exact mechanism of action of STS is unknown – interference with calcium phosphate crystal formation and anti-inflammatory actions are among the options [26, 27]. Nausea, vomiting, thrombophlebitis, headache, and hypocalcemia may occur with fast STS infusion. A central venous catheter might be necessary. Physicians should take the additional sodium load induced by STS into account, which might aggravate thirst and weight gain. The biological impact of STS-induced metabolic acidosis is unclear and appears to be a limited problem in dialysis patients with regular monitoring of blood pH [28]. Overall, the evidence to treat CUA patients with STS is low. We cannot exclude publication bias regarding STS failure.

Two recent uncontrolled retrospective case series (n=27 [6] and n=172 [29]) nicely summarize local experiences with STS. In both studies STS was not a singular study drug but part of an interdisciplinary, multimodal approach. STS application scheme was similar in both studies: Infusion of 25 g STS solution during the last hour of hemodialysis or shortly after each dialysis session. The overall length of treatment was weeks to several months, which is also our recommended application regimen. STS may also be given via alternative routes such as orally, intraperitoneally or via topical application directly to the wound surface.

Outcome data with STS regarding the local clinical findings are impressive at first sight: Zitt et al. reported complete remission in 52 % and partial remission in 19 % of their patients [6]. Nigwekar et al. reported complete remission in 26 %, marked improvement in 19 %, and some improvement in 28 % [29]. However, looking at survival data CUA conditions were apparently much more severe in the smaller Austrian cohort: 52 % patients died during a median follow up of 101 days in [6], whilst 1-year mortality was reported as only 35 % in the US cohort [29]. Moreover Nigwekar et al. cautiously speculated about survival improvement with STS application. The authors compared their 1-year survival data in STS treated patients (=35 %) [29] with a historical cohort described by Mazhar et al. characterized by a mortality rate of 55 % without STS [11] However, this comparison is dubious based on the remarkable imbalance in disease severity: All patients were stable outpatients in the Nigwekar et al. cohort [29] whereas the Mazhar study recruited mainly hospitalized patients [11]. Consequently, comparing CUA outpatients with hospitalized patients represents a clinically meaningful selection bias. In both studies no systematic outcome assessment regarding wound size was performed but efficacy solely relied on subjective assessment by the treating physician. So we are still far away from any clear message regarding survival improvement with STS application in CUA patients.

The optimal duration of STS application is unknown. If within the first weeks some improvement is detectable e.g. as evidenced by wound healing and pain relief ongoing STS application is indicated. However, preliminary data indicate that in some patients bone demineralization occurs with (long-term) STS treatment. Animal data from Pasch et al. obtained in adenine-induced chronic renal failure rats as well as in rats without renal failure [30] show that STS application lowered the mechanical load which was necessary to fracture the femur. A human study with dialysis patients who received STS in a trial investigating STS effects upon coronary artery calcification [31], also investigated bone mineral density development. Twenty-five percent STS (12.5 g), was given intravenously over 15–20 min after HD treatment was completed twice a week for a period of at least 4 months. This regimen led to a significant drop in total hip bone mineral density in the treatment group compared to controls. Facing the life-threatening prognosis of CUA patients we consider STS as a part of a multimodal treatment approach, in which, however, the specific contribution of each particular intervention is difficult to establish. Costs regarding STS application play an important role in the decision if and how long CUA patients should receive it. Large discrepancies exist between countries regarding costs and in contrast to North America the low price of STS in Germany and Europe helps treating physicians with a liberal application scheme.

22.10   International Registry Initiatives

Several groups world-wide address CUA and the yet unsolved issues around the disease with systematic registry approaches. Collecting patient related data through these registries will significantly increase our understanding of the disease. The European EuCalNet initiative will record detailed data upon therapy prior to disease outbreak hence providing novel insights into the potential role of (active) vitamin D treatment as potential CUA challenging factor (Table 22.4).

Table 22.4 Currently recruiting CUA registries

UK Calciphylaxis Study	http://www.gmann.co.uk/website/trials/iccn/home.cfm
EuCalNet (including the German registry)	http://www.calciphylaxis.net/
Kansas University registry	https://www2.kumc.edu/calciphylaxisregistry/
Australian Calciphylaxis Registry	http://www.calciphylaxis.org.au/

Acknowledgements Financial support: The German calciphylaxis registry is supported by a grant from Amgen and Sanofi

References

1. Nigwekar SU, Solid CA, Ankers E, Malhotra R, Eggert W, Turchin A, Thadhani RI, Herzog CA. Quantifying a rare disease in administrative data: the example of calciphylaxis. J Gen Intern Med. 2014;29:S724.
2. Angelis M, Wong LL, Myers SA, Wong LM. Calciphylaxis in patients on hemodialysis: a prevalence study. Surgery. 1997;122(6):1083–9.
3. Selye H, Berczi I. The present status of calciphylaxis and calcergy. Clin Orthop Relat Res. 1970;69:28–54.
4. Weenig RH, Sewell LD, Davis MD, McCarthy JT, Pittelkow MR. Calciphylaxis: natural history, risk factor analysis, and outcome. J Am Acad Dermatol. 2007;56(4):569–79.
5. Brandenburg VM, Cozzolino M, Ketteler M. Calciphylaxis: a still unmet challenge. J Nephrol. 2011;24(2):142–8.
6. Zitt E, Konig M, Vychytil A, Auinger M, Wallner M, Lingenhel G, Schilcher G, Rudnicki M, Salmhofer H, Lhotta K. Use of sodium thiosulphate in a multi-interventional setting for the treatment of calciphylaxis in dialysis patients. Nephrol Dial Transplant. 2013;28(5):1232–40.
7. Brandenburg VM, Sinha S, Specht P, Ketteler M. Calcific uraemic arteriolopathy: a rare disease with a potentially high impact on chronic kidney disease-mineral and bone disorder. Pediatr Nephrol. 2014;29:2289.
8. Nigwekar SU, Wolf M, Sterns RH, Hix JK. Calciphylaxis from nonuremic causes: a systematic review. Clin J Am Soc Nephrol. 2008;3(4):1139–43.
9. Hayashi M, Takamatsu I, Kanno Y, Yoshida T, Abe T, Sato Y. A case-control study of calciphylaxis in Japanese end-stage renal disease patients. Nephrol Dial Transplant. 2011;27(4):1580–4.
10. Fine A, Zacharias J. Calciphylaxis is usually non-ulcerating: risk factors, outcome and therapy. Kidney Int. 2002;61(6):2210–7.
11. Mazhar AR, Johnson RJ, Gillen D, Stivelman JC, Ryan MJ, Davis CL, Stehman-Breen CO. Risk factors and mortality associated with calciphylaxis in end-stage renal disease. Kidney Int. 2001;60(1):324–32.
12. Nigwekar SU, Bhan I, Turchin A, Skentzos SC, Hajhosseiny R, Steele D, Nazarian RM, Wenger J, Parikh S, Karumanchi A, Thadhani R. Statin use and calcific uremic arteriolopathy: a matched case-control study. Am J Nephrol. 2013;37(4):325–32.
13. Price PA, Williamson MK, Nguyen TM, Than TN. Serum levels of the fetuin-mineral complex correlate with artery calcification in the rat. J Biol Chem. 2004;279(3):1594–600.
14. Selye H, Sister Adrian M, Jean P. Systemic and topical factors involved in the production of experimental cutaneous calcinosis. J Invest Dermatol. 1961;37:7–12.
15. Nigwekar SU, Kroshinsky D, Nazarian RM, Goverman J, Malhotra R, Jackson VA, Kamdar MM, Steele DJ, Thadhani RI. Calciphylaxis: risk factors, diagnosis, and treatment. Am J Kidney Dis. 2015;66:133.
16. Cozzolino M, Brandenburg V. Paricalcitol and outcome: a manual on how a vitamin D receptor activator (VDRA) can help us to get down the "U". Clin Nephrol. 2009;71(6):593–601.
17. Rivet J, Lebbe C, Urena P, Cordoliani F, Martinez F, Baglin AC, Aubert P, Aractingi S, Ronco P, Fournier P, Janin A. Cutaneous calcification in patients with end-stage renal disease: a regulated process associated with in situ osteopontin expression. Arch Dermatol. 2006;142(7):900–6.
18. Chertow GM, Block GA, Correa-Rotter R, Drueke TB, Floege J, Goodman WG, Herzog CA, Kubo Y, London GM, Mahaffey KW, Mix TC, Moe SM, Trotman ML, Wheeler DC, Parfrey PS. Effect of cinacalcet on cardiovascular disease in patients undergoing dialysis. N Engl J Med. 2012;367(26):2482–94.

19. Floege J, Kubo Y, Floege A, Chertow GM, Parfrey PS. The effect of cinacalcet on calcific uremic arteriolopathy events in patients receiving hemodialysis: the EVOLVE trial. Clin J Am Soc Nephrol. 2015;10(5):800–7.

20. Luo G, Ducy P, McKee MD, Pinero GJ, Loyer E, Behringer RR, Karsenty G. Spontaneous calcification of arteries and cartilage in mice lacking matrix GLA protein. Nature. 1997;386(6620):78–81.

21. Beazley KE, Deasey S, Lima F, Nurminskaya MV. Transglutaminase 2-mediated activation of beta-catenin signaling has a critical role in warfarin-induced vascular calcification. Arterioscler Thromb Vasc Biol. 2012;32(1):123–30.

22. Krueger T, Westenfeld R, Schurgers L, Brandenburg V. Coagulation meets calcification: the vitamin K system. Int J Artif Organs. 2009;32(2):67–74.

23. Cozzolino M, Brandenburg V. Warfarin: to use or not to use in chronic kidney disease patients? J Nephrol. 2010;23(6):648–52.

24. Kruger T, Floege J. Vitamin k antagonists: beyond bleeding. Semin Dial. 2014;27(1):37–41.

25. Kruger T, Brandenburg V, Schlieper G, Marx N, Floege J. Sailing between Scylla and Charybdis: oral long-term anticoagulation in dialysis patients. Nephrol Dial Transplant. 2013;28(3):534–41.

26. O'Neill WC, Hardcastle KI. The chemistry of thiosulfate and vascular calcification. Nephrol Dial Transplant. 2012;27:521–6.

27. O'Neill WC. Sodium thiosulfate: mythical treatment for a mysterious disease? Clin J Am Soc Nephrol. 2013;8(7):1068–9.

28. Vedvyas C, Winterfield LS, Vleugels RA. Calciphylaxis: a systematic review of existing and emerging therapies. J Am Acad Dermatol. 2011;67(6):253–60.

29. Nigwekar SU, Brunelli SM, Meade D, Wang W, Hymes J, Lacson Jr E. Sodium thiosulfate therapy for calcific uremic arteriolopathy. Clin J Am Soc Nephrol. 2013;8(7):1162–70.

30. Pasch A, Schaffner T, Huynh-Do U, Frey BM, Frey FJ, Farese S. Sodium thiosulfate prevents vascular calcifications in uremic rats. Kidney Int. 2008;74(11):1444–53.

31. Adirekkiat S, Sumethkul V, Ingsathit A, Domrongkitchaiporn S, Phakdeekitcharoen B, Kantachuvesiri S, Kitiyakara C, Klyprayong P, Disthabanchong S. Sodium thiosulfate delays the progression of coronary artery calcification in haemodialysis patients. Nephrol Dial Transplant. 2010;25(6):1923–9.

Chapter 23
Vitamin D and Anemia in Chronic Kidney Disease

Fenna van Breda and Marc G. Vervloet

Abstract A considerable proportion of patients with chronic kidney disease develop anemia. Several factors are known to contribute to this renal anemia, like EPO deficiency, EPO hyporesponsiveness and functional iron deficiency due to increasing concentrations of hepcidin. Recent studies showing an association in abnormalities of the vitamin D system with low hemoglobin (Hb) levels and erythropoietin stimulating agent (ESA) resistance suggest cross-talk between the vitamin D system and erythropoiesis. The administration of either inactive or active vitamin D has been associated with an improvement of anemia and reduction in EPO hyporesponsiveness. Potential links between the vitamin D system and erythropoiesis are described in this chapter.

Keywords Chronic kidney disease • Anemia • EPO resistance • Inflammation • Hepcidin • Vitamin D deficiency • Vitamin D supplementation

23.1 Definition and Prevalence of Anemia

Anemia of chronic kidney disease (CKD) is a common complication among patients with CKD. There is much variability in the hemoglobin (Hb) threshold used to define anemia. According to the most recent definition in the Kidney Disease: Improving Global Outcomes (KDIGO) guidelines, anemia is diagnosed when there is a Hb concentration <13.0 g/dL for adult males and postmenopausal women and an Hb <12.0 g/dL for premenopausal women. A large U.S. survey observed Hb levels <12 g/dL in more than one in four with relative mild CKD (stage 1 and 2),

F. van Breda, MD, MSc
Department of Nephrology and Institute for Cardiovascular Research,
VU University Medical Center, Amsterdam, The Netherlands

M.G. Vervloet, MD, PhD, FERA (✉)
Department of Nephrology, VU University Medical Center, Amsterdam, The Netherlands
e-mail: M.Vervloet@vumc.nl

© Springer International Publishing Switzerland 2016   391
P.A. Ureña Torres et al. (eds.), *Vitamin D in Chronic Kidney Disease*,
DOI 10.1007/978-3-319-32507-1_23

Table 23.1 Symptoms of anemia

Signs and symptoms of anemia
Breathlessness
Chronic fatigue and weakness
Palpitations and tachycardia
Dizziness
Paleness
Loss of appetite
Depression
Irritability
Decreased muscle function
Impaired cognition
Loss of libido

increasing to more than half of those with severe CKD (stage 4) [1]. The prevalence of anemia in patients with chronic kidney disease is a contributing factor in many symptoms associated with reduced kidney function, including tiredness, fatigue, reduced exercise tolerance and dyspnea (Table 23.1). Anemia has consistently been associated with cardiovascular consequences like left ventricular hypertrophy (LVH) and left ventricular dysfunction [2] and with increased risk of morbidity and mortality due to cardiac disease and stroke [3, 4]. However, a definite cause-effect relationship has not been proven, so these associations may reflect confounding underlying comorbid conditions and severity of illness that contribute to both the severity of anemia and poor outcomes. This chapter will focus on the different causes of renal anemia and especially on the role of vitamin D in this common complication of patients with CKD.

23.2 Causes of Anemia in Patients with CKD

The causes of anemia in patients with CKD are various but clinically non-CKD related causes need to be ruled out. To diagnose anemia of chronic kidney disease requires careful examination of the degree of anemia in relation to the degree of renal impairment. The evaluation of anemia in CKD patients should include, besides careful history taking and physical exam, a complete blood count with red blood cell indices (mean corpuscular Hb concentration (MCHC), mean corpuscular volume (MCV)), white blood cell count (including differential), reticulocytes and platelet count. Deficiency of iron, vitamin B12 or folate should be ruled out, especially in case of macrocytic anemia for the latter two causes. It is important to recognize other causes of anemia because it can reflect nutritional deficits, systemic illness or other conditions that require diagnosis and specific treatment. In this chapter, we focus on renal anemia, which is typically a normochromic, normocytic anemia without changes in leukocytes and platelets. The causes of renal anemia are summarized in Table 23.2. Recently, several experimental in vivo and observational

Table 23.2 Causes of renal anemia

1. Iron deficiency
Abnormal iron absorption
Increased loss, especially in hemodialysis
Limited availability due to increased hepcidin concentrations
2. EPO deficiency
3. EPO resistance
4. Abnormal HIF metabolism
5. Hyperparathyroidism
6. Anemia of chronic inflammation
7. CKD related bone marrow suppression

clinical studies suggest that vitamin D deficiency might be an additional co-factor of renal anemia. How vitamin D influences these different causes of anemia is discussed below.

23.3 Association Between Anemia and Vitamin D

It is widely acknowledged that vitamin D plays an important role in bone and mineral metabolism. However, latest insights into the biological functions of vitamin D increased the interest in other clinical consequences of vitamin D deficiency. General population studies indicated a strong correlation between vitamin D deficiency and mortality and morbidity in patients with end-stage kidney failure treated with long-term hemodialysis [5, 6]. Moreover, vitamin D emerges as potentially important factor in erythropoiesis.

In hemodialysis population, vitamin D deficiency has been independently associated with erythropoietin hyporesponsiveness and anemia [7]. In addition, several studies have shown that the administration of vitamin D or its analogues has been associated with an improvement of anemia and/or a decrease in EPO requirements. Also in patients with chronic kidney disease not on dialysis, these associations are present [8]. However, despite the clear epidemiological association between vitamin D and anemia, the mechanism underlying this relationship has not been fully explained and several hypothesis are formulated how this link may be explained.

23.4 Iron Deficiency and the Role of Vitamin D

The small polypeptide hepcidin is an important factor in the development of renal anemia. Hepcidin is the main regulatory protein of systemic iron metabolism and is mainly produced in the liver. It binds to ferroportin, a cellular iron exporter, which is located on the basolateral surface of gut enterocytes, the plasma membrane of reticuloendothelial cells (macrophages) and hepatocytes. Binding of hepcidin results in internalization and degradation of ferroportin limiting the amount of iron release in the blood. The two major stimuli that are known to increase hepcidin levels are iron overload and (chronic) inflammation (Fig. 23.1). Since renal failure can be considered as a state of chronic inflammation, patients with chronic kidney disease frequently have high levels of hepcidin resulting in so called 'functional' iron deficiency.

Recently, hepcidin concentrations were found to have an inverse association with vitamin D levels in CKD patients and a negatively association with hemoglobin and iron concentration [9, 10]. Given this link, several studies have been designed to explore the possible role for vitamin D in iron homeostasis. In vitro, Bacchetta et al. demonstrated that both in monocytes and hepatocytes, vitamin D is an important regulator of hepcidin expression [11]. Treatment of cultured hepatocytes and mono-cytes with either prohormone 25-hydroxyvitamin D or active 1.25 dihydroxyvita-min D suppressed the expression of hepcidin and increased the expression of ferroportin. This in vitro effect was clinically studied by supplementing seven healthy volunteers with a single oral dose of vitamin D. Hepcidin levels decreased with 34 % within 24 h of vitamin D supplementation. The fact that vitamin D directly downregulates hepcidin expression can be explained on a molecular level by the presence of a VDR binding site on the human hepcidin promotor, suggesting a gene suppressing effect. Further evidence for a role of vitamin D on hepcidin expression comes from a study done by Zughaier et al. [12]. This in vitro experi-ment showed an association between vitamin D and decreased hepcidin expression in THP-1 (macrophage-like monocytic) cells in the presence of an inflammatory stimulus. Concurrently, vitamin D resulted in a dose dependent decrease in cyto-kines that increase hepcidin expression, like IL-6 and IL-1β. In vivo, vitamin D decreased systemic circulating hepcidin levels in humans with early stage CKD. Based on the current literature, one can conclude that high dose vitamin D therapy suppresses hepcidin expression directly, and indirectly by reducing hepcidin-inducing inflammatory cytokines IL-6 and IL-1β.

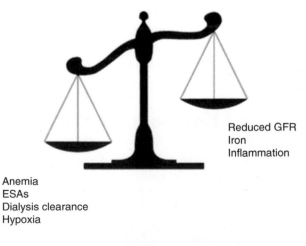

Fig. 23.1 Different factors influencing the amount of hepcidin levels in blood. Conditions at the left suppress hepcidin, while those on the right increase it

23.5   Erythropoietin Deficiency, Resistance and the Role of Vitamin D

The red cell life span and the rate of red cell production are reduced in CKD and ideally the bone marrow compensates for this by increasing erythropoiesis. However, EPO-dependent compensatory mechanism is impaired due to failure to excrete the kidney-derived EPO in higher amounts leading to partial or complete erythropoietin deficiency. There are no endogenous stores of EPO.

Despite the treatment of renal anemia with iron and erythropoietin stimulating agents (ESA), many patients still remain anemic due to EPO hyporesponsiveness/resistance, defined as inability to meet the specified targets of Hb despite higher than usual doses of ESA's. The main causes for suboptimal response to ESA therapy are summarized in Table 23.3.

Five to 10 % of EPO-treated patients exhibit an inadequate response to ESA's. It is well known that EPO hyporesponsiveness has an association with poor clinical outcomes, including cardiovascular morbidity, faster progression to end stage renal disease and all-cause mortality. Identification of factors that influence EPO responsiveness can optimize the management of anemia.

23.6   Erythropoiesis and Vitamin D

Erythropoiesis is a complex process in the bone marrow resulting in the formation of mature red blood cells (RBCs). This process is highly regulated so that, in non-disease states, the production of RBCs is equal to the destruction ensuring a constant red cell mass. Erythropoiesis is initiated when a pluripotent stem cell undergoes a series of subsequent differentiation steps in the hematopoietic

Table 23.3 Causes for suboptimal responses to EPO therapy	Causes for suboptimal response to ESA therapy
	Iron deficiency (absolute and functional)
	Infection/inflammation
	Bleeding/hemolysis
	Inadequate dialysis dose
	Malignancy
	Non-adherence with treatment therapies
	Secondary hyperparathyroidism (SHPT)
	Malnutrition
	Bone marrow disorders/hemoglobinopathies
	Vitamin B12/folate deficiency
	Hypothyroidism
	ACEi/ARB

ACEi angiotensin converting enzyme inhibitor, *ARB* angiotensin receptor blocker

Fig. 23.2 Histopathological morphology of (**a**) normal bone marrow with a normal erythropoietic cascade and (**b**) bone marrow of a CKD (stage 5D) patient with increased markers of inflammation, anemia and EPO resistance. An increase in stromal cells (adipocytes) is seen instead of hematopoietic cells (Courtesy N. Bravenboer, VU university medical center)

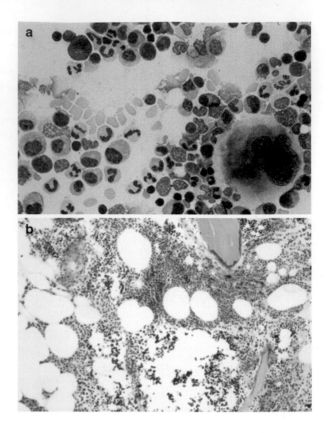

environment. Stem cells and erythroid precursors are in intimate contact with stromal cells (adipocytes, fibroblasts, macrophages and endothelial cells), accessory cells (monocytes, T-lymphocytes) and the extracellular matrix. These stromal and accessory cells create a micro-environment in which the erythron cascade is regulated by growth factors and cytokines which have stimulatory or augmented effects on erythroid progenitors. This process can be negatively influenced under pathological conditions, such as inflammation, in which suppressive cytokines derives from accessory cells (tumour necrosis factor-alpha (TNF-α), interferon-gamma (IFN-γ) and interleukin-6 (IL-6)) suppress the differentiation and proliferation (Fig. 23.2). Evidence for the effect of vitamin D on erythropoiesis comes from a study in which EPO was combined with or without vitamin D in cultured cells of patients with chronic uremia and in patients on chronic hemodialysis [13]. In vitro, vitamin D increased the proliferation of erythroid precursors with a synergistic action when combined with EPO. This result was confirmed in ten hemodialysis patients and seemed to be dose –dependent, synergistic with EPO but independent of iPTH suppression (Fig. 23.3).

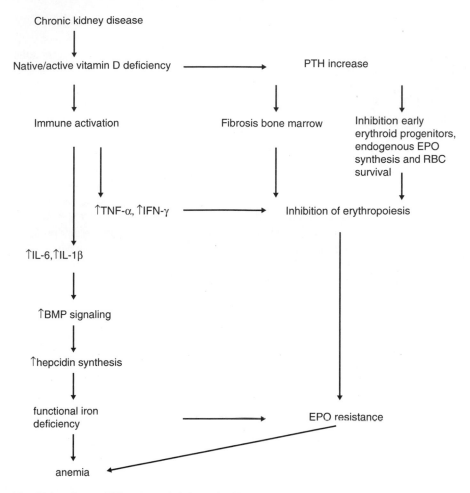

Fig. 23.3 Effects of Vitamin D deficiency in CKD on the immune system and EPO-resistant anaemia

23.7   The Role of Vitamin D on HIF Metabolism

Hypoxia-inducible factor (HIF-1) is a heterodimeric transcription factor and regulate expression of genes in response to reduced oxygen tension, including genes required for erythropoiesis and iron metabolism. HIF consists of two subunits, HIF-1-α and HIF-1-β. At normal oxygen concentrations, the regulatory subunits are modified by iron-dependent prolyl hydroxylases (PHDs) resulting in rapid degradation of HIF-1-α. As oxygen tension decreases, the activity of PHDs are diminished and HIF-1-α accumulates and translocates into the nucleus, where it dimerizes with

HIF-1-β. This leads to activation of transcriptional programs in response to hypoxia, resulting in increased production of erythropoietin and increased production of various proteins needed for effective iron transport, absorption and export from cells. These events, in conjunction with reduced hepcidin levels, enhance erythropoiesis.

The role of vitamin D in the HIF-1 pathway was described by Wong et al. [14]. While HIF-1-α is important in the activation of EPO expression, this study showed that vitamin D increased HIF-1-α through binding to its promotor in angiogenic myeloid cells of healthy volunteers. The effect of vitamin D on HIF-1-alpha in renal cells have never been tested, but clearly a vitamin D responsive element (VDRE) exist in the promotor region of HIF. Since vitamin D activation and EPO production all occur in close proximity, conceivably a paracrine cross-talk between these systems may be at hand. Indeed, the recently published study concerning the effect of roxadustat, an orally bioavailable HIF-PH inhibitor, confirmed the hypothesis that anemia in incident dialysis patients improves after administration of this protease inhibitor [15]. Based on these studies, one could speculate that vitamin D supplementation can be used to partially restore renal anemia by suppression of HIF-PH inhibitor, or increasing the expression of HIF-1-alpha. On the other hand, a study performed in various human cancer cells showed that vitamin D reduced the protein expression of HIF-1-α subunit and inhibited HIF-1 transcriptional activity [16]. However, cancer cells are genetic abnormal and behave in a different way, which could explain these discrepant findings.

Besides involved in EPO expression, HIF-1-alpha might also couple iron sensing to iron regulation, as shown in an in vivo study in which iron deficient mice reveal an induction of HIF-1 and a decrease of hepcidin [17]. The authors suggest that HIF-1-alpha may also bind to the hepcidin promotor as a gene suppressor, leading to decreased levels of hepcidin and consequently mobilizing iron to support erythrocyte production. HIF mobilizes iron to support erythrocyte production through a coordinated downregulation of hepcidin and upregulation of erythropoietin and ferroportin. A role for vitamin D in this mechanism has never been tested.

23.8   Vitamin D and Inflammation

The majority of studies regarding vitamin D and renal anemia suggest a central role of inflammation in the mechanism underlying this association. Chronic low-grade inflammation is a hallmark of CKD, and produced inflammatory cytokines affect erythropoiesis. Vitamin D appears to modulate the level of systemic cytokine production resulting in attenuated severity of anemia of chronic disease. Detailed information about the relation between vitamin D and inflammation is beyond the scope of this chapter and we refer to Chap. 21: Vitamin D and inflammation in CKD. In vivo and in vitro studies have demonstrated that calcitriol reduces cytokine production [18]. Briefly summarized, vitamin D shows anti-inflammatory properties that improve responsiveness to EPO through the reduced production of hepcidin and pro-inflammatory cytokines. Immune cells express the vitamin D receptor

(VDR) which, when activated, inhibits the expression of inflammatory cytokines like IL-1, IL-6, TNF-α and IFN-γ in accessory cells and in the serum. Additionally, VDR activation up-regulates the release of IL-10 from lymphocytes, which is an anti-inflammatory cytokine. It has been shown that calcitriol reduces cytokines production in human subjects as well [18] and in CKD patients vitamin D replacement could reduce this cytokine production leading to improved responsiveness to erythropoietin.

23.9 Vitamin D, Vitamin D Receptor and the EPO Receptor

Calcitriol exerts its functions by binding to the vitamin D receptor (VDR), a member of receptors present in several tissues, that includes stromal and accessory cells in the bone marrow. The calcitriol-VDR complex binds transcriptional cofactors which are able to interact with vitamin D responsive elements in gene promotor regions and regulate gene transcription. The uremic state in CKD affect the expression of VDR and VDR binding to vitamin D-responsive element in DNA [19]. In addition, the VDR genotype also may influence all steps in the biological actions of calcitriol. Because calcitriol is involved in hematopoiesis, the question arises whether specific VDR receptor genotypes, might influence EPO responsiveness of CKD patients. Indeed, some VDR gene polymorphisms turned out to be protective against anemia and EPO hyporesponsiveness in hemodialysis patients [20, 21]. Erytropoietin receptor (EpoR) expression and activation are required for development of erythroid progenitor cells. The effect of $1,25(OH)_2D_3$ and EPO on stem cell proliferation was studied by Alon et al. [23]. Calcitriol directly increased EpoR expression and synergistically stimulates cell proliferation along with EPO. There is evidence that vitamin D plays a role in EpoR expression, however the intracellular mechanisms by which $1,25(OH)_2D_3$ upregulates the expression of EpoRs is not elucidated yet.

More evidence for a link between VDR and anemia comes from a study performed by Amato et al. [22]. This study evaluated the association between VDR polymorphisms and iron indices in 88 hemodialysis patients. They showed a significant association between a specific VDR allele and low transferrin saturation. Despite the fact that underlying mechanisms are not elucidated yet, these associations suggest a regulatory role of the vitamin D system in erythropoiesis and iron homeostasis.

23.10 Vitamin D and PTH

Since observational studies demonstrated a clear association between high levels of PTH and EPO resistance [24], the hypothesis emerged that hyperparathyroidism plays a role in the development of renal anemia. Since secondary hyperparathyroidism can in part be a consequence of vitamin D deficiency, PTH may indirectly contribute to the role of vitamin D deficiency in renal anemia. It is however somewhat controversial if excessive parathyroid activity per se causes anemia or alternatively is just a confounding feature of low levels of vitamin D, which then is the actual contributing factor to anemia. Four possible explanations have been proposed as to how SHPT might directly influence hemoglobin levels.

The most acknowledged effect of PTH on bone marrow cellularity is the induction of marrow fibrosis (osteitis fibrosa) which limits the space for red marrow and reduces the number of erythroid precursors. In a cross sectional study of 18 HD patients who had received EPO therapy for 1–3 years, bone histomorphometry was performed [25]. The authors concluded that the dialysis patients with high doses of EPO needed to achieve an adequate hematocrit response had significant higher PTH concentrations, higher percentages of osteoclastic and eroded bone surfaces and higher degree of bone marrow fibrosis. In contrast, Mandolfo et al. showed that improvement of hemoglobin levels after parathyroidectomy (PTX) seems not to be related to improvement of marrow fibrosis but to the abrupt fall in PTH itself after surgery [26]. Currently, discussion is still going on whether myelofibrosis is reversible after PTX and if so, at what time interval this can be expected. Because bone biopsy, necessary to diagnose bone marrow fibrosis, is an invasive method its use is generally restricted to a limited number of clinical indications in just a few dedicated clinical centers.

Another potential explanation for the relationship between SHPT and anemia could be the inhibitory effect of PTH on EPO concentrations. Observations that plasma erythropoietin levels increase dramatically after parathyroidectomy point to a suppressive effect of parathyroid hormone on the already reduced endogenous erythropoietin production in CKD [27]. Washio et al. suggested the role of both an abrupt fall in PTH and ionized calcium in the elevation of EPO, since partial parathyroidectomy did not affect EPO levels [28]. Currently, it is not clear whether PTH directly suppresses EPO production or the release of EPO in CKD.

The normal life span of a red blood cell (RBC) is approximately 100 days, but in CKD patients this life span is reduced. One of the causes could be the increased osmotic fragility of the RBC's in this patient group. RBC osmotic fragility is the diminished resistance to hemolysis due to osmotic changes and this is used to evaluate RBC friability. Wu et al. found a significant relationship between increased iPTH levels and RBC fragility in hemodialysis patients (Wu, 1998, red blood cell osmotic fragility in chronically hemodialyzed patients). This could implicate that, in addition to dialysis therapy to improve uremic state, PTH reduction may improve the life span of the red blood cell and improve anemia.

Circulating EPO in the blood stream binds to EPO receptors on erythroblasts which is necessary for normal RBC development. It is speculated that PTH has direct effect on this growth of RBC's, but evidence for the inhibitory effect of PTH on bone marrow erythropoiesis is sparse and contradictory. Better underpinned is the direct effect of vitamin D on erythropoiesis as discussed above.

23.11 Treatment of Renal Anemia

Treatment of renal anemia should be started based on individual patient symptoms and Hb concentrations. Since the development of recombinant human erythropoietin (epoetin alfa, EPO) and its derivatives in the 1980s followed by its approval by the US Food and Drug Administration (FDA), this has become the standard treatment of anemia employed in most patients with advanced CKD or end stage renal disease (ESRD). Initially it was assumed that near-normal levels of Hb would be advantageous. However, three landmark trials, i.e. CREATE [29] and CHOIR study [30] published in 2006 and the TREAT study [31] published in 2009, showed no superiority of full anemia correction by ESA. Conversely, these studies revealed an increased risk of progression to renal replacement therapy with a higher risk of mortality and cardiovascular morbidity and an increase in venous trombo-embolic events. Secondary analyses of these trials showed that these risks may be especially present in patients with EPO hyporesponsiveness [32]. Since iron depletion is one of the main causes of hyporesponsiveness to ESA as outlined above, the KDIGO guideline on 2012 recommends that iron therapy should be used to correct iron deficiency before initiating ESA therapy.

Currently, there is no international consensus regarding which route of administration of iron therapy is more appropriate to treat iron deficient anemia in CKD patients. To explore the optimal route of administration and dosing for iron therapy for the management of iron deficient anemia in patients with CKD not on dialyses, with or without concomitant ESA therapy, the FIND-CKD study was performed [33]. This multicenter, prospective and randomized study was performed among 626 patients who received intravenous ferric carboxymaltose (FCM) targeting a higher (400–600 μg/L) or lower (100–200 μg/L) ferritin or oral iron therapy. The authors concluded that, compared with oral iron, IV FCM targeting a ferritin of 400–600 μg/L was superior to oral iron in delaying and/or reducing the need for other anemia management including ESA during this 12 month study. This study was not powered to assess safety end points, however, high ferritin FCM was well tolerated with no important adverse events.

Several small studies show that the administration of vitamin D or its analogues are associated with an improvement of anemia or a reduction in EPO requirements. Calcitriol improved Hb levels and reduced the need for EPO in CKD patients and HD patients [13, 34], while alfacalcidol [35], cholecalciferol and ergocalciferol induced higher levels of Hb in hemodialysis patients [36]. However, large and randomized trials aiming to improve anemia in CKD as primary endpoint, using any form of vitamin D are still lacking. The largest randomized trial in this field was performed in 60 CKD patients stage 3B-5 and anemia to determine whether paricalcitol, compared to calcitriol, improved anemia [37]. These patients, with normal PTH levels and without signs of clinical inflammation, were randomized in two groups to receive low doses calcitriol or paricalcitol for 6 months. During this period, paricalcitol resulted in a significant increase in Hb levels, without a change in iron balance, inflammatory markers and PTH plasma concentration. However, patients treated with calcitriol showed a decrease in Hb levels. Due to the lack of a control group in this study, it is impossible to draw conclusions about the role of vitamin D in the overall management of anemia in patients with CKD.

23.12 Conclusions

In conclusion, epidemiological data and biological mechanisms suggest that active vitamin D could have a positive effect on renal anemia. Currently however, the clinical relevance of this in unsure. In our opinion, it is too early to conclude that vitamin D administration improves renal anemia in CKD patients. It is conceivable though, that it may be considered in patients with unexplained EPO-hyporesponsiveness.

References

1. McClellan W, Aronoff SL, Bolton WK, Hood S, Lorber DL, Tang KL, et al. The prevalence of anemia in patients with chronic kidney disease. Curr Med Res Opin. 2004;20(9):1501–10.
2. Levin A, Thompson CR, Ethier J, Carlisle EJ, Tobe S, Mendelssohn D, et al. Left ventricular mass index increase in early renal disease: impact of decline in hemoglobin. Am J Kidney Dis. 1999;34(1):125–34.
3. Sarnak MJ, Tighiouart H, Manjunath G, Macleod B, Griffith J, Salem D, et al. Anemia as a risk factor for cardiovascular disease in The Atherosclerosis Risk in Communities (ARIC) study. J Am Coll Cardiol. 2002;40(1):27–33.
4. McClellan WM, Flanders WD, Langston RD, Jurkovitz C, Presley R. Anemia and renal insufficiency are independent risk factors for death among patients with congestive heart failure admitted to community hospitals: a population-based study. J Am Soc Nephrol. 2002;13(7):1928–36.
5. Wolf M, Shah A, Gutierrez O, Ankers E, Monroy M, Tamez H, et al. Vitamin D levels and early mortality among incident hemodialysis patients. Kidney Int. 2007;72(8):1004–13.
6. Matias PJ, Ferreira C, Jorge C, Borges M, Aires I, Amaral T, et al. 25-Hydroxyvitamin D3, arterial calcifications and cardiovascular risk markers in haemodialysis patients. Nephrol Dial Transplant. 2009;24(2):611–8.
7. Kiss Z, Ambrus C, Almasi C, Berta K, Deak G, Horonyi P, et al. Serum 25(OH)-cholecalciferol concentration is associated with hemoglobin level and erythropoietin resistance in patients on maintenance hemodialysis. Nephron Clin Pract. 2011;117(4):c373–8.
8. Patel NM, Gutierrez OM, Andress DL, Coyne DW, Levin A, Wolf M. Vitamin D deficiency and anemia in early chronic kidney disease. Kidney Int. 2010;77(8):715–20.
9. Carvalho C, Isakova T, Collerone G, Olbina G, Wolf M, Westerman M, et al. Hepcidin and disordered mineral metabolism in chronic kidney disease. Clin Nephrol. 2011;76(2):90–8.
10. Perlstein TS, Pande R, Berliner N, Vanasse GJ. Prevalence of 25-hydroxyvitamin D deficiency in subgroups of elderly persons with anemia: association with anemia of inflammation. Blood. 2011;117(10):2800–6.
11. Bacchetta J, Zaritsky JJ, Sea JL, Chun RF, Lisse TS, Zavala K, et al. Suppression of iron-regulatory hepcidin by vitamin D. J Am Soc Nephrol. 2014;25(3):564–72.
12. Zughaier SM, Alvarez JA, Sloan JH, Konrad RJ, Tangpricha V. The role of vitamin D in regulating the iron-hepcidin-ferroportin axis in monocytes. J Clin Transl Endocrinol. 2014;1(1):19–25.

13. Aucella F, Scalzulli RP, Gatta G, Vigilante M, Carella AM, Stallone C. Calcitriol increases burst-forming unit-erythroid proliferation in chronic renal failure. A synergistic effect with r-HuEpo. Nephron Clin Pract. 2003;95(4):c121–7.
14. Wong MS, Leisegang MS, Kruse C, Vogel J, Schurmann C, Dehne N, et al. Vitamin D promotes vascular regeneration. Circulation. 2014;130(12):976–86.
15. Besarab A, Chernyavskaya E, Motylev I, Shutov E, Kumbar LM, Gurevich K, et al. Roxadustat (FG-4592): correction of anemia in incident dialysis patients. J Am Soc Nephrol. 2016;27:1225–33.
16. Ben-Shoshan M, Amir S, Dang DT, Dang LH, Weisman Y, Mabjeesh NJ. 1alpha,25-dihydroxyvitamin D3 (Calcitriol) inhibits hypoxia-inducible factor-1/vascular endothelial growth factor pathway in human cancer cells. Mol Cancer Ther. 2007;6(4):1433–9.
17. Peyssonnaux C, Zinkernagel AS, Schuepbach RA, Rankin E, Vaulont S, Haase VH, et al. Regulation of iron homeostasis by the hypoxia-inducible transcription factors (HIFs). J Clin Invest. 2007;117(7):1926–32.
18. Blazsek I, Farabos C, Quittet P, Labat ML, Bringuier AF, Triana BK, et al. Bone marrow stromal cell defects and 1 alpha,25-dihydroxyvitamin D3 deficiency underlying human myeloid leukemias. Cancer Detect Prev. 1996;20(1):31–42.
19. Glorieux G, Vanholder R. Blunted response to vitamin D in uremia. Kidney Int Suppl. 2001;78:S182–5.
20. Sezer S, Tutal E, Bilgic A, Ozdemir FN, Haberal M. Possible influence of vitamin D receptor gene polymorphisms on recombinant human erythropoietin requirements in dialysis patients. Transplant Proc. 2007;39(1):40–4.
21. Erturk S, Kutlay S, Karabulut HG, Keven K, Nergizoglu G, Ates K, et al. The impact of vitamin D receptor genotype on the management of anemia in hemodialysis patients. Am J Kidney Dis. 2002;40(4):816–23.
22. Amato M, Pacini S, Aterini S, Punzi T, Gulisano M, Ruggiero M. Iron indices and vitamin D receptor polymorphisms in hemodialysis patients. Adv Chronic Kidney Dis. 2008;15(2):186–90.
23. Alon DB, Chaimovitz C, Dvilansky A, Lugassy G, Douvdevani A, Shany S, et al. Novel role of 1,25(OH)(2)D(3) in induction of erythroid progenitor cell proliferation. Exp Hematol. 2002;30(5):403–9.
24. Falko JM, Guy JT, Smith RE, Mazzaferri EL. Primary hyperparathyroidism and anemia. Arch Intern Med. 1976;136(8):887–9.
25. Rao DS, Shih MS, Mohini R. Effect of serum parathyroid hormone and bone marrow fibrosis on the response to erythropoietin in uremia. N Engl J Med. 1993;328(3):171–5.
26. Mandolfo S, Malberti F, Farina M, Villa G, Scanziani R, Surian M, et al. Parathyroidectomy and response to erythropoietin therapy in anaemic patients with chronic renal failure. Nephrol Dial Transplant. 1998;13(10):2708–9.
27. Urena P, Eckardt KU, Sarfati E, Zingraff J, Zins B, Roullet JB, et al. Serum erythropoietin and erythropoiesis in primary and secondary hyperparathyroidism: effect of parathyroidectomy. Nephron. 1991;59(3):384–93.
28. Washio M, Iseki K, Onoyama K, Oh Y, Nakamoto M, Fujimi S, et al. Elevation of serum erythropoietin after subtotal parathyroidectomy in chronic haemodialysis patients. Nephrol Dial Transplant. 1992;7(2):121–4.
29. Drueke TB, Locatelli F, Clyne N, Eckardt KU, Macdougall IC, Tsakiris D, et al. Normalization of hemoglobin level in patients with chronic kidney disease and anemia. N Engl J Med. 2006;355(20):2071–84.
30. Singh AK, Szczech L, Tang KL, Barnhart H, Sapp S, Wolfson M, et al. Correction of anemia with epoetin alfa in chronic kidney disease. N Engl J Med. 2006;355(20):2085–98.
31. Pfeffer MA, Burdmann EA, Chen CY, Cooper ME, de Zeeuw D, Eckardt KU, et al. A trial of darbepoetin alfa in type 2 diabetes and chronic kidney disease. N Engl J Med. 2009;361(21):2019–32.
32. Kilpatrick RD, Critchlow CW, Fishbane S, Besarab A, Stehman-Breen C, Krishnan M, et al. Greater epoetin alfa responsiveness is associated with improved survival in hemodialysis patients. Clin J Am Soc Nephrol. 2008;3(4):1077–83.

33. Macdougall IC, Bock AH, Carrera F, Eckardt KU, Gaillard C, Van WD, et al. FIND-CKD: a randomized trial of intravenous ferric carboxymaltose versus oral iron in patients with chronic kidney disease and iron deficiency anaemia. Nephrol Dial Transplant. 2014;29(11):2075–84.
34. Goicoechea M, Vazquez MI, Ruiz MA, Gomez-Campdera F, Perez-Garcia R, Valderrabano F. Intravenous calcitriol improves anaemia and reduces the need for erythropoietin in haemodialysis patients. Nephron. 1998;78(1):23–7.
35. Albitar S, Genin R, Fen-Chong M, Serveaux MO, Schohn D, Chuet C. High-dose alfacalcidol improves anaemia in patients on haemodialysis. Nephrol Dial Transplant. 1997;12(3):514–8.
36. Saab G, Young DO, Gincherman Y, Giles K, Norwood K, Coyne DW. Prevalence of vitamin D deficiency and the safety and effectiveness of monthly ergocalciferol in hemodialysis patients. Nephron Clin Pract. 2007;105(3):c132–8.
37. Riccio E, Sabbatini M, Bruzzese D, Capuano I, Migliaccio S, Andreucci M, et al. Effect of paricalcitol vs calcitriol on hemoglobin levels in chronic kidney disease patients: a randomized trial. PLoS ONE. 2015;10(3), e0118174.

Chapter 24
Vitamin D and Mortality Risk in Chronic Kidney Disease

John Cunningham

Abstract Our perception of vitamin D as a therapy in human disease has gone through three phases but only in the last has the possibility that vitamin D might have an important bearing on mortality been considered. The first phase encompassed the period following the discovery of vitamin D as an antirachitic substance and the role of sun exposure and certain foodstuffs in the maintenance of supply. It was discovered later that even in vitamin D resistant states such as chronic kidney disease (CKD) useful therapeutic responses could be obtained from the administration of extremely large doses of native vitamin D. The discovery of 1,25-dihydroxyvitamin D (calcitriol) as the hormonal form of vitamin D ushered in the second phase as these compounds were used to treat CKD patients with hyperparathyroidism. The third phase came with the realisation that vitamin D action is more widespread than originally thought and that the 1α-hydroxylase enzyme is expressed widely, as also is the vitamin D receptor. A range of experimental laboratory work and large observational studies supported the view that vitamin D may have beneficial effects on the main killers in CKD, namely cardiovascular disease and cancer. Because chronic kidney disease, at all levels of severity, carries a substantial burden of co-morbid conditions and increased mortality, the implications for this at the personal, family and broad socio-economic levels are enormous. Any management strategy or therapeutic intervention that could bring genuine benefits to this scenario is one that merits careful analysis and evaluation.

Keywords Calcidiol • Calcitriol • End-Stage Renal Disease • Dialysis • Survival • Calcium • Phosphate • PTH

J. Cunningham, MD
Centre for Nephrology, CL Medical School, Royal Free Campus, London, UK
e-mail: drjohncunningham@gmail.com

© Springer International Publishing Switzerland 2016   405
P.A. Ureña Torres et al. (eds.), *Vitamin D in Chronic Kidney Disease*,
DOI 10.1007/978-3-319-32507-1_24

24.1   Introduction

I shall review briefly the history of vitamin D in human medicine as a therapy that might have a bearing on survival outcomes. Detailed presentation of vitamin D biology is presented elsewhere in this book and will not be discussed in detail here. This review will extend to native vitamin D (cholecalciferol and ergocalciferol), and active vitamin D compounds (Vitamin D Receptor Activators – VDRA's) by which is meant compounds that either bind directly to the vitamin D receptor (VDR) or undergo efficient extrarenal bioactivation to generate directly active compounds. The effect of these agents on particular diseases that may influence mortality will be discussed, though the reader will also be referred to more detailed discussion of these matters in other chapters. The current state of play will be reviewed along with description of on going clinical trials and an outline of future needs.

24.2   Historical Issues

The chronology of vitamin D use in the CKD population is a long one, and in the general population is much longer still. Earlier reports of cholecalciferol and ergocalciferol as effective treatments for rickets and osteomalacia paid little heed to the level of kidney function and even less to mortality as an outcome. These native vitamin D compounds were used at very high dose in the treatment of patients with various "vitamin D resistant" states, including CKD. In the pre-dialysis era, patients with "renal rickets" and other forms of renal osteodystrophy who were treated in this way showed significant responses to heroic doses of native vitamin D. These responses included healing (or at least partial healing) of rickets and significant improvement of some patient level outcomes, essentially all of them musculoskeletal. The treatment was hazardous in that the doses required were so high that severe hypercalcaemia was a significant risk and with the benefit of hindsight we can see that vascular pathology was almost certainly accelerated substantially in some patients subjected to those treatments. Thus the early era of native vitamin D use in CKD resulted in mixed outcomes with some patients experiencing significant musculoskeletal benefits and others almost certainly suffering accelerated cardiovascular attrition and mortality.

   The discovery of calcitriol, the appreciation of its role as a vitamin D hormone, and of its apparently unique biosynthesis in the kidneys, dramatically changed the approach to treating disordered bone and mineral metabolism in advanced CKD [1]. By that time maintenance haemodialysis had already entered the clinical arena and was expanding rapidly. Calcitriol appeared dramatically effective in the treatment of hyperparathyroidism and hypocalcaemia in these patients and for at least two decades that remained essentially the sole therapeutic focus of nephrologists using calcitriol and related VDRA's [2]. Initially treatment was restricted largely to the haemodialysis population, but extended quickly to patients treated with peritoneal dialysis and to those with pre-dialysis CKD. In all cases the principal indication was 2^0 hyperparathyroidism, with or without hypocalcaemia.

24.3 A Broader Physiological Role for Vitamin D

In 2003 the first of a series of studies drew attention to an apparent reduction of mortality in dialysed patients who had received VDRA treatment compared with those who had not [3]. There is now a large body of epidemiological information attesting to a survival advantage in dialysis patients treated with compound that activate the vitamin D receptor (VDR) [4–6]. These studies are largely of historical cohort design and the early ones appeared to show a greater benefit with some of the newer VDRA's such as paricalcitol (compared with the physiological ligand, calcitriol) [3]. Most subsequent studies have not shown these differential effects, although the survival advantage seen with all VDRA's remains quite consistent [7]. The positive signal is similar if the active vitamin D compounds are given orally [6, 8, 9] and applies in both predialysis and dialysis populations.

The work reviewed below has provided three principal types of evidence supporting a role for vitamin D therapies in determining mortality outcomes in CKD. Broadly, these are better understanding of the cellular basis of vitamin D action in both "classical" and "non classical" targets, epidemiological data from the general population and observational data from particular sectors of the general population, as well as pre-dialysis CKD and dialysed populations. In these sectors, studies reporting positive outcomes greatly outnumber those reporting negative ones, but this must be taken with the caveat of possible investigator, editorial and other biases that may have distorted the balance of positive and negative publications. As will be seen, demonstration of a causal link between treatments with native vitamin D, or active VDRAs, and patient level clinical outcomes remains elusive.

24.4 Biological Plausibility

Studies have demonstrated expression of the vitamin D receptor in an increasingly wide range of tissues with co expression of CYP27B1 (25-hydroxyvitamin D 1α-hydroxylase) in a similarly wide range of tissues such that many cell types possessed the machinery needed to make calcitriol and also to respond to it. This enables autocrine/paracrine functions in addition to classical endocrine ones. These findings support the view that VDRAs may have actions in many "non classical" target tissues (so called pleiotropic effects), and also that adequate availability of precursor vitamin D compounds, in particular cholecalciferol, might be important in the maintenance of these effects by supporting local synthesis of active ligand and thereby locally driven activation of the VDR.

Epidemiological studies in the general population have consistently shown negative patient level outcomes in relation to a wide range of diseases, including mortality, in association with low 25-hydroxyvitamin D availability [10, 11]. Furthermore there is an exceptionally high prevalence of low 25-hydroxyvitamin D in chronic disease populations in general, including CKD [12] and there are abundant data linking adverse outcomes with low 25-hydroxyvitamin D concentrations in those populations.

24.5   Consequences of Vitamin D Deficiency and CKD

In the general population there are strong associations between vitamin D deficiency and malignant disease, cardiovascular disease, certain infections and all cause mortality [13]. A recent meta-analysis drawing data from approximately 850,000 subjects yielded pooled relative risk (RR) of 1.35 for all cause mortality, 1.14 for cancer death, and 1.35 for cardiovascular death. All three associations were highly significant [14].

In the CKD population, the principal causes of death are cardiovascular disease, cancer and infections. Vitamin D may have bearing on all of these.

24.6   Cardiovascular Disease

The widespread expression of the VDR includes important components of the cardiovascular system – the renin-angiotensin system (RAAS), vascular smooth muscle cells and cardiac myocytes. Important areas of activity of the vitamin D system, outside the traditional bone and mineral domains, are

1. Inhibiting vascular calcification
2. Reduction of systemic and vascular inflammation
3. Down regulation of the RAAS

Individually and collectively these actions may partake in the pathogenesis of local vascular health, blood pressure, and renal health.

24.7   Endothelial Dysfunction and Vascular Stiffness
         and Vascular Calcification

Vitamin D deficiency strongly predicts endothelial dysfunction in adults [15–19] and children [20, 21] with CKD. Associations also exist between poor vitamin D status and vascular calcification in patients of all ages [20, 22, 23] and also with vascular stiffness [18], all of which further predict cardiovascular events and mortality (Table 24.1). There is evidence that systemically administered active vitamin D may exert a bimodal effect on vascular calcification. This view is speculative, but is supported by observations in ex vivo arteries from children with ESRD in whom calcitriol/alfacalcidol exposure at the highest and lowest extremes was associated

Table 24.1 Coronary calcification (CAC) by eGFR and 25-hydroxyvitamin D concentration

GFR < 60 ml/min			GFR > 60 ml/min	
	25(OH)D >15 ng/ml	25(OH)D <15 ng/ml	25(OH)D >15 ng/ml	25(OH)D <15 ng/ml
Cumulative incidence of CAC (%)	18	32	21	29

Table made roughly from data of figure 1 of De Boer Iet al. [22]
Three-years cumulative incidence of CAC, by eGFR and 25(OH)D concentration, adjusted for age, gender, and race/ethnicity. N = 1370 participants: 394 with and 976 without chronic kidney disease (eGFR <60 ml/min per 1.73 m²)
GFR estimated glomerular filtration, *CAC* coronary artery calcification, *25(OH)D* circulating 25 hydroxy vitamin D concentration

with increased calcification [20]. A potential, but not established, mechanism for this observation is the potent suppression of 1a-hydroxylase as a result of exposure of cells to calcitriol raising the possibility that intermittent systemic exposure down regulates local production of calcitriol, thereby facilitating vascular calcification. These calcification scores were matched by carotid intima-media thickness measurements and at the lower end, with elevated CRP [20]. A prospective study examining the effect of supplementary native vitamin D on vascular stiffness is underway [24].

24.8 Hypertension, Cardiac Morphology and Progression of CKD

Studies suggest links between vitamin D status and vascular disease an the general population as well as in various chronic disease groups, including CKD [15, 17, 25–27]. The association of low UVB exposure with hypertension, based on analysis of blood pressure in relation to latitude of residence, has led to the hypothesis that increased UVB exposure may have salutary effects on blood pressure [28]. A very small intervention study of patients with untreated essential hypertension showed a reduction of blood pressure in those given UVB three times per week for 6 weeks, associated with significant increases of the level of 25-hydroxyvitamin D. In contrast, UVA exposure had no effect on either vitamin D status or blood pressure [29]. In the case of cholecalciferol, Pfeiffer randomised 148 vitamin D deficient women to receive 1.2 g of calcium or 1.2 g of calcium plus 800 u of cholecalciferol daily. After 8 weeks systolic, but not diastolic, blood pressure fell in both groups, though by 7.4 mmHg more in the calcium plus vitamin D group. This is consistent with the study of Krause using UVB as the vitamin D source. This is consistent with known effects of the VDR mediating the down regulation of the RAAS [30]. Genetically modified animals that do not express either the VDR [31], or the 1 alpha hydroxylase enzyme [32], express a substandard cardiovascular phenotype that includes up regulation of the RAAS, cardiac hypertrophy and hypertension. In the case of 1 alpha hydroxylase knockout animals, these changes are ameliorated by treatment with

VDR activators, though not by manipulation of dietary calcium and phosphorous such as to normalise the circulating concentrations of these minerals [32]. This remains an incomplete story, though the available data, still lacking positive outcomes in patients enrolled in to RCT's, has led some to propose hypertension as another indication for vitamin D replacement [33].

Cardiac morphology is floridly deranged in many subjects with CKD and this has prompted investigation of the effects of vitamin D on this potentially critical aspect of cardiovascular health. In children Patange et al. showed by multiple regression analyses that 25-hydroxyvitamin D and systolic blood pressure were independent predictors of increased left ventricular mass index [34]. The same authors had previously shown an association between low 25-hydroxyvitamin D and arterial stiffness, providing a plausible explanation the cardiac changes described a year later [21]. A small prospective study of 26 non diabetic subjects with CKD brachial artery flow mediated dilation and pulse wave velocity and documented favourable effects on both in response to two large doses of cholecalciferol [18]. The PRIMO study was an RCT designed to probe the effects of paricalcitol on cardiac structure as assessed by MRI and found no influence on the primary endpoint, namely left ventricular mass index [35]. In a post hoc analysis of the same study it was reported that paricalcitol treated patients apparently benefited from reduced left atrial volume and attenuated brain natriuretic peptide rises [36]. A different type of study in children looked at associations between nutritional vitamin D status and structural cardiac parameters, including left ventricular mass index (LVMI) and identified 25-hydroxyvitamin D as an independent predictor of LVMI [34].

de Borst et al. [37] reviewed studies examining an important related matter, namely renal protection. This is relevant because local RAAS activation is a major determinant of renal damage. The surrogate examined was proteinuria and randomised controlled trials of active vitamin D compounds in patients with CKD reporting effects on proteinuria were included, provided the samples size was greater than 50. Of 904 citations retrieved, only 6 were ultimately included (4 using paricalcitol and 2 calcitriol) providing data on a total of 688 patients. Most patients (84 %) received RAAS blockade throughout the study. Active vitamin D compounds reduced proteinuria by a mean of 16 % (95 % CI of 13–18 %), with no effect seen in controls. There was no evidence of superiority of either one of the studied active compounds, calcitriol and paricalcitol, over the other. Nor did studies using higher doses of paricalcitol show any additional benefit. There was a fairly good level of consistency across the studies with no evidence of a greater or lesser effect in diabetic nephropaths. Examination of the relationship between vitamin D parameters (25-hydroxyvitamin D and calcitriol) showed that low concentrations of either were associated with increased odds of having albuminuria [16] and in a prospective observational study investigators found that treatment of diabetics with nephropathy with cholecalciferol significantly decreased albuminuria and urinary TGF-β1 at 2 and 4 months [38]. A similar phenomenon was also seen in the VITAL study in which Type 2 diabetics with secondary hyperparathyroidism and albuminuria were treated with 1–2 mcg of paricalcitol, or placebo, per day for 24 weeks [39]. Subjects on the higher dose showed the expected reduction of parathyroid hormone (PTH) and also an 18% reduction of albuminuria (p<0.014). A post hoc analysis of in children (Effect of Strict Blood Pressure Control and ACE Inhibition on Progression of CKD in Paediatric Patients (ESCAPE) suggested that vitamin D sufficiency is associated with less proteinuria and slower progression compared with those with lower 25-hydroxyvitamin D concentrations [40]. These concepts are important because hypertension, proteinuria and level of GFR all provide potentially important links between vitamin D status and cardiovascular outcomes in normal and CKD populations [41, 42].

24.9   Cardiovascular Events and Mortality

Most deaths in CKD patients have a cardiovascular aetiology and in many of the studies suggesting beneficial non classical effects of vitamin D treatment in CKC, parallel improvements in total mortality, cardiovascular mortality, and non fatal cardiovascular events are seen. This adds weight to the general notion that the effects of vitamin D on survival are likely to be mediated by its actions on the cardiovascular system. A role for reduction of PTH is plausible, but not well supported by the data in which the apparent benefit of VDRA treatment was seen across the full range of PTH, calcium and phosphate, thereby including subgroups of patients in whom a relative contra-indication to VDRA treatment exists [4, 9]. Furthermore, effective lowering of PTH in response to calcimimetic treatment has not been convincingly associated with mortality reductions, at least in the ESRD population [43]. These observations support the view that any survival gain attributable to vitamin D is mediated by other means, possibly by direct action on cardiovascular and other tissues expressing the VDR [13].

After the initial publications showing apparently beneficial effects of active VDRA compounds [3, 4], there was a profusion of reports showing similar findings. Some of these were in incident dialysis populations [5] and others in pre-dialysis CKD subjects [8]. For example, patients with CKD stage III and IV treated with calcitriol and mild hyperparathyroidism exhibited a 26% mortality reduction compared to those who were not treated. Again, the baseline PTH, did not appear to influence this effect, even where PTH was low and there was a greater risk of hypercalcaemia [8, 9]. These and similar studies implied, somewhat counterintuitively, that perceived contraindications to vitamin D therapy, namely over suppressed PTH, high calcium and high phosphate, were either wrong, or overwhelmed by the other positive consequences of VDR activation. In one study of orally administered vitamin D metabolites, there was an inverse dose response relationship between vitamin D administered and beneficial outcome [6]. The result of these publications was to galvanise the nephrology community into considering vitamin D treatments as potentially going far beyond the traditional focus on calcium, phosphorous and calcium regulating hormones [13, 27, 44–49]. The apparent mortality reductions were dramatic – in the order of 20–30%, and even higher in some studies [4, 6, 8, 9]. Thus the stage was set for a rapidly expanding research effort to shed light on the credibility of these early observations, their potential applicability in the clinical arena, and also to potential underlying mechanisms.

Several authors sounded a note of caution however. Despite the profusion of studies purporting to show beneficial effects of active vitamin D compounds on survival in CKD patients, this finding is by no means universal and the inherent weaknesses in much of the published work, most of which falls short of any convincing demonstration of genuine cause and effect, is a matter for concern. These study designs are vulnerable to various confounders and not all have yielded positive results [7, 50, 51].

A large meta-analysis of randomised controlled studies (RCT's) by Mann et al. [52] examined the effects of oral vitamin D compounds (native and active) on cardiovascular outcomes in patients across the range of CKD stages. The intention of the authors was to include in a meta-analysis only placebo RCT's reporting original data of oral vitamin D compounds given as supplementation to adult patients at all stages of CKD. Transplanted subjects were excluded. The results are telling 4246 abstracts were identified leading to 107 manuscripts initially judged suitable, ultimately leading to only 13 studies (0.3 % of the potentially relevant abstracts) in which the RCT design was deemed eligible for inclusion. In the subsets of all cause mortality, cardiovascular mortality and serious cardiovascular events, the relative risks were respectively 0.84, 0.79 and 1.20, none of them coming close to statistical significance. Stratification by CKD stage, choice of vitamin D compound, and proportion of diabetics, had no bearing on all cause mortality. A similar analysis restricted to pre dialysis patients identified five RCT's comparing active vitamin D treatment with a placebo or no treatment in which the study outcome included cardiovascular events, blood pressure, cardiac structure and function and proteinuria [53]. Excluded were non RCT's, studies using native vitamin D and studies involving dialysis patients. From a total of 780 records screened, only seven ultimately met the criteria set by the authors. Five compared paricalcitol with control and two compared calcitriol with control. The results of these analysis showed a striking reduction of cardiovascular events in vitamin D treated subjects (RR 0.27; 95 % CI 0.13–0.59), and increased the likelihood of reduction of proteinuria (RR 1.9; 95 % CI 1.34–2.71). There were no effects on other cardiac parameters including LV mass index and systolic function. Blood pressure was not significantly altered. When considering the different outcome of these two analyses, a crucial question is the choice of subjects. In the study of Mann et al. nearly a third of the patients were receiving dialysis. Furthermore, in many of the studies reviewed, the design was principally aimed at measurement of biochemical and other surrogates and patient level cardiovascular and mortality outcomes, though available, had not been predefined.

Another meta-analysis examining the effect on mortality of vitamin D treatment in CKD patients was conducted by Duranton et al. [54]. These were observational studies, either prospective or retrospective with no blinding or randomisation. For inclusion the studies required a minimum follow up of 6 months, and sufficient data to calculate the RR's and CI's of all cause and cardiovascular mortality between treated and untreated subjects. Ultimately 14 articles met the criteria relating to all cause mortality (extracted from 13 studies including nearly 200,000 patients) and cardiovascular mortality (from 6 studies and approximately 78,000 patients). The vitamin D compounds given were calcitriol, paricalcitol, alfacalcidol and doxercalciferol. These agents were given orally or parentally and exposure was defined as receiving any dose of one of these compounds during follow up. The results favoured patients who had received active vitamin D, whether established on haemodialysis or predialysis significantly reduced the risk of all-cause mortality (relative risk 0.73, 95 % CI 0.65–0.82). The risk reduction was greatest in patients with the highest PTH levels (p=0.01).

A further review of prospective observational studies [55] examined 10 studies comprising a total of 6853 patients with CKD. There was a higher relative risk of mortality in subjects with low levels of 25-hydroxyvitamin D. The "dose response" reduction of mortality was 0.86 (95 % CI 0.82–0.91) with each increase of 25 nmol/L in the concentration of 25-hydroxyvitamin D. This study examined observational data only – one nested case control study and nine prospective cohort studies. A large majority of the patients included were at CKD stage V, although a considerable heterogeneity was evident. Furthermore, in many of the studies reviewed, the design was aimed principally at measurement of biochemical and other surrogates. Patient level cardiovascular and mortality outcomes, though available, had not been predefined.

24.10   Infections

A large body of data, almost all of association type, points to deficiency of vitamin D as a risk for infection. Empirically the use of tuberculosis (TB) sanatoria was consistent with this view, which is supported further by the demonstration that phagocytic microbial killing depended on vitamin D dependent regulation of cathelicidin [56]. The association with infection is particularly clear in regard to tuberculosis where certain polymorphisms of the vitamin D binding protein (DBP) gene or the VDR gene have greater susceptibility to mycobacterial infection. Increasing evidence indicates that vitamin D has important roles in the regulation of both the innate and adaptive immune systems. This has implications for infection and auto-immunity [57]. In several small studies in patients with CKD the administration of cholecalciferol or calcitriol has improved parameters of immune responsiveness and/or resolution of infection [58, 59]. These studies are mixed, not all showing significant responses [60, 61].

24.11   Cancer

The evidence that malignancy is influenced by vitamin D status is largely indirect, but quite persuasive [10]. Vitamin D sufficiency is associated with reduced instance of colon cancers, prostate cancer and breast cancer [62], though not all studies support this view [63]. Some haematological malignancies may also be influenced by vitamin D status. Epidemiological studies (prospective and retrospective) indicate that levels of 25-hydroxyvitamin D below 50 nmol/l are associated with a 30–50 % increased risk of incident colon [64] and other cancers. Mortality from these cancers is higher when vitamin D stores are low. A small study by Lappe et al. showed lower breast cancer recurrence rates in vitamin D + calcium supplemented patients than in those given calcium alone [65].

Support for this link also comes from in vitro studies which have shown potentially anti-oncogenic effects resulting from the binding of calcitriol to the VDR. Several mechanisms appear to be involved and are discussed in more detail in Chap. 10 and reviewed by Dusso et al. [66] and by Fleet et al. [67]. In the nephrology world, cancer has been considered normal or even low in CKD populations, and high following transplantation [68]. A recent larger study of 16,400 incident haemodialysis patients confirmed a very high prevalence of vitamin D deficiency/insufficiency with cancer prevalence also high at 22.1 % [69]. These frequencies were similar in patients with high and low 25-hydroxyvitamin D levels and the findings are therefore at variance with other studies in non-renal populations.

24.12   Which Vitamin D Should We Use? Native Vitamin D or Active VDRA Compound? D2 or D3?

Our understanding of vitamin D biology raises the important possibility that the requirement of cells for local production of calcitriol capable of activating the VDR in an autocrine or paracrine fashion might not be satisfied by normal concentrations of hormonal calcitriol, or for that matter, by the sort of calcitriol concentrations achieved during therapy with active vitamin D compounds [10, 70]. If true, this would mandate attention to, and treatment of, deficiency or insufficiency of native vitamin D in CKD patients, including those receiving active vitamin D compounds. Studies comparing prevailing 25-hydroxyvitamin D concentration with calcitriol concentration as predictors of mortality have suggested that vitamin D status as assessed by 25-hydroxyvitamin D is a better predictor of early mortality in haemodialysis patients [5] and for both early mortality and likelihood of progression to end stage renal disease in predialysis patients [25]. Certainly the body of data concerning 25-hydroxyvitamin D is greater than that of 1,25-dihydroxyvitamin D, although this may reflect no more than the relative abundance of 25-hydroxyvitamin D measurements in the data sets examined [55].

Little attention has been given to the choice of D3 over D2, or vice versa, and it is apparent that, certainly in the case of native vitamin D, the choice has been determined largely by local availability and licencing considerations. There is some evidence that D3 may increase the 25-hydroxylated product more than D2, but this seems unlikely to have practical implications beyond choice of dose [71].

24.13   Unmet Need

Studies capable of demonstrating a positive effect of treatment with vitamin D compounds at the patient level are difficult to undertake if sufficiently robust. Thus virtually all of the available data to hand at the moment fall some way short of being able to establish clear cut cause and effect in regard to mortality, and also in regard to specific patient level outcomes that are themselves likely to impact on mortality. Thus far interventional studies have focused largely on biochemical end points, although some have examined other surrogates such as mortality and morbid events that may be closer to the holy grail of patient level outcomes that really matter. Nevertheless we still lack convincing data from randomized intervention controlled trials demonstrating that any formulation of vitamin D results in improved patient level outcomes, although some are planned or are in progress. To be set against this negative view are the background plausibility as outlined above, and the experimental data and the extensive observational clinical data currently available.

The same limitations apply when it comes to making recommendations in regard to the indications for vitamin D treatment beyond the classical ones related to bone and mineral metabolism. This somewhat negative and cautious conclusion that applies to patients with CKD is close to that drawn by the Institute of Medicine when making recommendations regarding vitamin D supplementation [72]. That organisation considered how to ensure that the vitamin D requirements of the general population should be met and concluded that there was sufficiently robust evidence of beneficial effects in relation to classical bone mineral and skeletal indications to justify current strategies, albeit at slightly higher dose than historically recommended. The Institute of Medicine stopped short of recommending higher doses such as have been considered in the setting of the pleiotropic actions of cholecalciferol and also stopped short of routinely recommending treatment with vitamin D for indications related to infection, autoimmunity or cancer.

For the nephrologist one thing is clear. We need patient level outcome data from properly designed intervention studies capable of establishing, or refuting, cause and effect. Less clear is what we should do in the meantime [73]. A pragmatic view, based on the principle of "do good if you can, provided you do no harm", is to use active vitamin D compounds in appropriate pharmacological doses, often supraphysiological, for established indications based on the classical actions of vitamin D on the parathyroids, bone and mineral metabolism. This then leaves two important unanswered questions. First, should all CKD patients, whether or not manifesting an established indication, be offered **physiological** doses of active vitamin D in the hope of reaping the benefit implied in the results of the many large observational studies already published? Second, should generous supplementation with native vitamin D be offered to all CKD patients with the aim of supporting widespread extra renal generation of calcitriol and facilitating the putative pleiotropic effects of vitamin D that could mitigate some of the cardiovascular and other attrition faced by these patients (Fig. 24.1)? Such an approach appears extraordinarily unlikely to do harm and so, for the time being at least, a cautious and provisional "yes" to both questions appears justified.

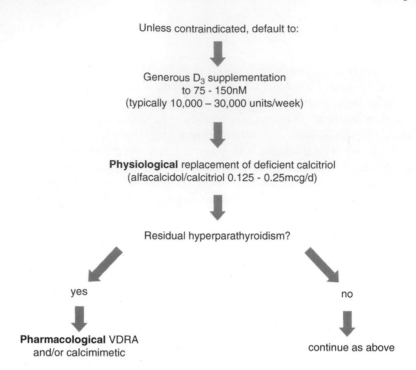

Fig. 24.1 An approach to vitamin D management in CKD. This presumes that the clinician is willing to make a decision on the basis of likely risk vs. possible, but unproven, benefit. It reflects widely adopted clinical practice. It is not based on hard evidence or current published guidance

References

1. Holick MF, Schnoes HK, DeLuca HF. Identification of 1,25-dihydroxycholecalciferol, a form of vitamin D3 metabolically active in the intestine. Proc Natl Acad Sci U S A. 1971;68(4):803–4.
2. Brickman AS, Coburn JW, Norman AW. Action of 1,25-dihydroxycholecalciferol, a potent, kidney-produced metabolite of vitamin D, in uremic man. N Engl J Med. 1972;287(18): 891–5.
3. Teng M, Wolf M, Lowrie E, Ofsthun N, Lazarus JM, Thadhani R. Survival of patients undergoing hemodialysis with paricalcitol or calcitriol therapy. N Engl J Med. 2003;349(5):446–56.
4. Teng M, Wolf M, Ofsthun MN, Lazarus JM, Hernán MA, Camargo CA, Thadhani R. Activated injectable vitamin D and hemodialysis survival: a historical cohort study. J Am Soc Nephrol. 2005;16(4):1115–25.
5. Wolf M, Shah A, Gutierrez O, Ankers E, Monroy M, Tamez H, et al. Vitamin D levels and early mortality among incident hemodialysis patients. Kidney Int. 2007;72(8):1004–13.
6. Naves-Díaz M, Alvarez-Hernández D, Passlick-Deetjen J, Guinsburg A, Marelli C, Rodriguez-Puyol D, Cannata-Andía JB. Oral active vitamin D is associated with improved survival in hemodialysis patients. Kidney Int. 2008;74(8):1070–8.
7. Tentori F, Hunt WC, Stidley CA, Rohrscheib MR, Bedrick EJ, Meyer KB, et al. Mortality risk among hemodialysis patients receiving different vitamin D analogs. Kidney Int. 2006;70(10): 1858–65.
8. Shoben AB, Rudser KD, de Boer IH, Young B, Kestenbaum B. Association of oral calcitriol with improved survival in nondialyzed CKD. J Am Soc Nephrol. 2008;19(8):1613–9.

9. Kovesdy CP, Ahmadzadeh S, Anderson JE, Kalantar-Zadeh K. Association of activated vitamin D treatment and mortality in chronic kidney disease. Arch Intern Med. 2008;168(4): 397–403.
10. Holick MF. Vitamin D deficiency. N Engl J Med. 2007;357(3):266–81.
11. Schottker B, Jorde R, Peasey A, Thorand B, Jansen EHJM, Groot LD, et al. Vitamin D and mortality: meta-analysis of individual participant data from a large consortium of cohort studies from Europe and the United States. BMJ. 2014;348:g3656.
12. Mehrotra R, Kermah D, Budoff M, Salusky IB, Mao SS, Gao YL, et al. Hypovitaminosis D in chronic kidney disease. Clin J Am Soc Nephrol. 2008;3(4):1144–51.
13. Chonchol M, Kendrick J, Targher G. Extra-skeletal effects of vitamin D deficiency in chronic kidney disease. Ann Med. 2011;43(4):273–82.
14. Chowdhury R, Kunutsor S, Vitezova A, Oliver-Williams C, Chowdhury S, Kiefte-de-Jong JC, et al. Vitamin D and risk of cause specific death: systematic review and meta-analysis of observational cohort and randomised intervention studies. BMJ. 2014;348:g1903.
15. London GM, Guérin AP, Verbeke FH, Pannier B, Boutouyrie P, Marchais SJ, Mëtivier F. Mineral metabolism and arterial functions in end-stage renal disease: potential role of 25-hydroxyvitamin D deficiency. J Am Soc Nephrol. 2007;18(2):613–20.
16. Isakova T, Gutiérrez OM, Patel NM, Andress DL, Wolf M, Levin A. Vitamin D deficiency, inflammation, and albuminuria in chronic kidney disease: complex interactions. J Ren Nutr. 2011;21(4):295–302.
17. Chitalia N, Recio-Mayoral A, Kaski JC, Banerjee D. Vitamin D deficiency and endothelial dysfunction in non-dialysis chronic kidney disease patients. Atherosclerosis. 2012;220(1):265–8.
18. Chitalia N, Ismail T, Tooth L, Boa F, Hampson G, Goldsmith D, et al. Impact of vitamin D supplementation on arterial vasomotion, stiffness and endothelial biomarkers in chronic kidney disease patients. PLoS ONE. 2014;9(3), e91363.
19. Dreyer G, Tucker AT, Harwood SM, Pearse RM, Raftery MJ, Yaqoob MM. Ergocalciferol and microcirculatory function in chronic kidney disease and concomitant vitamin d deficiency: an exploratory, double blind, randomised controlled trial. PLoS ONE. 2014;9(7), e99461.
20. Shroff R, Egerton M, Bridel M, Shah V, Donald AE, Cole TJ, et al. A bimodal association of vitamin D levels and vascular disease in children on dialysis. J Am Soc Nephrol. 2008;19(6): 1239–46.
21. Patange AR, Valentini RP, Du W, Pettersen MD. Vitamin D deficiency and arterial wall stiffness in children with chronic kidney disease. Pediatr Cardiol. 2012;33(1):122–8.
22. de Boer IH, Kestenbaum B, Shoben AB, Michos ED, Sarnak MJ, Siscovick DS. 25-hydroxyvitamin D levels inversely associate with risk for developing coronary artery calcification. J Am Soc Nephrol. 2009;20(8):1805–12.
23. Razzaque MS. The dualistic role of vitamin D in vascular calcifications. Kidney Int. 2011; 79(7):708–14.
24. Levin A, Perry T, De Zoysa P, Sigrist MK, Humphries K, Tang M, Djurdjev O. A randomized control trial to assess the impact of vitamin D supplementation compared to placebo on vascular stiffness in chronic kidney disease patients. BMC Cardiovasc Disord. 2014;14:156.
25. Melamed ML, Muntner P, Michos ED, Uribarri J, Weber C, Sharma J, Raggi P. Serum 25-hydroxyvitamin D levels and the prevalence of peripheral arterial disease: results from NHANES 2001 to 2004. Arterioscler Thromb Vasc Biol. 2008;28(6):1179–85.
26. Wang TJ, Pencina MJ, Booth SL, Jacques PF, Ingelsson E, Lanier K, et al. Vitamin D deficiency and risk of cardiovascular disease. Circulation. 2008;117(4):503–11.
27. Vaidya A, Forman JP. Vitamin D and vascular disease: the current and future status of vitamin D therapy in hypertension and kidney disease. Curr Hypertens Rep. 2012;14(2):111–9.
28. Rostand SG. Ultraviolet light may contribute to geographic and racial blood pressure differences. Hypertension. 1997;30(2):150–6.
29. Krause R, Bühring M, Hopfenmüller W, Holick MF, Sharma AM. Ultraviolet B and blood pressure. Lancet. 1998;352(9129):709–10.
30. Li YC, Kong J, Wei M, Chen Z-F, Liu SQ, Cao L-P. 1,25-dihydroxyvitamin D3 is a negative endocrine regulator of the renin-angiotensin system. J Clin Investig. 2002;110(2):229–38.

31. Xiang W, Kong J, Chen S, Cao L-P, Qiao G, Zheng W, et al. Cardiac hypertrophy in vitamin D receptor knockout mice: role of the systemic and cardiac renin-angiotensin systems. Am J Physiol Endocrinol Metab. 2005;288(1):E125–32.
32. Zhou C, Lu F, Cao K, Xu D, Goltzman D, Miao D. Calcium-independent and 1,25(OH)2d3-dependent regulation of the renin-angiotensin system in 1alpha-hydroxylase knockout mice. Kidney Int. 2008;74(2):170–9.
33. Pilz S, Tomaschitz A, Ritz E, Pieber TR. Vitamin D status and arterial hypertension: a systematic review. Nat Rev Cardiol. 2009;6(10):621–30.
34. Patange AR, Valentini RP, Gothe MP, Du W, Pettersen MD. Vitamin D deficiency is associated with increased left ventricular mass and diastolic dysfunction in children with chronic kidney disease. Pediatr Cardiol. 2013;34(3):536–42.
35. Thadhani R, Appelbaum E, Pritchett Y, Chang Y, Wenger J, Tamez H, et al. Vitamin D therapy and cardiac structure and function in patients with chronic kidney disease: the PRIMO randomized controlled trial. JAMA. 2012;307(7):674–84.
36. Tamez H, Zoccali C, Packham D, Wenger J, Bhan I, Appelbaum E, et al. Vitamin D reduces left atrial volume in patients with left ventricular hypertrophy and chronic kidney disease. Am Heart J. 2012;164(6):902–9.e2.
37. de Borst MH, Hajhosseiny R, Tamez H, Wenger J, Thadhani R, Goldsmith DJA. Active vitamin D treatment for reduction of residual proteinuria: a systematic review. J Am Soc Nephrol. 2013;24(11):1863–71.
38. Kim MJ, Frankel AH, Donaldson M, Darch SJ, Pusey CD, Hill PD, et al. Oral cholecalciferol decreases albuminuria and urinary tgf-β1 in patients with type 2 diabetic nephropathy on established renin-angiotensin-aldosterone system inhibition. Kidney Int. 2011;80(8):851–60.
39. De Zeeuw D, Agarwal R, Amdahl M, Audhya P, Coyne D, Garimella T, et al. Selective vitamin D receptor activation with paricalcitol for reduction of albuminuria in patients with type 2 diabetes (VITAL study): a randomised controlled trial. Lancet. 2010;376(9752):1543–51.
40. Shroff R, Aitkenhead H, Costa N, Trivelli A, Litwin M, Picca S, et al. Normal 25-hydroxyvitamin D levels are associated with less proteinuria and attenuate renal failure progression in children with CKD. J Am Soc Nephrol. 2016;27(1):314–22.
41. Andress DL. Vitamin D, in chronic kidney disease: a systemic role for selective vitamin D receptor activation. Kidney Int. 2006;69(1):33–43.
42. Shroff R, Wan M, Rees L. Can vitamin D slow down the progression of chronic kidney disease? Pediatr Nephrol. 2012;27(12):2167–73.
43. Chertow GM, Block GA, Correa-Rotter R, Drüeke TB, Floege J, Goodman WG, et al. Effect of cinacalcet on cardiovascular disease in patients undergoing dialysis. N Engl J Med. 2012;367(26):2482–94.
44. Cunningham J, Zehnder D. New vitamin D analogs and changing therapeutic paradigms. Kidney Int. 2011;79(7):702–7.
45. de Boer IH, Kestenbaum B. Vitamin D in chronic kidney disease: is the jury in? Kidney Int. 2008;74(8):985–7.
46. Kovesdy CP, Kalantar-Zadeh K. Vitamin D receptor activation and survival in chronic kidney disease. Kidney Int. 2008;73(12):1355–63.
47. Cozzolino M, Ketteler M, Zehnder D. The vitamin D system: a crosstalk between the heart and kidney. Eur J Heart Fail. 2010;12(10):1031–41.
48. Kovesdy CP. Survival benefits with vitamin D receptor activation: new insights since 2003. Clin J Am Soc Nephrol. 2010;5(9):1704–9.
49. Heaf JG, Joffe P, Marckmann P. Vitamin d and stage 5 chronic kidney disease: a new paradigm? Semin Dial. 2012;25(1):50–8.
50. Tentori F, Albert JM, Young EW, Blayney MJ, Robinson BM, Pisoni RL, et al. The survival advantage for haemodialysis patients taking vitamin D is questioned: findings from the dialysis outcomes and practice patterns study. Nephrol Dial Transplant. 2009;24(3):963–72.

51. Nigwekar SU, Thadhani RI. Shining light on vitamin D trials in chronic kidney disease. Kidney Int. 2013;83(2):198–200.
52. Mann MC, Hobbs AJ, Hemmelgarn BR, Roberts DJ, Ahmed SB, Rabi DM. Effect of oral vitamin D analogs on mortality and cardiovascular outcomes among adults with chronic kidney disease: a meta-analysis. Clin Kidney J. 2015;8(1):41–8.
53. Li X-H, Feng L, Yang Z-H, Liao Y-H. The effect of active vitamin D on cardiovascular outcomes in predialysis chronic kidney diseases: a systematic review and meta-analysis. Nephrology (Carlton). 2015;20(10):706–714.
54. Duranton F, Rodriguez-Ortiz ME, Duny Y, Rodriguez M, Daurès J-P, Argilés A. Vitamin D treatment and mortality in chronic kidney disease: a systematic review and meta-analysis. Am J Nephrol. 2013;37(3):239–48.
55. Pilz S, Iodice S, Zittermann A, Grant WB, Gandini S. Vitamin D status and mortality risk in CKD: a meta-analysis of prospective studies. Am J Kidney Dis. 2011;58(3):374–82.
56. Liu PT, Stenger S, Li H, Wenzel L, Tan BH, Krutzik SR, et al. Toll-like receptor triggering of a vitamin d-mediated human antimicrobial response. Science. 2006;311(5768):1770–3.
57. Yamshchikov AV, Desai NS, Blumberg HM, Ziegler TR, Tangpricha V. Vitamin D for treatment and prevention of infectious diseases: a systematic review of randomized controlled trials. Endocr Pract. 2009;15(5):438–49.
58. Gombart AF, Bhan I, Borregaard N, Tamez H, Camargo CA, Koeffler HP, Thadhani R. Low plasma level of cathelicidin antimicrobial peptide (hcap18) predicts increased infectious disease mortality in patients undergoing hemodialysis. Clin Infect Dis. 2009; 48(4):418–24.
59. Alvarez JA, Zughaier SM, Law J, Hao L, Wasse H, Ziegler TR, Tangpricha V. Effects of high-dose cholecalciferol on serum markers of inflammation and immunity in patients with early chronic kidney disease. Eur J Clin Nutr. 2013;67(3):264–9.
60. Moe SM, Zekonis M, Harezlak J, Ambrosius WT, Gassensmith CM, Murphy CL, et al. A placebo-controlled trial to evaluate immunomodulatory effects of paricalcitol. Am J Kidney Dis. 2001;38(4):792–802.
61. Sterling KA, Eftekhari P, Girndt M, Kimmel PL, Raj DS. The immunoregulatory function of vitamin D: implications in chronic kidney disease. Nat Rev Nephrol. 2012;8(7): 403–12.
62. Bolland MJ, Grey A, Gamble GD, Reid IR. Calcium and vitamin D supplements and health outcomes: a reanalysis of the women's health initiative (WHI) limited-access data set. Am J Clin Nutr. 2011;94(4):1144–9.
63. Gallicchio L, Moore LE, Stevens VL, Ahn J, Albanes D, Hartmuller V, et al. Circulating 25-hydroxyvitamin D and risk of kidney cancer: cohort consortium vitamin D pooling project of rarer cancers. Am J Epidemiol. 2010;172(1):47–57.
64. Lee JE, Li H, Chan AT, Hollis BW, Lee I-M, Stampfer MJ, et al. Circulating levels of vitamin D and colon and rectal cancer: the physicians' health study and a meta-analysis of prospective studies. Cancer Prev Res (Phila). 2011;4(5):735–43.
65. Lappe JM, Travers-Gustafson D, Davies KM, Recker RR, Heaney RP. Vitamin D and calcium supplementation reduces cancer risk: results of a randomized trial. Am J Clin Nutr. 2007;85(6):1586–91.
66. Dusso A, González EA, Martin KJ. Vitamin D in chronic kidney disease. Best Pract Res Clin Endocrinol Metab. 2011;25(4):647–55.
67. Fleet JC, DeSmet M, Johnson R, Li Y. Vitamin D and cancer: a review of molecular mechanisms. Biochem J. 2012;441(1):61–76.
68. Birkeland SA, Storm HH. Cancer risk in patients on dialysis and after renal transplantation. Lancet. 2000;355(9218):1886–7.
69. Marquardt P, Krause R, Schaller M, Bach D, von Gersdorff G. Vitamin D status and cancer prevalence of hemodialysis patients in Germany. Anticancer Res. 2015;35(2):1181–7.
70. Gröber U, Spitz J, Reichrath J, Kisters K, Holick MF. Vitamin D: update 2013: from rickets prophylaxis to general preventive healthcare. Dermatoendocrinology. 2013;5(3):331–47.

71. Trang HM, Cole DE, Rubin LA, Pierratos A, Siu S, Vieth R. Evidence that vitamin D3 increases serum 25-hydroxyvitamin D more efficiently than does vitamin D2. Am J Clin Nutr. 1998;68(4):854–8.
72. Ross AC, Manson JE, Abrams SA, Aloia JF, Brannon PM, Clinton SK, et al. The 2011 report on dietary reference intakes for calcium and vitamin D from the institute of medicine: what clinicians need to know. J Clin Endocrinol Metab. 2011;96(1):53–8.
73. Goldsmith DJA, Cunningham J. Mineral metabolism and vitamin D in chronic kidney disease – more questions than answers. Nat Rev Nephrol. 2011;7(6):341–6.

Part IV
Kidney Transplantation

Chapter 25
Vitamin D in Kidney Transplantation

Pieter Evenepoel

Abstract Renal transplantation restores renal functional mass and corrects metabolic and hormonal disturbances underlying the altered vitamin D metabolism in chronic kidney disease. As a consequence, concentrations of 1,25 dihydroxyvitamin D rapidly recover after successful renal transplantation. Remarkably however, concentrations remain often at the lower range in the early posttransplant period despite the presence of hyperparathyroidism and hypophosphatemia, conditions known to stimulate increased calcitriol synthesis. Also 25-hydroxyvitamin D concentrations increase following transplantation but, overall, these increases are modest. 25-hydroxyvitamin D deficiency and insufficiency thus remain very common among renal transplant recipients. Hypovitaminosis D may contribute to persistent hyperparathyroidism and posttransplant bone and vascular disease. Limited epidemiological evidence also suggest that hypovitaminosis D may foster malignancies and infections in renal transplant recipients. Disappointingly, intervention studies with vitamin D supplementations studies are scanty. They moreover did not yield unequivocal results. Hard endpoint intervention studies are lacking at all.

Keywords Vitamin D • Renal transplantation • CKD-MBD

25.1 Introduction

For patients with end stage renal disease, kidney transplantation undoubtedly is the best treatment option. Worldwide, the numbers of transplanted kidneys rise steadily. In the US alone, more than 17,500 kidneys are transplanted annually. The development of novel immunosuppressive therapies has led to a tremendous increase in the 1-year survival rates of renal allografts [1]. Accordingly, improving the long-term survival and quality of life for renal transplant recipients has become a major focus

P. Evenepoel, MD
Division of Nephrology, Dialysis and Renal Transplantation, Department of Medicine,
University Hospital Leuven, Leuven, Belgium
e-mail: Pieter.Evenepoel@uzleuven.be

© Springer International Publishing Switzerland 2016
P.A. Ureña Torres et al. (eds.), *Vitamin D in Chronic Kidney Disease*,
DOI 10.1007/978-3-319-32507-1_25

of post-transplantation patient care and includes prevention of cardiovascular complications, diabetes mellitus, infections, cancer, and fractures associated with bone disease. The increased awareness that vitamin D deficiency, being common among renal transplant recipients may be involved in the pathogenesis of each of these complications, fueled interest in posttransplant vitamin D metabolism and triggered several interventional studies specifically exploring the pivotal benefits of vitamin D supplementation on bone metabolism and beyond. The present review aims to present a state of the art on vitamin D metabolism and its association with non-renal outcomes in kidney transplant recipients.

25.2   Vitamin D Metabolism in Health, Chronic Kidney Disease and Renal Transplantation

25.2.1   Vitamin D Metabolism in Health

Vitamin D is a steroid hormone whose primary function is to regulate calcium homeostasis and bone mineralization; however, it is increasingly thought to exert important effects on other tissues such as vascular endothelium and cells of the immune system. It is a unique vitamin in that it can be sourced from the diet or synthesized in the skin by ultraviolet B (UVB) sunlight. Most people depend on solar synthesis of vitamin D to achieve adequate body stores, with dietary vitamin D normally contributing only 10–20 % of the recommended intake. The formation of fully active vitamin D out of the prohormones ergocalciferol (vitamin D2) and cholecalciferol (vitamin D3) requires a further two-step hydroxylation process. Hepatocytes mediate the first hydroxylation on carbon 25 (by the action of CYP2R1) to produce 25-hydroxyvitamin D (25(OH)D), also known as calcidiol), which binds the vitamin D receptor (VDR) with only a modest affinity. The complete activation of vitamin D requires further hydroxylation on carbon 1 by the enzyme CYP27B1, resulting in the formation of calcitriol or 1,25 dihydroxyvitamin D (1,25(OH)$_2$D). This last step takes place mainly in the proximal tubular cells of the kidney. Both 25(OH)D and 1,25(OH)$_2$D undergo catabolism via multiple side chain hydroxylations. Vitamin D catabolism is mediated mainly by renal CYP24A1. Evidence suggests that CYP3A4, i.e. the most abundant cytochrome P450 enzyme in the liver, may also be involved. The quantitative contribution of CYP3A4 to vitamin D catabolism, compared to CYP24A1, is poorly defined.

Production and catabolism of 1,25(OH)$_2$D by the kidney is tightly regulated through a complex system of hormones that together maintain calcium and phosphorus homeostasis. These hormones include parathyroid hormone (PTH), fibroblast growth factor 23 (FGF23), and 1,25(OH)$_2$D itself. While 1,25(OH)$_2$D is considered the biologically active form of vitamin D, 25(OH)D is the major circulating form and is considered the more reliable measure of vitamin D status.

25.2.2 Vitamin D Metabolism in Chronic Kidney Disease

In CKD, 1,25(OH)$_2$D production is reduced owing to alterations in CYP abundances, CYP activity, and delivery of substrate to CYP enzymes (for review see [2]). PTH and FGF23 exert opposite effect on CYP27B1 expression. The net effect is uncertain, as evidenced by experimental and clinical data. Impaired delivery of 25(OH)D to CYP27B1 and/or decreased CYP27B1 activity may prove more important than decreased enzymatic mass in CKD. Circulating 25(OH)D levels in CKD patients are often low as a result of low sun exposure, decreased cutaneous synthesis, and limited dietary intake. Moreover, reabsorption of filtered 25(OH)D in the proximal tubule may be impaired in CKD as a consequence of decreased megalin expression. CKD also disrupts vitamin D catabolism. PTH suppresses, while FGF23 stimulates CYP24A1 expression and activity. The net effect remains, as for CYP27B1, incompletely understood. Most recent data suggest that CKD should be considered a state of stagnant vitamin D metabolism characterized by reduced vitamin D catabolism and turnover in addition to reduced 1,25(OH)$_2$D production. In this paradigm, competing effects of PTH and FGF23 on the expression of CYP27B1 and CYP24A1 either balance each other or are superseded by a general decrease in vitamin D metabolic function of the kidney, caused either by impaired uptake of 25(OH)D, diminished metabolic activity of proximal tubular cells, or a simple reduction in the number of functioning nephrons (for review see [2]).

25.2.3 Vitamin D Metabolism in Renal Transplant Recipients

Renal transplantation restores, at least partly, renal functional mass and corrects metabolic and hormonal disturbances underlying the altered vitamin D metabolism in CKD [3].

25.2.3.1 25(OH)D Levels in Renal Transplant Recipients

Following renal transplantation, serum 25(OH)D levels commonly follow a biphasic pattern characterized by an early decrease followed by a modest recovery [4–8]. Several mechanisms may be hypothesized to contribute to the early decline [9]; first, tubular dysfunction (related to ischemia-reperfusion injury) associates with overload proteinuria which may result in substantial urinary losses of the Vitamin D- Vitamin D binding protein complex. Second, vitamin D catabolism may be enhanced in the posttransplant period, due to upregulation of CYP24A1 either by inappropriately high FGF23 levels [10] or by glucocorticoids [11]. Despite a slight recovery of 25(OH)D levels later on, 25(OH)D levels remain significantly lower compared with controls [12] and 25(OH)D deficiency and insufficiency remain very common among renal transplant recipients (see below). Sun avoidance behavior undoubtedly contributes to the high prevalence of low 25(OH)D levels among renal transplant recipients. Due to increased risk of skin cancers, renal transplant recipients are routinely advocated to limit sun exposure or to use sun blockers.

Vitamin D insufficiency, defined by a total 25(OH)D level below 30 ng/mL, is observed in 75–97 % of the renal transplant recipients [7, 9, 12–17]. Latitude, season, race, gender, comorbidity, diabetes, nutrition, body mass index, and time since transplantation correlate with serum 25(OH)D levels [15, 17, 18]. In a recent cohort study, 25(OH)D levels were independently and inversely associated with calcineurin inhibitor (CNI) exposure [17]. This observation argues against a prominent role of CYP3A4 in the catabolism of 25(OH)D, as CNI are well established competitive inhibitors of this enzyme.

The increased awareness of the many beneficial pleiotropic (nonskeletal) effects of 25-hydroxyvitamin D as well as the consistency of observational data showing a direct association between vitamin D deficiency and poor cardiovascular outcomes caused a vitamin D hype in recent years [19], not only in the general population but also in the transplant community. Supplementation of nutritional vitamin D has become routine practice in many dialysis and transplant units. As a consequence, vitamin D deficiency nowadays seems to be less common among renal transplant candidates and recipients (Evenepoel, unpublished data).

25.2.3.2   1,25(OH)₂D Levels in Renal Transplant Recipients

Serum $1,25(OH)_2D$ levels show a steady increase following successful transplantation [5, 20], parallel to the recovery of renal function. Remarkably however, concentrations remain often at the lower range in the early posttransplant period despite the presence of hyperparathyroidism and hypophosphatemia (see below), conditions known to stimulate increased calcitriol synthesis [5, 6, 21, 22]. Again, a diminished enzymatic function, perhaps related to redox imbalance being common in the early posttransplant period, may be involved. By 1 year after transplantation, calcitriol deficiency, defined by $1,25(OH)_2D$ concentrations below 20 ng/L, however is a rare finding, as long as eGFR >30 ml/min per 1.73 m² [5]. In a cross-sectional study, low PTH and high FGF23 levels associated with low calcitriol levels, independent of renal function [14, 23]. This observation confirms the opposing actions of FGF23 and PTH on CYP27B1 [14, 24]. The CNI cyclosporin increases the synthesis of $1,25(OH)_2D$ in rodents [25]. Clinical studies exploring the link between cyclosporine exposure and circulating levels of $1,25(OH)_2D$ are lacking. Finally, prospective data show that increments of calcitriol in the early posttransplant period are highest in patients who are able to maintain their 25(OH)D stores, emphasizing the importance of substrate availability [14, 26] (Fig. 25.1).

25.3   Vitamin D and Non-renal Outcomes in Renal Transplant Recipients

25.3.1   *Vitamin D and Mortality in Renal Transplant Recipients*

In agreement with observations in the general population and in CKD patients [27], low 25(OH)D levels in renal transplant recipients were recently shown to associate with increased (all-cause) mortality [28]. Whether restoring 25(OH)D levels reduces the risk of mortality, as suggested by a recent meta-analysis of randomized controlled trials [29], remains to be formally proven (Fig. 25.2).

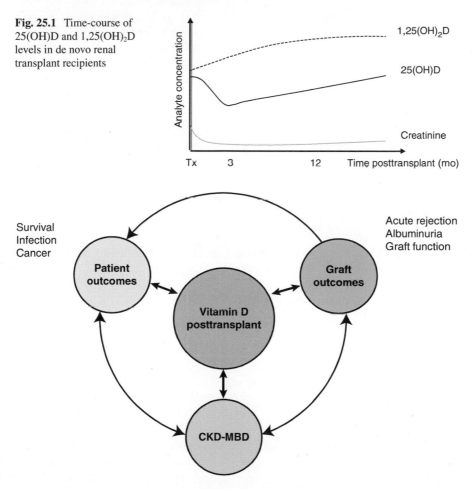

Fig. 25.1 Time-course of 25(OH)D and 1,25(OH)$_2$D levels in de novo renal transplant recipients

Fig. 25.2 Vitamin D and outcomes in renal transplant recipients

25.3.2   Vitamin D and Bone Health in Renal Transplant Recipients

25.3.2.1   Epidemiology of BMD Loss and Fractures in Renal Transplantation

Patients receiving a kidney transplant experience rapid bone loss [30, 31] and increased fracture risk [32], especially in the early posttransplant period. On the long term, BMD either recovers, further deteriorates at a slower pace or stabilizes [33–36]. Fracture risk in renal transplant recipients is fourfold higher than in healthy individuals [37–39]. Compared with dialysis patients on the waiting list, the relative risk of hip fracture in transplant recipients is 34 % higher during the first 6 months posttransplantation and decreases by ~1 % each month thereafter [40]. However, 10 years after transplantation, the fracture risk still is twofold higher than in controls [37]. Although posttransplantation fractures occur both peripherally and centrally, most studies demonstrate more fractures occurring at peripheral sites. Importantly, BMD loss and fracture risk is lower in more recent renal transplant cohorts [41]. This decrease may reflect either decreased cumulative steroid exposure, improved mineral metabolism control, or a combination of both [42–45]. This observation led some to conclude that the threat of postransplantation bone loss may have come to an end [46]. Dual-energy x-ray (DXA) is used in the routine to analyze bone mass. The reliability of DXA in CKD and, by extension, in renal transplantation has long been questioned [47]. Recent bone biopsy findings [48] and prospective observational data [49–52], however, clearly indicate that DXA may be as valuable in predicting osteoporosis and incident and prevalent fractures in CKD patients (including renal transplant recipients) as it is in the general population (Fig. 25.3).

25.3.2.2   Risk Factors and Pathophysiology of BMD Loss and Fractures in Renal Transplant Recipients

The factors contributing to bone loss and increased fracture risks are multiple with glucocorticoids and hyperparathyroidism being most prominent [3, 53–56]. **Glucocorticoids**, an integral component of the immunosuppressive regimen in renal transplantation, are believed to play a major role in compromising bone strength [57]. Glucocorticoids directly decrease bone formation through increasing apoptosis of osteoblasts and impairing osteogenesis. Glucocorticoids also directly reduce osteoclast production but, in contrast to the increase of osteoblast apoptosis, the lifespan of osteoclasts is prolonged. Therefore, with long-term therapy, osteoclast number are usually maintained in the normal range, whereas osteoblasts and bone formation decrease [58]. Glucocorticoids also indirectly decrease bone formation and mineralization through decreasing intestinal calcium absorption and increasing renal calcium secretion, thereby inducing a negative calcium balance [59]. The net result of glucocorticoid usage is loss of both cortical and cancellous bone. Finally, glucocorticoids also trigger osteocyte apoptosis.

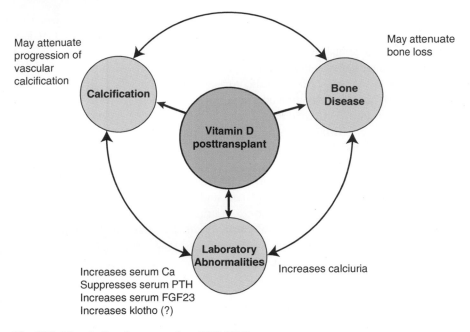

Fig. 25.3 Vitamin D and posttransplant CKD-MBD

Glucocorticoid-induced osteocyte apoptosis could account for the loss of bone strength that occurs before loss of BMD and the resultant mismatch between bone quantity and quality in patients with glucocorticoid-related osteoporosis [58]. The adverse effect of steroids primarily affect the axial (central) skeleton [32, 33, 60, 61]. The observation that fracture risk is substantially higher in renal transplant recipients than in recipients of other solid organs [62] suggest the involvement of specific risk factors. Available evidence points to pre-existing (renal) bone disease and persistent hyperparathyroidism as important culprits [3, 62]. **Persistent hyperparathyroidism** is common among renal transplant recipients, with reported prevalence rates ranging between 10 % and 66 %. Unique to the transplant setting is the combination of high PTH levels with low phosphate levels. High PTH and low phosphate levels have divergent effects on osteoblasts; low phosphate is associated with increased apoptosis, whereas high PTH is associated with preserved survival of osteoblasts [63]. Hypophosphatemia may be at least partly responsible for the uncoupling of bone resorption and formation and explain why low bone turnover is a frequent observation in renal transplant recipients with persistent hyperparathyroidism [64]. The bone phenotype of persistent hyperparathyroidism may thus be characterized by low bone volume in combination with either low, normal or high bone turnover. Most, but not all [30, 33, 42] epidemiological data in renal transplant populations show a direct association between PTH levels, (cortical) bone mineral density loss [61, 65, 66], and fracture risk [8, 67, 68]. Even in the absence of long-term corticosteroids exposure, high PTH levels may accelerate bone loss [69].

Besides glucocorticoids, pre-existing bone disease, and persistent hyperparathyroidism, older age, female sex [70], white race, deceased kidney donation, diabetes [70], hypogonadism, metabolic acidosis [71], high FGF23 level [42], increased time elapsed since transplantation and frequent falls (either related to postural instability, decreased visual acuity, peripheral neuropathy or myopathy) have been identified as risk factors for posttransplantation bone loss and fractures [32, 39, 55, 57].

Whether **vitamin D deficiency**, similar to as in the ageing general population [72] associates with BMD loss and fractures in renal transplant recipients has so far not been investigated. In combination with a low dietary calcium intake and glucocorticoids, vitamin D deficiency may induce a negative calcium balance, which, in turn may trigger or accentuate hyperparathyroidism and as such promote (cortical) bone resorption. Formal calcium balance studies are lacking in renal transplant recipients, but isotope studies and low 24 h-urinary calcium excretion at least lend support to the thesis of calcium malabsorption in renal transplant recipients [73]. Vitamin D deficiency, furthermore, may cause muscle weakness and postural instability and thereby increase the risk of falling [72].

25.3.2.3 Implications of Low BMD and Fractures in Renal Transplant Recipients

Low BMD and fractures confer important risks, not at the least an increased mortality. Hip fractures are the most devastating; the risk of death is approximately three times higher for individuals in the year after a hip fracture. In renal transplant recipients, mortality risk increases by another 60 % [38]. In addition to increased mortality due to low BMD, there is a detrimental effect on quality of life and a considerable financial burden.

25.3.2.4 Efficacy of Vitamin D Supplementation in Preserving Bone Health in Renal Transplant Recipients

Vitamin D supplementation is widely recommended and implemented in the prevention and treatment of both senile and glucocorticoid induced osteoporosis and fractures [74, 75], whether or not as an adjunct to specific pharmacologic agents and nonpharmacologic therapies [55]. Current evidence indicates that vitamin D plus calcium, as opposed to vitamin D alone, may prevent hip or any type of fracture [76, 77]. The need for calcium supplementation in addition to vitamin D is supported by experimental data showing that under conditions of calcium malabsorption exogenous vitamin D may actually decrease mineralization [78]. Interestingly, individuals in the older age groups having low baseline vitamin D status and low calcium intake seem to benefit most from vitamin D and calcium supplementation [72].

Due to the heterogeneity of bone changes after transplantation, osteoporosis treatment recommendations in the general population, including those related to vitamin D, may not be transferable to the specialized setting of renal transplantation.

Fortunately, a body of randomized data emerged in recent years specific to the treatment of bone disease with vitamin D in solid organ transplant recipients, including kidney transplant recipients. Among these studies, several investigated vitamin D (and calcium) vs. placebo [6, 79–83] or vitamin D and calcium vs calcium [4, 84–86]. Not surprisingly, vitamin D therapy suppresses PTH levels [6, 80, 87]. Vitamin D, conversely increases FGF23, which may explain why phosphorus concentrations tend to decrease in vitamin D treated patients [88]. Most, but not all [6, 81] controlled studies evaluating BMD by DEXA showed higher bone gains in the active treatment group, both at the lumbar spine and femoral neck. Studies comparing vitamin D to bisphosphonates showed mixed results with some investigators showing superiority of bisphosphonates [89, 90] and others showing equal efficacy [43]. Of note, no study was powered to show a reduction in risk for fracture at any site after transplantation.

Discrepancy between study results can be explained by differences in timing of intervention, baseline vitamin D status, baseline BMD, treatment regimen (dose, agent), or vitamin D receptor genotype. The VDR genotype polymorphisms affects the bone density of renal transplants via its effects on the severity of hyperparathyroidism [67, 91]. It has been suggested that a decreased transcriptional activity or stability of the VDR mRNA in patients with the bb haplotype could explain the decreased effects of calcitriol on the parathyroid gland [92]. Type of vitamin D agent and dose may matter as well [75, 93]. Both native vitamin D and active vitamin D (analogues) have been evaluated, but formal head to head comparisons are non-existing. A recent meta-analysis of RCTs including organ transplantation studies suggests superiority of active vitamin D (analogues) over native vitamin D [93]. The advantage of administrating active vitamin D (or its analogues) is that potential disturbances in hepatic and renal vitamin D metabolism do not have to be accounted for. However, in addition to their higher cost use of active vitamin D (or analogues) is associated with a higher risk of hypercalcemia and hypercalciuria compared to native vitamin D supplementation.

The optimal dose to replenish and maintain vitamin D stores are difficult to define. There is no such "one size fits all" regimen. Factors to be considered include the magnitude of the deficit and desired velocity of correction. Overall, high doses may be required, i.e. up to 100,000 IU every 2 weeks to correct vitamin D deficiency, and up to 50,000 IU every 4 weeks to maintain vitamin D sufficiency [15, 87, 94]. A recent meta-analysis indicate that vitamin D_3 is more efficacious in raising 25(OH)D concentrations compared to vitamin D_2 [95].

25.3.2.5 Safety of Vitamin D Supplementation in Renal Transplant Recipients

Vitamin D supplementation increases serum calcium levels and calciuria [87, 88]. Hypercalcemia is common in incident renal transplant recipients, even in those not receiving calcium or vitamin D supplements, with prevalence rates reported in literature varying between 5 and 66 % [13, 20, 96–100]. This wide variation may be explained, at least partly, by case-mix (variable interval since transplantation and study era) and differences in diagnostic criteria [101]. The pathophysiological mechanisms underlying the hypercalcemia in renal transplant recipients remain incompletely understood. PTH mediated calcium release from the bone, renal calcium retention and/or calcium-sensing receptor downregulation may all be speculated to be involved [97, 99]. The fear of triggering or aggravating hypercalcemia impedes the widespread implementation of vitamin D and calcium supplementation in the prevention of bone loss in incident renal transplant recipients. This fear may prove unjustified. Indeed, vitamin D and calcium supplementation may be hypothezised to be especially beneficial in the setting of persistent hypercalcemic hyperparathyroidism by reverting the main calcium influx from bone to the gastrointestinal tract. Awaiting additional data confirming or refuting this hypothesis, clinicians should be less reluctant to initiate vitamin D and calcium in incident renal transplant recipients and to decrease or stop vitamin D in the advent of mild hypercalemia.

Besides inducing hypercalcemia, vitamin D may cause a mild decline of measured creatinine clearance. This may related to suppression of PTH [102]. PTH has vasodilatory effects on pre-glomerular vessels, while efferent arterioles are constricted, presumably secondary to renin release [103]. Alternatively, it may be related to a reduced tubular secretion of creatinine [104].

25.3.3 Vitamin D and Vascular Calcification in Renal Transplant Recipients

Cardiovascular (CV) disease is the leading cause of premature death in renal transplant recipients with a 3.5–5 % annual risk of fatal or nonfatal CV events [105]. Vascular calcification burden, and even more so vascular calcification progression are potent predictors of future cardiovascular events in RTRs [106–108], likewise in the general population [109] and in CKD patients [110]. Most, but not all clinical data suggest that vitamin D may confer vascular benefits; a negative association has been observed between vitamin D level and vascular calcification [111–113], and pulse wave velocity [114], in CKD patients across stages of disease. Moreover, a positive and independent association has been observed between 25(OH)D [114, 115] and 1,25(OH)$_2$D [114] level and brachial artery distensability and flow-mediated dilation, both in dialysis patients [114] and renal transplant recipients [115]. Finally, high baseline 25(OH)D levels were associated with attenuated progression of vascular calcification in prevalent renal transplant recipients [116]. In aggregate, these results support an association between 25(OH)D and 1,25(OH)$_2$D deficiency and endothelial dysfunction, arteriosclerosis and arterial calcification. Nevertheless, randomized controlled trials remain mandatory to definitely proof the benefits of vitamin D treatment on cardiovascular outcomes both in the general population as in the setting of renal transplantation, especially since intervention trial in animals yielded discrepant findings [117]. The latter discrepancy most probably reflects differences in experimental conditions with dose and type of agent being important variables [118, 119]. The pathophysiological mechanisms underlying the putative beneficial effects of vitamin D on vascular health remain incompletely understood. Experimental evidence indicates that vitamin D may interact at the vascular tissue level both with Wnt/β-catenin [118], PTH [120], and FGF23/klotho signaling pathway [121]. Again, findings are dose and agent specific. Martinez-Moreno et al. for example, demonstrated that procalcifying Wnt signaling in VSMCs is suppressed by paricalcitol, but activated by calcitriol. Lim et al. demonstrated that calcitriol can restore klotho levels in procalcific environments, thereby rendering VSMCs again FGF-23 responsive, with proliferation and calcification inhibitory effects. Of note, similar results were obtained with calcidiol, suggesting that the VSMC 1α-hydroxylase enzyme is involved in mediating supportive autocrine/paracrine effects in the regulation of klotho [121]. It should be emphasized that these studies are debated [122] and need confirmation by independent investigators.

25.3.4 Vitamin D and Non-MBD Effects in Renal Transplant Recipients

Vitamin D status does not exclusively affect mineral and bone metabolism. Mounting evidence indicates that hypovitaminosis D may also be involved in the pathogenesis of oncologic, metabolic, and infectious diseases, all common in renal transplantation. The role of vitamin D in transplant immunology and the relationship between vitamin D levels, renal transplant rejection, function and survival are discussed elsewhere in this book. Herein, we summarize current evidence on the link between vitamin D, infections and cancer in renal transplant recipients.

25.3.4.1 Vitamin D and Infections in Renal Transplant Recipients

Vitamin D has emerged as a central player in the immune system, affecting T and B cells, macrophages and dendritic cells [123]. Contrary to the suppressive effects on the immune system, vitamin D also has a protective effect against infections. This was first shown in tuberculosis, where the traditional treatments with sunlight and cod liver oil, rich in vitamin D, are viewed in a new light after the discovery of antimicrobial peptides induced by vitamin D. The two antimicrobial peptides under the influence of vitamin D are LL-37 (cathelicidin) and β-defensin [124], which have activity against several bacteria, as well as viruses [125] and fungi [126]. Epidemiological studies have linked 25(OH)D deficiency to viral as well as bacterial infections in the general population (for review see [127]).

Infections are a common complication among renal transplant recipients. Clinical data on the association between vitamin D stores and infectious complications in transplant patients are scare. Severe vitamin D deficiency (25(OH)D3 <10ng/mL) was observed to be an independent predictor of urinary tract infections after renal transplantation [128]. In a cohort of 166 patients, who underwent allogeneic hematopoietic stem cell transplantation, low serum levels of 25(OH)D before transplantation significantly correlated to posttransplant cytomegalovirus (CMV) disease. Studies investigating the association between 25(OH)D deficiency and viral disease (including polyomavirus associated nephropathy (PVAN) and CMV disease) in renal transplant recipients have yielded conflicting results [129, 130]. Intervention studies in renal transplant recipients powered for infectious endpoints are non-existing.

25.3.4.2 Vitamin D and Cancer in Renal Transplant Recipients

In the past three decades, an increasing body of evidence has emerged on the role of vitamin D in cell differentiation. The data suggest that vitamin D has a potent antiproliferative action on various cell types, including bone marrow, skin, muscle, and intestine [131]. Serum level of 25(OH)D has been shown to inversely correlate with the incidence of various types of cancers (breast, prostate, and colon) in the general population [132]. The incidence of cancer considerably increases after organ transplantation [133]. Recent data suggest that the rates of cancer in renal transplant recipients are similar to nontransplanted population who are 20–30 years older [133]. Elevated cancer risk after transplantation is thought to result from the interplay of several factors including chronic uremic state, cumulative exposure to immunosuppressive drugs, and viral infections. Studies investigating the association between vitamin D status an incident malignancies in incident renal transplant recipients so far yielded discrepant findings with some investigators observing an inverse [134] and others observing no relationship [16].

25.4 Conclusions

Both 25(OH)D and 1,25(OH)$_2$D levels are inappropriately low in a substantial proportion of renal transplant recipients. As in the general population and CKD patients, low vitamin D levels overall associate with increased mortality, and confer an increased risk of fractures, infections and malignancy. It should be emphasized that epidemiological evidence is limited and not universally unequivocal. Intervention studies with vitamin D supplementation in renal transplant recipients showed higher bone gains in the active treatment group, both at the lumbar spine and femoral neck. None of the studies, however, was powered to show a reduction in risk for fracture (Table 25.1). Awaiting the results of additional studies, native vitamin D supplementation, whether or not guided by 25(OH)D levels, should be considered in renal transplant recipients.

Table 25.1 Comparison of population, duration, and treatment findings among four studies

Author	Duration (months)	Population	Treatment	Comparator	Main finding
Torres et al. [86]	12	Adult, de novo RTRs, n=86	aVitD 0,5 µg/2 days, 3 months + eCa 0,5 g/day, 12 months	eCa 0,5 g/day, 12 months	Better preservation aBMD total hip; better control HPT
De Sévaux et al. [4]	6	Adult, de novo RTRs, n=111	aVitD 0,25 µg/day	–	Better preservation a BMD lumbar spine
Wissing et al. [6]	12	Adult, de novo RTRs, n=90	nVitD 25,000 U/month + eCa 0,4 g/day	eCa 0,4 g/day	No significant benefit aBMD; better control HPT
El-Husseini et al. [83]	12	Children and adolescents, de novo RTRs, n=30	aVit D 0,5 µg/day	–	Increase aBMD at lumbar spine; better control HPT

RTR renal transplant recipient, *aVitD* active vitamin D, *nVitD* nutritional vitamin D, *eCa* elementary calcium, *HPT* hyperparathyroidism, *aBMD* areal bone mineral density (by DXA)

Acknowledgements The author thanks D. Vanderschueren, MD, PhD and S. Pauwels, MD for critical reading of the manuscript.

References

1. Sayegh MH, Carpenter CB. Transplantation 50 years later – progress, challenges, and promises. N Engl J Med. 2004;351:2761–6.
2. Bosworth C, de Boer IH. Impaired vitamin D metabolism in CKD. Semin Nephrol. 2013;33:158–68.
3. Evenepoel P. Recovery versus persistence of disordered mineral metabolism in kidney transplant recipients. Semin Nephrol. 2013;33:191–203.
4. de Sevaux RGL, Hoitsma AJ, Corstens FHM, Wetzels JFM. Treatment with vitamin D and calcium reduces bone loss after renal transplantation: a randomized study. J Am Soc Nephrol. 2002;13:1608–14.
5. Evenepoel P, Meijers BKI, De Jonge H, et al. Recovery of hyperphosphatoninism and renal phosphorus wasting one year after successful renal transplantation. CJASN. 2008;3:1829–36.
6. Wissing KM, Broeders N, Moreno-Reyers R, et al. A controlled study of vitamin D3 to prevent bone loss in renal-transplant patients receiving low doses of steroids. Transplantation. 2005;79:108–15.
7. Bienaime F, Girard D, Anglicheau D, et al. Vitamin D status and outcomes after renal transplantation. J Am Soc Nephrol. 2013;24:831–41.
8. Smets YF, de Fijter JW, Ringers J, et al. Long-term follow-up study on bone mineral density and fractures after simultaneous pancreas-kidney transplantation. Kidney Int. 2004;66:2070–6.
9. Sadlier DM, Magee CC. Prevalence of 25(OH) vitamin D (calcidiol) deficiency at time of renal transplantation: a prospective study. Clin Transplant. 2007;21:683–8.
10. Helvig CF, Cuerrier D, Hosfield CM, et al. Dysregulation of renal vitamin D metabolism in the uremic rat. Kidney Int. 2010;78:463–72.
11. Akeno N, Matsunuma A, Maeda T, et al. Regulation of vitamin D-1alpha-hydroxylase and -24-hydroxylase expression by dexamethasone in mouse kidney. J Endocrinol. 2000;164:339–48.
12. Querings K, Girndt M, Geisel J, et al. 25-hydroxyvitamin D deficiency in renal transplant recipients. J Clin Endocrinol Metab. 2006;91:526–9.
13. Stavroulopoulos A, Cassidy MJD, Porter CJ, et al. Vitamin D status in renal transplant recipients. Am J Transplant. 2007;7:2546–52.
14. Evenepoel P, Naesens M, Claes K, et al. Tertiary 'hyperphosphatoninism' accentuates hypophosphatemia and suppresses calcitriol levels in renal transplant recipients. Am J Transplant. 2007;7:1193–200.
15. Beique LC, Kline GA, Dalton B, et al. Predicting deficiency of vitamin D in renal transplant recipients in northern climates. Transplantation. 2013;95:1479–84.
16. Marcen R, Jimenez S, Fernandez-Rodriguez A, et al. Are low levels of 25-hydroxyvitamin D a risk factor for cardiovascular diseases or malignancies in renal transplantation? Nephrol Dial Transplant. 2012;27 Suppl 4:iv47–52.
17. Filipov JJ, Zlatkov BK, Dimitrov EP, Svinarov D. Relationship between vitamin D status and immunosuppressive therapy in kidney transplant recipients. Biotechnol Biotechnol Equip. 2015;29:331–5.
18. Stein EM, Shane E. Vitamin D in organ transplantation. Osteoporos Int. 2011;22:2107–18.
19. Maxmen A. Nutrition advice: the vitamin D-lemma. Nature. 2011;475:23–5.
20. Reinhardt W, Bartelworth H, Jockenhövel F, et al. Sequential changes of biochemical bone parameters after kidney transplantation. Nephrol Dial Transplant. 1998;13:436–42.
21. Fleseriu M, Licata AA. Failure of successful renal transplant to produce appropriate levels of 1,25-dihydroxyvitamin D. Osteoporos Int. 2007;18:363–8.

22. de Sevaux RG, Hoitsma AJ, van Hoof HJ, et al. Abnormal vitamin D metabolism and loss of bone mass after renal transplantation. Nephron Clin Pract. 2003;93:C21–8.

23. Ewers B, Gasbjerg A, Moelgaard C, et al. Vitamin D status in kidney transplant patients: need for intensified routine supplementation. Am J Clin Nutr. 2008;87:431–7.

24. Bhan I, Shah A, Holmes J, et al. Post-transplant hypophosphatemia: tertiary 'Hyper-Phosphatoninism'? Kidney Int. 2006;70:1486–94.

25. Stein B, Halloran BP, Reinhardt T, et al. Cyclosporin-A increases synthesis of 1,25-dihydroxyvitamin D3 in the rat and mouse. Endocrinology. 1991;128:1369–73.

26. Barros X, Fuster D, Rodriguez N, et al. Rapid calcitriol increase and persistent calcidiol insufficiency in the first 6 months after kidney transplantation. Nucl Med Commun. 2015;36:489–93.

27. Wolf M, Thadhani R. Vitamin D in patients with renal failure: a summary of observational mortality studies and steps moving forward. Steroid Biochem Mol Biol. 2007;103:487–90.

28. Keyzer CA, Riphagen IJ, Joosten MM, et al. Associations of 25(OH) and 1,25(OH)2 vitamin D with long-term outcomes in stable renal transplant recipients. J Clin Endocrinol Metab. 2015;100:81–9.

29. Autier P, Gandini S. Vitamin D supplementation and total mortality: a meta-analysis of randomized controlled trials. Arch Intern Med. 2007;167:1730–7.

30. Julian B, Laskow D, Dobovsky E, et al. Rapid loss of vertebral mineral density after renal transplantation. N Engl J Med. 1991;325:544–50.

31. Heaf JG. Bone disease after renal transplantation. Transplantation. 2003;75:315–25.

32. Nikkel LE, Hollenbeak CS, Fox EJ, et al. Risk of fractures after renal transplantation in the United States. Transplantation. 2009;87:1846–51.

33. Casez JP, Lippuner K, Horber FF, et al. Changes in bone mineral density over 18 months following kidney transplantation: the respective roles of prednisone and parathyroid hormone. Nephrol Dial Transplant. 2002;17:1318–26.

34. Marcen R, Caballero C, Pascual J, et al. Lumbar bone mineral density in renal transplant patients on neoral and tacrolimus: a four-year prospective study. Transplantation. 2006;81:826–31.

35. Westeel FP, Mazouz H, Ezaitouni F, et al. Cyclosporine bone remodeling effect prevents steroid osteopenia after kidney transplantation. Kidney Int. 2000;58:1788–96.

36. Brandenburg VM, Politt D, Ketteler M, et al. Early rapid loss followed by long-term consolidation characterizes the development of lumbar bone mineral density after kidney transplantation. Transplantation. 2004;77:1566–71.

37. Vautour LM, Melton III LJ, Clarke BL, et al. Long-term fracture risk following renal transplantation: a population-based study. Osteoporos Int. 2004;15:160–7.

38. Abbott KC, Oglesby RJ, Hypolite IO, et al. Hospitalizations for fractures after renal transplantation in the United States. Ann Epidemiol. 2001;11:450–7.

39. Palmer SC, Strippoli GFM, McGregor DO. Interventions for preventing bone disease in kidney transplant recipients. Am J Kidney Dis. 2005;45:638–49.

40. Ball AM, Gillen DL, Sherrard D, et al. Risk of hip fracture among dialysis and renal transplant recipients. JAMA. 2002;288:3014–8.

41. Sukumaran NS, Lenihan CR, Montez-Rath ME, et al. Temporal trends in the incidence, treatment and outcomes of hip fracture after first kidney transplantation in the United States. Am J Transplant. 2014;14:943–51.

42. Kanaan N, Claes K, Devogelaer JP, et al. Fibroblast growth factor-23 and parathyroid hormone are associated with post-transplant bone mineral density loss. Clin J Am Soc Nephrol. 2010;5:1887–92.

43. Smerud KT, Dolgos S, Olsen IC, et al. A 1-year randomized, double-blind, placebo-controlled study of intravenous ibandronate on bone loss following renal transplantation. Am J Transplant. 2012;12:3316–25.

44. Naylor KL, Jamal SA, Zou G, et al. Fracture incidence in adult kidney transplant recipients. Transplantation. 2016. 100(1):167–75

45. Stein EM, Ortiz D, Jin Z, et al. Prevention of fractures after solid organ transplantation: a meta-analysis. J Clin Endocrinol Metab. 2011;96:3457–65.
46. Brandenburg VM, Floege J. Transplantation: an end to bone disease after renal transplantation? Nat Rev Nephrol. 2013;9:5–6.
47. Kidney Disease: Improving Global Outcomes (KDIGO) CKD-MBD Work Group. KDIGO clinical practice guideline for the diagnosis, evaluation, prevention, and treatment of Chronic Kidney Disease-Mineral and Bone Disorder (CKD-MBD). Kidney Int Suppl. 2009;113: S1–130.
48. Adragao T, Herberth J, Monier-Faugere MC, et al. Low bone volume – a risk factor for coronary calcifications in hemodialysis patients. Clin J Am Soc Nephrol. 2009;4:450–5.
49. Iimori S, Mori Y, Akita W, et al. Diagnostic usefulness of bone mineral density and biochemical markers of bone turnover in predicting fracture in CKD stage 5D patients – a single-center cohort study. Nephrol Dial Transplant. 2012;27:345–51.
50. West SL, Lok CE, Langsetmo L et al. Bone mineral density predicts fractures in chronic kidney disease. J Bone Miner Res. 2015. 30(5):913–9.
51. Nickolas TL, Cremers S, Zhang A, et al. Discriminants of prevalent fractures in chronic kidney disease. J Am Soc Nephrol. 2011;22:1560–72.
52. Akaberi S, Simonsen O, Lindergard B, Nyberg G. Can DXA predict fractures in renal transplant patients? Am J Transplant. 2008;8:2647–51.
53. Kodras K, Haas M. Effect of kidney transplantation on bone. Eur J Clin Invest. 2006;36: 63–75.
54. Weisinger JR, Carlini RG, Rojas E, Bellorin-Font E. Bone disease after renal transplantation. Clin J Am Soc Nephrol. 2006;1:1300–13.
55. Alshayeb HM, Josephson MA, Sprague SM. CKD-mineral and bone disorder management in kidney transplant recipients. Am J Kidney Dis. 2013;61:310–25.
56. Sperschneider H, Stein G. Bone disease after renal transplantation. Nephrol Dial Transplant. 2003;18:874–7.
57. Nikkel LE, Mohan S, Zhang A, et al. Reduced fracture risk with early corticosteroid withdrawal after kidney transplant. Am J Transplant. 2012;12:649–59.
58. Weinstein RS. Glucocorticoid-induced osteoporosis and osteonecrosis. Endocrinol Metab Clin N Am. 2012;41:595–611.
59. Lee GS, Choi KC, Jeung EB. Glucocorticoids differentially regulate expression of duodenal and renal calbindin-D9k through glucocorticoid receptor-mediated pathway in mouse model. Am J Physiol Endocrinol Metab. 2006;290:E299–307.
60. van den Ham EC, Kooman JP, Christiaans ML, van Hooff JP. The influence of early steroid withdrawal on body composition and bone mineral density in renal transplantation patients. Transpl Int. 2003;16:82–7.
61. Terpstra AM, Kalkwarf HJ, Shults J, et al. Bone density and cortical structure after pediatric renal transplantation. J Am Soc Nephrol. 2012;23:715–26.
62. Ghanekar H, Welch BJ, Moe OW, Sakhaee K. Post-renal transplantation hypophosphatemia: a review and novel insights. Curr Opin Nephrol Hypertens. 2006;15:97–104.
63. Rojas E, Carlini RG, Clesca P, et al. The pathogenesis of osteodystrophy after renal transplantation as detected by early alterations in bone remodeling. Kidney Int. 2003;63:1915–23.
64. Borchhardt KA, Sulzbacher I, Benesch T, et al. Low-turnover bone disease in hypercalcemic hyperparathyroidism after kidney transplantation. Am J Transplant. 2007;7:2515–21.
65. Akaberi S, Lindergard B, Simonsen O, Nyberg G. Impact of parathyroid hormone on bone density in long-term renal transplant patients with good graft function. Transplantation. 2006;82:749–52.
66. Heaf J, Tvedegaard E, Kanstrup IL, Fogh-Andersen N. Hyperparathyroidism and long-term bone loss after renal transplantation. Clin Transplant. 2003;17:268–74.
67. Giannini S, Sella S, Silva NF, et al. Persistent secondary hyperparathyroidism and vertebral fractures in kidney transplantation: role of calcium-sensing receptor polymorphisms and vitamin D deficiency. J Bone Miner Res. 2010;25:841–8.

68. Perrin P, Caillard S, Javier RM, et al. Persistent hyperparathyroidism is a major risk factor for fractures in the five years after kidney transplantation. Am J Transplant. 2013;13:2653–63.
69. Iyer SP, Nikkel LE, Nishiyama KK, et al. Kidney transplantation with early corticosteroid withdrawal: paradoxical effects at the central and peripheral skeleton. J Am Soc Nephrol. 2014;25:1331–41.
70. Nisbeth U, Lindh E, Ljunghall S, et al. Increased fracture rate in diabetes mellitus and females after renal transplantation. Transplantation. 1999;67:1218–22.
71. Starke A, Corsenca A, Kohler T, et al. Correction of metabolic acidosis with potassium citrate in renal transplant patients and its effect on bone quality. Clin J Am Soc Nephrol. 2012;7:1461–72.
72. Lips P, Gielen E, van Schoor NM. Vitamin D supplements with or without calcium to prevent fractures. Bonekey Rep. 2014;3:512.
73. Yu RW, Faull RJ, Coates PT, Coates PS. Calcium supplements lower bone resorption after renal transplant. Clin Transplant. 2011;26:292–9.
74. Recommendations for the prevention and treatment of glucocorticoid-induced osteoporosis: 2001 update. American College of Rheumatology Ad Hoc Committee on Glucocorticoid-Induced Osteoporosis. Arthritis Rheum. 2001;44:1496–03.
75. Bischoff-Ferrari HA, Willett WC, Orav EJ, et al. A pooled analysis of vitamin D dose requirements for fracture prevention. N Engl J Med. 2012;367:40–9.
76. Avenell A, Mak JC, O'Connell D. Vitamin D and vitamin D analogues for preventing fractures in post-menopausal women and older men. Cochrane Database Syst Rev. 2014; 4, CD000227.
77. Bauer DC. Clinical practice. Calcium supplements and fracture prevention. N Engl J Med. 2013;369:1537–43.
78. Lieben L, Masuyama R, Torrekens S, et al. Normocalcemia is maintained in mice under conditions of calcium malabsorption by vitamin D-induced inhibition of bone mineralization. J Clin Invest. 2012;122:1803–15.
79. Koc M, Tuglular S, Arikan H, et al. Alendronate increases bone mineral density in long-term renal transplant recipients. Transplant Proc. 2002;34:2111–3.
80. Trillini M, Cortinovis M, Ruggenenti P, et al. Paricalcitol for secondary hyperparathyroidism in renal transplantation. J Am Soc Nephrol. 2015;26:1205–14.
81. Cueto-Manzano AM, Konel S, Freemont AJ, et al. Effect of 1,25-dihydroxyvitamin D3 and calcium carbonate on bone loss associated with long-term renal transplantation. Am J Kidney Dis. 2000;35:227–36.
82. Josephson MA, Schumm LP, Chiu MY, et al. Calcium and calcitriol prophylaxis attenuates posttransplant bone loss. Transplantation. 2004;78:1233–6.
83. El-Husseini AA, El-Agroudy AE, El-Sayed M, et al. A prospective randomized study for the treatment of bone loss with vitamin d during kidney transplantation in children and adolescents. Am J Transplant. 2004;4:2052–7.
84. Talalai M, Gradowska L, Marcinowska-Suchowierska E, et al. Efficiency of preventive treatment of glucocorticoid-induced osteoporosis with 25-hydroxyvitamin D3 and calcium in kidney transplant patients. Transplant Proc. 1996;28:3485–7.
85. El-Agroudy AE, El-Husseini AA, El-Sayed M, et al. A prospective randomized study for prevention of postrenal transplantation bone loss. Kidney Int. 2005;67:2039–45.
86. Torres A, Garcia S, Gomez A, et al. Treatment with intermittent calcitriol and calcium reduces bone loss after renal transplantation. Kidney Int. 2004;65:705–12.
87. Courbebaisse M, Thervet E, Souberbielle JC, et al. Effects of vitamin D supplementation on the calcium-phosphate balance in renal transplant patients. Kidney Int. 2009;75:646–51.
88. Amer H, Griffin MD, Stegall MD, et al. Oral paricalcitol reduces the prevalence of posttransplant hyperparathyroidism: results of an open label randomized trial. Am J Transplant. 2013;13:1576–85.
89. Walsh SB, Altmann P, Pattison J, et al. Effect of pamidronate on bone loss after kidney transplantation: a randomized trial. Am J Kidney Dis. 2009;53:856–65.

90. Jeffery JR, Leslie WD, Karpinski ME, et al. Prevalence and treatment of decreased bone density in renal transplant recipients: a randomized prospective trial of calcitriol versus alendronate. Transplantation. 2003;76:1498–502.

91. Messa P, Sindici C, Cannella G, et al. Persistent secondary hyperparathyroidism after renal transplantation. Kidney Int. 1998;54:1704–13.

92. Bover J, Bosch RJ. Vitamin D receptor polymorphisms as a determinant of bone mass and PTH secretion: from facts to controversies. Nephrol Dial Transplant. 1999;14:1066–8.

93. Kandula P, Dobre M, Schold JD, et al. Vitamin D supplementation in chronic kidney disease: a systematic review and meta-analysis of observational studies and randomized controlled trials. Clin J Am Soc Nephrol. 2011;6:50–62.

94. Alshayeb HM, Wall BM, Showkat A, et al. Chronic kidney disease and diabetes mellitus predict resistance to vitamin D replacement therapy. Am J Med Sci. 2013;345:314–20.

95. Tripkovic L, Lambert H, Hart K, et al. Comparison of vitamin D2 and vitamin D3 supplementation in raising serum 25-hydroxyvitamin D status: a systematic review and meta-analysis. Am J Clin Nutr. 2012;95:1357–64.

96. Evenepoel P, Claes K, Kuypers D, et al. Natural history of parathyroid function and calcium metabolism after kidney transplantation: a single-centre study. Nephrol Dial Transplant. 2004;19:1281–7.

97. Cundy T, Kanis JA, Heynen G, et al. Calcium metabolism and hyperparathyroidism after renal transplantation. QJM. 1983;52:67–78.

98. Schwartz GH, David DS, Riggio RR, et al. Hypercalcemia after renal transplantation. Am J Med. 1970;49:42–51.

99. Evenepoel P, Van Den Bergh B, Naesens M, et al. Calcium metabolism in the early posttransplantation period. Clin J Am Soc Nephrol. 2009;4:665–72.

100. Vezzoli G, Elli A, Palazzi P, et al. High plasma ionized calcium with normal PTH and total calcium levels in normal-function kidney transplant recipients. Nephron. 1986;42:290–4.

101. Evenepoel P, Bammens B, Claes K, et al. Measuring total blood calcium displays a low sensitivity for the diagnosis of hypercalcemia in incident renal transplant recipients. Clin J Am Soc Nephrol. 2010;5:2085–92.

102. Evenepoel P, Claes K, Kuypers D, et al. Impact of parathyroidectomy on renal graft function, blood pressure and serum lipids in kidney transplant recipients: a single centre study. Nephrol Dial Transplant. 2005;20:1714–20.

103. Massfelder T, Parekh N, Endlich K, et al. Effect of intrarenally infused parathyroid hormone-related protein on renal blood flow and glomerular filtration rate in the anaesthetized rat. Br J Pharmacol. 1996;118:1995–2000.

104. Goodman WG, Coburn JW. The use of 1,25-dihydroxyvitamin D3 in early renal failure. Annu Rev Med. 1992;43:227–37, 227–237.

105. Cianciolo G, Capelli I, Angelini ML, et al. Importance of vascular calcification in kidney transplant recipients. Am J Nephrol. 2014;39:418–26.

106. Nguyen PT, Henrard S, Coche E, et al. Coronary artery calcification: a strong predictor of cardiovascular events in renal transplant recipients. Nephrol Dial Transplant. 2010;25:3773–8.

107. DeLoach SS, Joffe MM, Mai X, et al. Aortic calcification predicts cardiovascular events and all-cause mortality in renal transplantation. Nephrol Dial Transplant. 2009;24:1314–9.

108. Claes KJ, Heye S, Bammens B, et al. Aortic calcifications and arterial stiffness as predictors of cardiovascular events in incident renal transplant recipients. Transpl Int. 2013;26:973–81.

109. Budoff MJ, Hokanson JE, Nasir K, et al. Progression of coronary artery calcium predicts all-cause mortality. JACC Cardiovasc Imaging. 2010;3:1229–36.

110. Noordzij M, Cranenburg EM, Engelsman LF, et al. Progression of aortic calcification is associated with disorders of mineral metabolism and mortality in chronic dialysis patients. Nephrol Dial Transplant. 2011;26:1662–9.

111. de Boer IH, Kestenbaum B, Shoben AB, et al. 25-hydroxyvitamin D levels inversely associate with risk for developing coronary artery calcification. J Am Soc Nephrol. 2009;20:1805–12.

112. Kasiske BL, Guijarro C, Massy ZA, et al. Cardiovascular disease after renal transplantation. J Am Soc Nephrol. 1996;7:158–65.

113. Garcia-Canton C, Bosch E, Ramirez A, et al. Vascular calcification and 25-hydroxyvitamin D levels in non-dialysis patients with chronic kidney disease stages 4 and 5. Nephrol Dial Transplant. 2011;26:2250–6.
114. London GM, Guerin AP, Verbeke FH, et al. Mineral metabolism and arterial functions in end-stage renal disease: potential role of 25-hydroxyvitamin D deficiency. J Am Soc Nephrol. 2007;18:613–20.
115. Yildirim T, Yilmaz R, Altindal M, et al. Endothelial dysfunction in renal transplant recipients: role of vitamin D and fibroblast growth factor-23. Transplant Proc. 2015;47:343–7.
116. Marechal C, Coche E, Goffin E, et al. Progression of coronary artery calcification and thoracic aorta calcification in kidney transplant recipients. Am J Kidney Dis. 2012;59:258–69.
117. Mathew S, Lund RJ, Chaudhary LR, et al. Vitamin D receptor activators can protect against vascular calcification. J Am Soc Nephrol. 2008;19:1509–19.
118. Martinez-Moreno JM, Munoz-Castaneda JR, Herencia C, et al. In vascular smooth muscle cells paricalcitol prevents phosphate-induced Wnt/beta-catenin activation. Am J Physiol Renal Physiol. 2012;303:F1136–44.
119. Lopez I, Mendoza FJ, Guilera-Tejero E, et al. The effect of calcitriol, paricalcitol, and a cal-cimimetic on extraosseous calcifications in uremic rats. Kidney Int. 2007;73:300–7.
120. Jono S, Nishizawa Y, Shioi A, Morii H. Parathyroid hormone-related peptide as a local regulator of vascular calcification: its inhibitory action on in vitro calcification by bovine vascular smooth muscle cells. Arterioscler Thromb Vasc Biol. 1997;17:1135–42.
121. Lim K, Lu TS, Molostvov G, et al. Vascular Klotho deficiency potentiates the development of human artery calcification and mediates resistance to FGF-23. Circulation. 2012;125:2243–55.
122. Mencke R, Harms G, Mirkovic K, et al. Membrane-bound Klotho is not expressed endogenously in healthy or uraemic human vascular tissue. Cardiovasc Res. 2015;108:220–31.
123. Maruotti N, Cantatore FP. Vitamin D and the immune system. J Rheumatol. 2010;37:491–5.
124. Wang TT, Nestel FP, Bourdeau V, et al. Cutting edge: 1,25-dihydroxyvitamin D3 is a direct inducer of antimicrobial peptide gene expression. J Immunol. 2004;173:2909–12.
125. Wilson SS, Wiens ME, Smith JG. Antiviral mechanisms of human defensins. J Mol Biol. 2013;425:4965–80.
126. Vandamme D, Landuyt B, Luyten W, Schoofs L. A comprehensive summary of LL-37, the factotum human cathelicidin peptide. Cell Immunol. 2012;280:22–35.
127. Pludowski P, Holick MF, Pilz S, et al. Vitamin D effects on musculoskeletal health, immunity, autoimmunity, cardiovascular disease, cancer, fertility, pregnancy, dementia and mortality-a review of recent evidence. Autoimmun Rev. 2013;12:976–89.
128. Kwon YE, Kim H, Oh HJ, et al. Vitamin D deficiency is an independent risk factor for urinary tract infections after renal transplants. Medicine (Baltimore). 2015;94, e594.
129. Lee JR, Dadhania D, August P, et al. Circulating levels of 25-hydroxyvitamin D and acute cellular rejection in kidney allograft recipients. Transplantation. 2014;98:292–9.
130. Rech MA, Fleming JN, Moore CL. 25-hydroxyvitamin D deficiency and opportunistic viral infections after kidney transplant. Exp Clin Transplant. 2014;12:95–100.
131. Nagpal S, Na S, Rathnachalam R. Noncalcemic actions of vitamin D receptor ligands. Endocr Rev. 2005;26:662–87.
132. Holick MF. Vitamin D deficiency. N Engl J Med. 2007;357:266–81.
133. Webster AC, Craig JC, Simpson JM, et al. Identifying high risk groups and quantifying absolute risk of cancer after kidney transplantation: a cohort study of 15,183 recipients. Am J Transplant. 2007;7:2140–51.
134. Ducloux D, Courivaud C, Bamoulid J, et al. Pretransplant serum vitamin D levels and risk of cancer after renal transplantation. Transplantation. 2008;85:1755–9.

Chapter 26
Vitamin D in Acute and Chronic Rejection of Transplanted Kidney

Marie Courbebaisse

Abstract Due to its nephroprotective and immunomodulatory properties, vitamin D is susceptible to have a protective role against acute and chronic renal graft rejection. Regarding acute rejection (AR), experimental studies have shown that vitamin D receptor (VDR) agonists attenuate CD4+ and CD8+ T-cell proliferation and their cytotoxic activity, decrease plasma cell differentiation, B-cell proliferation, IgG secretion and differentiation, as well as maturation and immunostimulatory capacity of dendritic cells (DCs). By limiting adaptative immune response and down-regulating DC, VDR agonists are thus susceptible to help in preventing AR. The immunomodulatory capacity of calcitriol observed in vitro has been confirmed in several animal models of transplantation without increasing the risk of infection. Some observational studies and small interventional trials in renal transplant recipients (RTR) support the potential protective role of active vitamin D against AR. Regarding chronic rejection, in addition to potentially inducing tolerogenic DCs, VDR agonists could also inhibit the production of chemokines, responsible for leukocytes infiltration in vessels allograft, and may down-regulate TGF-β pathway, which has a profibrotic activity. Other renoprotective effects of vitamin D, such as inhibition of renin angiotensin system and of NF-kB activation, may participate in the prevention of chronic allograft rejection. Although several studies have highlighted the potential nephroprotective role of vitamin D sufficiency and of VDR agonists in humans, very few studies have been performed in RTR. Three ongoing randomized controlled trials are testing native vitamin D in RTR and should help to precise the role of the vitamin D pathway in reducing (or not) the risk of acute and chronic allograft rejection.

Keywords Cholecalciferol • Calcium • Phosphate • Parathyroid hormone • Kidney transplantation • Graft rejection • Vitamin D

M. Courbebaisse, MD, PhD
Functional Renal Explorations Service, Department of Physiology,
Georges Pompidou European Hospital, Paris, France
e-mail: marie.courbebaisse@egp.aphp.fr; marie.courbebaisse@aphp.fr

© Springer International Publishing Switzerland 2016 443
P.A. Ureña Torres et al. (eds.), *Vitamin D in Chronic Kidney Disease*,
DOI 10.1007/978-3-319-32507-1_26

26.1   Introduction

Traditionally, vitamin D has been associated with mineral and bone health; its deficiency leads to rickets in children and osteomalacia in adults, and increases the risk of osteoporosis. More recently, vitamin D sufficiency has been associated with a reduced risk of many diseases including cardiovascular disease, type 2 diabetes mellitus, cancers, infections, and chronic kidney disease (CKD). All these diseases are more likely to occur in renal transplant recipients (RTR) than in the general population. Moreover, due to its nephroprotective and immunomodulatory properties, vitamin D seems to have a protective role against acute and chronic graft rejection. Currently, the active form of vitamin D is currently used after kidney transplantation for the prevention of post-transplant bone loss [1] and the treatment of normocalcemic persistent secondary hyperparathyroidism [2–4]. Treatment with active vitamin D or its analogues will not compensate for inadequate 25-hydroxyvitamin D (25(OH)D) however. 25(OH)D is a substrate for 1α-hydroxylase (CYP27B1) in the kidney, and also in several extrarenal tissues, and these extrarenal tissues are dependent on sufficient circulating levels of 25(OH)D to ensure adequate local calcitriol production. Although there is no current consensus, vitamin D insufficiency is usually defined as serum 25(OH)D levels lower than 30 ng/ml (or <75 nmol/l) [5], because this limit is associated with a decrease in active intestinal calcium absorption [6] and with an increase in the serum levels of parathormone (PTH), which is involved in the maintenance of normal serum calcium levels [5]. Furthermore, in all interventional studies showing positive effects of vitamin D supplementation on biochemical parameters and clinical outcomes, the serum 25(OH)D levels reached in the treated groups have been generally higher than 30 ng/ml [7]. This implies that, using this threshold, actually vitamin D insufficiency is present in more than 85 % of adult RTR [8].

The main causes of such high incidence of vitamin D insufficiency include: (1) insufficient vitamin D supplementation before and after renal transplantation; (2) increased 25(OH)D catabolism induced by immunosuppressive drugs [9] and by post-transplant persistent high serum fibroblast growth factor-23 concentration, which inhibits calcitriol synthesis and stimulates vitamin D catabolism [10]; and (3) the reduced sun exposure recommended to RTR to prevent skin cancers [11]. As a result, RTR are now systematically advised to protect themselves from exposure to solar or artificial ultraviolet (UV) radiation. This represents a serious dilemma, as 80–90 % of the human body's requirements for vitamin D result from photosynthesis of the vitamin from 7-dehydrocholesterol in the skin by the action of UVB radiation. Therefore, careful monitoring of vitamin D status and oral supplementation to ensure that vitamin D insufficiency does not occur is of great importance for RTR.

Despite the high prevalence of vitamin D insufficiency in RTR, there is no general consensus regarding vitamin D supplementation before and following kidney transplantation. In one study, it was shown that high doses of vitamin D_3 (100,000 IU cholecalciferol every other week for 2 months, equivalent to 6,600 IU/day) were able to correct 25(OH)D insufficiency in RTR without significant side effects, and this regimen was also associated with a significant decrease in serum PTH concentration. However, this study also indicated that the dose of cholecalciferol used during the maintenance phase (100,000 IU every other month from months 6 to 12 post-transplantation) was insufficient to maintain serum 25(OH)D concentration above 30 ng/ml in half of the patients [12]. Another study showed that 25,000 IU of oral cholecalciferol once a month failed to correct vitamin D insufficiency in RTR, suggesting that a higher dose of cholecalciferol is necessary to maintain adequate serum 25(OH)D levels after kidney transplantation [13]. The optimal dosage scheme was simulated from the data of a previous study [12] using a population pharmacokinetic approach. In order to maintain serum 25(OH)D concentrations between 30 and 80 ng/ml during the first year after renal transplantation, it was estimated that cholecalciferol dosing should be 100,000 IU once a month once correction of vitamin D insufficiency has been achieved [14].

26.2   Vitamin D and Kidney Graft Rejection

Even though the incidence has been greatly reduced, acute rejection (AR) and chronic allograft deterioration remain important issues after renal transplantation.

26.2.1   Acute Kidney Allograft Rejection

In retrospective case-control studies, it was reported that osteoporotic RTR experienced fewer AR after calcitriol treatment induction [15] and needed fewer pulse steroid doses [16]. More recently, it was reported in a retrospective observational study, including 351 RTR who had serum levels of 25(OH)D measured within the first 30 days of the renal transplantation, that biopsy-confirmed acute cellular rejection during the first year was more frequent in the vitamin D-deficient group than in the sufficient group (10.2 % vs. 3.7 %, P=0.04). By multivariable Cox regression analysis, vitamin D deficiency was an independent risk factor for AR (Hazard Ratio: 3.3, P=0.02). In this study, vitamin D deficiency was defined as a circulating level of 25(OH)D ≤20 ng/mL and was observed in 216 (61.5 %) of the RTR [17]. The authors confirmed that 1,25-dihydroxyvitamin D_3 supplementation initiated within the first 90 days of transplantation was associated with a lesser incidence of AR compared to no treatment with 1,25-dihydroxyvitamin D3 (5.1 % vs. 13.0 %, P=0.099). A Japanese monocentric observational study, including of 264 RTR with a baseline serum 25(OH)D concentration of 17.1±6.5 ng/mL, showed that vitamin D deficiency predicts a higher need for the use of intravenous (i.v.) methylprednisolone (as an index of AR episodes) at less than 10 years after renal transplantation [18].

Several experimental studies also support this effect. First, calcitriol inhibits the expression of IL-2 and interferon-γ mRNA and protein in T cells and attenuates CD4+ and CD8+ T-cell proliferation and their cytotoxic activity [19–21]. Vitamin D receptor (VDR) expression in T cells is not constitutive but only upregulated after activation by its own agonists [22]. Calcitriol also decreases plasma cell differentiation, B-cell proliferation, and IgG secretion [23]. Second, calcitriol inhibits the expression of major histocompatibility complex class II, CD40, CD80, and CD86, thus decreasing differentiation, maturation, and immunostimulatory capacity of dendritic cells (DCs) [24–26], which constitutively express VDR and CYP27B1 [24]. Even though DCs are not the most important cells implicated with the alloimmune response, their role has been emphasized [27]. Calcitriol also down-regulates IL-12 synthesis and simultaneously stimulates IL-10 production by DCs [25]. The net result is a decrease in T helper 1-cell responses and a possible induction of IL-10 producing T-regulatory type 1 cells. By limiting adaptive immune response and down-regulating DCs proliferation and activity, VDR agonists are, thus, susceptible to help in preventing AR [28]. The immunomodulatory capacity of calcitriol observed in vitro has been confirmed in several animal models of organ transplantation. Calcitriol or its analogs prolonged the survival of murine cardiac allograft [29], increased survival in a rat model of liver transplantation [30], delayed autoimmune disease recurrence after syngeneic islet transplantation in non-obese diabetic mice [31] and also reduced short- and long-term renal allograft rejection in the rat [32]. Importantly, Cantorna et al. [33] showed that calcitriol prolonged graft survival in animal models without increasing the risk of fungal or viral infection.

In a small prospective study, Ardalan et al. investigated the effect of calcitriol therapy which was started in the donor and continued in recipient side (nine donors, who all received calcitriol at a dose of 0.5 μg/day orally for 5 days before donation and nine RTR who were treated with the same regimen for 1 month post-transplant and thereafter received 0.25 μg/day for 5 months compared to ten controls with conventional treatment). Although only 19 RTR were included, a significant expansion of CD4+ CD25+ regulatory T cells in the calcitriol-treated group could be demonstrated, providing strong evidence of the immunomodulatory properties of active vitamin D after transplantation [34]. In another small prospective clinical trial, 24 uremic patients transplanted 6–18 months before the study were treated with calcitriol at a dose of 0.5 μg/day during 4 weeks. A decrease in HLA-DR, CD28, CD86, and CD40 expression on white blood cells was found after calcitriol treatment [35]. Altogether, VDR agonists could be used as potentially immunomodulatory agents in RTR. Currently, besides calcitriol, other VDR activators such as paricalcitol, which may exert immunomodulation without inducing hypercalcemia and hyperphosphatémia, could be potentially useful in RTR [36].

26.2.2 Chronic Renal Allograft Rejection and Renoprotective Effects of Vitamin D After Renal Transplantation

Chronic rejection is currently the most prevalent cause of renal transplant failure. Clinically, chronic rejection presents by chronic transplant dysfunction, characterized by a slow loss of renal function, often in combination with proteinuria and arterial hypertension. The histopathology is not specific in most cases but transplant glomerulopathy and multilayering of the peritubular capillaries are highly characteristic. Several risk factors have been identified such as young recipient age, black race, pre-sensitization, histo-incompatability, and acute rejection episodes, especially vascular rejection episodes and rejections that occur late after renal transplantation. Chronic rejection develops in grafts that undergo intermittent or persistent damage from cellular and humoral responses resulting from indirect recognition of alloantigens. Progression factors such as advanced donor age, renal dysfunction, hypertension, proteinuria, hyperlipidemia, and smoking accelerate deterioration of renal function.

A number of observational clinical studies have highlighted the potent renoprotective and antiproteinuric effects of vitamin D and its analogs [37, 38]. Importantly, serum 25(OH)D level was found to be inversely associated with the prevalence of albuminuria [39] and to be an independent inverse predictor of the progression to dialysis in patients with stage 2–5 CKD [40]. After renal transplantation, vitamin D insufficiency was significantly associated with the degree of proteinuria [38] and another retrospective study suggested a beneficial effect of calcitriol therapy on renal graft function [41]. More recently, a Japanese monocentric observational study cited above showed that vitamin D deficiency predicts a rapid decline in estimated GFR at less than 10 years after renal transplantation [18]. Polymorphism of genes encoding components of the vitamin D pathway including VDR and vitamin D binding protein (VDBP) have been explored due to the complex role played by vitamin D in renal transplant outcomes. It was reported that VDBP polymorphisms were associated with allograft survival (or AR) among 502 RTR; however, the authors found no association between polymorphic markers in the VDR gene and the renal allograft outcomes [42]. Inversely, another study conducted in 379 RTR showed that there was a significantly improved allograft survival for patients who were homozygous or heterozygous for the VDR FokI T allele [43].

Experimental data support these clinical observations. The potential protective role of VDR agonists against chronic renal allograft rejection is supported by many arguments. In addition to potentially inducing tolerogenic DCs, VDR agonists could also inhibit the production of chemokines, responsible for leukocytes infiltration in vessels allograft, and may down-regulate TGF-β pathway, which has a profibrotic activity [44]. Other renoprotective effects of vitamin D may participate in the prevention of chronic allograft rejection: calcitriol and analogs inhibit the renin-angiotensin-aldosterone system (RAAS), which has a pivotal role in glomerular and tubulo-interstitial damages, glomerular hypertension, and proteinuria [45]. It has also been shown that vitamin D inhibits NF-kB activation [46], which is known to play an important role in renal diseases by promoting inflammation and fibrogenesis. Many animal models of CKD have demonstrated the renoprotective effects of vitamin D analogs. They are able to attenuate tubulo-interstitial fibrosis and glomerulosclerosis, reduce proteinuria, repress extracellular matrix production, decrease epithelial-to-mesenchymal transition (EMT) markers, and inhibit TGF-β signaling pathway [47–49]. These effects were independent of PTH [48, 49] and at least in part dependent of RAAS inhibition [50]. Of interest, losartan or paricalcitol alone moderately improved kidney injury in a model of diabetic mice, whereas the combination of both molecules prevented albuminuria and reduced glomeruloscle-rosis [51]. Despite its benefits as a potent immunosuppressive agent, the use of ciclosporine A (CsA) is limited by its nephrotoxic properties after renal transplanta-tion. Interestingly, in a rat model, paricalcitol appears to attenuate CsA-induced nephropathy by suppression of inflammatory, pro-fibrotic, and apoptotic factors through inhibition of the NF-kB, Smad, and mitogen-activated protein kinase sig-naling pathways [52]. In addition, active compounds of vitamin D were shown to protect from chronic allograft rejection in a rat model of renal transplantation [53].

In humans, a recent randomized placebo-controlled, double-blind trial showed that addition of 2 µg/day paricalcitol to RAAS inhibition safely lowers residual albuminuria in patients with diabetic nephropathy [54] but the effects of vitamin D and analogs on renal transplant outcomes have not yet been reported in randomized controlled trials.

Very few studies investigated the potential nephroprotective role of vitamin D after renal transplantation. In a recent study, GFR measurement using iohexol plasma clearance, urinary procollagen III aminoterminal propeptide excretion, epithelial phe-notypic changes as markers of EMT and Banff scores at 3 and 12 months after renal transplantation were analyzed in 64 RTR with or without cholecalciferol supplemen-tation between months 3 and 12. The scheme of cholecalciferol treatment used in the treated group was described previously [12]. In the treated group, cholecalciferol supplementation did not prevent EMT, interstitial fibrosis, tubular atrophy, or renal function deterioration. These results challenged the experimental data, suggesting that vitamin D-analog supplementation confers nephroprotection. However, these negative results should be interpreted with caution because of the limited follow-up, the small size of the population and the lack of efficiency of the maintenance treat-ment to maintain serum 25(OH)D level above 30 ng/mL in the treated group [55].

26.3   Ongoing Clinical Trials Aiming at Studying the Effects of Vitamin D₃ on Extra-Osseous Criteria After Renal Transplantation, Including Graft Function and Rejection

The VITALE study [56] (VITamine D Supplementation in RenAL Transplant Recipients; ClinicalTrials.gov Identifier: NCT01431430) is a prospective, multicen-tre, double-blind, randomized, controlled trial with two parallel groups that will include a total of 640 RTR. RTR with vitamin D insufficiency (defined as circulat-ing 25OHD levels of less than 30 ng/ml), will be randomized between 12 and 48 months after renal transplantation to blinded groups to receive vitamin D₃ (cho-lecalciferol) either at high or low dose (respectively, 100,000 UI or 12,000 UI every 2 weeks for 2 months then monthly for 22 months) with a follow-up of 2 years. The primary objective of the study is to evaluate the benefit/risk ratio of high-dose ver-sus low-dose cholecalciferol on a composite endpoint consisting of de novo diabe-tes mellitus; major cardiovascular events; de novo cancer; and patient death. Secondary endpoints will include *the incidence of acute rejection episodes*; *renal allograft function using estimated glomerular filtration rate*; *proteinuria*; *graft survival*; blood pressure control; the incidence of infection; echocardiography findings; bone mineral density; the incidence of fractures; and biological relevant parameters of mineral metabolism. The VITA-D study [57] (Vitamin D_3 Substitution in Vitamin D Deficient Kidney Transplant Recipients; ClinicalTrials.gov Identifier: NCT00752401) is a double-blind, randomized, placebo-controlled study of RTR deficient in vitamin D, focusing on the impact of cholecalciferol substitution on *graft function (MDRD eGFR)*, *incidence of acute rejection episodes*, and posttransplant infections within the first year after renal transplantation. In total, 200 RTR with serum 25(OH)D level of less than 20 ng/ml at time of transplantation will be randomized to receive either cholecalciferol (6,800 IU/day during 1 year) or placebo. The CANDLE-KIT study (Correcting Anemia and Native Vitamin D Supplementation in Kidney Transplant Recipients; ClinicalTrials.gov Identifier: NCT01817699) is an open-label randomized controlled trial with four arms: (1) no intervention: low haemoglobin (Hb) target (Hb level: ≥ 9.5 and <10.5 g/dL) without cholecalciferol; (2) low Hb target with cholecalciferol 1,000 IU/day; (3) high Hb target (Hb level: ≥ 12.5 and <13.5 g/dL) without cholecalciferol, and (4) the experimental arm: high Hb target with cholecalciferol 1,000 IU/day. This study will recruit 324 RTR, who are at least 1 year post-transplantation. The primary endpoint will *be the change in allograft kidney function using MDRD estimated GFR*. Among the secondary endpoints are *urinary markers of kidney injury*, the dose of methoxy-polyethylene glycol epoetin β required to maintain the target Hb level, blood pressure, cardiac biomarkers, left ventricular mass index, *acute cellular rejection*, bone-turnover markers, intact PTH, bone mineral density, cardiovascular events, all-cause death, and cancer development or recurrence.

26.4   Conclusions

Further studies in RTR will help to elucidate if VDR activation, directly through administration of active vitamin D compounds or indirectly via administration of native vitamin D, might protect long-term graft function by reducing acute rejection episodes, proteinuria and renal fibrosis. We are awaiting the results of ongoing interventional clinical trials, which should help us answer this question.

References

1. Palmer SC, McGregor DO, Strippoli GF. Interventions for preventing bone disease in kidney transplant recipients. Cochrane Database Syst Rev. 2007;(18):CD005015.
2. De Sevaux RG, Hoitsma AJ, Corstens FH, Wetzels JF. Treatment with vitamin D and calcium reduces bone loss after renal transplantation: a randomized study. J Am Soc Nephrol. 2002;13:1608–14.
3. El-Agroudy AE, El-Husseini AA, El-Sayed M, Mohsen T, Ghoneim MA. A prospective randomized study for prevention of postrenal transplantation bone loss. Kidney Int. 2005;67:2039–45.

4. Torres A, Garcia S, Gomez A, Gonzalez A, Barrios Y, Concepcion MT, Hernandez D, Garcia JJ, Checa MD, Lorenzo V, Salido E. Treatment with intermittent calcitriol and calcium reduces bone loss after renal transplantation. Kidney Int. 2004;65:705–12.
5. Dawson-Hughes B, Heaney RP, Holick MF, Lips P, Meunier PJ, Vieth R. Estimates of optimal vitamin D status. Osteoporos Int. 2005;16:713–6.
6. Heaney RP. Vitamin D, depletion and effective calcium absorption. J Bone Miner Res. 2003;18:1342–3.
7. Bischoff-Ferrari HA, Giovannucci E, Willett WC, Dietrich T, Dawson-Hughes B. Estimation of optimal serum concentrations of 25-hydroxyvitamin D for multiple health outcomes. Am J Clin Nutr. 2006;84:18–28.
8. Courbebaisse M, Souberbielle JC, Thervet E. Potential nonclassical effects of vitamin D in transplant recipients. Transplantation. 2010;89:131–7.
9. Pascussi JM, Robert A, Nguyen M, Walrant-Debray O, Garabedian M, Martin P, Pineau T, Saric J, Navarro F, Maurel P, Vilarem MJ. Possible involvement of pregnane X receptor-enhanced CYP24 expression in drug-induced osteomalacia. J Clin Invest. 2005;115:177–86.
10. Bhan I, Shah A, Holmes J, Isakova T, Gutierrez O, Burnett SM, Juppner H, Wolf M. Post-transplant hypophosphatemia: tertiary 'hyper-phosphatoninism'? Kidney Int. 2006;70:1486–94.
11. Reichrath J. Dermatologic management, sun avoidance and vitamin D status in organ transplant recipients (OTR). J Photochem Photobiol B. 2012;101:150–9.
12. Courbebaisse M, Thervet E, Souberbielle JC, Zuber J, Eladari D, Martinez F, Mamzer-Bruneel MF, Urena P, Legendre C, Friedlander G, Prie D. Effects of vitamin D supplementation on the calcium-phosphate balance in renal transplant patients. Kidney Int. 2009;75:646–51.
13. Wissing KM, Broeders N, Moreno-Reyes R, Gervy C, Stallenberg B, Abramowicz D. A controlled study of vitamin D3 to prevent bone loss in renal-transplant patients receiving low doses of steroids. Transplantation. 2005;79:108–15.
14. Benaboud S, Urien S, Thervet E, Prié D, Legendre C, Souberbielle JC, Hirt D, Friedlander G, Treluyer JM, Courbebaisse M. Determination of optimal cholecalciferol treatment in renal transplant recipients using a population pharmacokinetic approach. Eur J Clin Pharmacol. 2013;69:499–506.
15. Tanaci N, Karakose H, Guvener N, Tutuncu NB, Colak T, Haberal M. Influence of 1,25-dihydroxyvitamin D3 as an immunomodulator in renal transplant recipients: a retrospective cohort study. Transplant Proc. 2003;35:2885–7.
16. Sezer S, Uyar M, Arat Z, Ozdemir FN, Haberal M. Potential effects of 1,25-dihydroxyvitamin D3 in renal transplant recipients. Transplant Proc. 2005;37:3109.
17. Lee JR, Dadhania D, August P, Lee JB, Suthanthiran M, Muthukumar T. Circulating levels of 25-hydroxyvitamin D and acute cellular rejection in kidney allograft recipients. Transplantation. 2014;98(3):292–9.
18. Obi Y, Hamano T, Ichimaru N, Tomida K, Matsui I, Fujii N, Okumi M, Kaimori JY, Yazawa K, Kokado Y, Nonomura N, Rakugi H, Takahara S, Isaka Y, Tsubakihara Y. Vitamin D deficiency predicts decline in kidney allograft function: a prospective cohort study. J Clin Endocrinol Metab. 2014;99(2):527–35.
19. Lemire JM, Adams JS, Kermani-Arab V, Bakke AC, Sakai R, Jordan SC. 1,25-Dihydroxyvitamin D3 suppresses human T helper/inducer lymphocyte activity in vitro. J Immunol. 1985;134: 3032–5.
20. Reichel H, Koeffler HP, Tobler A, Norman AW. 1 alpha, 25-Dihydroxyvitamin D3 inhibits gamma-interferon synthesis by normal human peripheral blood lymphocytes. Proc Natl Acad Sci U S A. 1987;84:3385–9.
21. Rigby WF, Yirinec B, Oldershaw RL, Fanger MW. Comparison of the effects of 1,25-dihydroxyvitamin D3 on T lymphocyte subpopulations. Eur J Immunol. 1987;17:563.
22. Veldman CM, Cantorna MT, DeLuca HF. Expression of 1, 25-dihydroxyvitamin D(3) receptor in the immune system. Arch Biochem Biophys. 2000;374:334.
23. Chen S, Sims GP, Chen XX, Gu YY, Chen S, Lipsky PE. Modulatory effects of 1, 25-dihydroxyvitamin D3 on human B cell differentiation. J Immunol. 2007;179:1634–47.

24. Fritsche J, Mondal K, Ehrnsperger A, Andreesen R, Kreutz M. Regulation of 25-hydroxyvitamin D3-1 alpha-hydroxylase and production of 1 alpha,25-dihydroxyvitamin D3 by human dendritic cells. Blood. 2003;102:3314–6.
25. Penna G, Adorini L. 1 Alpha,25-dihydroxyvitamin D3 inhibits differentiation, maturation, activation, and survival of dendritic cells leading to impaired alloreactive T cell activation. J Immunol. 2000;164:2405–11.
26. Griffin MD, Lutz W, Phan VA, Bachman LA, McKean DJ, Kumar R. Dendritic cell modulation by 1alpha,25 dihydroxyvitamin D3 and its analogs: a vitamin D receptor-dependent pathway that promotes a persistent state of immaturity in vitro and in vivo. Proc Natl Acad Sci U S A. 2001;98:6800.
27. Chen W. The role of plasmacytoid dendritic cells in immunity and tolerance. Curr Opin Organ Transplant. 2005;10:181.
28. Mora JR, Iwata M, von Andrian UH. Vitamin effects on the immune system: vitamins A and D take centre stage. Nat Rev Immunol. 2008;8:685.
29. Lemire JM, Archer DC, Khulkarni A, Ince A, Uskokovic MR, Stepkowski S. Prolongation of the survival of murine cardiac allografts by the vitamin D3 analogue 1,25-dihydroxy-delta 16-cholecalciferol. Transplantation. 1992;54:762–3.
30. Zhang AB, Zheng SS, Jia CK, Wang Y. Effect of 1,25-dihydroxyvitamin D3 on preventing allograft from acute rejection following rat orthotopic liver transplantation. World J Gastroenterol. 2003;9:1067.
31. Casteels K, Waer M, Laureys J, Valckx D, Depovere J, Bouillon R, Mathieu C. Prevention of autoimmune destruction of syngeneic islet grafts in spontaneously diabetic nonobese diabetic mice by a combination of a vitamin D3 analog and cyclosporine. Transplantation. 1998;65:1225–32.
32. Kallio E, Häyry P, Pakkala S. MC1288, a vitamin D analogue, reduces short- and long-term renal allograft rejection in the rat. Transplant Proc. 1996;28(6):3113.
33. Cantorna MT, Hullett DA, Redaelli C, Brandt CR, Humpal-Winter J, Sollinger HW, Deluca HF. 1,25-Dihydroxyvitamin D3 prolongs graft survival without compromising host resistance to infection or bone mineral density. Transplantation. 1998;66:828.
34. Ardalan MR, Maljaei H, Shoja MM, Piri AR, Khosroshahi HT, Noshad H, Argani H. Calcitriol started in the donor, expands the population of CD4+CD25+ T cells in renal transplant recipients. Transplant Proc. 2007;39:951–3.
35. Ahmadpoor P, Ilkhanizadeh B, Ghasemmahdi L, Makhdoomi K, Ghafari A. Effect of active vitamin D on expression of co-stimulatory molecules and HLA-DR in renal transplant recipients. Exp Clin Transplant. 2009;7:99–103.
36. van Etten E, Mathieu C. Immunoregulation by 1, 25-dihydroxyvitamin D3: basic concepts. J Steroid Biochem Mol Biol. 2005;97:93.
37. Agarwal R, Acharya M, Tian J, Hippensteel RL, Melnick JZ, Qiu P, Williams L, Batlle D. Antiproteinuric effect of oral paricalcitol in chronic kidney disease. Kidney Int. 2005;68: 2823–8.
38. Lee DR, Kong JM, Cho KI, Chan L. Impact of vitamin D on proteinuria, insulin resistance, and cardiovascular parameters in kidney transplant recipients. Transplant Proc. 2011;43(10): 3723–9.
39. de Boer IH, Ioannou GN, Kestenbaum B, Brunzell JD, Weiss NS. 25-Hydroxyvitamin D levels and albuminuria in the Third National Health and Nutrition Examination Survey (NHANES III). Am J Kidney Dis. 2007;50:69–77.
40. Ravani P, Malberti F, Tripepi G, Pecchini P, Cutrupi S, Pizzini P, Mallamaci F, Zoccali C. Vitamin D levels and patient outcome in chronic kidney disease. Kidney Int. 2009;75:88.
41. O'Herrin JK, Hullett DA, Heisey DM, Sollinger HW, Becker BN. A retrospective evaluation of 1,25-dihydroxyvitamin D(3) and its potential effects on renal allograft function. Am J Nephrol. 2002;22:515–20.
42. Vu D, Sakharkar P, Tellez-Corrales E, Shah T, Hutchinson I, Min DI. Association of vitamin D binding protein polymorphism with long-term kidney allograft survival in hispanic kidney transplant recipients. Mol Biol Rep. 2013;40(2):933–9.

43. Lavin PJ, Laing ME, O'Kelly P, Moloney FJ, Gopinathan D, Aradi AA, Shields DC, Murphy GM, Conlon PJ. Improved renal allograft survival with vitamin D receptor polymorphism. Ren Fail. 2007;29(7):785–9.
44. Adorini L, Amuchastegui S, Daniel KC. Prevention of chronic allograft rejection by vitamin D receptor agonists. Immunol Lett. 2005;100:34–41.
45. Brewster UC, Perazella MA. The renin-angiotensin-aldosterone system and the kidney: effects on kidney disease. Am J Med. 2004;116:263.
46. Sun J, Kong J, Duan Y, Szeto FL, Liao A, Madara JL, Li YC. Increased NF-kappaB activity in fibroblasts lacking the vitamin D receptor. Am J Physiol Endocrinol Metab. 2006;291:E315.
47. Tan X, Li Y, Liu Y. Paricalcitol attenuates renal interstitial fibrosis in obstructive nephropathy. J Am Soc Nephrol. 2006;17:3382.
48. Schwarz U, Amann K, Orth SR, Simonaviciene A, Wessels S, Ritz E. Effect of 1,25 (OH)2 vitamin D3 on glomerulosclerosis in subtotally nephrectomized rats. Kidney Int. 1998;53:1696.
49. Kuhlmann A, Haas CS, Gross ML, Reulbach U, Holzinger M, Schwarz U, Ritz E, Amann K. 1,25-Dihydroxyvitamin D3 decreases podocyte loss and podocyte hypertrophy in the subtotally nephrectomized rat. Am J Physiol Renal Physiol. 2004;286:F526.
50. Freundlich M, Quiroz Y, Zhang Z, Zhang Y, Bravo Y, Weisinger JR, Li YC, Rodriguez-Iturbe B. Suppression of renin-angiotensin gene expression in the kidney by paricalcitol. Kidney Int. 2008;74:1394–402.
51. Zhang Z, Sun L, Wang Y, Ning G, Minto AW, Kong J, Quigg RJ, Li YC. Renoprotective role of the vitamin D receptor in diabetic nephropathy. Kidney Int. 2008;73:163.
52. Park JW, Bae EH, Kim IJ, Ma SK, Choi C, Lee J, Kim SW. Paricalcitol attenuates cyclosporine-induced kidney injury in rats. Kidney Int. 2010;77(12):1076–85.
53. Hullett DA, Laeseke PF, Malin G, Nessel R, Sollinger HW, Becker BN. Prevention of chronic allograft nephropathy with vitamin D. Transpl Int. 2005;18:1175–86.
54. de Zeeuw D, Agarwal R, Amdahl M, Audhya P, Coyne D, Garimella T, Parving HH, Pritchett Y, Remuzzi G, Ritz E, Andress D. Selective vitamin D receptor activation with paricalcitol for reduction of albuminuria in patients with type 2 diabetes (VITAL study): a randomised controlled trial. Lancet. 2010;376(9752):1543–51.
55. Courbebaisse M, Xu-Dubois YC, Thervet E, Prié D, Zuber J, Kreis H, Legendre C, Rondeau E, Pallet N. Cholecalciferol supplementation does not protect against renal allograft structural and functional deterioration: a retrospective study. Transplantation. 2011;91(2):207–12.
56. Courbebaisse M, Alberti C, Colas S, Prié D, Souberbielle JC, Treluyer JM, Thervet E. VITamin D supplementation in renAL transplant recipients (VITALE): a prospective, multicentre, double-blind, randomized trial of vitamin D estimating the benefit and safety of vitamin D3 treatment at a dose of 100,000 UI compared with a dose of 12,000 UI in renal transplant recipients: study protocol for a double-blind, randomized, controlled trial. Trials. 2014;15:430.
57. Thiem U, Heinze G, Segel R, Perkmann T, Kainberger F, Mühlbacher F, Hörl W, Borchhardt K. VITA-D: cholecalciferol substitution in vitamin D deficient kidney transplant recipients: a randomized, placebo-controlled study to evaluate the post-transplant outcome. Trials. 2009;10:36.

Chapter 27
Nutrition and Dietary Vitamin D in Chronic Kidney Disease

Jean-Claude Souberbielle

Abstract Although the main source of vitamin D is not nutritional, some foods contain significant amounts of vitamin D. Fatty fish liver oil such as cod liver and fatty fish are the main natural source of dietary vitamin D3. White fish, offal (liver, kidney), egg yolk, and to a lesser extent meat (muscle) also contain significant amounts of vitamin D3, while dairy products (non fortified) contain very small amounts of vitamin D3 with the exception of butter that has significant amounts of vitamin D3 due to its high fat content. Mushrooms seem to be the only significant source of vitamin D2, and are the only non-animal-based foods containing vitamin D. As it has been demonstrated that some animal foods (meat, offal, egg yolk) contain 25(OH)D, and that 25(OH)D is better and more quickly absorbed than native vitamin D, it is now accepted that this metabolite contributes significantly to the vitamin D status. Food fortification is a good way to eradicate severe vitamin D deficiency (i.e. 25(OH)D <12 ng/mL) in the general population assuming staple foods are supplemented taking into account the nutritional habits and the diversity of consumption. In CKD patients however, the higher target serum 25(OH)D concentration makes that individualized pharmacological supplementation (i.e. adapting the dosage with the help of serum 25(OH)D measurement) should probably be preferred.

Keywords Vitamin D • Cholecalciferol • Ergocalciferol • 25-hydroxyvitamin D • Calcitriol • Food sources • Food fortification • Biofortification • Chronic kidney disease

27.1 Introduction

The term vitamin D refers to two different molecules, ergocalciferol, or vitamin D2, of plant origin, and cholecalciferol, or vitamin D3, of animal/human origin. These two secosteroids are chemically close from each other, vitamin D2 differing from

J.-C. Souberbielle, MD
Laboratoire d'explorations fonctionnelles, Hôpital Necker-Enfants Malades, Paris, France
e-mail: jean-claude.souberbielle@nck.aphp.fr

© Springer International Publishing Switzerland 2016   453
P.A. Ureña Torres et al. (eds.), *Vitamin D in Chronic Kidney Disease*,
DOI 10.1007/978-3-319-32507-1_27

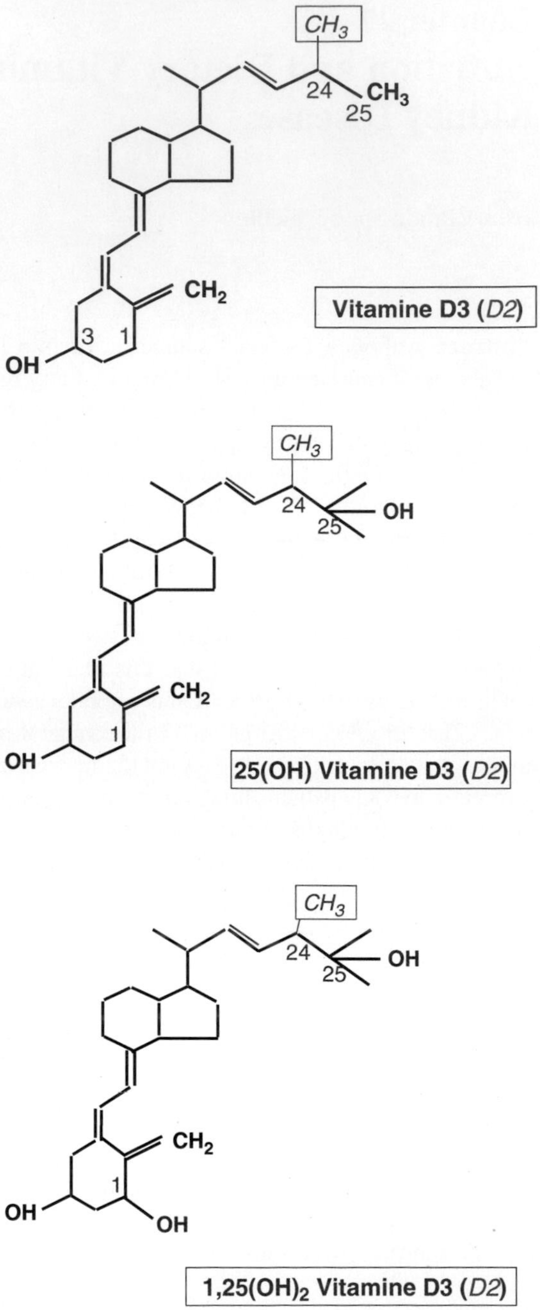

Fig. 27.1 Simplified representation of vitamin D, 25-hydroxyvitamin D molecules, and 1,25-dihydroxyvitamin D molecules

vitamin D3 only by having a double bond between C22 and C23, and a methyl residue in C24 as represented in Fig. 27.1. To become fully active, vitamin D, either D2 or D3, needs to be hydroxylated twice. A first hydroxylation occurs in the liver to form 25-hydroxyvitamin D [25(OH)D], which has a long half-life and whose serum concentration is the consensual marker of the vitamin D status. A second hydroxylation occurs in the proximal tubule of the kidney as well as in many other tissues to form 1,25-dihydroxyvitamin D [1,25(OH)$_2$D], also called calcitriol, the active metabolite. The renal production of 1,25(OH)$_2$D is tightly regulated, mainly stimulated by parathyroid hormone (PTH) and inhibited by Fibroblast Growth Factor 23 (FGF23). 1,25(OH)$_2$D produced by the proximal tubular cells is released into the bloodstream and binds, in distant target tissues, to a specific receptor, the VDR, to exert genomic effects. It can thus be considered as a hormone.

Vitamin D is not a vitamin *stricto sensu* (i.e. a "vital" compound that the body is not able to produce), as its main source comes from the synthesis by the skin when we expose ourselves to UVB-rays. However, vitamin D (D2 or D3) is also a vitamin in some way as a few natural dietary sources exist, and as pharmacological supplementation and/ or food fortification with vitamin D are commonly available, at least in some countries.

The aim of this chapter is to present the various dietary sources of vitamin D, and to discuss their capacity to improve the vitamin D status of the general population as well as of CKD patients.

27.2   Dietary Sources of Vitamin D2 and Vitamin D3

In the following paragraphs, vitamin D intakes/contents are expressed in µg. To convert into international units (IU), multiply the µg by 40 (1 µg = 40 IU).

Reviewing the relevant literature leads to the remark that evaluating the exact vitamin D content of a given natural food is far from an easy task. First, the analytical methods that have been used to measure vitamin D in foods, mostly HPLC or mass spectrometry, are not standardized (i.e. do not use the same calibrator) and differ sometimes greatly in their extraction step [1, 2]. Second, for a given mass (say 100 g) of a given animal species, the vitamin D content varied greatly in the published reports, depending on the fat content of the studied piece of food [3], whether the animal lived indoor or outdoor, and, for those living outdoor, on the season the animal has been sacrificed [4], and whether the animal has been supplemented with vitamin D [4, 5] or has a diet rich in vitamin D (a good example is the twice higher vitamin D content in wild salmon compared to farmed salmon [6]).

Having said that, it is clear that fatty fish liver oil such as cod liver oil [7] (seldom consumed outside the high latitude countries such as Norway, Iceland, or Greenland), and fatty fish are the main natural source of dietary vitamin D3 [8, 9]. White fish, offal (liver, kidney), egg yolk, and to a lesser extent meat (muscle) also contain significant amounts of vitamin D3, while dairy products (non fortified) contain very small amounts of vitamin D3 (with the exception of butter that has significant amounts of vitamin D3 due to its high fat content) [1].

Concerning vitamin D2, only mushrooms seem to be a significant source, and are the only non-animal-based food containing vitamin D. Vitamin D2 contents are large in many wild mushrooms such as the *chanterelle*, and in mushrooms that are cultivated outdoors, while the total content of vitamin D2 in mushrooms that are cultivated indoors depends whether the mushrooms have been irradiated by UVB rays [10]. While it has been suggested that vitamin D2 is insignificant in the human diet, it was calculated from a recent nutrition survey that the median vitamin D2 intake of the Irish general population was close to 2 µg/day [11]. Interestingly, it was recently shown that some mushrooms such as the shiitake mushroom are able to produce vitamin D4, a form of vitamin D, produced from the irradiation of 22,23-dihydroergocalciferol, that is similar to vitamin D3, but with a methyl group on carbon 24 of the vitamin D3 side chain [12]. Although the exact potency of vitamin D4 in humans is unknown, it has been shown to be approximately 60% as active as vitamin D3 in healing rickets in the rat [10].

27.3 25(OH)D as a Dietary a Source of Vitamin D

While the mean vitamin D intake that is usually calculated from food frequency questionnaires (FFQs) in the general population during various nutrition surveys is in the range of 3–4 µg [13–15], it has been recently hypothesized that the food inputs of vitamin D3 are in fact probably larger [16]. Indeed, despite discrepancies in the evaluation of the increase in serum 25(OH)D concentration for each µg of ingested vitamin D 3 (considered to be of approximately 1 nmol/L in mean with a huge inter-individual variability by some authors [17, 18], and approximately 2 nmol/L by others [19]), this apparent intake of 3–4 µg seems too low to explain the mean measured 25(OH)D concentration of approximately 50 nmol/L that is observed in winter in some populations living at latitude higher than 40° (i.e. when vitamin D3 skin synthesis is absent), who do not consume vitamin D-fortified foodstuffs or pharmacological supplements. As it has been demonstrated that some animal foods contain 25(OH)D, and that 25(OH)D is better and more quickly absorbed than native vitamin D [20], it is now accepted that this metabolite contributes significantly to the 25(OH)D serum concentration of certain persons [21]. Indeed, while 25(OH)D contents are very low in dairy and fish, it has been reported to be between 0.15 and 0.5 µg/100 g in meat and offal and between 0 and 4 µg/100 g in egg yolk depending on the supply of dietary vitamin D3 or 25(OH)D$_3$ to the laying hen, with a mean content of 1 µg/100 g [2, 20]. Furthermore, intervention studies showed that 25(OH)D$_3$ is about five times more effective in raising serum 25(OH)D levels than an equivalent amount of vitamin D3, 1 µg 25(OH)D corresponding thus to approximately 5 µg vitamin D (200 IU) [22]. According to these data, it may thus be assumed that consuming one egg may correspond to ingesting approximately 1 µg vitamin D3 and 0.2 µg 25(OH)D$_3$ (one egg yolk weights approximately 20 g) corresponding thus to approximately 2 µg vitamin D3 equivalents, while consuming one 150 g beefsteak would correspond to approximately 2–2.5 µg vitamin D3 equivalents essentially through the ingestion of 25(OH)D$_3$. In addition to the vitamin D content of some foods, the 25(OH)D content has now been taken into account in some food composition tables but not in all.

A summary of the content in vitamin D and 25(OH)D of different foods is presented in Table 27.1

Table 27.1 Natural vitamin D3 and 25(OH)D3 content in some animal foods

	Vitamin D3 (µg/100 g)	25(OH)D3 (µg/100 g)
Fish		
Cod liver oil	600	ND
Salmon	21.4 (0.6 [farmed]–32.5 [wild])	ND
Eel		ND
Trout	18.6 (14–27)	ND
Herring	10.8 (7.6–15)	ND
Pilchard	17.1–27.5	ND
Tuna	9.8–13.6	ND
Cod	3.7–10.1	ND
Egg	1.8–6.9	
Whole		0.7 (0.4–0.9)
Yolk	2.2 (0.08–3.4)	1.0 (0.05–1.3)
Meat	0.5 (0.4–0.6)	
Beef (muscle)		0.25 (0.0.5)
Beef (offal: liver, kidney)	0.3 (0–1)	0.5 (0.1–2.3)
Pork (muscle)	0.8 (0–1.5)	0.1
Pork (liver)	0.4 (0.05–1.4)	0.44
Lamb (muscle)	0.4–1.3	0.9 (0.6–1.2)
Chicken/duck	0.05 (0–0.09)	ND
Butter	4.8 (0–2.3)	1.0 (0.05–1.3)
	0.5 (0.4–0.6)	

Data are mean (minimum-maximum) as calculated from Schmid and Walther [1] (in some cases, only one or two data were available for one category of food). The (sometimes huge) variability of the reported vitamin D3/25(OH)D3 content for each food category is related to the variability in the analytical methods used to measure vitamin D3 and 25(OH)D3, to the fat content of the studied piece of food, to the fact that the sacrificed animal was raised indoor or outdoor or was wild or farmed, and whether it was supplemented with vitamin D3. (*ND* no data). Data are given in µg. To convert µg into International Units (IU), multiply µg by 40 (1 µg=40 IU). One µg 25(OH)D3 is thought to correspond to (approximately) 5 µg vitamin D3. In other words, a piece of food (100 g) that contains (for example) 1 µg vitamin D3 and 1 µg 25(OH)D3 would contain 6 µg vitamin D3 equivalent

27.4 Food-Fortification with Vitamin D or Dietary Supplements

It is widely recognized that, when only natural foods are taken into account, current dietary vitamin D intakes, even when considering 25(OH)D intakes, are usually not sufficient to maintain an adequate serum 25(OH)D concentration all-year round. Several intervention studies have shown that consumption of fortified foodstuffs and/or oil-based supplements such as cod liver oil may increase significantly the serum 25(OH)D concentration [18, 19]. There are however huge differences across countries in the use of dietary supplements as well as in fortification policies. Indeed, cod liver and cod liver oil supplements are essentially consumed in northern countries such as Scandinavia, Greenland, and Iceland, and rarely in more southern countries. Some countries such as the USA, Canada, Nordic countries, have mandatory fortification policies while in (many) other countries; vitamin D fortification is voluntary (commercial).

Foods/foodstuffs that are most frequently vitamin D-fortified are milk/dairy and oil/butter/margarine. However, this will only benefit, in terms of vitamin D status, to those who consume that kind of products. On the contrary, the risk of overdosing in those who consume very high quantities of these foods needs to be evaluated [23], even if it seems highly unlikely that they could attain the tolerable upper intake level of 100 μg/day that has been established by the Institute of Medicine expert panel [24]. A challenge would thus be to propose vitamin D fortification of varied staple foods, encompassing a large spectrum of consumers, and taking into account the cultural and dietary habits of the different countries. Other vehicles for fortification that have been tested beyond milk/dairy include orange juice, breakfast cereals, and bread. Another complementary option is to encourage "biofortification", that is addition of vitamin D or 25(OH)D to the livestock feeds (this concerns cultured fish, beef, pork, lamb and chicken), and embrace the practice of UVB-irradiation of mushrooms and baker's yeast.

27.5   Can We Evaluate the Effect of Nutrition on Vitamin D Status of Healthy Subjects and of CKD Patients?

While skin synthesize is recognized as the main natural source of vitamin D, many data suggest that nutrition is important for maintaining an optimal vitamin D status. An excellent example is the huge decrease of the serum 25(OH)D levels of Greenlandic Inuit population between 1987 and 2005–2010 while, during this period, the traditional diet containing large quantities of fish and sea mammals has been largely substituted by imported foodstuffs in this country [25]. Also interesting was the fact that, contrary to other areas in the world, the highest serum 25(OH)D levels were observed in the oldest group of Inuit individuals, correlating with the highest intake of traditional food in this age group. Also in favour of a significant effect of nutrition on vitamin D status is the fact that the mean serum 25(OH)D serum concentration of Scandinavian populations and of Mediterranean populations are quite similar to the vitamin D status despite much less days with sunshine in Scandinavia [13]. The high amount of fatty fish consumption and the more frequent fortification of foods in high latitude countries probably explain this lack of difference. Similarly, the mean serum 25(OH)D concentration in North America (USA, Canada) where fortification of some foods is mandatory is significantly higher than in Europe as summarized in Table 27.2 [26].

Having said that, it is obvious that natural food sources are not sufficient to maintain an optimal vitamin D status in many persons from the general population, at least during the part of the year when UVB rays are not present. According to the Institute of Medicine, a serum 25(OH)D concentration ≥20 ng/mL should be the target level in the general (healthy) population, and intakes of 15–20 μg/day of

Table 27.2 Estimation of the mean 25(OH)D concentration of the general population in various areas stratified by age categories

Area	25(OH)D Mean (ng/mL)	95 % CI of the mean 25(OH)D
Europe		
Children/adolescents (>1–17 years)	20.3	13.7–26.7
Adults (18–65 ans)	21.2	18.0–22.6
Elderly subjects (>65 ans)	20.7	18.3–23.1
North America		
Children/adolescents (>1–17 years)	31.3	23.8–39.9
Adults (18–65 years)	28.7	23.1–34.4
Elderly subjects (>65 years)	28.7	25.9–31.4
Asia/pacific		
Children/adolescents (>1–17 years)	12.8	10.0–15.5
Adults (18–65 years)	27.2	23.9–30.5
Elderly subjects (>65 years)	26.5	24.9–28.1
Middle-East/Africa		
Children/adolescents (>1–17 years)	30.2	22.6–37.8
Adults (18–65 years)	13.9	11.7–16.0
Elderly subjects (>65 years)	15.3	11.7–18.9

vitamin D are necessary to reach this concentration in most healthy subjects [24]. Other authors however found that higher intakes of 25 [27], or 28 [28] µg/day in Caucasians, or 42 µg/day in Black people [29] are more realistic to make that almost everybody has a serum 25(OH-)D concentration $\geq$20 ng/mL. With the exception of those consuming everyday one portion of (wild) fatty fish along with one or two eggs, nobody will obtain such intakes with natural foods, so that the importance of food fortification, or biofortification has been emphasized [30]. In a well-conducted controlled study, 782 Danish children and adults were randomly assigned to a diet containing vitamin D-fortified bread and milk (fortification group), or to a non-fortified diet (control group) between September 2010 and April 2011 [31]. At the end of the study, the mean serum 25(OH)D concentration in the fortification group was 27.0 ng/mL while it was 16.7 ng/mL in the control group, and <1 %, and 16 % of the subjects in the fortification group had a serum 25(OH)D concentration <12 ng/mL (considered as a cut-off below which symptomatic vitamin D deficiency is possible) and <20 ng/mL respectively, while the figure was of 25 % and 65 % in the control group. The mean daily total vitamin D intake in the fortification group was close to 10 µg, while it was close to 2 µg in the control group. Even if these results may appear very encouraging, some limitations must be underlined. First, the mean serum 25(OH)D concentration of the studied population at the beginning of the study (i.e. at the end of summer) was approximately 29 ng/mL, a value that is somewhat higher than what is found in other European populations at the end summer. It is thus unclear whether such favourable results would have been found in subjects with a lower post-summer serum 25(OH)D level. Second, the participants of this study were included on the basis of their daily consumption of bread and milk and did not change their diet habits throughout the study. The observance to the fortified diet was thus excellent, which may not be the case in a real-life setting in subjects with less regular consumption. Based on this study [31], but also on the results of the different trials of food fortification that have been combined in meta-analyses [18, 19], it is concluded that, if the dietary diversity is considered, food fortification or biofortification of different staple foods that add approximately 8–10 µg vitamin D to the usual diet will be able to almost eradicate severe (clinical) vitamin D deficiency (i.e. 25(OH)D ≤12 ng/mL) in the general population. A certain fraction of the general population will however keep a serum 25(OH)D concentration <20 ng/mL. The problem will be exacerbated in CKD patients. Even if they acknowledged that the level of evidence is moderate/weak, the KDIGO experts of the CKD-MBD field considered that correcting vitamin D deficiency/insufficiency is part of the first-line strategy to prevent secondary hyperparathyroidism [32]. Since the publication of the KDIGO guidelines in 2009, a systematic review published in 2011 [33] followed by more recent placebo-controlled randomized trials both in non dialyzed [34–37], and in dialyzed [38, 39] CKD patients have confirmed that supplementation with vitamin D or 25(OH)D decreases moderately but significantly the serum PTH concentration or delays the onset of secondary hyperparathyroidism [40]. In these studies, the mean serum 25(OH)D concentration in the vitamin D-treated groups was usually of 30 ng/mL or more. If this concentration of 30 ng/mL is the target level to be maintained in CKD patients as recommended by the Endocrine Society expert panel [41], it is clear that nutritional sources of vitamin D will not be sufficient, all the more that the nutritional recommendation is to limit, because of their high content in phosphorus, sodium, and/or potassium, the consumption of some foods that are naturally rich in vitamin D, or that are frequently vitamin D-fortified. My opinion is that, in CKD patients, pharmacological supplementation with native vitamin D is the best option, adapting the dosage to the individual needs by means of monitoring serum 25(OH)D concentration as suggested by us recently [42].

27.6   Conclusions

Although the main source of vitamin D is not nutritional, some foods contain significant amounts of vitamin D and 25(OH)D. Fatty fish liver oil such as cod liver and fatty fish are the main natural source of dietary vitamin D3. Food fortification of different staple foods may be a good way to eradicate severe vitamin D deficiency (i.e. 25(OH)D <12 ng/mL) in the general population. In CKD patients however, the higher target serum 25(OH)D concentration makes that individualized pharmacological supplementation (i.e. adapting the dosage with the help of serum 25(OH)D measurement) should probably be preferred.

References

1. Schmid A, Walther B. Natural vitamin D content in animal products. Adv Nutr. 2013;4:453–62.
2. Liu J, Arcot J, Cunningham J, Greenfield H, Hsu J, Padula D, Strobel N, Fraser D. New data for vitamin D in Australian foods of animal origin: impact on estimates of national adult vitamin D intakes in 1995 and 2011–2013. Asia Pac J Clin Nutr. 2015;24:464–71.
3. Clausen I, Jakobsen J, Leth T, Ovesen L. Vitamin D3 and 25-hydroxyvitamin D3 in raw and cooked pork cuts. J Food Compost Anal. 2003;16:575–85.
4. Mattila PH, Vakonen E, Valaja J. Effect of different vitamin D supplementations in poultry feed on vitamin D content of eggs and chicken meat. J Agric Food Chem. 2011;59:8298–303.
5. Wilborn B, Kerth C, Ovsley W, Jones W, Probish L. Improving pork quality by feeding supranutritional concentrations of vitamin D3. J Anim Sci. 2004;82:218–24.
6. Lu Z, Chen TC, Zhang A, Persons KS, Kohn N, Berkowitz R, Martinello S, Holick M. An evaluation of the vitamin D3 content in fish: is the vitamin D content adequate to satisfy the dietary requirement for vitamin D? J Steroid Biochem Mol Biol. 2007;103:642–4.
7. Brustad M, Sandanger T, Wilsgaard T, Aksnes L, Lund E. Change in plasma levels of vitamin D after consumption of cod-liver and fresh cod-liver oil as part of the traditional north Norwegian fish dish Molje. Int J Circumpolar Health. 2003;62:40–53.
8. Van der Meer I, Boeke J, Lips P, Grootjans-Geers I, Wuister J, Devillé W, Wielderst J, Bouter L, Middelkoop B. Fatty fish and supplements are the greatest modifiable contributors to the serum 25-hydroxyvitamin D concentration in a multiethnic population. Clin Endocrinol (Oxf). 2008;68:466–72.
9. Lehman U, Gjessing HR, Hirche F, Mueller-Belecke A, Gudbrandsen OA, Ueland PE, Mellgren G, Lauritzen L, Lindqvist H, Hansen AL, Erkkila A, Pot G, Stangl G, Dierkes J. Efficacy of fish intake on vitamin D status: a meta-analysis of randomized controlled trials. Am J Clin Nutr. 2015. doi:10.3945/ajcn.114.10/5395.
10. Keegan RJ, Lu Z, Bogusz J, Williams J, Holick M. Photobiology of vitamin D in mushrooms and its bioavailability in humans. Dermatoendocrinology. 2013;5:165–76.
11. Cashman K, Kinsella M, McNulty B, Walton J, Gibney M, Flynn A, Kiely M. Dietary vitamin D2-a potentially underestimated contributor to vitamin D nutritional status of adults? Br J Nutr. 2014;112:193–202.
12. Philipps K, Horst R, Koszewski N, Simon R. Vitamin D4 in mushrooms. PLoS One. 2012;7:e40702. doi:10.1371/journal.pone.0040702.
13. Spiro A, Buttriss JL. Vitamin D: an overview of vitamin D status and intake in Europe. Nutr Bull. 2014;39:322–50.
14. Touvier M, Deschassaux M, Montourcy M, Sutton A, Charmaux N, Kesse-Guyot E, Assmann K, Fezeu L, Latino-martel P, Druesne-Pecollo N, Guinot C, Latreille J, Malvy D, Galan P, Hercberg S, Le Clerc S, Souberbielle JC, Ezzedine K. Determinants of vitamin D status in Caucasian adults: influence of sun exposure, dietary intake, sociodemographic, lifestyle, anthropometric, genetic factors. J Invest Dermatol. 2015;135:378–88.
15. Rabenberg M, Scheidt-nave C, Busch M, Rieckman N, Hintzpeter B, Mensink G. Vitamin D status among adults in Germany health interview and examination survey for adults (DEGS1). BMC Public Health. 2015;15:641.
16. Heaney RP, Armas L, French C. All-source basal vitamin D inputs are greater than previously thought and cutaneous inputs are smaller. J Nutr. 2013;143:571–5.
17. Heaney RP, Davies K, Chen T, Holick M, Barger-Lux M. Human serum 25-hydroxycholecalciferol response to extended oral dosing with cholecalciferol. Am J Clin Nutr. 2003;77:204–10.
18. Black L, Seamans K, Cashman K, Kiely M. An updated systematic review and meta-analysis of the efficacy of vitamin D food fortification. J Nutr. 2012;142:1102–8.
19. Whiting S, Bonjour JP, Dontot Payen F, Rousseau B. Moderate amounts of vitamin D3 in supplements are effective in raising serum 25-hydroxyvitamin D from low baseline levels in adults: a systematic review. Nutrients. 2015;7:2311–23.

20. Ovesen L, Brot C, Jakobsen J. Food contents and biological activity of 25-hydroxyvitamin D: a vitamin D metabolite to reckoned with? Ann Nutr Metab. 2003;47:107–13.
21. Taylor C, Paterson K, Roseland J, Wise S, Merkel J, Pehrson P, Yetley E. Including food 25-hydroxyvitamin D in intake estimates may reduce the discrepancy between dietary and serum measures of vitamin D status. J Nutr. 2014;144:654–9.
22. Cashman K, Seamans K, Lucey A, Stöcklin E, Weber P, Kiely M, Hill T. Relative effectiveness of oral 25-hydroxyvitamin D3 and vitamin D3 in raising wintertime serum 25-hydroxyvitamin D3 in older adults. Am J Clin Nutr. 2012;95:1350–6.
23. Brown J, Sandmann A, Ignatius A, et al. New perspectives on vitamin D food fortification based on a modelling of 25(OH)D concentration. Nutr J. 2013;12:151.
24. Ross C, Manson JE, Abrams S, Aloia J, Brannon P, Clinton S, Durza-Arvizu R, Gallagher C, Gallo R, Jones G, Kovacs C, Mayne S, Rosen C, Shapes S. The 2011 report on dietary reference intakes for calcium and vitamin D from the Institute of Medicine: what clinicians need to know. J Clin Endocrinol Metab. 2011;96:53–8.
25. Nielsen N, Jorgensen M, Friis H, Melbye M, Soborg B, Jeppesen C, Lundqvist M, Cohen A, Hougaard D, Bjerregaard P. Decrease in vitamin D status in the Greenlandic adult population from 1987–2010. PloS One. 2014. doi:10.1371/journal.pone0112949.
26. Hilger J, Friedel A, Herr R, Rausch T, Roos F, Wahl DA, Pierroz DD, Weber P, Hoffmann K. A systematic review of vitamin D status in populations worldwide. Br J Nutr. 2014;111:23–45.
27. Cashman K, Wallace J, Horigan G, Hill T, Barnes M, Lucey A, Bonham M, Duffy E, Seamans K, Muldowney S, Fitzgerald A, Flynn A, Strain J, Kiely M. Estimation of the dietary requirement for vitamin D in free-living adults >=64 y of age. Am J Clin Nutr. 2008;88:1535–42.
28. Cashman K, Hill T, Lucey A, Taylor N, Seamans K, Muldowney S, Fitzgerald A, Flynn A, Barnes M, Horigan G, Bonham M, Duffy E, Strain J, Wallace J, Kiely M. Estimation of the dietary requirement for vitamin D in healthy adults. Am J Clin Nutr. 2009;89:1366–74.
29. Ng K, Scott J, Drake B, Chan A, Hollis B, Chandler P, Bennett G, Giovanucci E, Gonzalez-Suarez E, Meyerhardt J, Emmons K, Fuchs C. Dose response to vitamin D supplementation in African Americans: results of a 4-arm, randomized, placebo-controlled trial. Am J Clin Nutr. 2014;99:587–98.
30. Cashman K. Vitamin D: dietary requirements and food fortification as a means of helping achieve adequate vitamin d status. J Steroid Biochem Mol Biol. 2015;148:19–26.
31. Madsen K, Rasmussen L, Andersen R, Molgaard C, Jakobsen J, Bjerrun P, Andersen E, Mejborn H, Tetens I. Randomized controlled trial of the effects of vitamin D-fortified milk and bread on serum 25-hydroxyvitamin D concentrations in families in Denmark during winter: the VitmaD study. Am J Clin Nutr. 2013;98:374–82.
32. KDIGO. Clinical practice guideline for the diagnosis, evaluation, prevention, and treatment of chronic kidney disease-mineral and bone disorder (CKD-MBD). Kidney Int. 2009;79:S1–130.
33. Kandula P, Dobre M, Schold J, Schreiber M, Mehrotra R, Navaneethan S. Vitamin D supplementation in chronic kidney disease: a systematic review and meta-analysis of observational and randomized controlled trials. Clin J Am Soc Nephrol. 2011;6:50–62.
34. Markman P, Agerskov H, Thineshkumar S, Bladbjerg EM, Sidelman J, Jesperen J, NyBo M, Rasmussen L, Hansen D, Scholze A. Randomized controlled trial of cholecalciferol supplementation in chronic kidney disease patients with hypovitaminosis D. Nephrol Dial Transplant. 2012;27:3523–31.
35. Alvarez J, Low J, Cookley K, Zughaier S, Han L, Salles KS, Wasse H, Gutierrez O, Ziegler T, Tangpricha V. High-dose cholecalciferol reduces parathyroid hormone in patients with early chronic kidney disease: a pilot, randomized, double-blind, placebo-controlled trial. Am J Clin Nutr. 2012;96:672–9.
36. Molina P, Gorriz J, Molina M, Peris A, Beltran S, Kanter J, Escudero V, Romero R, Pallardo L. The effect of cholecalciferol for lowering albuminuria in chronic kidney disease: a prospective controlled study. Nephrol Dial Transplant. 2014;29:97–109.
37. Sprague S, Silva A, Al-Saghir F, Damle R, Tabash S, Petkovich M, Messner E, White J, Melnick J, Bishop C. Modified-release calcifediol effectively controls secondary hyperparathyroidism associated with vitamin D insufficiency in chronic kidney disease. Am J Nephrol. 2014;40:535–45.

38. Merino JL, Teruel JL, Fernandez-Lucas M, Villafruela JJ, Bueno B, Paraiso V, Quereda C. Effects of a single, high oral dose of 25-hydroxycholecalciferol on the mineral metabolism markers in hemodialysis patients. Ther Apher Dial. 2015;19:212–9.
39. Delanaye P, Weekers L, Warling X, Moonen M, Smelten N, Médart L, Krzesinski JM, Cavalier E. Cholecalciferol in haemodialysis patients: a randomized, double-blind, proof-of-concept and safety study. Nephrol Dial Transplant. 2013;28:1779–86.
40. Shroff R, Wan M, Gullett A, Lederman S, Shute R, Knott C, Wells D, Aitkenhead H, Manickavasagar B, van't Hoff W, Rees L. Ergocalciferol supplementation in children with CKD delays the onset of secondary hyperparathyroidism: a randomized trial. Clin J Am Soc Nephrol. 2012;7:216–23.
41. Holick M, Binkley N, Bischoff-Ferrari H, Gordon C, Hanley D, Heaney R, Murad M, Weaver C. Evaluation, treatment, and prevention of vitamin D deficiency: an Endocrine Society clinical practice guideline. J Clin Endocrinol Metab. 2011;96:1911–30.
42. Delanaye P, Bouquegneau A, Krzesinski JM, Cavalier E, Jean G, Urena-Torres P, Souberbielle JC. Native vitamin D in dialysis patients. Nephrol Ther. 2015;11:5–15.

Chapter 28
Natural Vitamin D in Chronic Kidney Disease

Carlo Basile, Vincent Brandenburg, and Pablo A. Ureña Torres

Abstract Vitamin D plays an essential role on bone and mineral metabolism. Its deficiency leads to bone demineralization, osteomalacia, skeletal fractures and skeletal deformation. The lack of vitamin D is also associated with an increased risk of developing arterial hypertension, cardiovascular diseases, diabetes, immune diseases, neurological disorders, malignancies, and other diseases. The supplementation of natural vitamin D usually corrects vitamin-deficiency-related mineral and bone disorders, however, the scientific evidences demonstrating any beneficial effect of natural vitamin D on non-classical target organs in the general population as well as in renal insufficient subjects are still inconsistent and await confirmation by large randomized clinical trials. Moreover, chronic kidney disease (CKD) beside its altered mineral and bone metabolism (MBD) is associated with low 25(OH)D (calcidiol), and low $1,25OH_2D_3$ (calcitriol) levels as well as vitamin D resistance. However, the major health care organizations worldwide have been unable to define a unique and consensual desirable circulating 25(OH)D values for the health population and for the CKD population. The aim of this chapter is to provide an update review of the sources and pharmacological characteristics of natural vitamin D compounds, their most important clinical uses and results obtained in CKD patients.

Keywords Cholecalciferol • Calcidiol • Calcitriol • Calcium • Phosphate • PTH • FGF23 • Uremia • Dialysis

C. Basile, MD (✉)
Division of Nephrology, Miulli General Hospital, Acquaviva delle Fonti, Italy
e-mail: basile.miulli@libero.it

V. Brandenburg
Department of Cardiology and Center for Rare Diseases (ZSEA), RWTH University Hospital, Aachen, Germany
e-mail: Vincent.Brandenburg@post.rwth-aachen.de

P.A. Ureña Torres, MD, PhD
Ramsay-Générale de Santé, Service de Néphrologie et Dialyse, Clinique du Landy, Saint Ouen, France

Department of Renal Physiology, Necker Hospital, University of Paris V, René Descartes, Paris, France
e-mail: urena.pablo@wanadoo.fr

© Springer International Publishing Switzerland 2016   465
P.A. Ureña Torres et al. (eds.), *Vitamin D in Chronic Kidney Disease*,
DOI 10.1007/978-3-319-32507-1_28

28.1   Introduction

Natural vitamin D2 and D3 are pre-hormones essential for an appropriate bone and mineral metabolism (Table 28.1). Their deficiency leads to severe defects in bone tissue mineralization defined as osteomalacia or rickets, skeletal fractures and deformation. There are now evidences that lack of vitamin D is also associated with a high risk of developing a variety of illnesses including arterial hypertension, cardiovascular diseases, diabetes, immune diseases, neurological disorders, malignancies, etc. (Table 28.1). The supplementation of natural vitamin D usually corrects all mineral and bone disorders, however, the scientific evidences demonstrating any beneficial effect of natural vitamin D on organs other than the skeleton in the

Table 28.1 Classical and non-classical biological effects of natural vitamin D

Classical	
Intestine	Stimulates calcium absorption
	Stimulates phosphate absorption
Bone	Stimulates FGF23 production
	Stimulates bone remodeling
	Improves bone mineralization in rickets/osteomalacia
	Increases bone release to normalize serum calcium levels
Parathyroid	Inhibits PTH synthesis and secretion
Non-classical	
Muscles	Maintains integrity and improves muscle strength
Kidney	Reduces proteinuria
	Decreases magnesium absorption
	Stimulates calcium and phosphate reabsorption
	Inhibits renin-angiotensin-aldosterone system
	Increases nephrin expression
	Reduces megalin and cubulin shedding
Cardiovascular	Inhibits renin-angiotensin-aldosterone system
	Decreases the risk of hypertension
	Decreased the risk of cardiovascular diseases
Immune system	Stimulates innate immunity
	Inhibits acquired and modulatory immunity
	Decreases inflammatory markers as C-reactive protein
	Decreases liver hepcidin expression
Cancer	May reduce the risk of certain cancers through its anti-proliferating and pro-differentiating properties
Pregnancy	Prevents against hypocalcemia and rickets
	May protect against preeclampsia, gestational diabetes, and premature birth
Diabetes	Improves insulin secretion and sensitivity
	May protect against diabetes

PTH parathyroid hormone, *FGF23* fibroblast growth factor 23

general population as well as in renal insufficient subjects are still inconsistent and need to be confirmed by large randomized clinical trials (RCTs).

Chronic kidney disease (CKD) is a growing global epidemic and is now recognized as a public health issue [1]. Disturbances in mineral and bone metabolism are one of the most common and important consequences of CKD development and progression. This systemic disorder is now referred to as CKD- mineral and bone disorder (CKD-MBD) [2]. Alteration in vitamin D metabolism is one of the key features of CKD-MBD that has major clinical and research implications. As well described in the literature, CKD is characterized by low 25(OH)D (calcidiol), low $1,25OH_2D_3$ (calcitriol) levels as well as vitamin D resistance [3]. CKD is definitely a state of vitamin D insufficiency or even deficiency. Numerous studies have reported varying prevalence rates of vitamin D deficiency in CKD with 70–80 % prevalence in some parts of the world [4, 5]. There is no consensus on how to exactly define vitamin D deficiency and this introduces significant difficulties in conducting epidemiological studies in this field [3]. The most widely accepted definition of vitamin D deficiency includes circulating serum 25(OH)D levels below 20 ng/ml (50 nmole/l), and patients with circulating serum 25(OH)D levels between 20 and 30 ng/ml (50 and 75 nmole/l) are referred to as vitamin D insufficient. However, the major health care organizations worldwide including WHO (World Health Organization), IOF (International Osteoporosis Foundation), IOM (Institute of Medicine), ES (Endocrine Society), AACE (American Association of Clinical Endocrinologists), and AEMD (the European Association of Medical Doctors) have reached different conclusions in term of defining the desirable circulating 25(OH)D values for the general population. Accordingly, no consensus has been reached for the CKD population. E.g., for the ES the desirable value of 25(OH)D has been set at 30 ng/ml whereas for the IOM it is of 20 ng/ml [6–8].

In spite of these discordances, the National Kidney Foundation-Kidney Disease Outcomes Quality Initiative (NKF/K-DOQI) guidelines currently recommend vitamin D supplementation in patients with stage 3–4 CKD with 25(OH)D levels <30 ng/ml [9]. The more recently released Kidney Disease Improving Clinical Outcomes (KDIGO) guidelines also recommend using vitamin D in patients with stage 3–5 CKD (not on dialysis) who are vitamin D deficient and who have parathyroid hormone (PTH) levels above the normal range [10].

Although this vitamin is mainly seen as a compound pivotal for bone physiology, it is also central to optimal functioning of other organ systems including the cardiovascular (CV), endocrine, and immune systems (Table 28.1). Mild to moderate vitamin D deficiency is associated with increased risk of cancer, hypertension, diabetes, and heart failure [11]. Such pleiotropic effects of vitamin D are of relevance to patients with CKD, particularly to those with end-stage renal disease (ESRD), a population where vitamin D insufficiency and/or low levels of the active form $1,25OH_2D_3$ is an almost universal finding. Furthermore, altered immune response, insulin resistance, vascular function, and cardiomyopathy [11] are all well documented clinical correlates of vitamin D deficiency in these patients.

The aim of this chapter is to provide the readers with an update review of the sources and pharmacological characteristics of natural vitamin D compounds, their most important clinical uses and results obtained in CKD patients.

28.2   Natural Vitamin D Compounds

The first use of natural vitamin D dates back to the nineteenth century where rickets patients were successfully treated and healed with fish oil. Then, in 1890 it was demonstrated that sun exposure was also an efficacious treatment of rickets. Later, in 1922, the anti-rachitic properties of liver-derived fish oils were linked to a lipo-soluble factor called for the first time vitamin D. Ergocalciferol, vitamin D2 or the vegetal vitamin D, was the first isolated and characterized natural vitamin D in 1931, followed by the isolation of its animal form cholecalciferol or vitamin D3 in 1936. Synthetic vitamin D2 and D3 compounds have been produced since 1952. In the 1960s, it was clearly demonstrated the vitamin D was a pro-hormone, and that it needed to undergo several stepwise conversions in the body, firstly in the skin, then in the circulating plasma, the liver, and finally in the kidney where 25(OH)D is transformed in calcitriol or $1,25OH_2D_3$, the active metabolite responsible for most of its biological activities. In 1969, the pleiotropic effects of vitamin D were rendered more plausible by the identification of the nuclear vitamin D receptor (VDR) in every cell type in the organism [12, 13]. Finally, in 1975 its transporter molecule, the vitamin D binding protein (DBP) was identified [14].

Vitamin D, either D2 or D3, circulates in the bloodstream bound to DBP. To become fully active, vitamin D needs to be transformed twice [15]. A first hydroxylation occurs in the liver to form 25-hydroxyvitamin D (25(OH)D). This liver hydroxylation is not tightly regulated and the more vitamin D is synthesized or ingested, the more 25(OH)D is produced. Circulating 25(OH)D, the most abundant vitamin D form, has a half-life of approximately 3 weeks, and its circulating concentration serves as the consensual marker of vitamin D status, reflecting the combined skin synthesis and dietary intake. It also binds to DBP. The 25(OH)D is hydroxylated by the 1α-hydroxylase (CYP27B1) in the kidney, within the cells of the proximal tubule, to form 1,25-dihydroxyvitamin D ($1,25OH_2D_3$, also called calcitriol), which is the active vitamin D metabolite. This renal hydroxylation is very tightly regulated, stimulated mainly by PTH and inhibited by calcium, phosphate, fibroblast growth factor 23 (FGF23), calcitonin, leptin, growth hormone, insulin growth factor 1, and calcitriol itself. Calcitriol is released into the bloodstream also bound to DBP, albeit with a lower affinity than 25(OH)D, and binds, in various distant tissues (i.e. intestine, bone, parathyroid cells), to the VDR. The VDR associates with the retinoic acid receptor (RXR) and the trimeric complex (calcitriol-VDR-RXR) binds to the DNA in special sites called "vitamin D responsive elements" (VDRE) to stimulate or inhibit the transcription of various genes. Calcitriol can thus be considered as a true hormone. It is of interest that 25(OH)D can be inactivated in the liver and in the kidney through a pathway involving a 24-hydroxylase whose expression is stimulated by FGF23 and calcitriol itself. The importance of this 24-hydroxylase has been highlighted recently with the demonstration that inactivating mutations of the gene (CYP24A1) coding for this enzyme induce hypersensitivity to vitamin D with severe neonatal hypercalcemia [16].

Both, the VDR and the enzymatic machinery that activates/inactivates vitamin D are expressed in a large number of tissues that are not involved in bone and/or calcium/phosphate metabolism. 25(OH)D enters these tissues and is locally transformed into calcitriol that binds to the VDR expressed in the cell and exerts various (non "calcemic") genomic effects. This locally produced calcitriol is thought to mainly stay within the producing tissue. However, even anephric patients exhibit some degree of circulating 1,25(OH)D levels [17]. The peripheral tissue production of 1,25(OH)D does not seem to be regulated by calciotropic hormones (PTH, calcitonin, and FGF23) and depends probably on the local 25(OH)D concentration in these tissues. This is the basis for the (commonly called) "non-classical" effects of vitamin D that can be considered as "intracrine and/or paracrine" by contrast with the endocrine above-mentioned classical effects. It is of note that a large number of genes contain VDRE and by consequence responsive to vitamin D. Circulating calcitriol can also exert non-genomic effects through the binding in some tissues to membrane proteins with subsequent modification of the intra-cellular calcium flux and stimulation of tyrosine-kinases [15, 18, 19].

All, vitamin D2, D3, 25(OH)D, and $1,25OH_2D_3$ are lipophilic, which favours their storage in adipose tissue for weeks and may explain why vitamin D intoxication is slow to resolve. The main classical effects of vitamin D through the endocrine action of calcitriol are to stimulate the absorption of calcium and phosphate by the intestine, to stimulate FGF23 production, to regulate bone metabolism and to exert a negative feedback on PTH secretion (Table 28.1). A severe deficiency in vitamin D may induce diseases characterized by bone mineralization defects, such as rickets in children and osteomalacia with spontaneous fractures in adults (Fig. 28.2). Less severe deficiency may favour/worsen osteoporosis, especially on cortical bone. Supplementation with vitamin D (800 IU/day at least) with calcium, but not vitamin D alone, significantly reduce the relative risk of hip fracture in subjects 60 years old and more, as demonstrated by a recent Cochrane review [20]. Correction of vitamin D deficiency/insufficiency is also a prerequisite before starting anti-osteoporotic drugs and lowering PTH agents, and specially bisphosphonates.

28.3 Biochemical and Pharmacological Characteristics of Cholecalciferol

Cholecalciferol, also called vitamin D3, is a 9, 10-seco-5,7,10(19)-cholestatriene-3β-ol, $C_{27}H_{44}O$, with a molecular weight of 384.6 Da and the structure depicted in Fig. 28.1. The biochemical and pharmacological characteristics of cholecalciferol are also summarized in Fig. 28.1. The main source of cholecalciferol comes from its synthesis from the cholesterol related product 7-dehydrocholesterol in the skin by keratinocyte cells under the effect of specific sunlight ultraviolet rays B (UVB, wavelength 280–315 nm, 0–10 % of the total solar UV radiation), and by a photolytic, non-enzymatic reaction, that transforms it in pre-vitamin D. This pre-vitamin D undergoes subsequently another non-enzymatic, thermal, isomerization in the skin to become vitamin D, either cholecalciferol or ergocalciferol [21]. The formation of pre-vitamin D is relatively rapid, reaching a maximum within hours. Both, the intensity of UVB and the type of skin

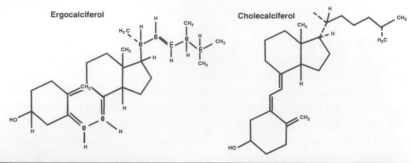

	Ergocalciferol	Cholecalciferol
Date of identification	1931	1936
Molecular weight	396.6 g/mol	384.6 g/mol
Normal circulating levels	30–75 ng/ml (75–187 nmol/l)	30–75 ng/ml (75–187 nmol/l)
Half life (T1/2)	Circulating : 2 days Functional: 2 months or less	Circulating : 19–25 h Functional: several weeks
Range of clinical dosage IU/day or mcg/day	800–2000 IU/day or 25,000 to 100,000 IU per week (200 IU = 5 mcg)	750–1000 IU/day to maximal of 4000 IU/day or 5000 IU once a week to 25,000–50,000 IU once a month (200 IU = 5 mcg)

Fig. 28.1 Cholecalciferol and ergocalciferol structural conformation and main chemical properties

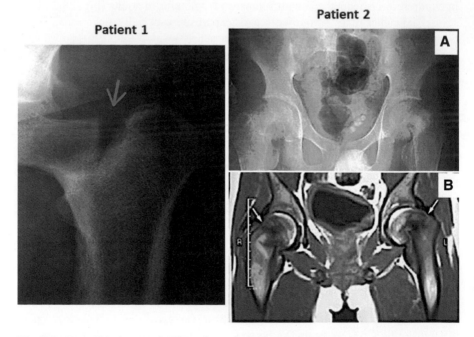

Fig. 28.2 Two clinical cases of CKD patients treated by hemodialysis with overt vitamin D deficiency (serum 25(OH)D levels <10 ng/ml or 25 nmole/l). Patients 1 had a low-kinetics fracture of her femoral neck as indicated by the arrow on the standard X-ray image. Patient 2 complained of progressive and mechanical walking pain. Standard X-ray image (*A*) showed a bilateral femoral neck deformation that where later confirmed by a magnetic resonance image (MRI). The MRI showed the fracture of both femoral necks (*white arrows*)

pigmentation regulate the rate of pre-vitamin D formation but not the maximal level achieved. With continuous sun exposure, pre-vitamin D is converted to biologically inactive lumisterol and tachysterol. The formation of lumisterol and tachysterol is reversible and can be converted back to pre-vitamin D in case of need. Thus, prolonged exposure to sunlight cannot produce toxic amounts of vitamin D because of this photo-conversion of pre-vitamin D to lumisterol and tachysterol. In addition, photo-conversion of vitamin D itself to suprasterols I and II, and 5,6 transvitamin D can also occur [22]. Inversely, administration of excessive doses of oral natural vitamin D can lead to vitamin D intoxication because of the lack of this counter-regulation.

Cholecalciferol is also found in some dietary products of animal origin, especially in meat, egg yolks, fishes, fish-liver oils, and fortified foods (margarine, cereals, milk). One international unit of vitamin D3 is equal to 0.025 mcg of cholecalciferol. More than 80 % of ingested cholecalciferol is absorbed from the gastro-intestinal tract, mainly in the small intestine, via chylomicrons of lymph and then binds to DBP. The intestinal absorption may be decreased in patients with hepatic, biliary, bariatric surgery or GI disease (e.g., Crohn's disease, Whipple's disease, sprue). Geriatric patients may also have a reduced intestinal absorption of physiological amount of vitamin D3. Pregnancy, CKD and macro-albuminuric patients may also require supra-physiological doses of vitamin D3 to achieve normal values. The use of some medications may also alter circulating 25(OH)D3 concentrations, for instance, compared with not treated subjects, subjects treated by statins exhibit lower 25(OH)D3 values and inversely subjects receiving renin-angiotensin inhibitors plus allopurinol have higher 25(OH)D3 values [23]. Similarly, the use of anticonvulsivants and corticosteroids are associated with lower 25(OH)D values. Certain dialysis techniques, such as online-hemodiafiltration may also lower systemic 25(OH)D levels by convective mechanisms [24]. The biological actions of cholecalciferol, namely its hypercalcemic action, are observed within the 10–24 h after its administration, with maximal effects observed 3–4 weeks later. Its mode of action has been described above. Cholecalciferol has a plasma half-life of 19–25 h and a terminal half-life of weeks to months. Calcifediol or 25(OH)D has an experimental elimination half-life of 19 days. It is catabolized by the liver 25-hydroxylation and by the degradation by microsomal enzymes as well as by the renal transformation in $1,25OH_2D_3$ and other inactive metabolites, then, most of the metabolites (96 %) are eliminated through the bile acids and the feces.

28.4   Biochemical and Pharmacological Characteristics of Ergocalciferol

Ergocalciferol, also called vitamin D2, is a 9, 10-secoergosta-5,7,10(19),22-tetraen-3ol, $C_{28}H_{44}O$, with a molecular weight of 396.65 Da and the structure depicted in Fig. 28.1. The biochemical and pharmacological characteristics of ergocalciferol are also summarized in Fig. 28.1. Together with ergocalciferol, there are more than ten substances belonging to a group of steroid compounds, classified as having vitamin D or antirachitic activity. The precursor ergosterol or pro-vitamin D_2 is found in plants and yeast and has no antirachitic activity. Ergocalciferol is a white, colorless crystal, insoluble in water, soluble in organic solvents, and slightly soluble in vegetable oils. It is affected by air and by light [25]. One international unit of vitamin D is equal to 0.025 mcg of ergocalciferol. More than 80 % of ingested ergocalciferol is absorbed from the gastro-intestinal tract, mainly in the small intestine, via chylomicrons of lymph and then binds to DBP. The intestinal absorption may be decreased in patients with hepatic, biliary, or GI disease (e.g., Crohn's disease, Whipple's disease, sprue). Geriatric patients may also have a reduced intestinal absorption of physiological amount of vitamin D2. Pregnancy, CKD and macro-albuminuric patients may also require supra-physiological doses of vitamin D2 to achieve normal values. The biological actions of ergocalciferol, namely its hypercalcemic action, are observed within the 10–24 h after its administration, with a maximal effect observed 3–4 weeks later. Its mode of action has been above described. It is catabolized by the liver 25-hydroxylation and by the degradation by microsomal enzymes as well as by the renal transformation in $1,25OH_2D_2$ and other inactive metabolites, and then most of the metabolites (96 %) are eliminated through the bile acids and the feces.

28.5   Differences Between Ergocalciferol and Cholecalciferol

Ergosterol in plants and 7-dehydrocholesterol in skin are the precursors for vitamin D2 and vitamin D3, respectively. UV light B breaks the B chain of each molecule to form the pre-D isomer, which then undergoes isomerization to vitamin D. Vitamin D2 and D3 differ only in the side chain in which D2 has a double bond between C22–C23 and a methyl group at C24. This difference between these two calciferols are thought to alter their binding affinities to DBP and VDR, as well as their liver metabolism, since vitamin D3 appears to be the preferred substrate for the liver 25-hydroxylase [25]. In addition, all the effects of these vitamin D compounds are partly influenced by the genetic environment. Indeed several single nucleotide polymorphisms of the genes coding for the DBP, the 1α-hydroxylase or the VDR exist with potential influence on circulating vitamin D2 and D3 concentrations as well as their active metabolites and their biological effects [26].

There are numerous clinical studies, and a large meta-analysis, demonstrating that vitamin 3 is more effective than vitamin D2 in terms of increase in calcidiol and PTH lowering in healthy volunteers as well as in CKD patients [27–30]. This is an important issue since most of negative results observed in North-American studies using vitamin D2 cannot be entirely transferred to Europe where the preferred prescribed vitamin D is the D3 [28, 29].

28.6   Natural Vitamin D Recommended Intake and Dosage in Clinical Practice

The recommended adequate intake of vitamin D for infants, children, and adults up to 50 years is currently 200 IU (5 mcg/day). In subjects older than 50 years, the recommended intakes vary between 600 and 800 IU according to the IOM, and between

600 and 2,000 IU according to the ES [6, 7]. Although the recommended intake during pregnancy and lactation is 200 IU/day, there is now evidence that increasing vitamin D intake up to 4,000 IU/day is safe and most effective in achieving sufficient values in pregnant women and their neonates regardless of ethnic origins. In the absence of sunlight, the recommended intake of vitamin D should be increased to 600–1,000 IU/day for some experts [31], and to 1,500–2,000 IU/day for others [6].

Which natural vitamin D should be used ergocalciferol or cholecalciferol? A recent meta-analysis assessing the effectiveness of ergocalciferol and cholecalciferol in the raising of serum 25(OH)D3 concentrations demonstrated that when given, as bolus dose, cholecalciferol was more efficient that ergocalciferol, but the difference disappeared with daily administration [30].

What would be the optimal dose, frequency, and route of administration of natural vitamin D compounds? Various approaches have been used for decades, including several types of vitamin D, dose intervals going from annual intramuscular injection to oral daily, weekly, monthly, every 3–4 months, etc. without a definitive clear-cut recommendation. While daily dosages seem more physiologic, spaced-out dosages are thought to favor adherence to supplementation. If intermittent dosages are chosen (most frequently in our practice), doses, and interval between doses should not be two large. Indeed, we currently have the demonstration that daily doses and the same cumulative doses administered weekly or monthly (i.e. 1,500 IU daily, 10,000 IU weekly, or 45,000 IU monthly) induce the same increase in the circulating 25(OH)D concentration [32, 33], while this is less obvious for larger intervals. Furthermore, in a recent 3-year RCT of 500,000 IU vitamin D3 versus placebo administered once a year to elderly women, more fractures and falls were recorded in the vitamin D group than in the placebo group [32, 33]. Interestingly, this excess in the number of falls and fractures was only observed during the 3 months following each yearly administration of this large dose of vitamin D.

Nevertheless, it is generally accepted that, as a rule of thumb, a daily oral administration of 1,000 IU of cholecalciferol or ergocalciferol increases serum 25(OH)D levels by 5–10 ng/mL [34] and is generally sufficient to keep 25(OH)D values above 20 ng/ml [31]. However, higher dosages are required in many patients if one targets a serum 25(OH)D level above 30 ng/mL [6].

28.7 Other Natural Vitamin D Products

28.7.1 25OH Vitamin D3

The 25(OH)D3 may be found in small quantities in some foods of animal origin (meat, liver…). There are doubts regarding whether dietary 25(OH)D3 can raise serum 25(OH)D as efficiently as the other natural vitamin D, cholecalciferol and ergocalciferol. It has now been clearly demonstrated, in a double-blind randomized clinical trial in healthy Caucasian subjects, that daily supplementation with 25(OH)D3 is four to five times more effective than vitamin D3 increasing serum 25(OH)D3 [35]. Intestinal absorption of 25(OH)D3 is faster compared to cholecalciferol or ergocalciferol, but it is however still unknown whether the bioavailability of 25(OH)D3 from meat and other foods is comparable to that from oral supplementation. The 25(OH)D3 can be considered as alternative to cholecalciferol/ergocalciferol therapy in patients with liver disease or malabsorption syndromes since in those patients 25(OH)D3 might be the superior substance for vitamin D replenishment [36].

28.7.2   Vitamin D4

It has recently demonstrated that the precursor of vitamin D2, the ergosta-5,7-dienol (22,23-dihydroerosterol) is present in almost all species of mushroom, and that another vitamin D compound (D4) (22,23-dihydroergocalciferol;9,10-seco(5Z,7E)-5,7,10(19)-ergostatriene-3β-ol), can also by produced after UV irradiation [37]. However, the contribution of vitamin D4 in the total vitamin D status remains to be determined.

28.8   Vitamin D Metabolism in CKD

As early as in stage 2 of CKD, serum 25(OH)D levels begin to significantly decline [38, 39]. Reduced sun exposure [40], impaired skin synthesis of cholecalciferol due to renal disease [41], hyperpigmentation seen in late CKD stages [42] and dietary restrictions that are commonly advised to CKD patients contribute to high prevalence of vitamin D deficiency. The intestinal absorption of dietary and supplemental vitamin D could also be reduced in CKD subjects as suggested by the results of experimental studies in uremic animals [43]. In addition, CKD patients with severe proteinuria also have high urinary losses of DBP leading to increased renal loss of vitamin D metabolites [43–45].

In addition to the reasons for calcidiol deficiency in CKD patients described above, CKD is also a state of calcitriol deficiency. Availability of renal 1-α hydroxylase, the key enzyme necessary for the conversion of calcidiol in calcitriol, is limited as the renal mass shrinks [46]. Renal 1α-hydroxylase is highly dependent on its substrate calcidiol; therefore, in CKD the reduced availability of calcidiol has an important role in calcitriol deficiency [47, 48]. Numerous factors can be responsible for the down-regulation of renal 1α-hydroxylase in CKD, including hyperphosphatemia, high FGF23, metabolic acidosis, hyperuricemia and uremia itself [49–52]. The 1α-hydroxylase is expressed almost ubiquitously, however, the effect of CKD on the 1α-hydroxylase enzymatic activity in many of the extra-renal tissues is still unclear [53]. The expression of renal tubular receptor, megalin, that is normally responsible for the uptake of calcidiol–DBP complex from the glomerular filtrate is also reduced in CKD. Furthermore, reduced filtration of calcidiol–DBP complex in the setting of reduced GFR further limits its delivery and uptake by renal tubular receptors [54, 55]. Additionally, SHPT and elevated FGF23 lead to degradation of 25(OH)D by promoting the enzyme 24-hydroxylase to form 24,25-dihydroxyvitamin D [56]. CKD is also characterized by vitamin D resistance, as there is a progressive loss of VDR in the parathyroid gland [57]. Low levels of active vitamin D lead to impairments in the binding of calcitriol to VDR-RXR as well as in the binding of trimeric calcitriol–VDR-RXR complex to the DNA in VDRE [58, 59].

Vitamin D status is generally measured in CKD patients using serum 25(OH)D levels as $1,25OH_2D_3$ does not appears to be a reliable measure of vitamin D status. Despite the central biological role of vitamin D in CKD–MBD, studies examining association between circulating 25(OH)D levels and biochemical abnormalities in calcium, phosphate and PTH in CKD have not shown consistent association between serum 25(OH)D levels and elevated serum PTH or lower serum calcium [44, 60]. One possible explanation for this is based on the free hormone hypothesis as 25(OH)D is a highly protein bound hormone and <1 % of circulating 25(OH)D exists in free form [61]. The majority (85–90 %) of 25(OH)D is tightly bound to DBP and a smaller amount (10–15 %) is loosely bound to albumin [62]. Bioavailable 25(OH)D (albumin-bound hormone combined with the free fraction) levels have been shown to have a better association with serum calcium and PTH concentrations than total 25(OH)D in ESRD patients [62]. Corresponding data in CKD are lacking and remain under investigation.

Studies of the association between circulating 25(OH)D levels, bone morphology, bone mineral density and bone fractures in CKD and/or ESRD are limited in number and robustness but very informative. Coen et al. conducted a retrospective study of 104 patients on maintenance hemodialysis. These patients (61 males, 43 females; mean age 52.9 ± 11.7 years) were not on any vitamin D supplements and underwent transiliac bone biopsy for histologic, histomorphometric and histodynamic evaluation [63]. Patients with serum 25(OH)D levels ≤15 ng/ml had lower bone formation rate and trabecular mineralization surface independent of serum PTH and calcitriol levels indicating an important role of 25(OH)D on bone health in ESRD patients.

Ambrus et al. retrospectively examined the association between fracture and vitamin D status in 130 patients on maintenance hemodialysis (HD) [64]. Patients with history of skeletal fractures had significantly lower serum 25(OH)D levels compared with patients without fractures and lower serum vitamin D levels were independently associated with increased risk of fracture in a multivariable analysis (OR 11.22, 95 % confidence interval 1.33–94.82). The same investigators also described low serum 25(OH)D levels associated with reduced mineral bone density (BMD) in maintenance hemodialysis patients. In another cross-sectional study by Mucsi et al. [65] serum 25(OH)D levels were positively correlated with radial BMD in maintenance hemodialysis patients ($r = 0.424$, $p < 0.01$) and with significant attenuation on quantitative bone ultrasound (beta $= 0.262$, $P < 0.05$). Moreover, lower 25(OH)D levels have been shown to be associated with increased subperiosteal resorption and also with reduced BMD at wrist and lumbar spine in ESRD patients [66, 67].

28.9   Natural Vitamin Supplementation in CKD: Case Reports, Clinical Observational Studies

The principal goal of supplementing natural vitamin D in CKD is to correct vitamin D insufficiency or deficiency in order to prevent or to treat SHPT and its clinical, biological and histological consequences. In the absence of liver failure, which may be the only indication for the prescription of 25(OH)D3, the two main types of treatment – ergocalciferol and cholecalciferol – may interchangeably be used. Supplementation with vitamin D compounds in the setting of CKD, has been reported as early as the 1950s [68]. One of the earliest reports on the role of 25(OH)D in ESRD patients was published by Fournier et al. over three decades ago [69]. In this study, bone matrix mineralization evaluated by histomorphometry increased in patients receiving natural 25(OH)D, whereas it did not change significantly in patients receiving calcitriol. However, this study was not a randomized trial and thus had limitations on its internal validity. Other interventional uncontrolled studies among CKD patients have shown that natural vitamin D supplementation improves biomarkers of bone and mineral metabolism, including a reduction of serum PTH levels, as well as other parameters of the non-classical actions of vitamin D such as a decrease in inflammatory markers, and improvement of glucose metabolism [3, 70–73].

Numerous interventional, uncontrolled and not randomized clinical studies, with natural vitamin D have been published, either using ergocalciferol or cholecalciferol over varying periods of time and with very different dosage protocols in CKD subjects. In most of them, the authors have found a significant increase in circulating 25(OH)D concentration [71, 74–77]. However, in many of these patients circulating 25(OH)D levels did not surpass the recommended threshold of 30 ng/ml, probably because of the differences in treatment protocols. Vitamin D supplementation had also a beneficial effect on the control of SHPT as illustrated by a significant decrease of serum PTH levels in dialysis patients without significant changes in serum calcium and phosphate levels [78–80].

The field has moved forward since then and multiple RCTs have been conducted to examine the role of active vitamin D compounds as well as nutritional vitamin D supplements in CKD and in dialysis. Many of these trials were not specifically designed to evaluate patient centered skeletal outcomes and had multiple methodological limitations including small sample size and short duration of follow-up [81].

28.10   Randomized Clinical Trials with Natural Vitamin D in CKD

Recently, Kandula et al. [3], performed a systematic review and meta-analysis including five RCTs evaluating nutritional vitamin D supplements (ergocalciferol or cholecalciferol) in CKD and ESRD [82–85]. In the pooled analyses of RCTs, there was a significant increase in serum 25(OH)D levels (mean difference 14 ng/ml) and an associated decline in serum PTH levels (mean decrease 31.5 pg/ml) with nutritional vitamin D supplements compared with placebo. A low incidence of mild and reversible hypercalcemia (up to 3 %) and hyperphosphatemia (up to 7 %) were reported with nutritional vitamin D supplements. However, none of the studies reported patient-centered outcomes related to bone pain, skeletal fractures or parathyroidectomy, and most trials were of low to moderate quality.

Very recently, a meta-analysis was conducted in order to assess whether vitamin D supplementation alters the relative risk of all-cause and cardiovascular mortality, as well as serious adverse cardiovascular events in patients with CKD, compared with placebo [86]. The study focused on patients with GFR $\leq$60 ml/min/1.73 m^2 including end-stage CKD requiring dialysis. The search identified 4,246 articles, of which 13 were included (in the latter, 5 studies had cholecalciferol as intervention, 4 paricalcitol, 2 doxercalciferol, 2 alfacalcidol). No significant treatment effect of vitamin D on all-cause mortality (RR: 0.84; 95 % CI: 0.47, 1.52), cardiovascular mortality (RR: 0.79; 95 % CI: 0.26, 2.28) or serious adverse cardiovascular events (RR: 0.79; 95 % CI: 0.26, 2.28) was observed [86]. As far the 5 RCTs (four of them double-blind, five of them placebo-controlled trials) evaluating cholecalciferol are concerned, the first one (double-blind, placebo-controlled trial) showed that 1-year treatment with oral cholecalciferol was safe and sufficient to maintain serum 25(OH)D levels within normal ranges and prevent vitamin D insufficiency in early CKD. Furthermore, serum PTH levels improved after cholecalciferol treatment, particularly in patients who had secondary hyperparathyroidism [87]. The second one (double-blind, placebo-controlled trial) showed that 1-year treatment with oral cholecalciferol was effective and safe and did not negatively affect calcium, phosphorus, PTH levels and vascular calcifications [78]. The third one (placebo-controlled trial) showed that 4-month treatment with oral cholecalciferol was able to increase serum 25(OH)D and 1,25OH$_2$D$_3$ levels, without increased calcium or phosphorus values. However, no effects were detected in muscle strength, functional capacity, pulse wave velocity and health-related quality of life [88]. The fourth one (double-blind, placebo-controlled trial) showed that 2-month treatment with oral cholecalciferol had favorable effects on 1,25OH$_2$D$_3$ and PTH levels in non-HD patients [89]. The fifth one (double-blind, placebo-controlled trial) showed that 3-week treatment with oral cholecalciferol was effective and safe in HD patients [80]. Finally, a very recent double-blind, placebo-controlled trial not included in the above-mentioned meta-analysis [86] showed that 6-month treatment with oral cholecalciferol did not improve 24-h blood pressure, arterial stiffness or cardiac function HD patients [90].

28.11 Effects of Natural Vitamin D Supplementation on Non-classic Target Organs

28.11.1 The Muscles

Vitamin D mediates protein synthesis and cellular ATP accumulation; vitamin D also increases troponin C, actin and sarcoplasmic protein expression in striated muscles. Vitamin D may also increase muscle mass by directly stimulating growth of type 2 muscle fibers [91–93]. It may also increase muscle strength via the release of intracellular calcium, which facilitates muscular contraction, after stimulating the intracellular phospholipase C and protein kinase C signaling pathway. The poor muscular performances associated with lack of vitamin D is also associated with a significant increase of fat infiltration in muscle [94, 95]. Such lipid infiltration may reduce muscle performances because of an impaired muscle mitochondrial activity and a decreased insulin-mediated glucose uptake, use and glycogen synthesis [96].

Numerous studies have evidenced that this muscular weakness can regress following natural vitamin D administration [97]. When the levels of vitamin D are increased from <5 to >16 ng/ml, after vitamin D supplementation (800 IU/day at least) with calcium, the performance in speed walking and proximal muscle strength are markedly and progressively improved until obtaining values of 40 ng/ml. The increased muscle capacity is clinically translated by a significant 22 % decrease in the risk of fall as demonstrated by the results of a large meta-analysis of five clinical trials [98, 99].

Muscle wasting and reduction in maximal exercise capacity have been reported at every CKD stage, their prevalence usually runs parallel with the progression of renal disease and affects more than half of patients undergoing dialysis therapy [100]. The clinical signs including sarcopenia, frailty as well as the morphological changes, which mainly affect type II muscle fibers, correlated with serum 25(OH)D levels [101]. Actually, vitamin D supplementation significantly improved muscle performance in the elderly, however, the results are more questionable in CKD patients and require definitive demonstration by large RCTs.

28.11.2   The Kidney and Nephroprotection

Experimental studies, using a variety of experimental models, including unilateral ureteral obstruction, anti-thy-1 glomerulonephritis, sub-total nephrectomy and diabetic nephropathy, have clearly demonstrated that vitamin D can be renoprotective against renal injury. Indeed, vitamin D exerts renal anti-inflammatory and immunomodulatory effects, inhibits the renin-angiotensin-aldosterone system, and inhibits the pathways leading to the stimulation of pro-fibrotic factors such as NF-kB and TGFβ. Vitamin D also decreases the renal expression of markers characteristics of the epithelia-mesenchymal transition, such as TGFβ, resulting in the attenuation of interstitial and glomerular renal fibrosis, as well as the degree of proteinuria [102, 103]. In human, most of the anti-proteinuric and renoprotection studies have been performed with active vitamin D analogs including calcitriol, 22-oxa-calcitriol, and paricalcitol [104–107] and no definitive scientific evidence exists showing that natural vitamin D2 or D3 could have renoprotection properties.

28.11.3   The Cardiovascular System

Vitamin D affects the cardiovascular system via direct effects, since cardiac and vascular cells express both the VDR and the 1a-hydroxylase, and also via indirect effects because calcitriol controls insulin secretion and sensitivity, inflammation, PTH, and renin, and thus blood pressure [108]. The vitamin D system is also linked to the FGF23-klotho axis, which also mediates left ventricular hypertrophy development. Epidemiological studies have demonstrated that people residing in higher latitudes and with low serum vitamin D levels have an increased risk of arterial hypertension and cardiovascular diseases [109]. Intervention studies, as reported by the results of a large meta-analysis including 18 randomized clinical trials, have also shown that natural vitamin D supplementation slightly but significantly decreased the risk of cardiovascular complications [110]. However, convincing results regarding the potential benefits of natural vitamin D supplementation in CKD subjects are still lacking. In addition, the recent PRIMO study (Paricalcitol capsule benefits in renal failure-induced cardiac morbidity) showed that 48-weeks treatment with paricalcitol did not improve let ventricular hypertrophy (LVH) or improve diastolic dysfunction in CKD patients [111]. Similarly, another RCT using paricalcitol was negative in term of cardiovascular endpoints – the OPERA study. This study failed to show reduction of LVH with paricalcitol in 60 CKD stage 3–5 patients [112].

28.11.4   The Immune System

Briefly summarized, vitamin D stimulates innate immunity with potential protective effects against some infectious diseases. In vitro treatment of monocyte/macrophage cells with natural vitamin D, through the VDR activation and the stimulation of Toll like 2 receptor, increases the expression of the antimicrobial molecule cathelicidin [113]. In vivo, only animal studies have demonstrated a protective effect of vitamin D treatment against mammary infection [114]. Although some trials have shown that, compared to placebo, vitamin D supplementation may reduce the incidence of some viral infections [115] or their outcomes [116], it remains to be confirmed in larger studies whether natural vitamin D supplementation reduce the frequency of viral, bacterial and parasite infections in the general population.

Regarding the adaptive immune system, vitamin D inhibits some part of the adaptive immunity, especially shifting Th1 and Th17 lymphocytes towards a Th2 and Treg phenotype, with potential protective effects on some autoimmune diseases [117]. It also suppresses T-cells proliferation, decreases the secretion of IL2 and IFNγ by TCD4, decreases the cytotoxicity of TCD8 cells. Through all these actions and the modulation of the acquired immune system, vitamin D has been suggest to protect against a variety of diseases such as tuberculosis, osteoarthritis, diabetes, seasonal flu, multiple sclerosis, and Crohn's disease [15]. No definitive scientific evidence exists demonstrating that natural vitamin D2 or D3 could improve immune response in CKD subjects.

28.12   Cancers

The cancer-protecting effects of vitamin D, in particular colon cancer, may be explained via its anti-proliferating properties and its pro-differentiating and pro-apoptotic effects. Vitamin D also inhibits angiogenesis and tumor growth. Moreover, vitamin D improves cell-to-cell contact, reinforces cell adherence and intercellular communication, decreasing by this way the risk of cell metastasis [118]. In human, several groups have reported contradictory findings, the Women's Health Initiative (WH) study did not find any cancer protecting effect of daily administration of 400 IU of vitamin D3 [119]. However, another study providing 1,100 IU/day of vitamin D observed a significant reduction in the risk of any cancer [120]. However, there is still a need of RCT in CKD demonstrating the anti-cancer effect of natural vitamin D supplementation.

28.13   Diabetes

There is a large body of experimental evidences demonstrating the protecting of natural vitamin D against diabetes and metabolic syndrome. Indeed, the VDR and the 1a-hydroxylase are expressed in pancreatic b-cells, and the insulin gene possesses the VRE in its promoter region. Thus, vitamin D stimulates insulin secretion, β-cell proliferation, glucose transport, and insulin sensitivity [121]. Epidemiological studies have found a significant association between low serum vitamin D levels and the prevalence of type 1 diabetes [122, 123]. However, there has not been clearly demonstrated that vitamin D supplementation prevents the occurrence of diabetes and/or improves glucose control in humans.

28.14   Potential Adverse Effects of Natural Vitamin D

As for most medication, some people can present signs of allergic reaction, which is mainly due to inactive ingredients contained in ergocalciferol formulations. The other potential side effects are related to calcium and phosphate metabolism and include   hypercalcemia   and   hyperphosphatemia   usually   secondary   to hypervitaminosis D, which has become very uncommon nowadays. The first cases were reported in 1992 from Boston, USA, where eight subjects had clinical and biological signs of hypervitaminosis D (mean serum 25(OH)D levels of 294 ng/ml) after having taken excessive vitamin D fortification of dairy milk [124]. Recently, seven cases of vitamin D intoxication occurred in Turkish children, who unintentionally received an estimated daily intake of vitamin D between 266,000 and 800,000 IU because of an erroneously manufactured vitamin D supplement from fish oil [125]. Hypervitaminosis D is extremely rare in the general population (<1 %) with current recommended dose range of 400–4,800 IU/day for up to 1 year [126, 127], and depends on numerous factors including the type of natural vitamin D compounds, the starting dosage, season, body mass index, baseline concentrations of 25(OH)D, calcium, and PTH, as well as genetic polymorphisms [126]. Similarly, oral administration of a dose up to 100,000 IU monthly of cholecalciferol maintained circulating 25(OH)D levels over 30 ng/ml in 90 % of CKD subjects without hypervitaminosis D. These values reached a plateau after the first 12 weeks of treatment and remained stable for next 3 months without any case of hypercalcemia or hyperphosphatemia [128].

The renal manifestation of hypervitaminosis D may be an impaired renal function with polyuria, polydipsia, hypercalciuria, reversible azotemia, nauseas, anorexia, constipation, arterial hypertension, anemia, weight loss, metabolic acidosis, nephrocalcinosis, generalized vascular calcification, irreversible renal failure and death. Excessive treatment with ergocalciferol has also been associated with the development of low bone remodeling in case of CKD patients, bone demineralization in adult osteoporotic patients. It has been also associated with a decline in the average rate of linear growth and an increased bone mineralization in children with dwarfism. Mental retardation has also been reported incase of hypervitaminosis D.

28.15   Conclusions

Assessment of vitamin D status in CKD patients is presently seen as a step for formulating appropriate treatment of SHPT and CKD-MBD. There is ample biological and observational data to support the importance of maintaining a normal vitamin D status in CKD. Ideally, changes in clinical practice should be based on experiments rather than on observational studies. Accordingly, RCTs with nutritional vitamin D compounds have demonstrated serum PTH reductions but with a possible increased risk of hypercalcemia and/or hyperphosphatemia. The size and quality issues of the existing trials limits conclusions that can be drawn regarding their effects on patient-level skeletal outcomes, and larger higher quality RCTs focused on skeletal and survival outcomes are needed, some of them are actually ongoing as listed on Table 28.2. Furthermore, future studies to further delineate role of bioavailable vitamin D in CKD are also needed.

Table 28.2 RCTs focused on skeletal and survival outcomes

Clinical trial name or sponsor	Country	Clinical trial number	Population	Number of patients and duration	Outcomes	Date end of study
DIVINE	USA	NCT00892099	Incident hemodialysis patients (HD)	36 patients treated by 50,000 IU Ergocalciferol weekly; 33 patients treated by 50,000 IU Ergocalciferol monthly; 36 patients treated by placebo	Cathelidicin-infection; achievement of vitamin D sufficeincy	2013
NUTRIVITA-D001	Italy	NCT01457001	Chronic hemodialysis patients	Number of patients not described. Two groups randomized to natural vitamin D versus placebo	Risk of myocardial infarction, stroke, sudden death, an death for other causes	2016
D2D	USA	NCT00535158	Chronic hemodialysis patients	Number of patients not described. Ergocalciferol (D2) 50,000 units once weekly for 8 weeks then every other week for 4 weeks versus placebo	Performance on muscle function tests	2011
TILLVAL-D	Sweden	NCT00893451	Chronic kidney disease stage 3–4	24 CKD patients, randomized, placebo-controlled, single-centre, two-way cross-over study with two treatment periods of 10 weeks separated by a washout period of 6 weeks. Cholecalciferol 3,200 IU/day versus placebo	Insulin secretion and insulin sensitivity determined by insulin-glucose clamp	2011
Melamed M.	USA	NCT01029002	Chronic kidney disease stage 3–4	75 patients with CKD stage 3–4. Randomized to 50,000 IU/month of ergocalciferol versus placebo for 3 months. Then open label for 3 more months	Effect of vitamin D on albuminuria	2014

Barts & The London NHS Trust	UK	NCT00882401	Chronic kidney disease stage 3–4	64 patients with CKD stage 3–4. Randomized to 50,000 IU/month of ergocalciferol versus placebo for 5 months	Effects of vitamin D therapy on endothelial function	2011
The Cleveland Clinic	USA	NCT01173848	Chronic kidney disease stage 3–4	90 patients with CKD stage 3–4. Randomized to either ergocalciferol or cholecalciferol 50,000 IU/week for 3 months and then every month for 3 additional months	Effect of vitamin D2 and D3 on serum 25(OH)D and PTH levels	2013
POSH-D	USA	NCT00781417	Chronic kidney disease stage 2–3	48 patients with CKD stage 2–3. Randomized to cholecalciferol 50,000 IU once a week for 12 weeks then every other week for 40 weeks versus placebo	Effect of vitamin D3 on serum 25(OH)D and PTH levels and on calciuria	2011
Atlanta VA Medical Center (2)	USA	NCT00427037	Chronic kidney disease stage 3–4	34 patients with CKD stage 3–4. Randomized to cholecalciferol 50,000 IU once a week for 12 weeks versus placebo	Effect of vitamin D3 on serum 25(OH)D and PTH levels and bone turnover markers (CTX and C-telopeptide)	2013
EVIDENCE	China	NCT01672047	Kidney transplant	250 patients with CKD stage 3–4 and 100 CKD stage 5. Randomized to ergocalciferol according to 25(OH)D level <12 nmol/L 50,000 IU/week × 12 week, 12–39 nmol/L 50,000 IU/week × 4 week then,50,000 IU/month, 40–75 nmol/L 50,000 IU/month, 75–116.75 nmol/L 25,000 IU/ month versus placebo, for 2 years	Progression of coronary calcification	2015

(continued)

Table 28.2 (continued)

Clinical trial name or sponsor	Country	Clinical trial number	Population	Number of patients and duration	Outcomes	Date end of study
St George's University of London	UK	NCT01323712	Chronic kidney disease stage 3b–4	50 patients with CKD stage 3b–4. Randomized to cholecalciferol Cholecalciferol 100,000 Units 6 doses; 0, 4, 8, 12, 24, 42 weeks versus placebo	Impact of vitamin D supplementation on cardiac hypertrophy and function	2014
D-FENCE	UK	NCT01532349	Children, between 1 and 21 years old, with CKD stage 2–5	28 children with CKD stage 2–5. Randomized to 2,000 IU/day of cholecalciferol or to cholecalciferol 400 IU/day for 3 months	Changes in serum hepcidin levels after vitamin D supplementation	2015
CHAMBER	Japan	NCT02214563	Hemodialysis patients	90 patients with CKD stage 5D	Impact of vitamin D supplementation on serum hepcidin levels	2015
University of Colorado, Denver	USA	NCT02360644	Chronic kidney disease stage 2–5	120 subjects divided in 5 groups: 30 CKD 1–2, 30 CKD 3, 30 CKD 4–5, and 30 control. Treated by 5,000 IU/day of cholecalciferol	Study of the two major phase I drug metabolizing enzymes (CYP2B6, CYP3A), and three transporters [P-gp, MRP2, and MATE1/2 K]. Also CYP450s responsible for vitamin D metabolism	2019
Indiana University	USA	NCT00749736	Chronic kidney disease stage 3–4	100 patients with CKD stage3–4, randomized to 4,000 IU/day of cholecalciferol or doxercalciferol for 6 months	Change in CD4+/CD8+ ratio, TH1/TH2 cytokine profile, and conversion from anergic to reactive skin testing	2012

University of Kansas	USA	NCT01835691	Chronic kidney disease stage 3–4	60 subjects divided in 2 groups: one treated by 50,000 IU/week of cholecalciferol and the other with 50,000 IU/week of ergocalciferol, for 12 weeks	Effect on vitamin D levels and inflammatory parameters	2015
NEPH-Cal-D	USA	NCT01325610	Chronic hemodialysis patients	37 hemodialysis patients treated by 20,000 IU/day of cholecalciferol. Open lable, for 12 weeks	Vitamin D status as measured by 25(OH)D levels, and calcium absorption	2012
Massachusetts General Hospital	USA	NCT01026363	Chronic kidrey disease stage 3–4	60 subjects divided in 2 groups: one treated by 50,000 IU every other day of calcitriol 0.25 mcg/day, for 14 days	Effect on vitamin D on cathelidicin (hCAP18) levels	2014
University of British Columbia	Canada	NCT01247311	Chronic kidney disease stage 3b–4	129 patients with CKD stage 3b–4, randomized to 5,000 IU 3 x week of cholecalciferol or calcitriol 0.50 mcg 3 × week or placebo for 3 6 months	Effect of vitamin D on pulse wave velocity, blood pressure control. Change in proteinuria, FGF23, PTH, phosphate, calcium and C-reactive protein	2014

References

1. Meguid El Nahas A, Bello AK. Chronic kidney disease: the global challenge. Lancet. 2005;365:331–40.
2. Moe S, Drueke T, Cunningham J, et al. Definition, evaluation, and classification of renal osteodystrophy: a position statement from Kidney Disease: Improving Global Outcomes (KDIGO). Kidney Int. 2006;69:1945–53.
3. Kandula P, Dobre M, Schold JD, Schreiber Jr MJ, Mehrotra R, Navaneethan SD. Vitamin D supplementation in chronic kidney disease: a systematic review and meta-analysis of observational studies and randomized controlled trials. Clin J Am Soc Nephrol. 2011;6:50–62.
4. Bhan I, Burnett-Bowie SA, Ye J, Tonelli M, Thadhani R. Clinical measures identify vitamin D deficiency in dialysis. Clin J Am Soc Nephrol. 2010;5:460–7.
5. LaClair RE, Hellman RN, Karp SL, et al. Prevalence of calcidiol deficiency in CKD: a cross-sectional study across latitudes in the United States. Am J Kidney Dis. 2005;45:1026–33.
6. Holick MF, Binkley NC, Bischoff-Ferrari HA, et al. Evaluation, treatment, and prevention of vitamin D deficiency: an Endocrine Society clinical practice guideline. J Clin Endocrinol Metab. 2011;96:1911–30.
7. Ross AC, Manson JE, Abrams SA, et al. The 2011 report on dietary reference intakes for calcium and vitamin D from the Institute of Medicine: what clinicians need to know. J Clin Endocrinol Metab. 2011;96:53–8.
8. Watts NB, Bilezikian JP, Camacho PM, et al. American Association of Clinical Endocrinologists Medical Guidelines for Clinical Practice for the diagnosis and treatment of postmenopausal osteoporosis. Endocr Pract: Off J Am Coll Endocrinol Am Assoc Clin Endocrinol. 2010;16 Suppl 3:1–37.
9. National KF. K/DOQI clinical practice guidelines for bone metabolism and disease in chronic kidney disease. Am J Kidney Dis. 2003;42:S1–201.
10. KDIGO. KDIGO clinical practice guideline for the diagnosis, evaluation, prevention, and treatment of Chronic Kidney Disease-Mineral and Bone Disorder (CKD-MBD). Kidney Int. 2009;(Suppl 113):S1–130.
11. Ravani P, Malberti F, Tripepi G, et al. Vitamin D levels and patient outcome in chronic kidney disease. Kidney Int. 2009;75:88–95.
12. Blunt JW, DeLuca HF, Schnoes HK. 25-hydroxycholecalciferol. A biologically active metabolite of vitamin D3. Biochemistry. 1968;7:3317–22.
13. Blunt JW, Tanaka Y, DeLuca HF. Biological activity of 25-hydroxycholecalciferol, a metabolite of vitamin D3. Proc Natl Acad Sci U S A. 1968;61:1503–6.
14. Haussler M, Whitfield G, Haussler C, et al. The nuclear vitamin D receptor: biological and molecular regulatory properties reealed. J Bone Min Res. 1998;13:325–49.
15. Holick MF. Vitamin D, deficiency. N Engl J Med. 2007;357:266–81.
16. Schlingmann KP, Kaufmann M, Weber S, et al. Mutations in CYP24A1 and idiopathic infantile hypercalcemia. N Engl J Med. 2011;365:410–21.
17. Dusso A, Lopez-Hilker S, Rapp N, Slatopolsky E. Extra-renal production of calcitriol in chronic renal failure. Kidney Int. 1988;34:368–75.
18. Holick MF. Optimal vitamin D status for the prevention and treatment of osteoporosis. Drugs Aging. 2007;24:1017–29.
19. Souberbielle JC, Body JJ, Lappe JM, et al. Vitamin D and musculoskeletal health, cardiovascular disease, autoimmunity and cancer: recommendations for clinical practice. Autoimmun Rev. 2010;9:709–15.
20. Avenell A, Mak JC, O'Connell D. Vitamin D and vitamin D analogues for preventing fractures in post-menopausal women and older men. Cochrane Database Syst Rev. 2014;4, CD000227.
21. Holick MF. Vitamin D: a D-Lightful health perspective. Nutr Rev. 2008;66:S182–94.
22. Holick MF, Uskokovic M, Henley JW, MacLaughlin J, Holick SA, Potts Jr JT. The photoproduction of 1 alpha,25-dihydroxyvitamin D3 in skin: an approach to the therapy of vitamin-D-resistant syndromes. N Engl J Med. 1980;303:349–54.

23. Yuste C, Quiroga B, Garcia de Vinuesa S, et al. The effect of some medications given to CKD patients on vitamin D levels. Nefrologia. 2015;35:150–6.
24. Uhlin F, Magnusson P, Larsson TE, Fernstrom A. In the backwater of convective dialysis: decreased 25-hydroxyvitamin D levels following the switch to online hemodiafiltration. Clin Nephrol. 2015;83:315–21.
25. Holick MF, Biancuzzo RM, Chen TC, et al. Vitamin D2 is as effective as vitamin D3 in maintaining circulating concentrations of 25-hydroxyvitamin D. J Clin Endocrinol Metab. 2008;93:677–81.
26. Powe CE, Evans MK, Wenger J, et al. Vitamin D-binding protein and vitamin D status of black Americans and white Americans. N Engl J Med. 2013;369:1991–2000.
27. Armas LA, Hollis BW, Heaney RP. Vitamin D2 is much less effective than vitamin D3 in humans. J Clin Endocrinol Metab. 2004;89:5387–91.
28. Lehmann U, Hirche F, Stangl GI, Hinz K, Westphal S, Dierkes J. Bioavailability of vitamin D(2) and D(3) in healthy volunteers, a randomized placebo-controlled trial. J Clin Endocrinol Metab. 2013;98:4339–45.
29. Logan VF, Gray AR, Peddie MC, Harper MJ, Houghton LA. Long-term vitamin D3 supplementation is more effective than vitamin D2 in maintaining serum 25-hydroxyvitamin D status over the winter months. Br J Nutr. 2013;109:1082–8.
30. Tripkovic L, Lambert H, Hart K, et al. Comparison of vitamin D2 and vitamin D3 supplementation in raising serum 25-hydroxyvitamin D status: a systematic review and meta-analysis. Am J Clin Nutr. 2012;95:1357–64.
31. Ross C, Manson JE, Abrams S, et al. The 2011 report on dietary reference intakes for calcium and vitamin D from the Institute of Medicine: what clinicians need to know. J Clin Endocrinol Metab. 1999;96:53–8.
32. Binkley N, Gemar D, Engelke J, et al. Evaluation of ergocalciferol or cholecalciferol dosing, 1,600 IU daily or 50,000 IU monthly in older adults. J Clin Endocrinol Metab. 2011;96:981–8.
33. Ish-Shalom S, Segal E, Salganik T, Raz B, Bromberg IL, Vieth R. Comparison of daily, weekly, and monthly vitamin D3 in ethanol dosing protocols for two months in elderly hip fracture patients. J Clin Endocrinol Metab. 2008;93:3430–5.
34. Heaney RP. Vitamin D, in health and disease. Clin J Am Soc Nephrol. 2008;3:1535–41.
35. Cashman KD, Seamans KM, Lucey AJ, et al. Relative effectiveness of oral 25-hydroxyvitamin D3 and vitamin D3 in raising wintertime serum 25-hydroxyvitamin D in older adults. Am J Clin Nutr. 2012;95:1350–6.
36. Brandenburg VM, Kruger T. Calcifediol – more than the stepchild of CKD-MBD therapy? Curr Vasc Pharmacol. 2014;12:286–93.
37. Phillips KM, Horst RL, Koszewski NJ, Simon RR. Vitamin D4 in mushrooms. PLoS One. 2012;7, e40702.
38. Rickers H, Christiansen C, Christensen P, Christensen M, Rodbro P. Serum concentrations of vitamin D metabolites in different degrees of impaired renal function. Estimation of renal and extrarenal secretion rate of 24,25-dihydroxyvitamin D. Nephron. 1985;39:267–71.
39. Urena-Torres P, Metzger M, Haymann JP, et al. Association of kidney function, vitamin D deficiency, and circulating markers of mineral and bone disorders in CKD. Am J Kidney Dis. 2011;58:544–53.
40. Del Valle E, Negri AL, Aguirre C, Fradinger E, Zanchetta JR. Prevalence of 25(OH) vitamin D insufficiency and deficiency in chronic kidney disease stage 5 patients on hemodialysis. Hemodial Int. 2007;11:315–21.
41. Jacob AI, Sallman A, Santiz Z, Hollis BW. Defective photoproduction of cholecalciferol in normal and uremic humans. J Nutr. 1984;114:1313–9.
42. Abdelbaqi-Salhab M, Shalhub S, Morgan MB. A current review of the cutaneous manifestations of renal disease. J Cutan Pathol. 2003;30:527–38.
43. Vaziri ND, Hollander D, Hung EK, Vo M, Dadufalza L. Impaired intestinal absorption of vitamin D3 in azotemic rats. Am J Clin Nutr. 1983;37:403–6.
44. Gonzalez EA, Sachdeva A, Oliver DA, Martin KJ. Vitamin D insufficiency and deficiency in chronic kidney disease. A single center observational study. Am J Nephrol. 2004;24:503–10.

45. Sato KA, Gray RW, Lemann Jr J. Urinary excretion of 25-hydroxyvitamin D in health and the nephrotic syndrome. J Lab Clin Med. 1982;99:325–30.
46. Mawer EB, Taylor CM, Backhouse J, Lumb GA, Stanbury SW. Failure of formation of 1,25-dihydroxycholecalciferol in chronic renal insufficiency. Lancet. 1973;1:626–8.
47. Ishimura E, Nishizawa Y, Inaba M, et al. Serum levels of 1,25-dihydroxyvitamin D, 24,25-dihydroxyvitamin D, and 25-hydroxyvitamin D in nondialyzed patients with chronic renal failure. Kidney Int. 1999;55:1019–27.
48. Nigwekar SU, Bhan I, Thadhani R. Ergocalciferol and cholecalciferol in CKD. Am J Kidney Dis. 2012;60:139–56.
49. Gutierrez O, Isakova T, Rhee E, et al. Fibroblast growth factor-23 mitigates hyperphosphatemia but accentuates calcitriol deficiency in chronic kidney disease. J Am Soc Nephrol. 2005;16:2205–15.
50. Hsu CH, Vanholder R, Patel S, De Smet RR, Sandra P, Ringoir SM. Subfractions in uremic plasma ultrafiltrate inhibit calcitriol metabolism. Kidney Int. 1991;40:868–73.
51. Kawashima H, Kraut JA, Kurokawa K. Metabolic acidosis suppresses 25-hydroxyvitamin in D3-1alpha-hydroxylase in the rat kidney. Distinct site and mechanism of action. J Clin Invest. 1982;70:135–40.
52. Takahashi S, Yamamoto T, Moriwaki Y, Tsutsumi Z, Yamakita J, Higashino K. Decreased serum concentrations of 1,25(OH)2-vitamin D3 in patients with gout. Adv Exp Med Biol. 1998;431:57–60.
53. Zehnder D, Bland R, Williams MC, et al. Extrarenal expression of 25-hydroxyvitamin d(3)-1 alpha-hydroxylase. J Clin Endocrinol Metab. 2001;86:888–94.
54. Nykjaer A, Dragun D, Walther D, et al. An endocytic pathway essential for renal uptake and activation of the steroid 25-(OH) vitamin D3. Cell. 1999;96:507–15.
55. Takemoto F, Shinki T, Yokoyama K, et al. Gene expression of vitamin D hydroxylase and megalin in the remnant kidney of nephrectomized rats. Kidney Int. 2003;64:414–20.
56. Shimada T, Kakitani M, Yamazaki Y, et al. Targeted ablation of Fgf23 demonstrates an essential physiological role of FGF23 in phosphate and vitamin D metabolism. J Clin Invest. 2004;113:561–8.
57. Fukuda N, Tanaka H, Tominaga Y, Fukagawa M, Kurokawa K, Seino Y. Decreased 1,25-dihydroxyvitamin D3 receptor density is associated with a more severe form of parathyroid hyperplasia in chronic uremic patients. J Clin Invest. 1993;92:1436–43.
58. Hsu CH, Patel SR. Altered vitamin D metabolism and receptor interaction with the target genes in renal failure: calcitriol receptor interaction with its target gene in renal failure. Curr Opin Nephrol Hypertens. 1995;4:302–6.
59. Patel SR, Ke HQ, Vanholder R, Koenig RJ, Hsu CH. Inhibition of calcitriol receptor binding to vitamin D response elements by uremic toxins. J Clin Invest. 1995;96:50–9.
60. London GM, Guerin AP, Verbeke FH, et al. Mineral metabolism and arterial functions in end-stage renal disease: potential role of 25-hydroxyvitamin D deficiency. J Am Soc Nephrol. 2007;18:613–20.
61. Mendel CM. The free hormone hypothesis: a physiologically based mathematical model. Endocr Rev. 1989;10:232–74.
62. Bhan I, Powe CE, Berg AH, et al. Bioavailable vitamin D is more tightly linked to mineral metabolism than total vitamin D in incident hemodialysis patients. Kidney Int. 2012;82:84–9.
63. Coen G, Mantella D, Manni M, et al. 25-hydroxyvitamin D levels and bone histomorphometry in hemodialysis renal osteodystrophy. Kidney Int. 2005;68:1840–8.
64. Ambrus C, Almasi C, Berta K, et al. Vitamin D insufficiency and bone fractures in patients on maintenance hemodialysis. Int Urol Nephrol. 2011;43:475–82.
65. Mucsi I, Almasi C, Deak G, et al. Serum 25(OH)-vitamin D levels and bone metabolism in patients on maintenance hemodialysis. Clin Nephrol. 2005;64:288–94.
66. Elder GJ, Mackun K. 25-hydroxyvitamin D deficiency and diabetes predict reduced BMD in patients with chronic kidney disease. J Bone Miner Res. 2006;21:1778–84.
67. Ghazali A, Fardellone P, Pruna A, et al. Is low plasma 25-(OH)vitamin D a major risk factor for hyperparathyroidism and Looser's zones independent of calcitriol? Kidney Int. 1999;55:2169–77.

68. Stanbury SW. Azotaemic renal osteodystrophy. Br Med Bull. 1957;13:57–60.
69. Fournier A, Bordier P, Gueris J, et al. Comparison of 1 alpha-hydroxycholecalciferol and 25-hydroxycholecalciferol in the treatment of renal osteodystrophy: greater effect of 25-hydroxycholecalciferol on bone mineralization. Kidney Int. 1979;15:196–204.
70. Blair D, Byham-Gray L, Lewis E, McCaffrey S. Prevalence of vitamin D [25(OH)D] deficiency and effects of supplementation with ergocalciferol (vitamin D2) in stage 5 chronic kidney disease patients. J Ren Nutr. 2008;18:375–82.
71. Jean G, Souberbielle JC, Chazot C. Monthly cholecalciferol administration in haemodialysis patients: a simple and efficient strategy for vitamin D supplementation. Nephrol Dial Transplant. 2009;24:3799–805.
72. Kooienga L, Fried L, Scragg R, Kendrick J, Smits G, Chonchol M. The effect of combined calcium and vitamin D3 supplementation on serum intact parathyroid hormone in moderate CKD. Am J Kidney Dis. 2009;53:408–16.
73. Stubbs JR, Idiculla A, Slusser J, Menard R, Quarles LD. Cholecalciferol supplementation alters calcitriol-responsive monocyte proteins and decreases inflammatory cytokines in ESRD. J Am Soc Nephrol. 2010;21:353–61.
74. Albalate M, de la Piedra C, Ortiz A, et al. Risk in dosing regimens for 25-OH vitamin D supplementation in chronic haemodialysis patients. Nephron Clin Pract. 2012;121:c112–9.
75. Buccianti G, Bianchi ML, Valenti G, Lorenz M, Cresseri D. Effects of calcifediol treatment on the progression of renal osteodystrophy during continuous ambulatory peritoneal dialysis. Nephron. 1990;56:353–6.
76. Daroux M, Shenouda M, Bacri JL, Lemaitre V, Vanhille P, Bataille P. Vitamin D2 versus vitamin D3 supplementation in hemodialysis patients: a comparative pilot study. J Nephrol. 2013;26:152–7.
77. Matias PJ, Jorge C, Ferreira C, et al. Cholecalciferol supplementation in hemodialysis patients: effects on mineral metabolism, inflammation, and cardiac dimension parameters. Clin J Am Soc Nephrol. 2010;5:905–11.
78. Delanaye P, Weekers L, Warling X, et al. Cholecalciferol in haemodialysis patients: a randomized, double-blind, proof-of-concept and safety study. Nephrol Dial Transplant. 2013;28:1779–86.
79. Massart A, Debelle FD, Racape J, et al. Biochemical parameters after cholecalciferol repletion in hemodialysis: results from the VitaDial randomized trial. Am J Kidney Dis. 2014;64:696–705.
80. Wasse H, Huang R, Long Q, Singapuri S, Raggi P, Tangpricha V. Efficacy and safety of a short course of very-high-dose cholecalciferol in hemodialysis. Am J Clin Nutr. 2012;95:522–8.
81. Palmer SC, McGregor DO, Macaskill P, Craig JC, Elder GJ, Strippoli GF. Meta-analysis: vitamin D compounds in chronic kidney disease. Ann Intern Med. 2007;147:840–53.
82. Chandra P, Binongo JN, Ziegler TR, et al. Cholecalciferol (vitamin D3) therapy and vitamin D insufficiency in patients with chronic kidney disease: a randomized controlled pilot study. Endocr Pract: Off J Am Coll Endocrinol Am Assoc Clin Endocrinol. 2008;14:10–7.
83. Dogan E, Erkoc R, Sayarlioglu H, Soyoral Y, Dulger H. Effect of depot oral cholecalciferol treatment on secondary hyperparathyroidism in stage 3 and stage 4 chronic kidney diseases patients. Ren Fail. 2008;30:407–10.
84. Oksa A, Spustova V, Krivosikova Z, et al. Effects of long-term cholecalciferol supplementation on mineral metabolism and calciotropic hormones in chronic kidney disease. Kidney Blood Press Res. 2008;31:322–9.
85. Wissing KM, Broeders N, Moreno-Reyes R, Gervy C, Stallenberg B, Abramowicz D. A controlled study of vitamin D3 to prevent bone loss in renal-transplant patients receiving low doses of steroids. Transplantation. 2005;79:108–15.
86. Mann MC, Hobbs AJ, Hemmelgarn BR, Roberts DJ, Ahmed SB, Rabi DM. Effect of oral vitamin D analogs on mortality and cardiovascular outcomes among adults with chronic kidney disease: a meta-analysis. Clin Kidney J. 2015;8:41–8.
87. Alvarez JA, Law J, Coakley KE, et al. High-dose cholecalciferol reduces parathyroid hormone in patients with early chronic kidney disease: a pilot, randomized, double-blind, placebo-controlled trial. Am J Clin Nutr. 2012;96:672–9.

88. Hewitt NA, O'Connor AA, O'Shaughnessy DV, Elder GJ. Effects of cholecalciferol on functional, biochemical, vascular, and quality of life outcomes in hemodialysis patients. Clin J Am Soc Nephrol. 2013;8:1143–9.
89. Marckmann P, Agerskov H, Thineshkumar S, et al. Randomized controlled trial of cholecalciferol supplementation in chronic kidney disease patients with hypovitaminosis D. Nephrol Dial Transplant. 2012;27:3523–31.
90. Mose FH, Vase H, Larsen T, et al. Cardiovascular effects of cholecalciferol treatment in dialysis patients – a randomized controlled trial. BMC Nephrol. 2014;15:50.
91. Harter HR, Birge SJ, Martin KJ, Klahr S, Karl IE. Effects of vitamin D metabolites on protein catabolism of muscle from uremic rats. Kidney Int. 1983;23:465–72.
92. Pointon JJ, Francis MJ, Smith R. Effect of vitamin D deficiency on sarcoplasmic reticulum function and troponin C concentration of rabbit skeletal muscle. Clin Sci (Lond). 1979;57: 257–63.
93. Francis MJ, Pointon JJ, Smith R, Mercola DA. Decreased troponin C concentrations in vitamin D-deficient rabbit skeletal muscle [proceedings]. Biochem Soc Trans. 1978;6:1273–4.
94. Gilsanz V, Kremer A, Mo AO, Wren TA, Kremer R. Vitamin D status and its relation to muscle mass and muscle fat in young women. J Clin Endocrinol Metab. 2010;95:1595–601.
95. Kremer R, Campbell PP, Reinhardt T, Gilsanz V. Vitamin D status and its relationship to body fat, final height, and peak bone mass in young women. J Clin Endocrinol Metab. 2009;94: 67–73.
96. Morino K, Petersen KF, Sono S, et al. Regulation of mitochondrial biogenesis by lipoprotein lipase in muscle of insulin-resistant offspring of parents with type 2 diabetes. Diabetes. 2012;61:877–87.
97. Stockton KA, Mengersen K, Paratz JD, Kandiah D, Bennell KL. Effect of vitamin D supplementation on muscle strength: a systematic review and meta-analysis. Osteoporos Int. 2011;22:859–71.
98. Bischoff-Ferrari HA, Borchers M, Gudat F, Durmuller U, Stahelin HB, Dick W. Vitamin D receptor expression in human muscle tissue decreases with age. J Bone Miner Res. 2004;19: 265–9.
99. Bischoff-Ferrari HA, Dawson-Hughes B, Willett WC, et al. Effect of vitamin D on falls: a meta-analysis. JAMA. 2004;291:1999–2006.
100. Clyne N, Jogestrand T, Lins LE, Pehrsson SK. Progressive decline in renal function induces a gradual decrease in total hemoglobin and exercise capacity. Nephron. 1994;67:322–6.
101. Gordon PL, Doyle JW, Johansen KL. Association of 1,25-dihydroxyvitamin D levels with physical performance and thigh muscle cross-sectional area in chronic kidney disease stage 3 and 4. J Ren Nutr. 2012;22:423–33.
102. Li J, Zhang Z, Wang D, Wang Y, Li Y, Wu G. TGF-beta 1/Smads signaling stimulates renal interstitial fibrosis in experimental AAN. J Recept Signal Transduct Res. 2009;29:280–5.
103. Zhang Y, Kong J, Deb DK, Chang A, Li YC. Vitamin D receptor attenuates renal fibrosis by suppressing the renin-angiotensin system. J Am Soc Nephrol. 2010;21:966–73.
104. Hirata M, Katsumata K, Endo K, Fukushima N, Ohkawa H, Fukagawa M. In subtotally nephrectomized rats 22-oxacalcitriol suppresses parathyroid hormone with less risk of cardiovascular calcification or deterioration of residual renal function than 1,25(OH)2 vitamin D3. Nephrol Dial Transplant. 2003;18:1770–6.
105. Makibayashi K, Tatematsu M, Hirata M, et al. A vitamin D analog ameliorates glomerular injury on rat glomerulonephritis. Am J Pathol. 2001;158:1733–41.
106. Zhang X, Zanello LP. Vitamin D receptor-dependent 1 alpha,25(OH)2 vitamin D3-induced anti-apoptotic PI3K/AKT signaling in osteoblasts. J Bone Miner Res. 2008;23:1238–48.
107. Zhang Z, Sun L, Wang Y, et al. Renoprotective role of the vitamin D receptor in diabetic nephropathy. Kidney Int. 2008;73:163–71.
108. Li YC. Vitamin D, regulation of the renin-angiotensin system. J Cell Biochem. 2003;88: 327–31.
109. Rostand SG. Vitamin D, blood pressure, and African Americans: toward a unifying hypothesis. Clin J Am Soc Nephrol. 2010;5:1697–703.

110. Hsia J, Heiss G, Ren H, et al. Calcium/vitamin D supplementation and cardiovascular events. Circulation. 2007;115:846–54.
111. Thadhani R, Appelbaum E, Pritchett Y, et al. Vitamin D therapy and cardiac structure and function in patients with chronic kidney disease: the PRIMO randomized controlled trial. JAMA. 2012;307:674–84.
112. Wang AY, Fang F, Chan J, et al. Effect of paricalcitol on left ventricular mass and function in CKD – the OPERA trial. J Am Soc Nephrol. 2014;25:175–86.
113. Liu PT, Stenger S, Li H, et al. Toll-like receptor triggering of a vitamin D-mediated human antimicrobial response. Science. 2006;311:1770–3.
114. Yamshchikov AV, Desai NS, Blumberg HM, Ziegler TR, Tangpricha V. Vitamin D for treatment and prevention of infectious diseases: a systematic review of randomized controlled trials. Endocr Pract: Off J Am Coll Endocrinol Am Assoc Clin Endocrinol. 2009;15:438–49.
115. Urashima M, Segawa T, Okazaki M, Kurihara M, Wada Y, Ida H. Randomized trial of vitamin D supplementation to prevent seasonal influenza A in schoolchildren. Am J Clin Nutr. 2010;91:1255–60.
116. Abu-Mouch S, Fireman Z, Jarchovsky J, Zeina AR, Assy N. Vitamin D supplementation improves sustained virologic response in chronic hepatitis C (genotype 1)-naive patients. World J Gastroenterol: WJG. 2011;17:5184–90.
117. Munger KL, Levin LI, Hollis BW, Howard NS, Ascherio A. Serum 25-hydroxyvitamin D levels and risk of multiple sclerosis. JAMA. 2006;296:2832–8.
118. Krishnan AV, Feldman D. Mechanisms of the anti-cancer and anti-inflammatory actions of vitamin D. Annu Rev Pharmacol Toxicol. 2011;51:311–36.
119. Wactawski-Wende J, Kotchen JM, Anderson GL, et al. Calcium plus vitamin D supplementation and the risk of colorectal cancer. N Engl J Med. 2006;354:684–96.
120. Lappe JM, Travers-Gustafson D, Davies KM, Recker RR, Heaney RP. Vitamin D and calcium supplementation reduces cancer risk: results of a randomized trial. Am J Clin Nutr. 2007;85:1586–91.
121. Pittas AG, Dawson-Hughes B. Vitamin D and diabetes. J Steroid Biochem Mol Biol. 2010;121:425–9.
122. Hypponen E, Laara E, Reunanen A, Jarvelin MR, Virtanen SM. Intake of vitamin D and risk of type 1 diabetes: a birth-cohort study. Lancet. 2001;358:1500–3.
123. Zipitis CS, Akobeng AK. Vitamin D supplementation in early childhood and risk of type 1 diabetes: a systematic review and meta-analysis. Arch Dis Child. 2008;93:512–7.
124. Jacobus CH, Holick MF, Shao Q, et al. Hypervitaminosis D associated with drinking milk. N Engl J Med. 1992;326:1173–7.
125. Kara C, Gunindi F, Ustyol A, Aydin M. Vitamin D intoxication due to an erroneously manufactured dietary supplement in seven children. Pediatrics. 2014;133:e240–4.
126. Gallagher JC, Sai A, Templin 2nd T, Smith L. Dose response to vitamin D supplementation in postmenopausal women: a randomized trial. Ann Intern Med. 2012;156:425–37.
127. Gallagher JC, Smith LM, Yalamanchili V. Incidence of hypercalciuria and hypercalcemia during vitamin D and calcium supplementation in older women. Menopause. 2014;21:1173–80.
128. Jean G, Souberbielle JC, Lechevallier S, Chazot C. Kinetics of serum 25-hydroxyvitamin D in haemodialysis patients treated with monthly oral cholecalciferol. Clin Kidney J. 2015;8:388–92.

Chapter 29
Which Vitamin D in Chronic Kidney Disease: Nutritional or Active Vitamin D? Or Both?

Armando Luis Negri, Elisa del Valle, and Francisco Rodolfo Spivacow

Abstract As vitamin D insufficiency is very common world-wide, vitamin D supplementation has generated much debate and subsequent research not only in the general population but also in patients with chronic kidney disease (CKD). Several observational and mechanistic studies have suggested that vitamin D's actions may be more broad and significant than originally appreciated, far exceeding bone and mineral metabolism. This is probably due to the fact that most tissues in the body express vitamin D receptors. As patients with kidney disease cannot convert 25-hydroxyvitamin D [25(OH)D] to its more active form, 1,25-dihydroxy vitamin D [1,25(OH)$_2$D] because of reduced activity of the enzyme 1α-hydroxylase in the kidneys to produce classic bone and mineral effects, nephrologists have traditionally replaced patients with kidney disease with active vitamin D, 1,25-dihydroxvitamin D, or related analogs. Multiple observational studies in patients with CKD have shown that they not only have low levels of 1,25(OH)$_2$D, but also low 25(OH)D levels. The fact that there is also extrarenal conversion of 25(OH) vitamin D to 1,25(OH)$_2$ vitamin D in CKD in multiple tissues leading to autocrine effects, has led to the speculation that CKD patients should also need to be supplemented with nutritional vitamin D. This chapter outlines the available evidence on the controversy about which vitamin D is better for patients with kidney disease: Active vitamin D, nutritional or both.

Keywords 25-hydroxyvitamin D • Nutritional vitamin D • Active vitamin D • Mineral metabolism • Extra skeletal effects • Chronic kidney disease (CKD) • Vitamin D deficiency • Vitamin D supplementation • Cardiovascular risk • Survival • Toxicity

A.L. Negri, MD, FACP (✉)
Instituto de Investigaciones Metabólicas, Buenos Aires, Argentina
e-mail: negri@casasco.com.ar; armando.negri@gmail.com

E. del Valle, MD • F.R. Spivacow, MD
IDIM Instituto de Investigaciones Metabólicas, Universidad del Salvador, Buenos Aires, Argentina
e-mail: spiva@idim.com.ar; frspivacow@gmail.com

© Springer International Publishing Switzerland 2016
P.A. Ureña Torres et al. (eds.), *Vitamin D in Chronic Kidney Disease*,
DOI 10.1007/978-3-319-32507-1_29

Table 29.1 Vitamin D sterols used in chronic kidney disease

Native vitamin D	
Vitamin D2	Ergocalciferol
Vitamin D3	Cholecalciferol
Vitamin D prohormones	
1 alfa (OH) D2	Doxercalciferol
1 alfa (OH) D3	Alfacalcidiol
Active vitamin D Sterols	
1,25(OH)$_2$D$_3$	Calcitriol
19-NOR-1,25(OH)$_2$D$_3$	Paricalcitol
22-OXA-1,25(OH)$_2$D$_3$	Maxacalcitol
1,25(OH)2-26,27-F6-D3	Falecalcitriol

29.1 Introduction

Vitamin D insufficiency is very common world-wide, especially in areas with increased latitude from the equator or during the winter months. Vitamin D supplementation has generated much debate and subsequent research not only in the general population but also in patients with CKD. As patients with kidney disease cannot convert 25-hydroxyvitamin D [25(OH)D] to its more active form, 1,25-dihydroxy vitamin D [1,25(OH)$_2$D] because of reduced activity of the enzyme 1-α hydroxylase (CYP27B1) in the kidneys, nephrologists have traditionally replaced patients with kidney disease with active vitamin D, 1,25-dihydroxvitamin D, or related analogs. As the presence of extra-renal 1-α hydroxylation has been appreciated since long time [1, 2], the potential use this extra-renal of 1α-hydroxylation of vitamin D for autocrine and paracrine signaling [3] has led nephrologists to consider replacing kidney disease patients with nutritional vitamin D, the inactive form, as well as with active vitamin D (Table 29.1). This chapter outlines the available evidence on the controversy about which vitamin D is better for patients with kidney disease.

29.2 Vitamin D Physiology

Vitamin D can be generated through cutaneous synthesis following sunlight exposure or acquired through diet consuming vitamin D–rich foods (oily fish, dairy products), fortified foods or supplements. Ultraviolet B radiation (UVB) in combination with heat catalyzes conversion of 7-dehydrocholesterol to D3 (cholecalciferol). Cholecalciferol is relatively inactive without further metabolism. The liver introduces hydroxylation at the 25th position, largely unregulated, that yields 25-hydroxyvitamin D (25(OH)D). With its long half-life (2–3 weeks), 25(OH)D is the most stable and widely used measure of vitamin D status. 25(OH)D circulates in nanogram per milliliter concentrations, which are 1,000-fold higher than concentrations of 1,25(OH)$_2$D. Although 25(OH)D stimulates the vitamin D receptor (at

100–150-fold higher concentrations than $1,25(OH)_2D$) in vitro [4, 5], it is unclear whether it has effects in vivo. Vitamin D is a highly protein-bound hormone with less than 1 % of circulating 25-(OH) D existing in its free form [6]. The majority of circulating 25(OH)D (85–90 %) is tightly bound to its specific vitamin D-binding protein and a smaller amount (10–15 %) is loosely bound to albumin. The CYP27B1 enzyme (1α-hydroxylase), primarily located in the kidney, converts 25(OH)D to 1,25-dihydroxyvitamin D $(1,25(OH)_2D)$. This more active form of vitamin D, has a $t_{1/2}$ of only 8–12 h and responds dynamically to changes in calcium and phosphate metabolism.

Circulating $1,25(OH)_2D$ enters the target cell, either in its free form or facilitated by megalin [7], and binds to the vitamin D receptor (VDR) in the cytoplasm which then translocates to the nucleus and heterodimerizes with the retinoic X receptor (RXR). The $1,25(OH)_2D$-VDR-RXR complex then binds to vitamin D response elements (VDRE) on DNA to increase transcription of vitamin D regulated genes. Classic functions regulated by vitamin D include genes important for mineralization of bone and calcium transport in the intestine [8]. Non-classic or novel functions of vitamin D under investigation include genes important for innate immunity, cancer proliferation, muscle (both skeletal and smooth) function and endothelial cell proliferation [3].

Finally, CYP24A1, 25-hydroxyvitamin D3 24-hydroxylase is the enzyme that converts the major circulating and active forms of vitamin D to inactive metabolites.

29.3 Vitamin D and CKD

Renal CYP27B1 activity declines along with glomerular filtration rate (GFR) in advancing CKD. Circulating $1,25(OH)_2D$ levels consequently decrease, resulting in reduced absorption of intestinal calcium, hypocalcemia and secondary hyperparathyroidism (SHPT). SHPT, characterized by elevated parathyroid hormone (PTH) levels, is associated with bone disease named renal osteodystrophy. Before the discovery of calcitriol, patients in dialysis with SHPT were treated with high doses of nutritional vitamin D [9]. Most studies performed were observational in nature and with small number of patients. Once calcitriol was introduced several small randomized control trials were performed [10–12]. Thus, replacement of vitamin D with calcitriol or one of its analogues has thus become standard therapy in CKD, aimed at normalizing serum calcium and mitigating bone disease caused by SHPT.

Multiple observational studies in patients with CKD and end-stage renal disease (ESRD) have shown that they not only have low levels of $1,25(OH)_2D$, but also low 25(OH)D levels [13, 14]. Many factors may account for the low levels of 25(OH)D in kidney disease, including loss of vitamin D binding protein in the urine [15], ineffective synthesis in the skin upon exposure to ultraviolet B radiation [16], and also reduced nutritional intake and sun exposure [17].

29.4 Classical and Non-classical Actions of Vitamin D

Several observational and mechanistic studies have suggested that vitamin D's actions may be more broad and significant than originally appreciated, far exceeding bone and mineral metabolism. This is probably due to the fact that most tissues in the body express vitamin D receptors [18]. These other actions of vitamin D, that are unrelated to its classical effects on bone mineralization and calcium and phosphate absorption, are called "non-classical actions". Interesting observations come from knockout mice for the vitamin D receptor. These mice develop elevated blood pressures and left ventricular hypertrophy [19] that occurs due to a rise in renin consequent to the loss of normal suppression of the renin-angiotensin system by vitamin D [20]. Vitamin D also plays a role in the innate immune system. The 25(OH)D enters the macrophage where it is transformed by local 1α-hydroxylase into active vitamin D, which increases the expression of cathelicidin, an antimicrobial peptide [21].

Non-classical effects are likely mediated by autocrine or paracrine stimulation of vitamin D receptors, following the local generation of 1,25(OH)$_2$D by extra-renal 1α-hydroxylase. This implies that adequate circulating 25(OH)D, rather than circulating 1,25(OH)$_2$D is essential for the expression of non-classical actions. There is experimental evidence to support this contention in some tissues, including lymphoid tissue and vascular smooth muscle [22–24].

29.5 Nutritional Vitamin D

29.5.1 Nutritional Vitamin D Deficiency Effects on Bone and Mineral Metabolism in CKD

Vitamin D status is generally measured in CKD patients using 25(OH) vitamin D levels as 1,25(OH)$_2$ vitamin D levels are not a reliable measure of vitamin D status. Despite the central biological role of vitamin D in CKD–MBD, studies examining association between 25 (OH) vitamin D levels and biochemical abnormalities in calcium, phosphorous and PTH in CKD have not shown consistent association between serum 25 (OH) vitamin D levels and elevated serum PTH or lower serum calcium [25] One possible explanation for this is based on free hormone hypothesis. As we explained in vitamin D physiology, 25 (OH) vitamin D is a highly protein bound prohormone and <1 % of circulating 25 (OH) vitamin D exists in free form [26] being the majority tightly bound to DBP and albumin. Bhan et al. have shown that bioavailable 25 (OH) vitamin D (albumin-bound prohormone combined with the free fraction) levels have a better association with serum calcium and PTH than total 25 (OH) vitamin D in ESRD patients [6]. Corresponding data in CKD are lacking and remain under investigation.

Studies of the association between 25(OH) vitamin D levels, bone morphology, bone mineral density and bone fractures in CKD and/or ESRD are limited in number but very informative. Coen et al. [27] conducted a retrospective study of 104 patients (61 males, 43 females; mean age 52.9 ± 11.7 years) on maintenance hemodialysis who were not receiving any vitamin D supplements and underwent transiliac bone biopsy for histomorphometric analysis. In those with serum 25-OHD levels <15 ng ml/1, bone formation rate and trabecular mineralization surface were lower, independent of PTH and calcitriol levels, indicating an important role that 25 (OH) vitamin D has in bone health in ESRD patients. Ambrus et al. performed a retrospective analysis of the association between fracture and vitamin D status in 130 patients on maintenance hemodialysis [28]. Patients with fractures had significantly lower 25 (OH) vitamin D levels compared with patients without fractures and lower vitamin D levels were independently associated with increased fracture risk in a multivariable analysis (OR 11.22, 95 % CI 1.33–94.82). The same investigators also described low 25 (OH) vitamin D levels associated with reduced bone mineral bone density in maintenance hemodialysis patients. In another cross-sectional study, Mucsi et al. [29] found that 25 (OH) vitamin D levels were positively associated with radial bone mineral density in maintenance hemodialysis patients and with significant attenuation on quantitative bone ultrasound. Lower 25 (OH) vitamin levels have been shown to be associated with increased subperiosteal resorption and also with reduced bone mineral density at wrist and lumbar spine in patients [30, 31].

29.5.2 Nutritional Vitamin D Supplementation Effects on Bone and Mineral Metabolism in CKD and ESRD

The use of vitamin D compounds in the setting of renal disease have been reported as early as the 1950s [32] One of the earliest reports on the role of 25 (OH) vitamin D in ESRD patients was published by Fournier et al. over three decades ago [33]. In this non-randomized trial, bone matrix mineralization evaluated by histomorphometry, increased in patients receiving 25 (OH) vitamin D, whereas it did not change significantly in patients receiving calcitriol.

Kandula et al. [34] recently in their systematic review and meta-analysis of identified five randomized trials evaluating nutritional vitamin D supplements (ergocalciferol or cholecalciferol) in CKD and ESRD. In the pooled analyses of randomized trials, there was a significant increase in serum 25 (OH) vitamin D levels (mean difference 14 ng ml/1) and an associated decline in PTH levels (mean decrease 31.5 pg ml/1) with nutritional vitamin D supplements compared with placebo. A low incidence of mild and reversible hypercalcemia (up to 3 %) and hyperphosphatemia (up to 7 %) were reported with nutritional vitamin D supplements. However, none of the studies reported patient centered outcomes related to bone fractures, bone pain or parathyroidectomy and most trials were of low to moderate quality.

29.5.3   Nutritional Vitamin D Deficiency Effects
on Non-classical Actions of Vitamin D

Several investigations have suggested potential beneficial effects of vitamin D on both cardiac function and immunity. This is particularly relevant to patients with ESRD as cardiovascular and infectious disease represent the leading causes of morbidity and mortality in this population. The mechanism for how vitamin D may improve cardiovascular disease outcomes are not completely clear; however, potential hypotheses include the down regulation of the renin-angiotensin-aldosterone system, direct effects on the heart and vasculature or improvement of glycemic control.

29.5.3.1   Epidemiological Evidence Evaluating Cardiovascular Risk
in Relation to Nutritional Vitamin D Status in the General
Population

Kendrick et al. reported that individuals surveyed in The National Health and Nutritional Examination Surveys (NHANES) 1988–1994 with vitamin D deficiency (25(OH)D <20 ng/mL) had higher prevalence of self-reported angina, myocardial infarction and heart failure compared to individuals with higher levels of vitamin D (OR (95 % CI) 1.20 (1.01–1.36)) [35]. Several cardiovascular risk factors were associated with lower vitamin D status including hypertension, diabetes, elevated body mass index (>30), elevated triglyceride level and microalbuminuria in NHANES 1988–1994 [36, 37]. In the most recent NHANES 2000–2004 survey, vitamin D deficiency was also associated with increased prevalence of self-reported coronary heart disease, heart failure and peripheral vascular disease [38].

Prevalence of peripheral arterial disease is also increased comparing lowest quartile of 25(OH)D to highest quartile of 25(OH)D [39]. Judd et al. determined in non-hypertensive individuals from NHANES 1988–1994, optimal vitamin D status (>32 ng/mL) provided a 20 % reduction in the rate of blood pressure rise with age [40].

Melamed et al. examined all-cause mortality by quartile of 25(OH)D and found that the lowest quartile of 25(OH)D had significantly increased adjusted mortality rate ratios (MRR (95 % CI) 1.28 (1.11–1.48) compared to individuals with the highest quartile of 25(OH)D [41]. There was a trend towards increased mortality rate in the lowest quartile of 25(OH)D due to cardiovascular mortality; however, this did not reach statistical significance (MRR (95 % CI) 1.22 (0.90–1.65)).

Several studies have prospectively evaluated long-term cardiovascular outcomes in subjects with no previous history of CVD in relation to their baseline vitamin D status. Men in the Health Professionals Follow-up Study (HPFS) without previous CVD who had vitamin D deficiency [(25(OH)D <15 ng/mL] exhibited a twofold increased rate of myocardial infarction during a 10 year follow-up period [42]. In the Framingham Offspring Study, subjects with no previous history of CVD and severe vitamin D deficiency [25(OH)D <10 ng/mL] experienced an increased hazard ratio for developing a first cardiovascular event after 5 years of follow-up (1.80; 95 % CI, 1.05–3.08) compared to subjects with higher levels of 25(OH)D (>15 ng/mL) [43].

Other studies have evaluated cardiovascular risk in relation to vitamin D status in subjects with established cardiovascular disease. In over 3,000 subjects undergoing coronary angiography, severe vitamin D deficiency [25(OH)D <10 ng/mL] had three to five times risk of dying from sudden cardiac death or heart failure over a 7 year follow-up period compared to optimal levels of vitamin D [25(OH)D >30 ng/mL] [44]. Further, in these same subjects, vitamin D deficiency imparted a 50 % increase in fatal stroke [45]. Subjects in the lowest quartile for 25(OH)D had increased hazard ratios for all cause and cardiovascular mortality compared to subjects in the highest quartile for 25(OH)D [46].

29.5.3.2 Epidemiological Evidence Evaluating Cardiovascular Risk in Relation to Nutritional Vitamin D Status in CKD Patients

Similar findings have been reported in subjects with CRF and in incident hemodialysis patients. All cause and cardiovascular mortality was evaluated in a cohort of 444 patients with eGFR <60 mL/min/1.73 m^2 from the Ludwigshafen Risk and Cardiovascular Health Study, during a median follow-up time of 9.4 years [47]. Multivariate adjusted hazard ratios in severely vitamin D-deficient [25(OH)D <10 ng/mL] compared to vitamin D-sufficient patients [25(OH)D ≥30 ng/mL] were 3.79 (1.71–8.43) for all-cause and 5.61 (1.89–16.6) for cardiovascular mortality with no significant interaction with serum PTH concentrations. In another cohort of patients at different CKD stages, the relationship between vitamin D serum levels, vascular calcification and stiffness, and the mortality risk was determined [48]. Patients with 25(OH)D ≤16.7 ng/ml had a significantly lower survival rate than patients above that level. Multivariate adjustments for confounders confirmed 25(OH)D level as an independent predictor of all-cause mortality. Low 25(OH)D levels affected mortality independently of vascular calcification and stiffness, suggesting that 25D may influence survival in CKD patients via additional pathways. In the prospective cohort study of incident dialysis patients in the Netherlands (the NECOSAD), all patients with measured 25(OH)D at 12 months after the start of dialysis were selected [49]. In 762 patients the impact of 25(OH)D levels on short-term (6 months of follow-up) and longer-term mortality (3 years of follow-up) was assessed. After adjustments for possible confounders, the hazard ratio for mortality was 2.0 (1.0–3.8) for short-term and 1.5 (1.0–2.1) for longer-term mortality when comparing patients with 25(OH)D levels ≤10 ng/mL with those presenting with 25(OH)D levels >10 ng/mL. Adjusted hazard ratios for cardiovascular mortality were 2.7 (1.1–6.5) and 1.7 (1.1–2.7) for short- and longer-term mortality, respectively. For non-cardiovascular mortality, there was no relevant association overall. In these patients, the impact of 25(OH)D levels on clinical events was modified by PTH status, with low 25(OH)D levels meaningfully affecting outcomes only in patients with PTH levels above the median of 123 pmol/L.

29.5.3.3 Nutritional Vitamin D Supplementation Effects on Non-classical Actions of Vitamin D

Nutritional Vitamin D supplementation and cardiovascular risk and infection reduction in the general population.

Very few studies have been conducted to evaluate vitamin D supplementation on risk of cardiovascular mortality. Two studies prospectively examined vitamin D supplementation on cardiovascular mortality. In the WHI, women randomized to vitamin D 400 IU daily and 1,000 mg of calcium had no difference in all cause or cardiovascular mortality [50]. In a European study by Trivedi et al. elderly individuals receiving a daily equivalent dose of 800 IU of vitamin D did not have improved cardiovascular survival compared to controls [51].

Wang et al. [52] assess whether vitamin D and calcium supplements reduce the risk for cardiovascular events in adults. They selected 17 prospective studies and randomized trials that examined vitamin D supplementation, calcium supplementation, or both and subsequent cardiovascular events. Results of secondary analyses in eight randomized trials showed a slight but statistically non-significant reduction in CVD risk (pooled relative risk, 0.90 [95 % CI, 0.77–1.05]) with vitamin D supplementation at moderate to high doses (approximately 1,000 IU/day) but not with calcium supplementation (pooled relative risk, 1.14 [CI, 0.92–1.41]), or a combination of vitamin D and calcium supplementation (pooled relative risk, 1.04 [CI, 0.92–1.18]) compared with placebo.

In a recent systematic review of vitamin D on cardiometabolic outcomes Pittas et al. [53] analyzed four trials on the effect of vitamin D supplementation on incident cardiovascular disease. None reported a statistically significant effect of vitamin D supplementation on various cardiovascular outcomes, including myocardial infarction, stroke and other cardiac and cerebrovascular outcomes.

Enhancing immunity represents another relevant and promising target for vitamin D therapy. Despite encouraging observational data and clear biological rationale, recent interventional studies have been less encouraging.

One study of 322 obese individuals who received either 40,000 or 20,000 IU of cholecalciferol weekly or placebo over a year found no association between 25(OH)D and inflammatory markers (such as IL-6 and TNF-α), even after combining the low and high-dose cholecalciferol groups [54]. Similarly, in the Vitamin D and Acute Respiratory Infection Study (VIDARIS) in New Zealand, high dose monthly cholecalciferol therapy failed to prevent the development of upper respiratory tract infections, or affect missed work days, duration of symptoms, or severity of illness [55].

29.5.3.4 Nutritional Vitamin D Supplementation and Cardiovascular Risk and Infection Reduction in CKD Patients

Although several interventional studies with nutritional vitamin D supplementation (with cholecalciferol or ergocalciferol) have been performed in CKD patients, none of them have analyzed CV risk and mortality [56–58]. As we mention previously a recent systematic review and meta-analysis of observational studies and randomized controlled trials (RCT) on Vitamin D supplementation in chronic kidney disease performed by Kandula et al. included 22 studies, 17 observational and 5 RCTs. There was a significant improvement in 25-hydroxyvitamin D and an associated decline in serum PTH levels among observational studies [34]. PTH reduction was higher in dialysis patients. Among RCTs, there was a significant improvement in 25-hydroxyvitamin D and an associated decline with a low incidence of hypercalcemia and hyperphosphatemia. As with skeletal effects of vitamin D supplementation no cardiovascular and infectious outcomes were studied.

With respect to infection reduction in CKD with vitamin D supplementation, The Dialysis Infection and Vitamin D In New England study (DIVINE; NCT00892099) is randomizing 120 incident hemodialysis patients to one of two ergocalciferol arms (60,000 IU weekly or 50,000 IU monthly) or to placebo over 12 weeks and following the response in serum 25(OH)D levels. Secondary outcomes include hospitalizations, changes in cytokines and immunologically active proteins such as cathelicidin [59].

29.6 Active Vitamin D

29.6.1 Active Vitamin D Administration Effects on Mineral and Skeletal Outcomes in CKD

Multiple randomized trials have been conducted to examine the role of active vitamin compounds in CKD and ESRD. Many of these trials were not specifically designed to evaluate patient centered skeletal outcomes and had multiple methodological limitations including small sample size and short duration of follow-up. Several trials have shown that intravenous calcitriol is an effective therapy for the reduction of serum PTH levels in long term studies [60, 61]. Despite this, very few studies have shown that this treatment reverses biopsy proven bone lesions as osteitis fibrosa in hemodialysis patients [62] (Table 29.2).

Palmer et al. [63] examined the evidence from randomized controlled trials regarding the efficacy of vitamin D compounds in CKD and ESRD patients. These investigators conducted a comprehensive literature search and included trials that investigated different vitamin D compounds including calcitriol, alfacalcidol, doxercalciferol, maxacalcitol, paricalcitol and falecalcitriol. They noted significant variation in PTH lowering effects of vitamin D compounds with newer active vitamin D compounds (doxercalciferol, maxacalcitol, paricalcitol and falecalcitriol) significantly lowering PTH compared with placebo [64–66] but no significant PTH reduction was noted with established vitamin D compounds such as calcitriol, alfacalcidol [67–72]. The more recently developed vitamin D analogues were associated with hypercalcemia (relative risk, but not hyperphosphatemia, with significant reductions in PTH serum levels. For suppression of PTH, intravenous administration was superior to oral vitamin D, but higher intravenous doses were used. In terms of

Table 29.2 Studies evaluating activated vitamin D and skeletal outcomes in CKD patients

Study	N	Examined treatments	Type of population	Results
Memmos et al. [67]	57	Oral calcitriol (0.25–0.5 µg) vs no treatment	Prevalent HD	Prevented the development of radiological erosions or reversed minimal erosions
Przedlacki et al. [72]	13	Oral calcitriol (0.25 µg) vs no treatment	CKD stage 4–5 not on dialysis	Increase in bone mineral density in the calcitriol group in femoral neck and lumbar spine
Hamdy et al. [73]	176	Alfacalcidol 0.25–1 µg	CKD stage 3–4	Histological indices of bone turnover significantly improved in patients given alfacalcidol vs controls
Baker et al. [74]	75	Oral calcitriol (0.25 µg) vs no treatment	Prevalent HD without biochemical or radiological evidence of bone disease	Calcitriol delays and may prevent the development of osteitis fibrosa
Andress et al. [62]	12	IV calcitriol (1.0–2.5 µg three times weekly)	Prevalent HD with refractory SHPT	Effective in ameliorating osteitis fibrosa

patient-level skeletal outcomes such as fractures, bone pain, requirement of surgical parathyroidectomy, no benefit was noted from the administration of vitamin D compounds [73–76] Table 29.2. However, most studies had inadequate power and insufficient follow-up to appropriately ascertain these outcomes. A more recent meta-analysis focused on paricalcitol in stage 2–5 CKD patients, confirmed that paricalcitol can effectively suppress PTH but did not address any patient-level outcomes [77].

In the recently published EVOLVE study with cinacalcet; the comparative arm was standard of care, namely vitamin D analogs. The calcimimetic arm achieved lower levels of serum calcium compared with standard care (median level 9.8 mgdl/1 vs 9.2 mgdl/1 at 4 months) [78]. Although there were no differences between the two arms in fractures (13 % vs 12 %), the incidence of parathyroidectomy was significantly lower in cinacalcet arm (7 % vs 14 %).

29.6.2 *Active Vitamin D Administration Effects on Non-classical Vitamin D Outcomes*

Mineral and bone disorders (MBD) are early and common complications of CKD, and progress as glomerular filtration rate declines. Kidney Disease: Improving Global Outcomes has defined chronic kidney disease-mineral and bone disorder (CKD-MBD) as a systemic syndrome characterized by: (1) abnormalities in serum calcium, phosphorus and PTH concentration and vitamin D metabolism, (2) abnormalities in bone turnover, but also in bone mass, quality and mineralization; and finally the presence of vascular calcifications [79]. This syndrome is common among CKD patients and has been associated with an increased risk of cardiovascular risk and mortality [80]. Multiple factors contribute to the development and maintenance of CKD-MBD, but principally involve phosphate retention and vitamin D metabolism abnormalities. As the lack of active vitamin D (calcitriol) is the principal vitamin D abnormality, great impetus has been given to explore if administration of active vitamin D derivatives can decrease cardiovascular and infectious complications in dialysis patients and increase survival.

29.6.2.1   Oral Calcitriol and Survival in CKD Patients

Three papers have shown that oral calcitriol even in low doses (less than 1 mcg) reduce overall and cardiovascular mortality in predialysis and hemodialyzed patients (Table 29.3). Kovesdy et al. [81] examined the association of oral calcitriol treatment with mortality and the incidence of dialysis in 520 old male US veterans with CKD stages 3–5 and not yet receiving dialysis with an estimated glomerular filtration rate of 30.8 ml/min. Associations were adjusted for age, race, and comorbidities. Two hundred fifty-eight of 520 subjects received treatment with calcitriol, 0.25–0.5 ucg/day, for a median duration of 2.1 years (range, 0.06–6.0 years). The incidence rate ratios for mortality and combined death and dialysis initiation were significantly lower in treated with oral calcitriol versus the untreated patients (p<0.001 for both in the fully adjusted models). A similar study evaluated associations of oral calcitriol use with mortality and dialysis dependence in 1,418 non-dialysis patients with CKD and hyperparathyroidism [82]. The authors abstracted the data from the Northwest Veterans' Affairs Consumer Health Information and Performance Sets (CHIPS) database. They focus on calcitriol as this medication is commonly prescribed in CKD and could be accurately ascertained from pharmacy records. Incident calcitriol users and nonusers were selected on the basis of stages 3–4 CKD, hyperparathyroidism, and the absence of hypercalcemia before calcitriol use and then were matched by age and estimated kidney function. During a median follow-up of 1.9 years, 408 (29%) patients died and 217 (16%) initiated long-term dialysis. After adjustment for demographics, comorbidities, estimated renal function, medications, and baseline levels of PTH, calcium, and phosphorous, oral calcitriol use was associated with a 26% lower risk for death (95% confidence interval 5–42% lower; p=0.016) and a 20% lower risk for death or dialysis (95% confidence interval 1–35% lower; p=0.038). The association of calcitriol with improved survival was not statistically different across baseline parathyroid hormone levels. The use of calcitriol was associated with a greater risk for hypercalcemia. The primary limitation of this study was the potential for confounding by indication, although the authors used a number of techniques to address this problem.

Table 29.3 Observational studies examining all cause and cardiovascular associated with treatment with activated vitamin D vs no treatment in CKD patients

Study	N	Examined treatments	Type of population	Results
Kovesdy et al. [81]	520	Oral calcitriol vs no treatment	CKD stage 2–5 not on dialysis	Lower all-cause mortality; trend to lower ESRF
Shoben et al. [82]	1,418	Oral calcitriol vs no treatment	CKD stage 3–4 with SHPT	26 % lower risk of death; 20 % lower risk of death or dialysis
Naves-Diaz et al. [83]	7,203 vs 8,801	Oral active vitamin D (calcitriol) vs no treatment	Prevalent HD CORES database	Lower all-cause mortality risk
Shoji et al. [84]	242	Oral alfa calcidiol vs no treatment	Prevalent HD	Lower CV similar all-cause mortality
Ogawa et al. [85]	190	Oral alfa calcidiol vs no treatment	Prevalent HD	Lower all-cause and CV mortality
Teng et al. [91]	51,037	Any activated IV vitamin D vs no treatment	Prevalent HD from single non-profit Dialysis chain	20 % lower all-cause mortality
Tentori et al. [92]	7,731	Any activated IV vitamin D vs no treatment	Prevalent HD from single non-profit Dialysis chain	Lower all-cause mortality

Finally, a recent paper addressed the use of oral calcitriol use on the survival of hemodialysis patients [83]. The authors determined the survival benefit of oral active vitamin D in hemodialysis patients from six Latin America countries (FME Register(R) as part of the CORES study) followed for a median of 16 months. Time-dependent Cox regression models, after adjustment for potential confounders, showed that the 7,203 patients who received oral active vitamin D had significant reductions in overall, cardiovascular, infectious and neoplastic mortality compared to the 8,801 patients that had not received vitamin D. Stratified analyses found a survival advantage in the group that had received oral active vitamin D in 36 of the 37 strata studied including that with the highest levels of serum calcium, phosphorus and PTH (Table 29.3). Here Multivariable adjusted analyses revealed that patients who received oral active vitamin D had a significant 45 % (HR 0.55; 95 % CI 0.49–0.63) lower mortality risk compared to patients who did not receive oral active vitamin D. Reductions in mortality risk were similar for cardiovascular, infectious, and neoplastic causes. The survival benefit of oral active vitamin D was seen in those patients receiving mean daily doses of less than 1 mcg with the highest reduction associated with the lowest dose (<0.25 mcg). The reduction in mortality risk was seen even in the lowest PTH tertile, where a tendency to a higher mortality has been described. Survival benefit was also seen in patients with high serum phosphorus levels, in which mortality have been shown to be higher. Survival results were consistent in all centers and across countries despite the differences in mortality rates among them. As in the previous study, the risk of confounding by indication cannot be ruled out.

29.6.2.2   Effect of Other Oral Active Vitamin D Analogues on Survival and Cardiovascular Outcomes in CKD Patients

Although alfacalcidol has been used extensively in Europe and Japan, there has been few communications of survival in hemodialysis using oral active vitamin D compounds. Shoji et al. [84] found in a small hemodialysis population that patients on a low-dose oral alfacalcidol had a significantly lower risk for cardiovascular death than those without vitamin D supplementation. More recently Ogawa et al. [85] collected demographic and clinical baseline data from 190 prevalent HD patients in a regional Japanese cohort. A 5-year survival analysis was performed according to whether the patients were receiving calcitriol analog therapy. Alfacalcidol therapy at a mean dose of 5.2 ± 1.8 μg/week was performed in 89 (46.8 %) of the 190 patients. Most patients took oral alfacacidol at a dose not higher than 1 ug per day. They recorded deaths and cardiovascular events during the follow-up period. A Kaplan-Meier analysis demonstrated that the alfacalcidol users had a significantly lower rate of all-cause mortality and cardiovascular mortality than the non-users.

Few studies have been performed with Doxercalciferol (1 alfa hydroxi D2) in predialysis patients for the control of secondary hyperparathyroidism, but without evidence on its effects on survival [64, 86]. The same has happened with oral paricalcitol, which have shown to produce reduction in albuminuria in patients with type 2 diabetes [87, 88]. With this agent two studies have tried to analyze its effects on cardiac structure and function. In the PRIMO study, 196 patients with chronic kidney disease (GFR 15–60 mL/min), mild to moderate left ventricular hypertrophy, and preserved ejection fraction were randomly assigned to 2 μg of oral paricalcitol or matching placebo for 48 weeks [89]. Over the study period, there was a significant decrease in left auricular volume although not in left ventricular mass in the paricalcitol group compared with the placebo group. Paricalcitol also attenuated the rise in levels of brain natriuretic. The OPERA trial [90] was a prospective, double-blind, randomized, placebo-controlled trial that tried to determine whether oral paricalcitol (1 μg) for 52 weeks could reduce left ventricular mass compared to placebo in patients with stages 3–5 CKD with LV hypertrophy. Change in LV mass index did not differ significantly between groups.

29.6.2.3   Effect of Parenteral Active Vitamin D Analogues on Survival and Cardiovascular Outcomes in CKD Patients

Parenteral vitamin D has been associated with improved survival among long-term hemodialyzed patients. In a retrospective study, patients who received injectable vitamin D (either calcitriol or paricalcitol) had a 20–25 % higher survival rate than those that did not received injectable vitamin D over the same period of time [91]. All-cause mortality, as well as cardiovascular mortality was less in the group receiving injectable vitamin D after adjusting for potential confounders. In another study Tentori et al. assessed mortality associated with different vitamin D analogs and with the lack of vitamin D therapy in patients who began HD [92]. In unadjusted models, mortality was lower in patients on doxercalciferol and paricalcitol versus calcitriol, but in adjusted models, this difference was not statistically significant. In all models mortality was higher for patients who did not receive vitamin D versus those who did.

29.7   Nutritional Vitamin D: Optimal Levels, Required Supplementation Dose and Toxicity

There has been a move to alter the definition of vitamin D sufficiency in the general population, so that it is no longer simply a 25(OH)D level that avoids rickets. This has led to a progressive rise in the minimum recommended level of 25(OH)D to 30 ng/ml or above to optimize bone density, falls prevention, calcium absorption, and PTH suppression. Applying this cut-off value to hemodialysis patients, the prevalence of vitamin D deficiency in very high, ranging from 50 to 98 % [49]. Deficiency appears to be both more severe and more common in peritoneal dialysis [93]. The K/DOQI and KDIGO guidelines have recommended testing for vitamin D insufficiency and deficiency in patients with CKD using the cut-off value of the general population, although there is no consensus on the definition of vitamin D insufficiency in CKD.

There are conflicting estimates for the dose necessary to achieve 25(OH)D level of 30 ng/ml (75 nmol/l) in hemodialysis patients. Published data use a variety of dosing intervals; however, Cholecalciferol given monthly at an oral dose of 100,000 IU during a 15-month period is usually sufficient to raise levels over 30 ng/ml in around 90 % of the patients without any evident mineral metabolism toxicity [94]. Saab et al. [95] have given ergocalciferol oral supplementation at 50,000 IU monthly to hemodialysis patients during for 6 months increasing 25(OH)D >30 ng/ml in 95 % of the patients, having none >100 ng/ml. In our own study we have found similar results with higher initial doses of ergocalciferol but lower maintenance doses [96].

Except in patients with autonomous 1α-hydroxylase activity, there are no compelling reports of vitamin D toxicity at 25(OH)D levels consistent with sun exposure alone (<111 ng/ml) or at doses in of vitamin D up to 10,000 U/day [97]. These doses generally result in serum 25(OH)D levels remaining below approximately 88 ng/ml (220 mmol/l) [98]. At this serum level 25(OH)D does not have a direct effect on gut calcium absorption [99] and hence should not by itself, be capable of causing hypercalcemia. At levels over approximately 120 ng/ml (300 mmol/l), 25(OH)D does directly affect calcium absorption [99]. Theoretically, toxicity could still occur at lower 25(OH)D if they result in an increase in free or total $1,25(OH)_2$ D levels. This is less probable because 24-hydroxylation degradation pathways are induced by $1,25(OH)_2D$ and FGF23 [100–102]. So any rise in free or total $1,25(OH)_2D$ would lead to an acceleration in the rate of degradation for both 25(OH)D and $1,25(OH)_2D$. As we said before, high levels 25(OH)D stimulate the vitamin D receptor [99], and the higher levels by itself would lead to protective acceleration of degradation. This could explain the trend toward a smaller relative increment in serum 25(OH)D when higher doses of vitamin D are given [103]. FGF23 levels tend to be high in dialysis patients. It has been postulated that FGF23 levels could stimulate 24-hydroxylase activity and explain in part very high prevalence of low 25(OH)D and 1,25(OH)$_2$D levels in dialysis patients. It has been recently shown that patients with CKD exhibit an decrease ability to increase serum 24,25(OH)$_2$D3 after cholecalciferol therapy, suggesting decreased 24-hydroxylase activity in CKD [104]. The observed relationship between baseline FGF23 and increments in 24,25(OH)$_2$D3 further refutes the idea that FGF23 directly contributes to 25(OH)D insufficiency in CKD through stimulation of 24-hydroxylase activity.

29.8 Conclusions

In addition to the endocrine effects of the vitamin D axis on bone and mineral metabolism, studies have demonstrated there is also extrarenal conversion of 25(OH) vitamin D to 1,25(OH)$_2$ vitamin D in multiple cells leading to autocrine effects. This advance has led to the speculation that CKD patients may also need to be supplemented with nutritional vitamin D (ergocalciferol or cholecalciferol). Unfortunately, to date, the majority of interventional studies have focused on biochemical end points. There are no randomized controlled trials demonstrating that therapy with any formulation of vitamin D results in improved patient level outcomes. Despite the physiologic importance of vitamin D in health and disease, more research is required to determine which vitamin D derivative is required for optimal health in CKD patients. Observational studies or even clinical trials in populations different from the one we are studying may not clearly inform the practicing physician of the correct treatment. Examples of this are hormone replacement therapy in women or statin use in dialysis patients. The real gold standard for clinical decision-making come from randomized clinical trials, conducted in the population we want to treat and with clinically meaningful end points. Unfortunately, this level of evidence does not exist for vitamin D therapy in CKD. There are no randomized controlled trials demonstrating that therapy with any formulation of vitamin D results in improved patient level outcomes. Without randomized clinical trials, causation cannot be inferred from observational studies. Because well designed clinical trials are expensive, evidence from animal studies, observational studies, and small pilot randomized trials with surrogate outcomes are needed to evaluate which therapies have the most potential for success to be tested in definitive clinical trials.

Multiple observational studies suggest an important role of vitamin D in patients with CKD and ESRD and potentially in the general population. There could be potentially different roles for nutritional and active vitamin D compounds, having nutritional vitamin D a preferred role in infections and cancer prevention, whereas active vitamin D compounds may play more of a role bone disease and mortality.

Both nutritional and active vitamin D, eventually activate the same vitamin D receptor; however, nutritional vitamin D has to undergo additional activation in other body sites distant from the kidney. Active vitamin D has been shown to decrease albuminuria, blood pressure, and eGFR in patients with diabetic kidney disease. There are current ongoing studies to test these outcomes with nutritional vitamin D compounds as well. It is important to mention that there are very few data about combining therapy with both nutritional and active vitamin D compounds; thus, caution should be used in clinical practice because of worry about possible vitamin D intoxication, manifested by hypercalcemia and possibly vascular calcifications.

Many questions remain unanswered. For example, do we need to measure 25(OH)D levels in all CKD patients, or can we replete knowing that of them most are deficient? Can we combine nutritional and active vitamin D or does this put patients at increased risk? Does vitamin D has to be replaced in renal transplant patients and does this affect graft function?

References

1. Dusso A, Lopez-Hilker S, Rapp N, Slatopolsky E. Extrarenal production of calcitriol in chronic renal failure. Kidney Int. 1988;34:368–75.
2. Weisman Y, Vargas A, Duckett G, Reiter E, Root AW. Synthesis of 1,25-dihydroxyvitamin D in the nephrectomized pregnant rat. Endocrinology. 1978;103:1992–6.
3. Holick MF. Vitamin D deficiency. N Engl J Med. 2007;357(3):266–81.
4. Raiszrummel CL, Holick MF. DeLucaHF:1,25dihydroxycholecalciferol: a potent stimulator of bone resorption in tissue culture. Science. 1972;175:768–9.
5. Brumbaugh PF, Haussler MR. 1 alpha,25-dihydroxycholecalciferol receptors in intestine. I. Association of 1 alpha,25-dihydroxycholecalciferol with intestinal mucosa chromatin. J Biol Chem. 1974;249:1251–7.
6. Bhan I, Powe CE, Berg AH, et al. Bioavailable vitamin D is more tightly linked to mineral metabolism than total vitamin D in incident hemodialysis patients. Kidney Int. 2012;82:84–9.
7. Rowling MJ, Kemmis CM, Taffany DA, Welsh J. Megalin-mediated endocytosis of vitamin D binding protein correlates with 25-hydroxycholecalciferol actions in human mammary cells. J Nutr. 2006;136(11):2754–9.
8. Pike JW, Zella LA, Meyer MB, Fretz JA, Kim S. Molecular actions of 1,25-dihydroxyvitamin D3 on genes involved in calcium homeostasis. J Bone Miner Res. 2007;22 Suppl 2:V16–9.
9. Recker R, Schenfeld P, Letteri J, Slatopolsky E, Goldsmith R, Brickman A. The efficacy of calcifediol in renal osteodystrophy. Arch Intern Med. 1978;138:857–63.
10. Memmos DE, Eastwood JB, Harris E, O'Grady A, de Wardener HE. Response of uremic osteoid to vitamin D. Kidney Int Suppl. 1982;11:S50–4.
11. Maxwell DR, Benjamin DM, Donahay SL, Allen MK, Hamburger RJ, Luft FC. Calcitriol in dialysis patients. Clin Pharmacol Ther. 1978;23(5):515–9.
12. Berl T, Berns AS, Hufer WE, Hammill K, Alfrey AC, Arnaud CD, Schrier RW. 1,25 dihydroxycholecalciferol effects in chronic dialysis. A double-blind controlled study. Ann Intern Med. 1978;88(6):774–80.
13. Gonzalez EA, Sachdeva A, Oliver DA, Martin KJ. Vitamin D insufficiency and deficiency in chronic kidney disease. A single center observational study. Am J Nephrol. 2004;24(5):503–10.
14. Bhan I, Burnett-Bowie SA, Ye J, Tonelli M, Thadhani R. Clinical measures identify vitamin D deficiency in dialysis. Clin J Am Soc Nephrol. 2010;5:460–7.

15. Koenig KG, Lindberg JS, Zerwekh JE, Padalino PK, Cushner HM, Copley JB. Free and total 1,25-dihydroxyvitamin D levels in subjects with renal disease. Kidney Int. 1992;41:161–5.

16. Jacob AI, Sallman A, Santiz Z, Hollis BW. Defective photoproduction of cholecalciferol in normal and uremic humans. J Nutr. 1984;114:1313–9.

17. Del Valle E, Negri AL, Aguirre C, Fradinger E, Zanchetta JR. Prevalence of 25(OH) vitamin D insufficiency and deficiency in chronic kidney disease stage 5 patients on hemodialysis. Hemodial Int. 2007;11(3):315–21.

18. Holick MF. Sunlight and vitamin D for bone health and prevention of autoimmune diseases, cancers and cardiovascular disease. Am J Clin Nutr. 2004;80:1678S–88.

19. Li YC, Kong J, Wei M, Chen S, Cao LP, Qiao G, Zheng W, Liu W, Li X, Gardner DG, Li YC. Cardiac hypertrophy in vitamin D receptor knockout mice: role of the systemic and the cardiac renin-angiotensin systems. Am J Physiol Endocrinol Metab. 2005;288:E125–32.

20. Li YC, Kong J, Wei M, Chen ZF, Liu SQ, Cao LP. 1,25Dihydroxyvitamin D83) is a negative regulator of the renin-angiotensin system. J Clin Invest. 2002;110:229–38.

21. Liu PT, Stenger S, Li H, Wenzel L, Tan BH, Krutzik SR, Ochoa MT, Schauber J, Wu K, Meinken C, Kamen DL, Wagner M, Bals R, Steinmeyer A, Zügel U, Gallo RL, Eisenberg D, Hewison M, Hollis BW, Adams JS, Bloom BR, Modlin RL. Toll-like receptor triggering of a vitamin D-mediated human antimicrobial response. Science. 2006;311 (5768):1770–3.

22. Zehnder D, Bland R, Chana RS, Wheeler DC, Howie AJ, Williams MC, Stewart PM, Hewison M. Synthesis of 1,25-dihydroxyvitamin D(3) by human endothelial cells is regulated by inflammatory cytokines: a novel autocrine determinant of vascular cell adhesion. J Am Soc Nephrol. 2002;13(3):621–9.

23. Segersten U, Correa P, Hewison M, Hellman P, Dralle H, Carling T, Akerström G, Westin G. 25-hydroxyvitamin D(3)-1alpha-hydroxylase expression in normal and pathological parathyroid glands. J Clin Endocrinol Metab. 2002;87(6):2967–72.

24. Somjen D, Weisman Y, Kohen F, Gayer B, Limor R, Sharon O, Jaccard N, Knoll E, Stern N. 25-hydroxyvitamin D3-1alpha-hydroxylase is expressed in human vascular smooth muscle cells and is upregulated by parathyroid hormone and estrogenic compounds. Circulation. 2005;111(13):1666–71.

25. London GM, Guerin AP, Verbeke FH, Pannier B, Boutouyrie P, Marchais SJ, et al. Mineral metabolism and arterial functions in end-stage renal disease: potential role of 25-hydroxyvitamin D deficiency. J Am Soc Nephrol. 2007;18:613–20.

26. Mendel CM. The free hormone hypothesis: a physiologically based mathematical model. Endocr Rev. 1989;10:232–74.

27. Coen G, Mantella D, Manni M, Balducci A, Nofroni I, Sardella D, et al. 25-hydroxyvitamin D levels and bone histomorphometry in hemodialysis renal osteodystrophy. Kidney Int. 2005;68:1840–8.

28. Ambrus C, Almasi C, Berta K, Deak G, Marton A, Molnar MZ, Nemeth Z, Horvath C, Lakatos P, Szathmari M, Mucsi I. Vitamin D insufficiency and bone fractures in patients on maintenance hemodialysis. Int Urol Nephrol. 2011;43(2):475–82.

29. Mucsi I, Almasi C, Deak G, Marton A, Ambrus C, Berta K, et al. Serum 25(OH)-vitamin D levels and bone metabolism in patients on maintenance hemodialysis. Clin Nephrol. 2005;64:288–94.

30. Ghazali A, Fardellone P, Pruna A, Atik A, Achard JM, Oprisiu R, et al. Is low plasma 25-(OH) vitamin D a major risk factor for hyperparathyroidism and Looser's zones independent of calcitriol? Kidney Int. 1999;55:2169–77.

31. Elder GJ, Mackun K. 25-hydroxyvitamin D deficiency and diabetes predict reduced BMD in patients with chronic kidney disease. J Bone Miner Res. 2006;21:1778–84.

32. Stanbury SW. Azotaemic renal osteodystrophy. Br Med Bull. 1957;13:57–60.

33. Fournier A, Bordier P, Gueris J, Sebert JL, Marie P, Ferriere C, et al. Comparison of 1 alpha-hydroxycholecalciferol and 25-hydroxycholecalciferol in the treatment of renal osteodystrophy: greater effect of 25-hydroxycholecalciferol on bone mineralization. Kidney Int. 1979;15:196–204.

34. Kandula P, Dobre M, Schold JD, Schreiber Jr MJ, Mehrotra R, Navaneethan SD. Vitamin D supplementation in chronic kidney disease: a systematic review and meta-analysis of observational studies and randomized controlled trials. Clin J Am Soc Nephrol. 2011;6(1):50–62.
35. Kendrick J, Targher G, Smits G, Chonchol M. 25-hydroxyvitamin D deficiency is independently associated with cardiovascular disease in the Third National Health and Nutrition Examination Survey. Atherosclerosis. 2009;205(1):255–60.
36. Martins D, Wolf M, Pan D, Zadshir A, Tareen N, Thadhani R, Felsenfeld A, Levine B, Mehrotra R, Norris K. Prevalence of cardiovascular risk factors and the serum levels of 25-hydroxyvitamin D in the United States: data from the Third National Health and Nutrition Examination Survey. Arch Intern Med. 2007;167(11):1159–65.
37. Scragg R, Sowers M, Bell C. Serum 25-hydroxyvitamin D, ethnicity, and blood pressure in the Third National Health and Nutrition Examination Survey. Am J Hypertens. 2007;20(7):713–9.
38. Kim DH, Sabour S, Sagar UN, Adams S, Whellan DJ. Prevalence of hypovitaminosis D in cardiovascular diseases (from the National Health and Nutrition Examination Survey 2001 to 2004). Am J Cardiol. 2008;102(11):1540–4.
39. Melamed ML, Muntner P, Michos ED, Uribarri J, Weber C, Sharma J, Raggi P. Serum 25-hydroxyvitamin D levels and the prevalence of peripheral arterial disease: results from NHANES 2001 to 2004. Arterioscler Thromb Vasc Biol. 2008;28(6):1179–85.
40. Judd SE, Nanes MS, Ziegler TR, Wilson PW, Tangpricha V. Optimal vitamin D status attenuates the age-associated increase in systolic blood pressure in white Americans: results from the third National Health and Nutrition Examination Survey. Am J Clin Nutr. 2008;87(1):136–41.
41. Melamed ML, Michos ED, Post W, Astor B. 25-hydroxyvitamin D levels and the risk of mortality in the general population. Arch Intern Med. 2008;168(15):1629–37.
42. Giovannucci E, Liu Y, Hollis BW, Rimm EB. 25-hydroxyvitamin D and risk of myocardial infarction in men: a prospective study. Arch Intern Med. 2008;168(11):1174–80.
43. Wang TJ, Pencina MJ, Booth SL, Jacques PF, Ingelsson E, Lanier K, Benjamin EJ, D'Agostino RB, Wolf M, Vasan RS. Vitamin D deficiency and risk of cardiovascular disease. Circulation. 2008;117(4):503–11.
44. Pilz S, März W, Wellnitz B, Seelhorst U, Fahrleitner-Pammer A, Dimai HP, Boehm BO, Dobnig H. Association of vitamin D deficiency with heart failure and sudden cardiac death in a large cross-sectional study of patients referred for coronary angiography. J Clin Endocrinol Metab. 2008;93(10):3927–35.
45. Pilz S, Dobnig H, Fischer JE, Boehm BO, März W. Low vitamin D levels predict stroke in patients referred to coronary angiography. Stroke. 2008;39:2611–3.
46. Dobnig H, Pilz S, Scharnagl H, Renner W, Seelhorst U, Wellnitz B, Kinkeldei J, Boehm BO, Weihrauch G, Maerz W. Independent association of low serum 25-hydroxyvitamin d and 1,25-dihydroxyvitamin d levels with all-cause and cardiovascular mortality. Arch Intern Med. 2008;168(12):1340–9.
47. Pilz S, Tomaschitz A, Friedl C, Amrein K, Drechsler C, Ritz E, Boehm BO, Grammer TB, März W. Vitamin D status and mortality in chronic kidney disease. Nephrol Dial Transplant. 2011;26(11):3603–9.
48. Barreto DV, Barreto FC, Liabeuf S, Temmar M, Boitte F, Choukroun G, Fournier A, Massy ZA. Vitamin D affects survival independently of vascular calcification in chronic kidney disease. Clin J Am Soc Nephrol. 2009;4(6):1128–35.
49. Drechsler C, Verduijn M, Pilz S, Dekker FW, Krediet RT, Ritz E, Wanner C, Boeschoten EW, Brandenburg V, NECOSAD Study Group. Vitamin D status and clinical outcomes in incident dialysis patients: results from the NECOSAD study. Nephrol Dial Transplant. 2011;26(3):1024–32.
50. Lacroix AZ, Kotchen J, Anderson G, Brzyski R, Cauley JA, Cummings SR, Gass M, Johnson KC, Ko M, Larson J, Manson JE, Stefanick ML, Wactawski-Wende J. Calcium plus vitamin D supplementation and mortality in postmenopausal women: the women's health initiative calcium-vitamin D randomized controlled trial. J Gerontol A Biol Sci Med Sci. 2009;64(5):559–67.

51. Trivedi DP, Doll R, Khaw KT. Effect of four monthly oral vitamin D3 (cholecalciferol) supplementation on fractures and mortality in men and women living in the community: randomized double blind controlled trial. BMJ. 2003;326(7387):469.
52. Wang L, Manson JE, Song Y, Sesso HD. Systematic review: vitamin D and calcium supplementation in prevention of cardiovascular events. Ann Intern Med. 2010;152(5):315–23.
53. Pittas AG, Chung M, Trikalinos T, Mitri J, Brendel M, Patel K, Lichtenstein AH, Lau J, Balk EM. Systematic review: vitamin D and cardiometabolic outcomes. Ann Intern Med. 2010;152(5):307–14.
54. Beilfuss J, Berg V, Sneve M, et al. Effects of a 1-year supplementation with cholecalciferol on interleukin-6, tumor necrosis factor-alpha and insulin resistance in overweight and obese subjects. Cytokine. 2012;60:870–4.
55. Murdoch DR, Slow S, Chambers ST, et al. Effect of vitamin D3 supplementation on upper respiratory tract infections in healthy adults: the VIDARIS randomized controlled trial. JAMA. 2012;308:7.
56. Alvarez JA, Law J, Coakley KE, et al. High-dose cholecalciferol reduces parathyroid hormone in patients with early chronic kidney disease: a pilot, randomized, double-blind, placebo controlled trial. Am J Clin Nutr. 2012;96:672–9.
57. Hewitt NA, O'Connor AA, O'Shaughnessy DV, et al. Effects of cholecalciferol on functional, biochemical, vascular, and quality of life outcomes in hemodialysis patients. Clin J Am Soc Nephrol. 2013;8:1143–9.
58. Marckmann P, Agerskov H, Thineshkumar S, et al. Randomized controlled trial of cholecalciferol supplementation in chronic kidney disease patients with hypovitaminosis D. Nephrol Dial Transplant. 2012;27:3523–31.
59. Bhan I, Tamez H, Thadhani R. Impact of new vitamin D data on future studies and treatment. Curr Opin Nephrol Hypertens. 2013;22(4):377–82.
60. Rodriguez M, Felsenfeld AJ, Williams C, Pederson JA, Llach F. The effect of long-term intravenous calcitriol administration on parathyroid function in hemodialysis patients. J Am Soc Nephrol. 1991;2(5):1014–20.
61. Malberti F, Corradi B, Cosci P, Calliada F, Marcelli D, Imbasciati E. Long-term effects of intravenous calcitriol therapy on the control of secondary hyperparathyroidism. Am J Kidney Dis. 1996;28(5):704–12.
62. Andress DL, Norris KC, Coburn JW, Slatopolsky EA, Sherrard DJ. Intravenous calcitriol in the treatment of refractory osteitis fibrosa of chronic renal failure. N Engl J Med. 1989;321(5):274–9.
63. Palmer SC, McGregor DO, Macaskill P, Craig JC, Elder GJ, Strippoli GF. Meta-analysis: vitamin D compounds in chronic kidney disease. Ann Intern Med. 2007;147:840–53.
64. Coburn JW, Maung HM, Elangovan L, Germain MJ, Lindberg JS, Sprague SM, et al. Doxercalciferol safely suppresses PTH levels in patients with secondary hyperparathyroidism associated with chronic kidney disease stages 3 and 4. Am J Kidney Dis. 2004;43:877–90.
65. Martin KJ, Gonzalez EA, Gellens M, Hamm LL, Abboud H, Lindberg J. 19-Nor-1-alpha-25-dihydroxyvitamin D2 (Paricalcitol) safely and effectively reduces the levels of intact parathyroid hormone in patients on hemodialysis. J Am Soc Nephrol. 1998;9:1427–32.
66. Moe SM, Zekonis M, Harezlak J, Ambrosius WT, Gassensmith CM, Murphy CL, et al. A placebo controlled trial to evaluate immunomodulatory effects of paricalcitol. Am J Kidney Dis. 2001;38:792–802.
67. Memmos DE, Eastwood JB, Talner LB, Gower PE, Curtis JR, Phillips ME, et al. Double-blind trial of oral 1,25-dihydroxy vitamin D3 versus placebo in asymptomatic hyperparathyroidism in patients receiving maintenance haemodialysis. Br Med J (Clin Res Ed). 1981;282:1919–24.
68. Watson AR, Kooh SW, Tam CS, Reilly BJ, Balfe JW, Vieth R. Renal osteodystrophy in children on CAPD: a prospective trial of 1-alpha hydroxycholecalciferol therapy. Child Nephrol Urol. 1988;9:220–7.

69. Baker LR, Abrams L, Roe CJ, Faugere MC, Fanti P, Subayti Y, et al. 1,25(OH)2D3 administration in moderate renal failure: a prospective double-blind trial. Kidney Int. 1989;35:661–9.

70. Moriniere P, Fournier A, Leflon A, Herve M, Sebert JL, Gregoire I, et al. Comparison of 1 alpha-OH-vitamin D3 and high doses of calcium carbonate for the control of hyperparathyroidism and hyperaluminemia in patients on maintenance dialysis. Nephron. 1985;39:309–15.

71. Coen G, Mazzaferro S, Manni M, Fondi G, Perruzza I, Pasquali M, et al. No acceleration and possibly slower progression of renal failure during calcitriol treatment in predialysis chronic renal failure. Nephrol Dial Transplant. 1994;9:1520.

72. Przedlacki J, Manelius J, Huttunen K. Bone mineral density evaluated by dual-energy X-ray absorptiometry after one-year treatment with calcitriol started in the predialysis phase of chronic renal failure. Nephron. 1995;69:433–7.

73. Hamdy NA, Kanis JA, Beneton MN, Brown CB, Juttmann JR, Jordans JG, et al. Effect of alfacalcidol on natural course of renal bone disease in mild to moderate renal failure. BMJ. 1995;310:358–63.

74. Baker LR, Muir JW, Sharman VL, Abrams SM, Greenwood RN, Cattell WR, et al. Controlled trial of calcitriol in hemodialysis patients. Clin Nephrol. 1986;26:185–91.

75. Llach F, Keshav G, Goldblat MV, Lindberg JS, Sadler R, Delmez J, et al. Suppression of parathyroid hormone secretion in hemodialysis patients by a novel vitamin D analogue: 19-nor-1,25-dihydroxyvitamin D2. Am J Kidney Dis. 1998;32 Suppl 2:S48–54.

76. Delmez JA, Kelber J, Norwood KY, Giles KS, Slatopolsky E. A controlled trial of the early treatment of secondary hyperparathyroidism with calcitriol in hemodialysis patients. Clin Nephrol. 2000;54:301–8.

77. Cheng J, Zhang W, Zhang X, Li X, Chen J. Efficacy and safety of paricalcitol therapy for chronic kidney disease: a meta-analysis. Clin J Am Soc Nephrol. 2012;7:391–400.

78. Chertow GM, Block GA, Correa-Rotter R, Drueke TB, Floege J, Goodman WG, et al. Effect of cinacalcet on cardiovascular disease in patients undergoing dialysis. N Engl J Med. 2012;367:2482–94.

79. Kidney disease improving global outcomes (KDIGO) CKD-MBD work group. KDIGO clinical guidelines for the diagnosis, evaluation, prevention, and treatment of chronic kidney disease mineral and bone disorder (CKD-MBD). Kidney Int. 2009;113:S1–130.

80. Streja E, Wang HY, Lau WL, Molnar MZ, Kovesdy CP, Kalantar-Zadeh K, Park J. Mortality of combined serum phosphorus and parathyroid hormone concentrations and their changes over time in hemodialysis patients. Bone. 2014;61:201–7.

81. Kovedsdy CP, Ahmadzadeh S, Anderson JE, Kalantar-Zadeh K. Association of activated vitamin D treatment and mortality in chronic kidney disease. Arch Intern Med. 2008;168(4):397–403.

82. Shoben AB, Rudser KDD, de Boer IH, Young B, Kestenbaum B. Association of oral calcitriol with improved survival in nondialyzed CKD. J Am Soc Nephrol. 2008;19(8):1613–9.

83. Naves-Díaz M, Alvarez-Hernández D, Passlick-Deetjen J, Guinsburg A, Marelli C, Rodríguez-Puyol D, Cannata-Andía JB. Oral active vitamin D is associated with improved survival in hemodialysis patients. Kidney Int. 2008;74(8):1070–8.

84. Shoji T, Shinohara K, Kimoto E, Emoto M, Tahara M, Koyama H, Inaba M, Fukumoto S, Ishimura E, Miki T, Tabata T, Nishizawa Y. Lower risk for cardiovascular mortality in oral 1alpha-hydroxy vitamin D3 users in a haemodialysis population. Nephrol Dial Transplant. 2004;19(1):179–84.

85. Ogawa M, Ogawa T, Inoue T, Otsuka K, Nitta K. Effect of alfacalcidol therapy on the survival of chronic hemodialysis patients. Ther Apher Dial. 2012;16(3):248–53.

86. Frazao JM, Elangovan L, Maung HM, et al. Intermittent doxercalciferol (1alpha-hydroxyvitamin D(2)) therapy for secondary hyperparathyroidism. Am J Kidney Dis. 2000;36:550–61.

87. Coyne D, Acharya M, Qiu P, et al. Paricalcitol capsule for the treatment of secondary hyperparathyroidism in stages 3 and 4 CKD. Am J Kidney Dis. 2006;47:263–76.

88. de Zeeuw D, Agarwal R, Amdahl M, et al. Selective vitamin D receptor activation with pari-calcitol for reduction of albuminuria in patients with type 2 diabetes (VITAL study): a ran-domized controlled trial. Lancet. 2010;376:1543–51.
89. Thadhani R, Appelbaum E, Pritchett Y, et al. Vitamin D therapy and cardiac structure and function in patients with chronic kidney disease: the PRIMO randomized controlled trial. JAMA. 2012;307(7):674–84.
90. Wang AY, Fang F, Chan J, et al. Effect of paricalcitol on left ventricular mass and function in CKD—The OPERA trial. J Am Soc Nephrol. 2014;25:175–86.
91. Teng M, Wolf M, Amdahl, et al. Activated injectable vitamin D and hemodialysis survival: a historical cohort study. J Am Soc Nephrol. 2005;16:1115–25.
92. Tentori F, Hunt WC, Stidley CA, Rohrscheib MR, Bedrick EJ, Meyer KB, Johnson HK, Zager PG, Medical Directors of Dialysis Clinic Inc. Mortality risk among hemodialysis patients receiving different vitamin D analogs. Kidney Int. 2006;70(10):1858–65.
93. Wang AY, Lam CW, Sanderson JE, Wang M, Chan IH, Lui SF, Sea MM, Woo J. Serum 25-hydroxyvitamin D status and cardiovascular outcomes in chronic peritoneal dialysis patients: a 3-y prospective cohort study. Am J Clin Nutr. 2008;87(6):1631–8.
94. Jean G, Souberbielle JC, Chazot C. Monthly cholecalciferol administration in haemodialysis patients: a simple and efficient strategy for vitamin D supplementation. Nephrol Dial Transplant. 2009;24(12):3799–805.
95. Saab G, Young DO, Gincherman Y, Giles K, Norwood K, Coyne DW. Prevalence of vitamin D deficiency and the safety and effectiveness of monthly ergocalciferol in hemodialysis patients. Nephron Clin Pract. 2007;105(3):c132–8.
96. Del Valle E, Negri AL, Fradinger E, Canalis M, Bevione P, Curcelegui M, Bravo M, Puddu M, Marini A, Ryba J, Peri P, Rosa Diez G, Sintado L, Gottlieb E. Weekly high-dose ergocal-ciferol to correct vitamin D deficiency/insufficiency in hemodialysis patients: a pilot trial. Hemodial Int. 2015;19(1):60–5.
97. Vieth R, Chan PC, MacFarlane GD. Efficacy and safety of vitamin D3 intake exceeding the lowest observed adverse effect level. Am J Clin Nutr. 2001;73:288–94.
98. Vieth R. Vitamin D supplementation, 25-hydroxyvitamin D concentrations, and safety. Am J Clin Nutr. 1999;69(5):842–56.
99. Heaney RP, Barger-Lux MJ, Dowell MS, Chen TC, Holick MF. Calcium absorptive effects of vitamin D and its major metabolites. J Clin Endocrinol Metab. 1997;82(12):4111–6.
100. Zierold C, Darwish HM, DeLuca HF. Two vitamin D response elements function in the rat 1,25-dihydroxyvitamin D 24-hydroxylase promoter. J Biol Chem. 1995;270(4):1675–8.
101. Perwad F, Zhang MY, Tenenhouse HS, Portale AA. Fibroblast growth factor 23 impairs phos-phorus and vitamin D metabolism in vivo and suppresses 25-hydroxyvitamin D-1alpha-hydroxylase expression in vitro. Am J Physiol Renal Physiol. 2007;293(5):F1577–83.
102. Sakaki T, Sawada N, Komai K, Ahiozawa S, Yamada S, Yamamoto K, Ohyama Y, Inouye K. Dual metabolic pathway of 25-hydroxyvitamin D3 catalyzed by human CYP24. Eur J Biochem. 2000;267(20):6158–65.
103. Aloia JF, Patel M, Dimaano R, Li-Ng M, Talwar SA, Mikhail M, Pollack S, Yeh JK. Vitamin D intake to attain a desired serum 25-hydroxyvitamin D concentration. Am J Clin Nutr. 2008;87(6):1952–8.
104. Stubbs JR, Zhang S, Friedman PA, Nolin TD. Decreased conversion of 25-hydroxyvitamin D3 to 24,25-dihydroxyvitamin D3 following cholecalciferol therapy in patients with CKD. Clin J Am Soc Nephrol. 2014;9(11):1965–73.

Chapter 30
Use of New Vitamin D Analogs in Chronic Kidney Disease

Riccardo Floreani and Mario Cozzolino

Abstract Vitamin D is a common treatment against secondary hyperparathyroidism in renal patients. However, the rationale for the prescription of vitamin D sterols in chronic kidney disease (CKD) is rapidly increasing due to the coexistence of growing expectancies close to unsatisfactory evidences, such as the lack of randomized controlled trials (RCTs) proving the superiority of any vitamin D sterol against placebo on patient-centered outcomes, the scanty clinical data on head-to-head comparisons between the multiple vitamin D sterols currently available, the absence of RCTs confirming the crescent expectations on nutritional vitamin D pleiotropic effects even in CKD patients and the promising effects of vitamin D receptors activators (VDRA) against proteinuria and myocardial hypertrophy in diabetic CKD cohorts. The present chapter arguments these issues focusing on the opened questions that nephrologists should consider dealing with the prescription and the choice of a VDRA.

Keywords VDRA • Alfacalcidol • Doxercalciferol • Paricalcitol • Cinacalcet • Secondary hyperparathyroidism • Albuminuria • Left ventricular hypertrophy • Left atrial dimension • Bone histology • Bone mineral density • Kidney transplantation

30.1 Introduction

Secondary hyperparathyroidism (SHPT) is recognized as a major complication of chronic kidney disease (CKD). Over the past decades, nephrologists have been encouraged to effectively control PTH due to the reported worrisome consequences

R. Floreani, MD
Renal and Dialysis Unit, San Paulo Hospital, Milan, Italy
e-mail: Riccardo.Floreani@unimi.it

M. Cozzolino, MD, PhD, FERA (✉)
Renal Division, Department of Health Sciences, San Paolo Hospital, University of Milan, Milan, Italy
e-mail: mario.cozzolino@unimi.it

© Springer International Publishing Switzerland 2016   515
P.A. Ureña Torres et al. (eds.), *Vitamin D in Chronic Kidney Disease*,
DOI 10.1007/978-3-319-32507-1_30

of SHPT as pruritus, bone pain, severe bone demineralization, skeletal fractures, brown tumors, severe cardiac hypertrophy, and calciphylaxis. Although repeated observational data described an independent association between serum PTH levels and unfavorable outcomes in CKD stage 3–5 as well as in end-stage renal disease (ESRD) patients, no randomized controlled trial (RCT) has still proven that an active reduction of PTH values could improve patient-centered outcomes as hospitalizations, cardiovascular events (CVE), CKD progression, and survival. Furthermore, the optimal targets of PTH levels are still uncertain in CKD as well as in ESRD cohorts. Thus, Kidney Disease-Improving Global Outcomes (KDIGO) guidelines provide a low-grade suggestion to maintain serum PTH levels into the range of normality in CKD 3–5 and between two and nine times the upper limit of normal range in ESRD.

Active vitamin D receptor activators (VDRA) (Table 30.1) are one of the classic therapies suggested to achieve those PTH targets. Emerging evidence of several pleiotropic effects related to the activation of the vitamin D receptor (VDR) is transforming the original world of vitamin D into a more complex scenario and affecting the use of vitamin D sterols among nephrologists. Different forms of vitamin D analogs are currently available in several countries, but clinical data on head-to-head comparisons between them are still scanty. Nonetheless, promising data suggest some beneficial effects of vitamin D analogs on proteinuria, myocardial hypertrophy in diabetic CKD cohorts, inflammation, and cardio-renal syndromes. Nutritional vitamin D replenishment is also receiving a growing interest for its potential autocrine-paracrine effects even in CKD patients, although its use is still based on observational rather than RCT data.

Table 30.1 Vitamin D sterols currently available as medical treatments in nephrology field

	Nutritional vitamin D		VDRA	
		Hydroxylation required to activate VDR		Hydroxylation required to activate VDR
Vitamin D2 and its analogs	Ergocalciferol	25-hydroxylation and 1-hydroxylation	Paricalcitol 19-nor1,25(OH)$_2$D$_2$	–
			Doxercalciferol 1α(OH)D$_2$	25-hydroxylation
Vitamin D3 and its analogs	Cholecalciferol	25-hydroxylation and 1-hydroxylation	Calcitriol 1,25(OH)$_2$D$_3$	–
	Calcifediol	1-hydroxylation	Alfacalcidol 1α(OH) D$_3$	25-hydroxylation
			Oxacalcitriol 22oxa1,25(OH)$_2$D$_3$	–

All the VDRA reported in the table are considered analogs with the exception of calcitriol, which corresponds to the natural form of 1,25(OH)$_2$D$_3$
VDRA vitamin D receptor activators, *VDR* vitamin D receptor

30.2   Alfacalcidol

30.2.1   Non-dialysis CKD: Effects on Bone Histology and Bone Mineral Density

A multicenter, prospective, double-blind, randomized, placebo-controlled trial was conducted on 176 non dialysis CKD patients (GFR 15–50 ml/min) with no baseline clinical, radiographic or biochemical signs of bone disease to test efficacy of a 2 year oral Alfacalcidol treatment (dose range 0.25 µg every other day to 1 µg a day) on bone histological pattern and quantitative changes in histomorphometric parameters [1]. Oral Alfacalcidol was administered in order to maintain serum calcium concentration at the upper limit of the normal laboratory reference range; calcium supplements were allowed (maximum 500 mg a day of elemental calcium), phosphorus restriction and phosphate binders were allowed to keep serum phosphate below 6.8 mg/dl.

All 176 patients underwent baseline bone biopsy, while only 134 (76%) received a second bone biopsy at the end of treatment (n = 124) or after premature withdrawal because of starting dialysis (n = 10). Reasons for premature withdrawal included need to start dialysis, default and death, while no patients withdrew for adverse events.

By definition, all 176 patients had normal serum calcium and alkaline phosphatase at baseline, while serum phosphate levels were high in 50 patients and PTH levels were high in 72 patients. Prevalence of histological abnormalities was high at baseline (132/176 patients), with those patients with no subclinical bone disease having a higher mean GFR. After randomization, no difference in baseline biochemical and bone disease pattern was found between treatment groups, except for PTH levels (93.6 pg/ml VS 58.2 pg/ml in Alfacalcidol group versus placebo, respectively).

Among 134 patients, 72 taking Alfacacidol and 62 taking placebo, whom paired bone biopsy specimens were available for analysis, 76% and 73% respectively had significant bone abnormalities at baseline. At the end of the study, proportion of patients with bone disease decreased to 54% in Alfacacidol group, while it increased to 82% in placebo group. When considering only patients with bone abnormalities at baseline, 42% of patients receiving Alfacalcidol treatment showed normal bone histology at the end of the study compared to only 4% receiving placebo. Among patients with apparently normal bone at baseline, no difference in bone histology was found between groups at the end of the study. When compared to placebo, Alfacalcidol treatment among patients with subclinical bone disease caused a statistical significant decrease in bone marrow fibrosis, bone turnover (bone resorption and bone formation) and osteomalacia indexes. Four of the six patients in Aflacalcidol group resolved adynamic bone disease (ABD) by the end of the study versus two out of the three patients taking placebo; by contrast eight versus four patients in Alfacalcidol and placebo group respectively developed ABD.

Mild hypercalcemia occurred in three patients given placebo versus ten patients given Alfacalcidol, severe hypercalcemia occurred only in one patient taking Alfacalcidol. Serum phosphate levels increased in both groups in a similar way. Serum PTH levels rapidly decreased among patients taking Alfacalcidol and then returned toward baseline levels by 24 month, while progressive increase of serum PTH levels was observed in placebo group. Serum total alkaline phosphatase levels showed a similar trend. Serum 25(OH) vitamin D levels were not assessed. There was a similar decline in glomerular filtration rate (GFR) decline between groups (P=0.94).

These results strongly support precocious use of Alfacalcidol among CKD patients in order to improve subclinical bone disease: benefits seem to overwhelm hazards in terms of developing ABD, hypercalcemia risk and fastening GFR decrease.

Results from this study were corroborated by another small prospective double blind placebo-controlled study which examined the effect of 18-month low dose Alfacalcidol treatment on bone mineral density (BMD) and markers of bone metabolism in early CKD (GFR 10–60 ml/min) [2]. Starting dose of 0.25 µg a day was increased in a 3-month period up to a maximum of 0.75 µg a day, while maintaining ionized serum calcium below 1.35 mmol/l and serum phosphate below 6.2 mg/dl. BMD was assessed in five sites: lumbar spine, femoral neck, total femur, distal forearm, and total body. ANOVA analysis with BMD as the dependent variable and treatment and time as independent variables suggested a significant effect of Alfacalcidol treatment on BMD in the hip, spine and total body sites. During treatment period, only one episode of hypercalcemia occurred among Alfacalcidol-treated subjects, serum phosphate levels were unaffected and a between-group difference in serum PTH levels was evident from week 3 onward, with lower levels among Alfacalcidol-treated subjects. Alfacalcidol-treated group showed a significant decrease over time of serum osteocalcin and bone alkaline phosphatase levels compared to placebo, while no statistical differences was observed in propeptide of type I collagen (PICP) – a marker of bone formation – and telopeptide of type I collagen (ICTP) – a marker of bone resorption. No difference in GFR decline rate was also found between groups.

30.2.2   Kidney Transplant Recipients: Effects on Bone Mineral Density

Bone disease after kidney transplantation is a complex matter with multiple contributing factors, including corticosteroid treatment, duration of prior chronic renal disease and dialysis, metabolic acidosis, vitamin D insufficiency/deficiency, hyperparathyroidism, hypophosphatemia, diabetes mellitus, etc. A few studies suggest beneficial effects of Alfacalcidol treatment among kidney transplant recipients.

A randomized study examined the effect of a 12 months course of low dose Alfacalcidol plus calcium versus calcium supplementation alone in pediatric renal transplant recipients with low baseline BMD at lumbar spine, femoral neck and for the whole body (z-score < −1.0 by DEXA) and a transplant vintage of more than 1 year [3]. High proportion of patients in both groups showed high serum PTH, low osteocalcin and elevated alkaline phosphatase levels at baseline. Alfacalcidol treatment was shown to significantly improve BMD at the lumbar spine, femoral neck and whole body and to reduce serum PTH and alkaline phosphatase levels.

Data from the same authors seem to suggest equal or superior efficacy of Alfacalcidol plus calcium treatment on BMD compared to alendronate or nasal spray calcitonin in a similar kidney transplant pediatric population [4].

Among adult population, De Sevaux et al. [5] found a beneficial effect of Alfacalcidol plus calcium (0.25 μg + 1,000 mg daily) versus placebo during the first 6 months after renal transplantation in terms of reduction of BMD loss in the lumbar spine and femoral neck.

Trabulus et al. [6] compared 1 year treatment with calcium plus either Alfacalcidol (0.5 μg daily), Alendronate (10 mg/daily) or a combination of both drugs on transplant recipients with a T-score equal or less than −1.0 at either lumbar spine (LS) or femoral neck (FN). The range of time since renal transplantation was 1–179 months. Combination therapy lead to an increase of BMD in the LS and FN of about 8 % from baseline. Alfacalcidol treatment alone failed to show significant effects in BMD of the LS, while it gave a small advantage in terms of lesser decrease in BMD of the FN compared to control group.

30.2.3   Comparison with Other VDRAs

Comparison studies of Alfacalcidol with other active forms of vitamin D are scanty.

El-Reshaid et al. [7] demonstrated comparable effects of i.v. Calcitriol and i.v. Alfacalcidol in terms of PTH suppression. Moe et al. [8] found that Calcitriol was superior to Alfacalcidol in a 6 week crossover study of PTH suppression in hemodialysis patients when both drugs were given orally at equal doses (PTH reduction 26.2 % in Calcitriol arm versus 6.2 % in Alfacalcicol arm). In contrast, Kiattisunthorn et al. [9] compared both drugs given orally after hemodialysis session for 24 weeks to control SHPT when administered Alfacalcidol dose was 1.5–2.0 times that of Calcitriol: both drugs gave analogous PTH suppression, with no significant difference in episodes of hypercalcemia and hyperphosphatemia.

Hansen et al. [10] conducted a multicenter randomized open label trial to compare i.v. Paricalcitol to i.v. Alfacalcidol in the treatment of SHPT in hemodialysis patient. The original study had a crossover design, but after first treatment period and a 6-week washout period, PTH values were significantly lower than at study baseline, suggesting a biological effect of both drugs lasting more than 6 weeks after treatment discontinuation. This fact led to decision of excluding data from crossover period from being analyzed.

Among 80 patients who concluded the first treatment period, baseline serum PTH levels were 571 ± 210 pg/ml versus 528 ± 176 pg/ml in Alfacalcidol and Paricalcitol group, respectively; there was no difference in biochemical and dialytic parameters at baseline. Paricalcitol and Alfacalcidol were administered at a starting dose of 9 µg/week and 3 µg/week, respectively, and subsequently titrated to reach a >30 % reduction of baseline serum PTH levels, while keeping serum ionized calcium concentration <1.35 mmol/l and serum phosphate levels <6.2 mg/dl. Hyperphosphatemia was treated by means of administration of calcium-free intestinal phosphate binders, dietary intervention and reevaluation of dialysis dose. After 16 weeks treatment, similar proportion of patients reached a 30 % reduction of baseline PTH (82 % and 93 %, for Alfacalcidol and Paricalcitol groups, respectively, P=0.18) and serum PTH levels less than 300 pg/ml (68 % and 83 %, respectively, P=0.188). Serum calcium, phosphate, total alkaline phosphatase at week 16 did not significantly differ; single episodes and repeated episodes of hypercalcemia were comparable. When correcting for baseline serum PTH levels, a significant interaction was found between baseline PTH values and effect of treatment, with Alfacalcidol effectively suppressing PTH throughout the entire range of PTH values, while Paricalcitol having a better efficacy on lower serum PTH levels than higher ones.

30.2.4   Doxercalciferol

30.2.4.1   Secondary Hyperparathyroidism Treatment in Non-dialysis CKD Patients

Couburn et al. [11] conducted a multicenter double-blinded randomized placebo-controlled trial to test efficacy and safety of Doxercalciferol treatment on SHPT in non-dialysis CKD patients.

After an 8-week washout period, 55 CKD patients (GFR range 13–47 ml/min) with a baseline PTH above 85 pg/ml received 24 week treatment with oral Doxercaciferol or placebo. Starting dose was 1 µg daily, subsequently titrated to reach 30 % of baseline PTH suppression while keeping serum calcium, serum phosphate and urinary calcium within the normal range. Moderate hypercalcemia (serum calcium >10.7 mg/dl), hypercalciuria (urinary calcium >200 mg/day) and PTH oversuppression (iPTH <15 pg/ml) lead to temporary discontinuation of study drug, while mild hypercalcemia (Ca 10.3–10.7 mg/dl) or hyperphosphatemia (serum phosphate >5.0 mg/dl) lead to the prescription of calcium-based intestinal phosphate binder or Doxecracliferol dose adjustment.

During treatment, serum PTH levels decreased from 219 ± 22 to 118 ± 17 pg/ml (-43 ± 7.6 %) at week 24 in Doxercalciferol group, while they remained unchanged in placebo group. Seventy-four percent of patients in Doxercalciferol group reached a 30 % or more reduction of baseline serum PTH levels during week 20–24, compared to only 7 % in placebo group. Serum calcium levels increased slightly in Doxercalciferol-treated patients from baseline, but no between-groups difference was found except than at week 20. Significant higher serum phosphate levels were also found in Doxercalciferol group compared to placebo at weeks 4 and 24. Doxercalciferol group experienced an increase in 24-h urinary calcium excretion from baseline onward, but no significant difference was found between groups at any time during treatment. Prevalence of hypercalcemia, defined as Ca >10.5 mg/dl, was not different between groups (2.6% versus VS 1.9% in Doxercalciferol and placebo groups, respectively, P=0.27), as no difference was found in prevalence of hyperphosphatemia defined as P>5.0 mg/dl (8.8% versus 6.5%, respectively, P=0.47). Mean GFR decline rate was similar between groups. Doxercalciferol leads to reduction of serum total alkaline phosphatase by 12% (P<005), bone-specific alkaline phosphatase by 27.9% (P<0.001) and osteocalcin by 22% (P<0.001) from baseline to week 24, compared to no reduction of either marker in the placebo group.

30.2.4.2   Secondary Hyperparathyroidism Treatment in Dialysis Patients

Oral intermittent Doxercalciferol administration for PTH suppression in hemodialysis patients was evaluated in a study conducted by Frazão et al. [12]. This study consisted in an 8-week washout period from previously calcitriol administration and a 24-week period, divided in a 16 week open-label treatment with Doxercalciferol for all patients and an 8-week randomized double-blind placebo-controlled Doxercalciferol administration.

After washout, patients should have baseline serum PTH levels above 400 pg/ml with no upper limit of severity, serum phosphate levels between 2.9 and 6.9 mg/dl and serum calcium levels below 10.6 mg/dl. Calcium based phosphate binders administration was allowed.

One hundred thirty-eight patients entered in the treatment period. During open-label treatment, Doxercalciferol was administered at a starting dose of 10 mg a day, subsequently titrated up to a maximum dose of 20 mg thrice weekly to reach serum PTH levels between 150 and 300 pg/ml, while avoiding development of hypercalcemia (Ca >11.2 mg/dl), repeated hyperphosphatemia (P>8.0 mg/dl) or elevated calcium x phosphorus product. During double-blind treatment, 50% of patients were switched to placebo with unchanged pill dose. Patients who developed serum phosphate levels above 6.9 mg/dl were excluded from primary efficacy analysis, which was conducted as per-protocol analysis.

Mean serum PTH levels decreased rapidly during open-label treatment and reached 44.7% reduction from baseline to week 16 (P<0.001). After switching to placebo, serum PTH levels remained suppressed only in Doxercalciferol-treated patients, while placebo-receiving patients experienced an increase in serum PTH levels, which did not differ from baseline by week 20. During blinded treatment the prevalence of hypercalcemia (defined as serum calcium >10.5 mg/dl) was 5.5% versus 15% in placebo and Doxercalciferol group, respectively. Prevalence of hyperphosphatemia (serum phosphate >6.9 mg/dl) was 9.7% versus 16.9% respectively. Efficacy analysis was also conducted after splitting patients into three groups depending on the baseline serum PTH levels: patients with more severe hyperparathyroidism needed a longer treatment with higher Doxercalciferol doses, in spite of comparable calcium and phosphate baseline levels.

Patients who completed open-label oral treatment were subsequently enrolled in another trial [13] aimed at comparing oral to intravenous (IV) administration route.

After an 8-week washout period, patients underwent a 12 week open-label Doxercalciferol treatment with the drug administered IV at the end of each hemodialysis session at 40 % of the oral dose previously received. Drug titration and/or temporary suspension followed the same rules of the oral administration trial [12].

Following washout period, only 70 patients entered the IV trial. Mean baseline serum PTH levels in this trial were slightly but significantly lower than in the oral trial (748 versus 950 pg/ml, p < 0.05), thus suggesting a prolonged treatment effect of Doxercalciferol previously administered orally.

Oral and IV routes gave comparable effects in terms of absolute PTH suppression, the proportion of patients achieving 30 and 50 % baseline PTH suppression, and PTH oversuppression (PTH <150 pg/ml). The average increase in serum calcium levels calculated over the 12 weeks treatment period was significantly greater during oral than IV Doxercalciferol therapy (+0.5 mg/dl versus +0.3 mg/dl, respectively, P < 0.02). Similar results were found with respect to the increase in serum phosphate levels (+0.89 mg/dl versus +0.5 mg/dl, respectively, P < 0.02). Proportion of patients experiencing hypercalcemia and hyperphosphatemia were not statistically different between the two trials, but absolute number of episodes of hypercalcemia and hyperphosphatemia were greater with the oral route of administration.

30.2.4.3   Comparison with Other VDRAs

Two small trials were conducted among HD patients to evaluate dose equivalency between Doxercalciferol and Paricalcitol in SHPT treatment.

Zisman et al. [14] switched 27 patients on stable Paricalcitol treatment to a 6-week Doxercalciferol treatment at three different doses, and found comparable PTH inhibition at a Doxercalciferol dose of 55–60 % previous Paricalcitol dose. Fadem et al. [15] converted 42 HD patients receiving a fixed Paricalcitol dose to Doxercalciferol treatment, at a starting dose of either 50 or 65 % of Paricalcitol dose, which was subsequently titrated to reach a serum PTH level between 150 and 300 pg/ml. Authors found comparable efficacy of both regimens on PTH suppression, with significant cost-saving effect with Doxercalciferol treatment compared to Paricalcitol.

30.3   Paricalcitol

30.3.1   Secondary Hyperparathyroidism Treatment in Non-dialysis CKD Patients

Coyne et al. [16] evaluated results from three independently performed prospective, double-blinded, multicenter trials in which 220 stage 3 and 4 CKD patients were randomized to receive either oral Paricalcitol (n = 107) or placebo (n = 113) to control SHPT (PTH >120 pg/ml). Paricalcitol was administered either daily (initial dose of 1 µg or 2 µg according to baseline PTH <500 pg/ml or >500 pg/ml) or thrice-weekly (2 µg or 4 µg according to the same baseline PTH cut-off). Mean baseline estimated GFR (eGFR) and PTH levels were 23.1 ml/min/1.73 m² and 265 pg/ml in Paricalcitol group and 23.0 ml/min/1.73 m² and 280 pg/ml in placebo group, respectively. After 24 weeks, 91 % of patients receiving Paricalcitol versus 13 % of patients receiving placebo (P<0.001) had two consecutive serum PTH levels reductions <30 % under the baseline levels. Both the regimens of Paricalcitol administration were equally effective in achieving PTH reduction; average daily Paricalcitol dose in either regimen was between 1.3 and 1.4 µg. Hypercalcemia (defined as two consecutive corrected calcium values >10.5 mg/dl [2.62 mmol/l]) was observed in 2 % of patients receiving Paricalcitol, but in none receiving placebo; hyperphosphatemia (serum phosphorus >5.5 mg/dl on two consecutive determinations) occurred similarly in both groups (10 % for Paricalcitol versus 12 % for placebo); urinary calcium excretion increased slightly in patients receiving Paricalcitol (from 39.6 mg/day to 42.0 mg/day) although no significant differences were observed between groups from baseline to final visit. Paricalcitol-treated subjects had also a significant reduction in serum levels of bone formation markers (bone-specific alkaline phosphatase and osteocalcin).

Only one randomized trial [17] compared efficacy and safety of Paricalcitol versus Calcitriol treatment in stage 3 and 4 CKD patients with SHPT. In this study 107 patients with a baseline PTH value >120 pg/ml were randomized to receive a starting daily dose of either Paricalcitol 1 µg (n=53) or Calcitriol 0.25 µg (n=54), subsequently titrated to reach PTH suppression of 40–60 % below baseline. Primary end point was the rate of confirmed hypercalcemia (calcium >10.5 mg/dl), and this was similar between treatment groups (5.7 % for Paricalcitol and 1.9 % for Calcitriol, P=0.36). Percentage 24 week reduction of PTH was similar between groups (−52 % in Paricalcitol group versus −46 % in Calcitriol group, P=0.17) even if baseline PTH values were slightly different, being higher in Calcitriol group (176 pg/ml [IQR 142–221] versus 209 pg/ml [IQR 158–287], respectively). After 24 weeks, a significant greater proportion of patients reached a >40 and >60 % percentage reduction of baseline PTH in Paricalcitol-treated compared to Calcitriol-treated subjects (98 % versus 87 %, P=0.03 and 83 % versus 52 %, P<0.001, respectively). Average daily Paricalcitol dose administered was 1.3 µg, while average daily Calcitriol dose was 0.5 µg. The study showed also a similar small increase in serum calcium levels, phosphate levels and reduction in total alkaline phosphatase between treatment groups (P = NS for all). Both drugs increased in a similar way urinary calcium excretion.

30.3.2   Albuminuria Reduction

GFR and albuminuria are important independent risk factors for kidney failure, acute kidney injury, and all-cause or cardiovascular mortality [18]. RAAS inhibitors, such as ACE inhibitors or angiotensin receptor blockers, are the treatment of choice in albuminuric CKD, because they may delay cardiovascular and renal disease as well as mortality. However, residual CV and renal risk can be high in patients treated with RAAS inhibitors, and this residual risk is positively associated to residual albuminuria [19, 20]: this underlines the role of albuminuria as a surrogate marker and a potential target for intervention in CKD patients.

Paricalcitol anti-albuminuric effect was first demonstrated in humans in a post hoc analysis [21] of a trial, which investigated Paricalcitol role in SHPT suppression in non-dialysis CKD patients. This antiproteinuric effect may be not specific for Paricalcitol, but it could be a class-effect of vitamin D compounds [22].

The VITAL study [23] was a multinational, placebo-controlled, double-blind trial specifically designed to test the anti-albuminuric effect of incremental doses of Paricalcitol on top of Renin-Angiotensin-Aldosterone System (RAAS) inhibition in patients affected by type 2 diabetes, albuminuria and CKD. Eligible patients had type 2 diabetes, a urinary albumin-to-creatinine ratio (UACR) 11–339 mg/mmol [100–3,000 mg/g], eGFR 15–90 ml/min and serum PTH concentration 35–500 pg/ml.

A total of 281 patients were randomly assigned to receive Paricalcitol 1 µg/day (n=93), Paricalcitol 2 µg/day (n=95), or placebo (n=93) for 24 weeks. Mean baseline eGFR and UACR were similar between groups being 40, 42 and 39 ml/min/1.73 m^2 and 101, 92 and 94 mg/mmol [894, 814 and 832 mg/g] for 1 µg Paricalcitol, 2 µg Paricalcitol and placebo, respectively. All patients, except 2 in 2 µg Paricalcitol group, received some form of RAAS inhibition (ACE inhibitors, ARB, other RAAS inhibitors or a combination of these drugs); as a rule, this regimen could not be changed after randomization. Patients in this trial were generally 25OH-vitamin D depleted, being mean baseline serum levels 40, 42 and 42 nmol/L [16, 17 and 17 ng/ml] for 1 µg Paricalcitol, 2 µg Paricalcitol and placebo, respectively.

The primary efficacy point was the percentage change in geometric mean UACR from baseline to the last measurement during treatment. When compared to placebo, combined Paricalcitol groups showed a trend to reduction of UACR (between-group difference −15 %, 95 % CI −28 % to +1 %; P=0.071). Further analysis of data suggested that UACR reduction could be dose-dependent, being difference between placebo and 2 µg Paricalcitol group closer to statistical significance (between-group difference −18 %, 95 % CI −32–0, P=0.053), while that between placebo and 1 µg Paricalcitol being not (P=0.23).

Secondary efficacy analysis seemed to confirm dose-dependency of Paricalcitol anti-albuminuric effect: a significant 24 urinary albumin reduction in 2 µg Paricalcitol group compared to placebo (between-group difference −28 %; 95 % CI −43 to −8, P=0.009) and a higher proportion of patients achieving a change in UACR of at last 15 % between baseline and the last measurement (55 % versus 40 %, P=0.038) were observed. UACR reduction (2 µg Paricalcitol versus placebo) was sustained during treatment, and reversible after treatment discontinuation. Degree of PTH reduction and rate of hypercalcemia reported were similar to previously published trials.

In a post-hoc analysis patients were stratified in tertiles according to their baseline 24 h urinary sodium excretion (<121 mmol; 121–178 mmol; >178 mmol). The greatest efficacy in UACR reduction was found in patients with the highest sodium intake receiving Paricalcitol 2 µg/day (−40 % versus placebo, P=0.005).

Interestingly, 43 % of patients in the study were receiving maximal recommended dose of RAAS inhibition but no interaction was found with UACR reduction during Paricalcitol treatment, suggesting the efficacy of this regimen irrespective to the degree of RAAS inhibition. No significant changes were found between treatment groups in plasma renin activity and aldosterone levels.

A recent randomized, double blinded, placebo-controlled, crossover study was conducted to investigate whether antialbuminuric Paricalcitol effect could be due to plasma renin suppression [24]. Twenty-six non diabetic stage 3 and 4 CKD patients with urinary albumin >30 mg/l received a 6 weeks treatment with either Paricalcitol 2 µg/day or placebo, while discontinuing all RAAS inhibitors. Patients received a standardized diet during the last 4 days of each 6 weeks period, before assessment of plasma renin concentration (PRC). Etiology of CKD included polycystic kidney disease (n = 3), glomerulonephritis (n = 6), chronic interstitial nephritis (n = 2) or was unknown (n = 15); average baseline albuminuria was 169 mg/l (IQR 59–489).

No difference was found in PRC at the end of 6 weeks treatment with Paricalcitol compared to placebo, no significant difference was also found in 24 h urinary albumin excretion during Paricalcitol treatment (−7 % versus placebo, 95 % CI −20–7, P = 0.12).

With a complex experimental procedure, investigators wanted also to test Paricalcitol effect on hemodynamic and biochemical parameters before and during infusion of L-NMMA, a nitric-oxide synthase (NOS) inhibitor, supposing a modulatory effect of Paricalcitol on renal nitric oxide bioavailability. They observed that while acute NOS inhibition induced an albuminuric effect in patients taking placebo, the albuminuric response was blunted in Paricalcitol-treated subjects.

30.3.3 Cardiac Structure and Function, Cardiovascular End-Points

Vitamin D deficiency is associated with hypertension, left ventricular hypertrophy (LVH) and heart failure, and animal models demonstrated that vitamin D therapy prevents the progression of LVH [25, 26]. Retrospective data suggested a beneficial role of Paricalcitol treatment in humans on diastolic function and LVH [27]. These suggestions were explored in some specifically designed prospective trials.

The PRIMO study [28] was a multinational, randomized, placebo-controlled trial to test Paricalcitol ability to reduce left ventricular mass index (LVMI) and ameliorate cardiac diastolic parameters in stage 3 and 4 CKD patients with echocardiographic evidence of mild to moderate LVH and preserved systolic function, with baseline PTH values 50–300 pg/ml.

Patients were randomized to receive either Paricalcitol 2 µg/day or placebo for 48 weeks, with pre-specified dose reduction to 1 µg/day in case of hypercalcemia (serum calcium >11 mg/dl). At 24 and 48 weeks patients underwent cardiovascular magnetic resonance (CMR) to assess LVMI and transthoracic echocardiography (TTE) to measure diastolic cardiac parameters (peak early diastolic lateral mitral annular tissue velocity (E'), isovolumetric relaxation time, ratio of early mitral inflow wave velocity E-wave (E) to E', E-wave deceleration time). PTH and B-natriuretic peptide (BNP) were measured throughout the study period. Cardiovascular hospitalization and deaths were also recorded.

Baseline mean GFR and albuminuria were similar between groups, diabetics accounted for about one-half of sample size (54.8 % in Paricalcitol versus 50.9 % in placebo-treated patients), blood pressure was well controlled in both groups (mean 135/76 mmHg in Paricalcitol versus 135/75 mmHg in placebo group). Baseline LVMI normalized to height to the 2.7th power and E' were similar between groups, consistent with mild to moderate LVH and diastolic dysfunction (LVMI 23.7 ± 7.3 g/m$^{2.7}$ versus 23.5 ± 8.3 g/m$^{2.7}$ and E' 8.2 ± 2.5 versus 8.4 ± 2.4 cm/s in Paricalcitol and placebo-treated subjects, respectively).

One hundred two patients receiving Paricalcitol and 94 patients receiving placebo were included in primary intention-to-treat efficacy analysis. No cardiac parameter was significantly different between groups after 24 and 48 weeks. A trend was observed towards LVMI reduction in placebo-treated subjects compared to Paricalcitol-treated ones. In a pre-specified analysis considering patients with more severe baseline LMVI (the upper three quartile of baseline LVMI, named "LVH population") LVMI increased slightly in the Paricalcitol group with borderline statistical significance (P=0.5).

Although all-cause hospitalization rate was similar between groups, Paricalcitol-treated patients had fewer cardiovascular hospitalizations compared to placebo (1 versus 8, P=0.03). Plasma brain natriuretic peptide (BNP) levels increased in both groups, with no difference after 48 weeks in the ITT population, while Paricalcitol showed a blunting effect on BPN increase among patients in LHV population: Paricalcitol +15 % VS Placebo +50 % from baseline, P=0.04).

As already seen in other studies, Paricalcitol treatment effectively decreased PTH levels compared to placebo, but in this study a higher rate of confirmed hypercalcemia during Paricalcitol treatment was observed than previously reported (prevalence of serum calcium >10.5 mg/dl in two consecutive determinations: 22.6 % VS 0.9 %, P<0.001).

The OPERA trial [29] was a randomized-controlled trial with a study design similar to PRIMO study. Sixty patients from Hong Kong population were included in this RCT to test efficacy of Paricalcitol on LVMI reduction and amelioration of diastolic cardiac indices in a stage 3–5 non dialysis CKD population with echocardiographic documented LVH. Patients received Paricalcitol (1 or 2 µg/day, depending on baseline PTH value <500 pg/ml or >500 pg/ml, subsequently titrated to avoid hypercalcemia) or placebo for 52 weeks. LVMI was assessed by means of CMR and diastolic function by means of TTE.

Patients had an overall good blood pressure control (mean Paricalcitol group 131/76 mmHg; mean placebo group 135/74 mmHg). Compared to PRIMO study, patients in this trial had a more severe LVH and worse diastolic dysfunction at baseline (LVMI 39.2 ± 7.3 g/m$^{2.7}$ versus 38.0 ± 8.5 g/m$^{2.7}$ and E' 6.8 ± 1.5 versus 6.7 ± 1.8 cm/s in Paricalcitol and placebo-treated subjects, respectively).

As already seen in PRIMO trial, there was no difference was found between groups in LVMI and diastolic parameters after 52 weeks. All-cause hospitalizations were fewer in Paricalcitol treated subjects (7 % versus 33 %, P=0.02), with all cardiovascular-hospitalization being in placebo group. Hypercalcemia was higher in Paricalcitol group (43.3 % versus 3.3 %, P<0.001), with a high proportion of patients being treated with calcium-based phosphate binders during hypercalcemic episodes (69.2 %). PTH suppression was similar to previously reported studies, even with a smaller daily Paricalcitol dose. No significant difference was found in 24 h urinary protein excretion between groups after 52 weeks treatment.

A post-hoc analysis of the PRIMO study [30] considered Paricalcitol effect on left atrium volume (LAV), which is considered a sensitive indicator of diastolic dysfunction severity, with added prognostic value above left ventricular morphology and function [31, 32].

LAV, assessed by biplane 2D echocardiography and indexed to body surface area (LAVi), at baseline showed a similar moderate enlargement in both groups (32.8 ± 9.8 ml/m^2 versus 35.4 ± 11.4 ml/m^2 in Paricalcitol group compared to placebo). Over the study period, LAVi demonstrated a significant decrease in Paricalcitol-treated patients compared with placebo-treated (-2.79 ml/m^2; 95 % CI -4.00 to -1.59 VS -0.7 ml/m^2; 95 % CI -1.93 to 0.53; P=0.002), which paralleled corresponding attenuation in the rise in plasma levels of BNP. Given the fact that diuretic use and body weight changes were similar between groups, Paricalcitol effect on LAVi seems to be independent from extracellular volume reduction, even if Paricalcitol-induced BNP-mediated natriuresis or increase in urinary calcium concentration could have a contributory role in subclinical extracellular volume reduction.

30.3.4 Secondary Hyperparathyroidism Treatment in Dialysis Patients

In 2003 Sprague et al. [33] conducted the first multicenter, prospective, controlled, double-blind, randomized study to compare the safety and effectiveness of intravenous Calcitriol and intravenous Paricalcitol in medically stable hemodialysis patients with SHPT (PTH >300 pg/ml after SHPT-controlling drugs suspension).

It is important to emphasize that investigators used a very high threshold to define hypercalcemia (serum calcium >11.5 mg/dl), reflecting nephrologists' practice of the early-to-mid 1990s: this level was used to initially define patients suitable to active vitamin D therapy and to manage vitamin D dose titration. Furthermore, except from aluminium-containing phosphate binders, which were a priori excluded from the trial, the only intestinal phosphate binders available at time were calcium-containing ones. All these aspects should be considered when analyzing these results and trying to translate them in today's clinical practice.

Two hundred sixty-three patients were randomized to receive either Paricalcitol 0.04 µg/kg (n = 130) or Calcitriol 0.01 µg/kg (n = 133) thrice weekly. Dose could be increased every 4 weeks to reach a 50 % reduction from baseline PTH without PTH oversuppression (PTH <150 pg/ml), dose reduction could be done at 1 week intervals in case of hypercalcemia or two consecutive elevated $Ca \times P$ products (>75 mg^2/dl^2). Investigators were instructed not to change phosphate binder prescription.

After a pre-treatment phase, in which previous SHPT-controlling drugs were discontinued and phosphate binder doses and dialysate bath calcium were adjusted, mean baseline PTH were 648 pg/ml VS 645 pg/ml, mean serum calcium 9.0 mg/dl VS 9.0 mg/dl, mean serum phosphorus 5.9 mg/dl VS 5.8 mg/dl for Paricalcitol and Calcitriol-treated patients, respectively. Dialysis vintage was variable, including subjects with 5 years or more in both groups (prevalence in both groups about 30 %). Treatment phase lasted 12–32 weeks for each patient.

Both treatment groups achieved the primary end point of 50 % reduction of mean PTH, although Paricalcitol-treated subjects reached the end point earlier (15 weeks versus 23 weeks). Proportion of patients achieving a 50 % reduction from baseline PTH at least once during treatment period was more than 80 % in both groups, while 4 weeks-sustained PTH suppression was more frequently achieved in Paricalcitol-treated patients (64 % versus 54 %).

Proportion of patients who experienced a single episode of hypercalcemia or elevated $Ca \times P$ product was comparable between groups (64 % versus 68 %, P = 0.52, for Paricalcitol and Calcitriol respectively), while incidence of confirmed hypercalcemia or elevated $Ca \times P$ product was higher in Calcitriol group (38 % versus 50 %, P = 0.034, respectively). Hyperphosphatemia was very common and comparable between groups; similar reduction in total alkaline phosphatase levels was observed with both drugs.

A recent small study compared oral Paricalcitol versus oral Calcitriol for SHPT treatment in a Malaysian population of dialysis patients [34], a small percentage of peritoneal dialysis patients was also included. Patients eligibility criteria included PTH >300 pg/ml and absence of hypercalcemia (defined as serum calcium above 11 mg/dl).

Initial doses of either drug were calculated from baseline PTH obtained after a 3 weeks wash out period from previous drugs. Starting doses were PTH/120 for Paricalcitol and PTH/360 for Calcitriol. Drugs were titrated every 3 week to achieve a 30 % reduction of baseline PTH, while keeping it in the range 150–300 pg/ml. If hypercalcemia or elevated $Ca \times P$ occurred, dose reduction was required. No change in phosphate binder dose or calcium concentration in the dialysate bath was allowed.

Thirty-six and 30 patients received Paricalcitol and Calcitriol treatment, respectively. Mean dialysis vintage was 8.7 VS 7.8 years and baseline PTH levels were 495.0 VS 558.5 pg/ml, in Paricalctol group and Calcitriol group respectively.

At the end of 24 weeks 61.1 % of Paricalcitol-treated subjects and 73.3 % of Calcitriol-treated subjects (P = 0.29) achieved the primary end point of 30 % PTH reduction from baseline. No difference in time of primary end point achievement was observed between groups. Median percentage PTH reduction from baseline to weeks 12 and 24 was similar between groups (54.3 % versus 57.4 % at 12 weeks, 48.4 % versus 41.9 % at 24 weeks, for Paricalcitol and Calcitriol, respectively).

Average weekly dose of Paricalcitol administered was 20.7 μg, average Calcitriol dose was 7.1 μg/week, with a ratio of about 3:1, similar to starting dose.

Serum calcium increased in a similar way in both groups, while serum phosphorus was minimally reduced in Paricalcitol-treated subjects compared to Calcitriol-treated ones (−0.37 mg/dl versus +0.47 mg/dl, P<0.01). Proportion of patients experiencing hypercalcemia was similar between groups (16.7 %); if the threshold for hypercalcemia definition had been lowered down to 10.2 mg/dl, incidence of hypercalcemia would have been significantly higher: 27.8 % for Paricalcitol and 33.3 % for Calcitriol. Both treatments reduced serum alkaline phosphatase, with greater reduction obtained by Calcitriol.

30.3.5   Treatment of Secondary Hyperparathyroidism: Comparison Between a Paricalcitol-Based and a Cinacalcet-Based Regimen

Hypercalcemia and hyperphosphatemia are known risk factors for vascular and soft tissue calcification. Acceptable levels of serum calcium and phosphate while treating CKD mineral and bone disease in dialysis patients were re-evaluated in 2003 NKF/K-DOQI (National Kidney Foundation/Kidney-Dialysis Outcome Quality Initiative) guidelines, which suggested to keep serum calcium and phosphate concentrations as close as possible to their normal range and to maintain $Ca \times P$ product below 55 mg^2/dl^2. Those levels were considerably lower than previously accepted in everyday clinical practice.

Moreover, 2009 KDIGO (Kidney Disease-Improving Global Outcomes) CKD-mineral bone disease (CKD-MBD) guidelines suggested to keep PTH between two and nine times the upper normal limit of the assay used, widening the range of previously accepted serum PTH levels of 150–300 pg/ml. While previous guidelines suggested tight PTH control to avoid low and high bone turnover disease, subsequent studies showed poor predictive value of this range with respect to bone histology in dialysis patients. Moreover, observational data suggested that a wider PTH range could be acceptable when considering patient-level outcomes (mortality, cardiovascular death and bone fractures).

After 2003 guidelines release, two trials were conducted to assess whether a Cinacalcet-based or a Vitamin D-based therapy was better to achieve the new targets advocated while treating CKD-MBD. These two trials gave somewhat conflicting results.

The ACHIEVE study [35] was a multicenter, open-label, RCT. Eligible subjects included HD patients already receiving vitamin D therapy (Paricalcitol or Doxercalciferol) without attaining PTH target levels (150–300 pg/ml) or $Ca \times P$ target levels (<55 mg^2/dl^2).

Patients were randomly assigned to receive either Cinacalcet plus low fixed doses of VDRA (Doxercalciferol 1 μg or Paricalcitol 2 μg i.v. thrice weekly) – named "Cinacalcet-D group" – or escalating doses of VDRA – named "Flexi-D group". Very tight rules were given to manage drug dosing, with respect to calcium, phosphate and PTH levels.

Cinacalcet-D patients (n=87) received a starting dose of 30 mg Cinacalcet, raised every 4 weeks up to 180 mg/day, if needed. Criteria for Cinacalcet reduction were hypocalcemia (Ca <7.5 mg/dl) and PTH oversuppression (<150 pg/ml) with low serum calcium. Criterion for VDRA suspension was oversuppression of PTH with a serum calcium level >8.4 mg/dl. VDRA was reduced if serum calcium exceeded 9.5 mg/dl or serum phosphate exceeded 5.5 mg/dl.

Flexi-D patients (n=86) received escalating doses of either Paricalcitol (starting dose 2 µg thrice weekly) or Doxercalciferol (1 µg thrice weekly): upwards titration was accomplished every 4 weeks. Criteria for vitamin D suspension were PTH oversuppression, hypercalcemia (Ca >10.2 mg/dl), hyperphosphatemia (P>5.5 mg/dl) or elevated Ca×P product. Vitamin D therapy could be subsequently resumed at a lower dose.

Dialysate calcium and phosphate binder doses could be adjusted throughout the study. Doxercalciferol and Paricalcitol were considered biologically equivalent with a 2:1 dosing ratio. The study had a 16-week titration phase and a 11 week efficacy assessment phase, during which no escalation of VDRA or Cinacalcet could be made.

Patients enrolled had a mean dialysis vintage of 46 months in both groups, with similar median baseline PTH levels (Cinacalcet-D 597 pg/ml, IQR 471–775 versus Flexi-D 621 pg/ml, IQR 463–883). Baseline calcium and phosphate levels were also similar. During assessment phase, Flexi-D patients received mean weekly dose of 13.9±10.4 µg Paricalcitol equivalents, while Cinacalcet-D patients received a Cinacalcet mean daily dose of 68.5±41.1 mg). Phosphate binder use (either calcium-free, calcium-containing or a combination of both) did not differ between study groups.

Notably, a high dropout rate (25 % overall) should be considered when analyzing study results.

The primary end point was the proportion of patients simultaneously reaching a PTH in the range 150–300 pg/ml and Ca×P product >55 mg^2/dl^2 during the assessment phase. Only a small minority of patients achieved the combined end point, with no statistical difference between groups (Cinacalcet-D 21 % versus Flexi-D 14 %, P=0.231), mainly for PTH oversuppression in Cinacalcet-D group. Patients simultaneously achieving serum calcium, phosphate, PTH and Ca×P product target levels suggested by KDOQI guidelines were even a smaller group (8 % versus 0 %, respectively, P=0.017).

When considering single parameters, PTH suppression was more pronounced in patients receiving Cinacalcet-based therapy with respect to median values achieved in assessment phase (Cinacalcet-D 320 pg/ml, IQR 211–589 versus Flexi-D 559 pg/ml, IQR 314–768). Median calcium levels significantly decreased in Cinacalcet-D patients compared to Flexi-D grop (assessment phase 8.9 mg/dl versus 9.7 mg/dl, respectively) while serum phosphate did not change appreciably (5.3 mg/dl for both).

The IMPACT SHPT study was a multicenter, international, RCT [36, 37]. Paricalcitol-based therapy was compared to Cinacalcet-based therapy in terms of efficacy of PTH suppression in HD patients. Vitamin D route of administration defined two strata (oral, in non-US sites, and intra-venous, in US and Russian sites), which were considered separately for randomization and efficacy analysis.

Patients eligible for the study were HD patients with a serum PTH between 300 and 800 pg/ml, normal serum calcium levels and phosphate levels below 6.5 mg/dl after discontinuation of previous assumed PTH suppressing drugs.

Paricalcitol group received a starting dose of 0.07 μg/kg IV thrice weekly or daily oral dose calculated from PTH/60 μg, according to stratum. It was subsequently titrated every 2 weeks, first according to $Ca \times P$ product (which must be maintained below 75 –IV stratum – or 70 – oral stratum mg^2/dl^2), then to serum calcium levels (<10.5 mg/dl), then to serum PTH levels to reach a value between 150 and 300 pg/ml. Cinacalcet could be co-administered as supplemental medication in case of confirmed hypercalcemia.

Cinacalcet group received oral drug plus small fixed doses of VDRA (either Doxercalciferol 1 μg thrice weekly – IV stratum – or Alfacalcidol 0.25 μg daily – oral stratum). Starting Cinacalcet dose was 30 mg, subsequently titrated according first to serum calcium levels and then to serum PTH levels, with the same target of 150–300 pg/ml. Oral calcium could be administered to maintain serum calcium between 8.4 and 10.5 mg/dl.

Two hundred seventy-two patients were randomized and 268 received one or more dose of study drug. Among 126 patients who constituted the IV stratum 62 received Paricalcitol and 64 received Cinacalcet, among 142 in the oral stratum 72 received Paricalcitol and 70 received Cinacalcet. Mean dialysis vintage was 3.7 ± 3.4 years and mean baseline PTH was 509 pg/ml. PTH, duration of dialysis and demographic characteristics were similar across treatment groups and strata.

Study design included a treatment period and an evaluation period (from week 21 to week 28). Only patients with two or more PTH assessments during evaluation period were included in primary efficacy analysis. Discontinuation rates, mainly due to adverse events, were quite high and ranged from 19.4 % in the Paricalcitol group/IV stratum to 31.1 % in the Cinacalcet group/IV stratum.

The proportion of patients achieving a PTH in the range 150–300 pg/ml (primary end point) was higher in Paricalcitol-treated patients compared to Cinacalcet-treated in both strata, although only in the IV stratum the difference was statistically significant (IV stratum 57.7 % versus 32.7, P=0.016; oral stratum 54.4 % versus 43.4 %, P=0.26). When the strata were combined in a subsequent analysis Paricalcitol was proven superior to Cinacalcet (P=0.01) in terms of achieving specific PTH target levels. Moreover the proportion of patients achieving a >30 and >50% reduction from baseline PTH was higher in the Paricalcitol group. Average doses administered were 3.5 ± 3.5 μg/day, 5.5 ± 3.7 μg thrice weekly, 31.8 ± 28.7 mg/day and 61.6 ± 44.8 mg for oral Paricalcitol, IV Paricalcitol, Cinacalcet in the oral stratum and Cinacalcet in the IV stratum, respectively.

Only a minority of patients received Cinacalcet while being treated with Paricalcitol (five patients per stratum): sensitivity analysis conducted excluding these subjects lead to similar conclusions. Phosphate binder use and doses increased in both treatment groups, consisting primarily in calcium-containing phosphate binders for Cinacalcet-receiving group and calcium-free compounds for

Paricalcitol-receiving group. While hypocalcemia was a frequent condition during the evaluation period among patients receiving Cinacalcet (46.9 % and 54.7 % in the IV stratum and oral stratum, respectively), hypercalcemia rarely occurred among patients receiving Paricalcitol (7.7 % and 0 % in the IV stratum and oral stratum, respectively).

A subsequent analysis [38] conducted on IMPACT study markers of bone mineral disease showed a decrease in total alkaline phosphatase and bone specific AP in the Paricalcitol centered group in both strata from baseline to week 28 (for AP: IV stratum 109.2–91.7 UI/L, oral stratum 95.6–81.2 UI/L). In contrast, AP and BSAP increased from baseline to the end of the study in the Cinacalcet centered groups (for AP: IV stratum 124–153 UI/L, oral stratum 104.5–108.9 UI/L).

Paricalcitol treatment was also associated with an increase of FGF23 (fibroblast growth factor 23) levels from baseline to subsequent assessments in both strata, while Cinacalcet administration was associated with minimal FGF23 levels reduction. In addition, while phosphate levels peaked early (week 5) among Paricalcitol treated patients and subsequently declined, Cinacalced treated subjects showed a minimal decrease in phosphate levels in the IV stratum, while in the oral stratum after an initial decrease serum phosphate levels returned to baseline levels.

30.4   Conclusions

An expanding body of evidence is rapidly enriching the rationale for vitamin D use in CKD-MBD. The traditional action of VDRAs on PTH suppression is now flanked by encouraging data on their pleiotropic effects on microalbuminuria and LVH. Furthermore, nutritional Vitamin D is receiving a growing interest as a preventive and treating strategy against SHPT as well as a protective intervention on immune responses, insulin resistance, and inflammation even in renal patients. However, further RCTs are advocated to investigate the many opened questions and uncertainties on the effects of VDRA and nutritional vitamin D on hard end points and their comparison with calcimimetic in CKD.

References

1. Hamdy NA, Kanis JA, Beneton MN, Brown CB, Juttmann JR, Jordans JG, Josse S, Meyrier A, Lins RL, Fairey IT. Effect of alfacalcidol on natural course of renal bone disease in mild to moderate renal failure. BMJ. 1995;310(6976):358–63.
2. Rix M, Eskildsen P, Olgaard K. Effect of 18 months of treatment with alfacalcidol on bone in patients with mild to moderate chronic renal failure. Nephrol Dial Transplant. 2004;19(4):870–6.
3. El-Husseini AA, El-Agroudy AE, El-Sayed M, Sobh MA, Ghoneim MA. A prospective randomized study for the treatment of bone loss with vitamin d during kidney transplantation in children and adolescents. Am J Transplant. 2004;4(12):2052–7.
4. El-Husseini AA, El-Agroudy AE, El-Sayed MF, Sobh MA, Ghoneim MA. Treatment of osteopenia and osteoporosis in renal transplant children and adolescents. Pediatr Transplant. 2004;8(4):357–61.

5. De Sévaux RG, Hoitsma AJ, Corstens FH, Wetzels JF. Treatment with vitamin D and calcium reduces bone loss after renal transplantation: a randomized study. J Am Soc Nephrol. 2002;13(6):1608–14.
6. Trabulus S, Altiparmak MR, Apaydin S, Serdengecti K, Sariyar M. Treatment of renal transplant recipients with low bone mineral density: a randomized prospective trial of alendronate, alfacalcidol, and alendronate combined with alfacalcidol. Transplant Proc. 2008;40(1):160–6.
7. El-Reshaid K, El-Reshaid W, Sugathan T, Al-Mohannadi S, Sivanandan R. Comparison of the efficacy of two injectable forms of vitamin D3 and oral one-alpha in treatment of secondary hyperparathyroidism in patients on maintenance hemodialysis. Am J Nephrol. 1997;17(6):505–10.
8. Moe S, Wazny LD, Martin JE. Oral calcitriol versus oral alfacalcidol for the treatment of secondary hyperparathyroidism in patients receiving hemodialysis: a randomized, crossover trial. Can J Clin Pharmacol. 2008;15(1):e36–43. Epub 2008 Jan 9.
9. Kiattisunthorn K, Wutyam K, Indranoi A, Vasuvattakul S. Randomized trial comparing pulse calcitriol and alfacalcidol for the treatment of secondary hyperparathyroidism in haemodialysis patients. Nephrology (Carlton). 2011;16(3):277–84.
10. Hansen D, Rasmussen K, Danielsen H, Meyer-Hofmann H, Bacevicius E, Lauridsen TG, Madsen JK, Tougaard BG, Marckmann P, Thye-Roenn P, Nielsen JE, Kreiner S, Brandi L. No difference between alfacalcidol and paricalcitol in the treatment of secondary hyperparathyroidism in hemodialysis patients: a randomized crossover trial. Kidney Int. 2011;80(8):841–50.
11. Coburn JW, Maung HM, Elangovan L, Germain MJ, Lindberg JS, Sprague SM, Williams ME, Bishop CW. Doxercalciferol safely suppresses PTH levels in patients with secondary hyperparathyroidism associated with chronic kidney disease stages 3 and 4. Am J Kidney Dis. 2004;43(5):877–90.
12. Frazão JM, Elangovan L, Maung HM, Chesney RW, Acchiardo SR, Bower JD, Kelley BJ, Rodriguez HJ, Norris KC, Robertson JA, Levine BS, Goodman WG, Gentile D, Mazess RB, Kyllo DM, Douglass LL, Bishop CW, Coburn JW. Intermittent doxercalciferol (1alpha-hydroxyvitamin D(2)) therapy for secondary hyperparathyroidism. Am J Kidney Dis. 2000;36(3):550–61.
13. Maung HM, Elangovan L, Frazão JM, Bower JD, Kelley BJ, Acchiardo SR, Rodriguez HJ, Norris KC, Sigala JF, Rutkowski M, Robertson JA, Goodman WG, Levine BS, Chesney RW, Mazess RB, Kyllo DM, Douglass LL, Bishop CW, Coburn JW. Efficacy and side effects of intermittent intravenous and oral doxercalciferol (1alpha-hydroxyvitamin D(2)) in dialysis patients with secondary hyperparathyroidism: a sequential comparison. Am J Kidney Dis. 2001;37(3):532–43.
14. Zisman AL, Ghantous W, Schinleber P, Roberts L, Sprague SM. Inhibition of parathyroid hormone: a dose equivalency study of paricalcitol and doxercalciferol. Am J Nephrol. 2005;25(6):591–5.
15. Fadem SZ, Al-Saghir F, Zollner G, Swan S. Converting hemodialysis patients from intravenous paricalcitol to intravenous doxercalciferol – a dose equivalency and titration study. Clin Nephrol. 2008;70(4):319–24.
16. Coyne D, Acharya M, Qiu P, Abboud H, Batlle D, Rosansky S, Fadem S, Levine B, Williams L, Andress DL, Sprague SM. Paricalcitol capsule for the treatment of secondary hyperparathyroidism in stages 3 and 4 CKD. Am J Kidney Dis. 2006;47:263–76.
17. Coyne DW, Goldberg S, Faber M, Ghossein C, Sprague SM. A randomized multicenter trial of paricalcitol versus calcitriol for secondary hyperparathyroidism in stages 3–4 CKD. Clin J Am Soc Nephrol. 2014;9(9):1620–6.
18. Komenda P, Rigatto C, Tangri N. Estimated glomerular filtration rate and albuminuria: diagnosis, staging, and prognosis. Curr Opin Nephrol Hypertens. 2014;23(3):251–7.
19. De Zeeuw D, Lambers Heerspink HJ, Gansevoort RT, Bakker SJL. How to improve renal outcome in diabetes and hypertension – the importance of early screening for and treatment of microalbuminuria. Eur Nephrol. 2009;3:13–5.
20. Eijkelkamp WB, Zhang Z, Remuzzi G, Parving HH, Cooper ME, Keane WF, Shahinfar S, Gleim GW, Weir MR, Brenner BM, de Zeeuw D. Albuminuria is a target for renoprotective

therapy independent from blood pressure in patients with type 2 diabetic nephropathy: post hoc analysis from the Reduction of Endpoints in NIDDM with the Angiotensin II Antagonist Losartan (RENAAL) trial. J Am Soc Nephrol. 2007;18(5):1540–6.

21. Agarwal R, Acharya M, Tian J, Hippensteel RL, Melnick JZ, Qiu P, Williams L, Batlle D. Antiproteinuric effect of oral paricalcitol in chronic kidney disease. Kidney Int. 2005;68(6):2823–8.

22. Liu LJ, Lv JC, Shi SF, Chen YQ, Zhang H, Wang HY. Oral calcitriol for reduction of proteinuria in patients with IgA nephropathy: a randomized controlled trial. Am J Kidney Dis. 2012;59(1):67–74.

23. De Zeeuw D, Agarwal R, Amdahl M, Audhya P, Coyne D, Garimella T, Parving HH, Pritchett Y, Remuzzi G, Ritz E, Andress D. Selective vitamin D receptor activation with paricalcitol for reduction of albuminuria in patients with type 2 diabetes (VITAL study): a randomised controlled trial. Lancet. 2010;376(9752):1543–51.

24. Larsen T, Mose FH, Bech JN, Pedersen EB. Effect of paricalcitol on renin and albuminuria in non-diabetic stage III–IV chronic kidney disease: a randomized placebo-controlled trial. BMC Nephrol. 2013;14:163.

25. Bae S, Yalamarti B, Ke Q, Choudhury S, Yu H, Karumanchi SA, Kroeger P, Thadhani R, Kang PM. Preventing progression of cardiac hypertrophy and development of heart failure by paricalcitol therapy in rats. Cardiovasc Res. 2011;91(4):632–9.

26. Pilz S, Tomaschitz A, Drechsler C, de Boer RA. Vitamin D deficiency and heart disease. Kidney Int Suppl. 2011;1:111–5.

27. Bodyak N, Ayus JC, Achinger S, Shivalingappa V, Ke Q, Chen YS, Rigor DL, Stillman I, Tamez H, Kroeger PE, Wu-Wong RR, Karumanchi SA, Thadhani R, Kang PM. Activated vitamin D attenuates left ventricular abnormalities induced by dietary sodium in Dahl salt-sensitive animals. Proc Natl Acad Sci U S A. 2007;104(43):16810–5.

28. Thadhani R, Appelbaum E, Pritchett Y, Chang Y, Wenger J, Tamez H, Bhan I, Agarwal R, Zoccali C, Wanner C, Lloyd-Jones D, Cannata J, Thompson BT, Andress D, Zhang W, Packham D, Singh B, Zehnder D, Shah A, Pachika A, Manning WJ, Solomon SD. Vitamin D therapy and cardiac structure and function in patients with chronic kidney disease: the PRIMO randomized controlled trial. JAMA. 2012;307(7):674–84.

29. Wang AY, Fang F, Chan J, Wen YY, Qing S, Chan IH, Lo G, Lai KN, Lo WK, Lam CW, Yu CM. Effect of paricalcitol on left ventricular mass and function in CKD – the OPERA trial. J Am Soc Nephrol. 2014;25(1):175–86.

30. Tamez H, Zoccali C, Packham D, Wenger J, Bhan I, Appelbaum E, Pritchett Y, Chang Y, Agarwal R, Wanner C, Lloyd-Jones D, Cannata J, Thompson BT, Andress D, Zhang W, Singh B, Zehnder D, Pachika A, Manning WJ, Shah A, Solomon SD, Thadhani R. Vitamin D reduces left atrial volume in patients with left ventricular hypertrophy and chronic kidney disease. Am Heart J. 2012;164(6):902–9.e2.

31. Tsang TS, Barnes ME, Gersh BJ, Bailey KR, Seward JB. Left atrial volume as a morphophysiologic expression of left ventricular diastolic dysfunction and relation to cardiovascular risk burden. Am J Cardiol. 2002;90(12):1284–9.

32. Patel RK, Jardine AG, Mark PB, Cunningham AF, Steedman T, Powell JR, McQuarrie EP, Stevens KK, Dargie HJ, Jardine AG. Association of left atrial volume with mortality among ESRD patients with left ventricular hypertrophy referred for kidney transplantation. Am J Kidney Dis. 2010;55(6):1088–96.

33. Sprague SM, Llach F, Amdahl M, Taccetta C, Batlle D. Paricalcitol versus calcitriol in the treatment of secondary hyperparathyroidism. Kidney Int. 2003;63(4):1483–90.

34. Ong LM, Narayanan P, Goh HK, Manocha AB, Ghazali A, Omar M, Mohamad S, Goh BL, Shah S, Seman MR, Vaithilingam I, Ghazalli R, Rahmat K, Shaariah W, Ching CH, Oral Paricalcitol in ESRD Study Group. Randomized controlled trial to compare the efficacy and safety of oral paricalcitol with oral calcitriol in dialysis patients with secondary hyperparathyroidism. Nephrology (Carlton). 2013;18(3):194–200.

35. Fishbane S, Shapiro WB, Corry DB, Vicks SL, Roppolo M, Rappaport K, Ling X, Goodman WG, Turner S, Charytan C. Cinacalcet HCl and concurrent low-dose vitamin D improves treatment of secondary hyperparathyroidism in dialysis patients compared with vitamin D alone: the ACHIEVE study results. Clin J Am Soc Nephrol. 2008;3(6):1718–25.
36. Ketteler M, Martin KJ, Cozzolino M, Goldsmith D, Sharma A, Khan S, Dumas E, Amdahl M, Marx S, Audhya P. Paricalcitol versus cinacalcet plus low-dose vitamin D for the treatment of secondary hyperparathyroidism in patients receiving haemodialysis: study design and baseline characteristics of the IMPACT SHPT study. Nephrol Dial Transplant. 2012;27(5):1942–9.
37. Ketteler M, Martin KJ, Wolf M, Amdahl M, Cozzolino M, Goldsmith D, Sharma A, Marx S, Khan S. Paricalcitol versus cinacalcet plus low-dose vitamin D therapy for the treatment of secondary hyperparathyroidism in patients receiving haemodialysis: results of the IMPACT SHPT study. Nephrol Dial Transplant. 2012;27(8):3270–8.
38. Cozzolino M, Ketteler M, Martin KJ, Sharma A, Goldsmith D, Khan S. Paricalcitol- or cinacalcet-centred therapy affects markers of bone mineral disease in patients with secondary hyperparathyroidism receiving haemodialysis: results of the IMPACT-SHPT study. Nephrol Dial Transplant. 2014;29(4):899–905.

Chapter 31
Interaction Between Vitamin D and Calcimimetics in Chronic Kidney Disease

Sandro Mazzaferro, Lida Tartaglione, Silverio Rotondi, and Marzia Pasquali

Abstract For many years vitamin D has been the only available drug to suppress parathyroid hormone (PTH) hypersecretion in patients with renal insufficiency. This effect is accomplished directly through activation of the vitamin D receptor (VDR) on parathyroid cells. However, vitamin D also stimulates intestinal absorption of calcium and phosphate, thus often resulting in hypercalcemia and hyperphosphatemia, both undesirable in renal patients. For this reason vitamin D analogs with less calcemic effects have been developed, with some improvement of this problematic effect. The discovery of calcium sensing receptor (CaSR) and the subsequent production of drugs capable of stimulating it, has allowed the introduction of calcimimetics as an alternative therapy to vitamin D. Cinacalcet, the first to be available for clinical uses, has been successfully employed to reduce serum PTH levels in patients with end stage renal disease. At variance with vitamin D, calcimimetics, while decreasing PTH, also decrease serum levels of calcium and phosphate. The effect on serum calcium is of such entity that symptomatic hypocalcemia may occur. As a consequence, vitamin D is frequently associated and instead of becoming an alternative, cinacalcet is mostly prescribed together with vitamin D. Importantly, we have clear experimental evidence that vitamin D administration increases the expression of CaSR on target cells and that, reciprocally, calcimimetics increase VDR expression. This interaction allows presuming potential clinical advantages to control secondary hyperparathyroidism. Further, since both VDR and CaSR are expressed also in tissues not involved with mineral metabolism, other still unpredicted clinical effects are possible.

Keywords Chronic Kidney Disease Mineral Bone Disorders (CKD-MBD) • Vitamin D • Vitamin D analogs • Paricalcitol • Calcimimetic • Cinacalcet • Secondary hyperparathyroidism • Chronic renal failure • Dialysis • Parathyroid hormone • Fibroblast growth factor 23

S. Mazzaferro (✉)
Department of Cardiovascular, Respiratory Nephrologic Anesthetic and Geriatric Sciences, Sapienza University, Nephrology and Dialysis Unit, Policlinico Umberto I, Rome, Italy
e-mail: sandro.mazzaferro@uniroma1.it

L. Tartaglione, MD • S. Rotondi, MD • M. Pasquali, MD, PhD
Department of Cardiovascular, Respiratory, Nephrologic and Geriatric Sciences,
Sapienza University of Rome, Rome, Italy

© Springer International Publishing Switzerland 2016
P.A. Ureña Torres et al. (eds.), *Vitamin D in Chronic Kidney Disease*,
DOI 10.1007/978-3-319-32507-1_31

31.1   Introduction

Vitamin D is the emblematic compound that fixes calcium into bone. However, the appreciation that its specific receptor is widely distributed in human tissues and that numerous different cell types can synthesize its active metabolites (pointing to auto- and/or paracrine actions), gives biologic plausibility to the so-called "pleiotropic effects" of vitamin D. We can better understand the biologic complexity of this vitamin considering that it is a very old and dynamic molecule. Evolution from a defensive-anti-inflammatory compound into a sophisticated endocrine system (the vitamin D endocrine system) deeply involved with both energy and extracellular mineral metabolism is now envisaged [1]. The potential clinical uses of vitamin D are numerous and the industry tries to synthesize vitamin D analog drugs to be employed for several different human diseases as different as infection, cancer or diabetic nephropathy. While the therapeutic use of vitamin D and of some analogues is now established to treat bone diseases like osteoporosis, rickets/osteomalacia and renal osteodystrophy, the molecular mechanisms of action of vitamin D are under evaluation in every possible detail aiming at recognizing further therapeutic indications. Interaction with others drugs obviously represent a further field of research.

Aim of this chapter is to recapitulate the interactions between vitamin D and calcimimetics in particular in chronic renal failure. Before examining the interactions, we will briefly recapitulate characteristics of the calcium sensing receptor (CaSR) and the properties of the compounds capable to stimulate it (calcimimetics). We will not examine vitamin D receptor or vitamin D metabolites, since they are widely described in other chapters of this book.

31.2   CaSR: Generalities and Mechanism of Action

31.2.1   Identification of CaSR

For many years calcium has been considered a simple divalent ion involved with mineral metabolism, and as such devoid of any regulatory role on intestinal and/or renal calcium transport. We knew that its extracellular concentration was maintained within a very narrow range thanks to a sensitive homeostatic mechanism involving kidney, intestine and bone [2]. We also knew that parathyroid glands secrete their hormone (parathyroid hormone, PTH) strictly dependent on extracellular calcium shifts, as illustrated by the inverse sigmoidal relationship existing between serum calcium and PTH in vitro and in vivo [3, 4]. All of this knowledge allowed hypothesizing the existence of a mechanism by which cells involved with calcium homeostasis could sense calcium concentrations. In fact, in 1993 Brown et al. [5] isolated and cloned a 5.3 kilobase DNA sequence encoding a protein described as the bovine parathyroid calcium receptor (BoPCaR). Soon after, the presence of such calcium sensing receptor (CaSR) was demonstrated in human parathyroid cells [6], thus proving the hypothesis that cells can sense calcium (Ca) concentration. Accordingly, we must now regard Ca ions not only as second intracellular messengers of cell communications but also as a first messenger, with hormone-like properties.

31.2.2 Structure of Human CaSR, Activators and Signal Transduction Pathways

CaSR is present in humans and in all vertebrates. Importantly, a high similarity of the amino acid sequences (>90%) is evident among different species, suggesting that this gene has a common ancestral origin and is evolutionarily conserved. Surprisingly, a CaSR gene is detectable also in animals without parathyroid glands (e.g. sharks) [7]. In these animals, CaSR can be found in kidney tubules and other osmoregulatory tissues (like rectal gland, intestine, stomach and olfactory epithelia) and this suggests that a salinity sensor role is possible besides that of calcium ion regulator [8]. Anyhow, CaSR is the major sensor involved with blood calcium levels control. It is a member of the G-protein coupled receptors (GPCR) family, in particular of the C group. The family includes several receptors (like metabotropic glutamate receptors and gamma-aminobutyric acid (GABA) type B receptors), which share at least 20% of their amino-acid sequence in the transmembrane domain [9].

Human CaSR structure shows a large 612 amino acid extracellular domain (ECD), a seven-helices transmembrane domain (TMD) and a carboxy-terminal, at last 216 amino-acid long, intracellular domain. Following intracellular synthesis, in the endoplasmatic reticulum, CaSR molecules homodimerize through two disulfide bonds involving cysteine 129 and 131 residues within each monomer [10]. Dimerization is essential for biologic activity and occurs even in the absence of disulfide bonds and in fact non-covalent dimers are present in the cell surface. Moreover, CaSR extracellular domain has nine potential sites of N-glycosylation, required for the normal expression of the receptor on cell surface [11]. The fully glycosylated protein has a MW of 150–160 KDa. In the biologically active form each monomer has two lobes (LB1 and LB2) separated by a cleft delineating the ligand-binding domain named "Venus flytrap" (VFT) [12]. The VFT contains five calcium-binding sites [12] located on the protein surface and characterized by clusters of neutral or negatively charged amino acids. Calcium ions bind to these specific sites to determine an inward bending of the two lobes and their final closure, with VFT rotation and the eventual activation of the receptor [13] (Fig. 31.1).

Notably, besides Ca ions also other molecules activate CaSR. Among cations, we find inorganic di- and trivalent ions (Mg^{2+}, Sr^{2+}, La^{3+}, Gd^{3+}) and organic compounds such as polyamines (spermine), aminoglycosides and other amino acids or peptides (polyarginine) [14]. All of these agonists bind the ligand site in the ECD and directly activate the receptor, even in the absence of Ca ions. These directly acting non-calcium dependent activators are termed type I agonists. Type I CaSR agonists include Ca ions

EXTRACELLULAR SPACE

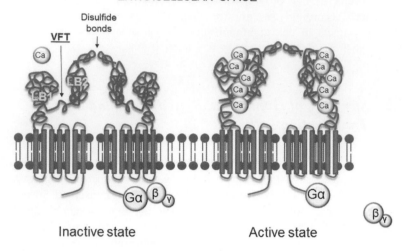

Fig. 31.1 Calcium sensing receptor structure: In the biologically inactive form (shown to the *left*) each monomer has two lobes (*LB1* and *LB2*) separated by a cleft delineating the ligand-binding domain named "Venus flytrap" (*VFT*). The VFT contains five calcium binding sites. When calcium ions bind to these specific sites (*right side* of the figure) determine an inward bending of the two lobes and their final closure, with VFT rotation and the eventual activation of G protein

as the ones with highest affinity. At variance, type II agonists require the presence of extracellular Ca ions to be active. As described later, type II agonists include pharmacological allosteric modulators of CaSR and several L-amino acids (Table 31.1).

Once bound to its receptor, calcium activates the G protein coupled pathway. The G-protein is bound to the inner surface of the cell membrane and consist of three subunits: Gα, Gβ and Gγ [15]. When the receptor is inactive, subunit Gα binds Guanosine Diphosphate (GDP). Following activation, a conformational change occurs in the receptor that leads to the exchange of GDP for Guanosine Triphosphate (GTP), thus facilitating dissociation of the Gα subunit from the Gβγ dimer. Both Gα and Gβγ dimer activate second messenger proteins that are capable of modulating cellular secretion, proliferation, differentiation, apoptosis and gene expression. Specifically, among the different subunits, CaSR couples with $G\alpha_{i/0}$ and $G\alpha_{q/11}$ proteins and possibly with $G\alpha_{12/13}$ [10, 16, 17].

Intracellular signaling activated by these three different Gα proteins leads respectively to decreased cAMP accumulation ($G\alpha_i$), activation of phospholipase C (PLC) with secondary generation of diacylglycerol and inositol triphosphate $IP_3(G\alpha_{q/11})$ and finally activation of Rho kinase ($G\alpha_{12/13}$) [16–18]. This, in turn, is associated with activation of several intracellular signaling systems, among which the most important is the initiation of mitogen activated protein kinases (MAPKs) such as extracellular signal-regulated kinases (ERK) 1 and 2, p38 MAPK and c-Jun N-terminal kinase (JNK) [19]. Of these MAPK pathways, the ERK/MAPK

Table 31.1 Orthosteric and allosteric modulators of CaSR

CaSR activators	
Orthosteric activators (calcimimetic type I)	Allosteric activators (calcimimetic type II)
Cations	Aromatic L aminoacids
Magnesium	L-phenylalanine
Lanthanum	L-tryptophane
Gadolinium	L-tyrosine
Aluminum	L-histidine
Barium	
Cadmium	
Nickel	
Cobalt	
Iron	
Polyamines	Drugs
Spermine,	Fendiline
Exaciclina	NPS R-568
Polylysine	NPS R-467
Polyarginine	AMG 073
Protamine	AMG 416
Aminoglycoside	
Neomycin	
Gentamicin	
Tobramycin	

Abbreviations: *CaSR* calcium-sensing receptor

subfamily is particularly important since it controls cell proliferation. Activation of ERK-1 and -2 is considered relevant for CaSR-mediated suppression of parathyroid cells proliferation and secretion.

31.2.3   CaSR Expression and Modulation in Tissues Involved with Mineral Metabolism

In humans CaSR is not only essential in maintaining calcium homeostasis but also in regulating several calcium-dependent secretion of different hormones, like adrenocorticotropic hormone (ACTH), growth hormone (GH), insulin, glucagon [20–22]. It is commonly recognized that CaSR is expressed not only in organs involved in mineral metabolism (kidney, intestine, bone and parathyroid glands) but also in many other organs like skin, stomach, colon, brain cells, pancreas. Table 31.2 shows the different tissues in which CaSR is expressed and its physiological role.

Mechanisms that modulate CaSR gene expression under different physiological or pathological conditions are not fully understood. We will briefly examine CaSR expression and actions in tissues involved with mineral metabolism.

31.2.3.1 CaSR and Parathyroid Glands

Under physiological conditions, high calcium inhibits PTH secretion, PTH gene expression and parathyroid cell proliferation; also it stimulates PTH molecule degradation. Studies on CaSR activators have shown that the secretion of PTH is strictly regulated by CaSR, and that activation of the receptor rapidly (few minutes) leads to inhibition of PTH secretion, both in vitro and in vivo [13]. This action is too fast to be dependent on the reduction PTH synthesis or degradation and is demonstrated to be linked to inhibition of the exocytosis process [23]. Moreover, CaSR activators

Table 31.2 Tissues in which CaSR is expressed and its physiological role

	Tissue	Cells type	Physiological role
Involved in Ca homeostasis	Parathyroid glands	Parathyroid cells	Inhibits PTH secretion
			Inhibits PTH gene expression
			Reduces parathyroid cellular proliferation
			Degrades active PTH
			Stimulates VDR expression
	Thyroid gland	C cells	Stimulates calcitonin secretion
			Stimulates calcitonin gene expression
	Kidney	PT cells	Decreases 1-alpha-hydroxylase activity and 1,25-dyhidroxyvitamin D synthesis (through VDR)
		cTAL cells	Inhibits paracellular calcium reabsorption
		DCT cells	Stimulates activity of TRPV5 and reabsorption of calcium
	Bone	Osteoclasts	Inhibits osteoclast-like cells formation
			Inhibits osteoclast activity and stimulate apoptosis
		Osteoblasts	Promotes proliferation, mineralization and expression of osteoblast differentiation markers
	Intestine	Enterocytes	Stimulates TRPV6 and calbindin expression only in
			VDR $^{-/-}$ / 1-Alpha $^{-/-}$ transgenic animals

Table 31.2 (continued)

Uninvolved in Ca homeostasis	Stomach	G cells	Stimulates gastrin secretion
		Parietal cells	Increases acid secretion through apical H$^+$-K$^+$-ATPase
	Small and large intestine	Crypt cells	Inhibits of intestinal fluid transport
		Smooth muscle nerve plexuses	Stimulates colon motility
		Colonic mucosa	Cell proliferation and differentiation
	Skin	Keratinocytes	Stimulates growth and differentiation
	Pancreas	Alpha cells	Inhibits glucagon secretion
		Beta cells	Stimulates insulin secretion
	Pituitary	Pituitary cells	Stimulates ACTH secretion
			Stimulates growth hormone secretion
	Kidney	Principal cells of the collecting duct	Attenuates AVP-induced AQP2 expression
		cTAL	Inhibits NaCl reabsorption directly through NKCC2 and indirectly through ROMK

CaSR calcium-sensing receptor, *VDR* vitamin D receptor, *PT* Proximal tubule, *cTAL* cortical thick ascending limb, *DCT* distal convolute tubule, *TRPV5* transient receptor potential cation channel subfamily V member 5, *AVP* arginine vasopressin, *AQP2* aquaporin-2, *NKCC2* Na$^+$ K$^+$ 2Cl$^-$ cotransporter, *ROMK* renal outer medullary K$^+$ channel

stimulate degradation of active PTH into its inactive and smaller fragments (e.g. PTH 7–84, PTH 35–84, PTH 1–34, and others) [24], but are also involved with reduction of transcription processes [25]. Studies in patients with inactivating mutations of CaSR and in CaSR gene knock-out mice [26, 27] strongly support the importance of CaSR in the regulation of parathyroid cellular proliferation: in both of these conditions, despite high calcium levels, polyclonal proliferation of parathyroid cell is increased.

In other pathological conditions, such as primary or secondary hyperparathyroidism (SHPT), CaSR expression in parathyroid cells is reduced [28, 29]. Interestingly, in experimental models of SHPT, down-regulation of CaSR occurs only after the development of hyperplasia [30] suggesting that the reduction is secondary to proliferation rather than to the primary cause. Anyhow, the observed reduction in CaSR is expected to lead to an increase of ionized Ca set point, which is a common finding in patients with uremic SHPT. Slatopolsky et al. [31] showed that high dietary calcium inhibits parathyroid growth in uremic rats. However, neither serum calcium increments nor administration of CaSR activators, do invariably result into an up-regulation of CaSR [32–34]. Therefore, the link between serum Ca and/or administration of CaSR activators and the expression of the receptor on parathyroid cells is not fully understood. At variance, all available studies in vitro and in vivo, invariably show that 1,25-dyhidroxyvitamin D3 administration increases the expression of CaSR in parathyroid cells [35]. Canaff et al. identified transcriptional promoters of the human CaSR gene and demonstrated the presence of Vitamin D Response Elements in these promoters [36]. Thus, $1,25(OH)_2D_3$ in the regulation of PTH secretion.

31.2.3.2 CaSR and Kidney

In 1995 CaSR was cloned from human kidney [37] and immunohistochemical studies showed large expression in the medullary and cortical parts of the Henle's loop thick ascending limb [38, 39]. Furthermore, CaSR expression was described in proximal convoluted tubule (PCT), distal convoluted tubule (DCT) and cortical collecting ducts (CCD) [40].

In proximal tubule, CaSR regulates activity of 1α-hydroxylase, the key enzyme involved with $1,25(OH)_2D_3$ synthesis. It is now evident that the inhibitory role of hypercalcemia on this enzyme and on the synthesis of $1,25(OH)_2D_3$ is direct and mediated by CaSR activation[41]. In fact, CaSR activation up regulates VDR expression, which in turn decreases 1α-hydroxylase activity and 1,25D synthesis [42]. Moreover, $1,25(OH)_2D_3$ increases CaSR expression in the kidney [36] further indicating the tight connection between CaSR and vitamin D.

CaSR expression in other segments of the kidney tubule is implicated in the modulation of several transepithelial transporters like Na/K ATP-ase [43], apical K channel [44], aquaporin expression [45] and transient receptor potential vanilloid member 5 (TRPV5) [46]. In particular, in the proximal tubule CaSR inhibits paracellular Ca transport, while in distal tubule it up-regulates TRPV5 thus favoring calcium reabsorption. Notably, TRPV5 expression in distal tubule is also increased by $1,25(OH)_2D_3$ through VDR activation [47]. It is interesting noticing that in different segments of the nephrons CaSR can be expressed either in the apical or basolateral portion of the tubular cells. In this way in different segments of the nephron CaSR activation may increase either resorption or secretion.

31.2.3.3 CaSR and Bone

Although not invariably, CaSR expression has been described in bone cells. Among cells of the osteoclast lineage, it seems to be expressed in osteoclast precursors [48], in multinucleated pre-osteoclasts and in mature osteoclasts [49]. In in-vitro studies, both high calcium levels and calcimimetics inhibit osteoclast-like cells formation, suggesting a modulatory role for the receptor [50]. Further, high levels of calcium inhibit osteoclast activity and stimulate apoptosis in vitro [48]. In vivo studies are thus warranted to better define the role of CaSR on bone resorption and osteoclastogenesis. Among cells of the osteoblastic lineage expressing CaSR, high calcium levels promote proliferation [51], mineralization [52] and expression of osteoblast differentiation markers such as osteocalcin, osteoprotegerin and collagen type I. Moreover, mice with selective knock-out of CaSR exon 7 in osteoblasts, show poor skeletal development, reduced mineralization and die within 3 weeks of birth [53]. Thus a role for CaSR in osteoblasts biology seems evident.

31.2.3.4 Factors Involved with CaSR Expression

As outlined in previous paragraphs, there is a significant relationship between parathyroid CaSR expression and serum levels of calcium and/or vitamin D. Clinical evidence is nonetheless available suggesting that also other factors may affect CaSR expression and function.

Patients with inflammatory disease, severe sepsis or brain injury experiment hypocalcemia generically referred to peripheral resistance to PTH and/or reduced PTH secretion [54]. Experimental studies show that interleukin 1β (IL-1β) increase CaSR expression in bovine parathyroid gland [55] and reduce serum PTH levels thus becoming a possible explanation for inflammation related hypocalcemia. By analogy, in rats, intraperitoneal injection of IL-1β increases CaSR expression in parathyroid, thyroid, and kidney [56]. Moreover Carlstedt et al. [57] showed *in* bovine parathyroid cells that IL-6 decreases PTH secretion. Canaff et al. demonstrated that IL-1β and IL-6 bind to the promoter of CaSR gene up-regulating its expression [56].

In addition, hyperphosphatemia has been claimed to exert a regulatory role on CaSR expression. In experimental SHPT, rats fed high phosphorus diet show reduced CaSR expression in parathyroid glands [58]; when switched to a low phosphate diet, CaSR expression increases and parathyroid cell proliferation is restored [59]. However, up-regulation of CaSR seems to occur only after reduction of parathyroid cell proliferation, suggesting that CaSR expression is more strictly linked to proliferation rate than to phosphorous intake.

31.3 Ca-Mimetics: Generalities and Types

As described previously, the CaSR has three major domains: a large extracellular portion (N-terminal), a seven transmembrane domain and an intracellular domain (C-terminal) (Fig. 31.1). Accordingly, it is possible that substances activating this receptor can bind to different portions of the molecule. In particular, those that bind the N-terminal portion of the receptor directly activate it and are called orthosteric or type I calcimimetics (CaM). Other substances that bind to the transmembrane portion and modify the sensitivity of the receptor to natural activators are called indirect allosteric, or type II CaSR activators. It might be useful to underline that the latter substances require the presence of natural activators, like Ca ions, to activate the receptor [60].

31.3.1   Orthosteric CaSR Activators (Type I, or Direct)

The first and most important orthosteric CaSR activator is, of course, ionized calcium (Ca^{2+}). This divalent ion directly binds the extracellular portion of the receptor to activate it [12]. Experimental in vitro studies with Human Embryonic Kidney cells (HEK) expressing a modified CaSR, deprived of the extra- and intra- cellular domains demonstrate that Ca^{2+} ions can still activate the intracellular Ca-signaling pathway, pointing to the peculiarity of this receptor and, eventually, to the importance of the transmembrane domain [13].

Other direct activators of CaSR with different activating ability include: Mg, Be, Ba, Sr, La, Gd and a list of organic polycations (spermine, exacyclin, polylysine, polyarginine, protamine, neomycin and gentamycin) (Table 31.1). Among these, magnesium and aminoglycoside antibiotics may have special clinical interest.

31.3.2   Magnesium

In experimental studies, magnesium directly binds and activates CaSR [11] on different cell types such as parathyroid and renal tubular cells. The link between Mg and CaSR could however be considered of limited clinical relevance since ionized Mg concentrations are definitely lower than that of Ca. However, in patients with inactivating mutation of CaSR, like Familial hypocalciuric hypercalcemia and Neonatal Severe Primary Hyperparathyroidism, hypercalcemia associates with hypermagnesemia, pointing to a significant role of the receptor in the physiologic regulation of Mg [61].

Further, in experimental severe hypomagnesemia the correlation between Mg and CaSR activity becomes inverse (lower Mg levels resulting in increased activity of CaSR) [62], possibly secondary to the reduction of the inhibitory role of intracellular Mg on the activity of the heterotrimeric G proteins. Therefore, the link between Mg and CaSR seems to involve also the intracellular magnesium fraction [62–64].

31.3.3   Aminoglycoside Antibiotics

Neomycin, gentamycin, and tobramycin (Fig. 31.2) are able to directly activate the CaSR in proportion to the number of amino groups present in their structure (five for gentamicin, and tobramycin, six for neomycin) [65]. Activation of CaSR by these antibiotics has a possible role in their nephrotoxicity. In vitro studies demonstrated that activation of CaSR by gentamycin in renal tubular cells involves the intracellular MAP-kinase pathway, which in turn promotes cell apoptosis [66].

Orthosteric or direct CaSR activators

Ions

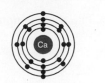

Aminoglycoside antibiotics

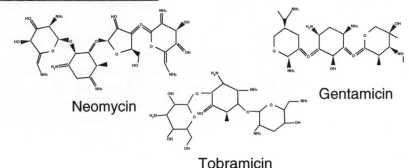

Neomycin

Gentamicin

Tobramicin

Allosteric or indirect CaSR activators

Aromatic L amino acids.

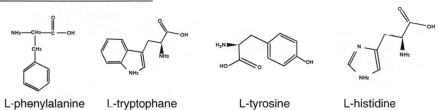

L-phenylalanine   L-tryptophane   L-tyrosine   L-histidine

Specific drugs

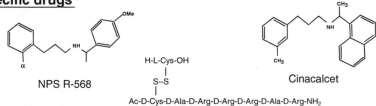

NPS R-568

H-L-Cys-OH
|
S--S
|
Ac-D-Cys-D-Ala-D-Arg-D-Arg-D-Arg-D-Ala-D-Arg-NH₂

Cinacalcet

AMG 416

Fig. 31.2 CaSR activators. *Top* Orthostatic or direct CaSR activators. *Bottom* Allosteric or indirect CaSR activators

31.3.4   Allosteric (or Indirect) CaSR Activators (Type II)

Allosteric modulators of CaSR can be divided into natural (aromatic amino acids), and artificial or pharmacologic.

31.3.4.1   Aromatic L Amino Acids

Aromatic L-amino acids with an allosteric modulation activity on CaSR include L-Phenylalanine, L-Tryptophan, L-Tyrosine, and L-Histidine (Fig. 31.2) [67]. Also, other non-aromatic amino acids (e.g. L-Leucine and poly L-Arginine) can bind the CaSR [68] and this points to the relationship between amino acids and calcium metabolism. Diets rich in aromatic L-amino acid lead to increased urinary calcium [69] while low amino acid diets promote the development of SHPT [70]. Also, in the gastrointestinal system, amino acids regulate gastric acid and cholecystokinin secretion through activation of intestinal CaSR [68, 70, 71].

31.3.4.2   Pharmacological Modulation

Small organic compounds with similarities to aromatic amino acids (aromatic ring and positive charges) are the drugs for pharmacologic activation of CaSR. These type II calcimimetic drugs increase the sensitivity of the receptor to orthosteric activators and thus require the presence of Ca to be active. Fendiline, which is characterized by the presence of a phenethyl group (C6H5CH2CH2), was among the first drugs with evident CaSR activation properties (Fig. 31.2). Starting from the structure of this small organic compound other more selective compounds were synthesized and dubbed CaM. The R enantiomer of these compounds binds the transmembrane portion of the CaSR, probably at the sixth and seventh transmembrane segments. The eventual change in the N terminal portion results in an increased sensitivity of the receptor to calcium [72].

31.3.5   R-568

R-568 (Fig. 31.2) is the first calcimimetic drug subjected to experimental and clinical research. It was capable of reducing PTH secretion and parathyroid cell proliferation with improvement of bone turnover in animal models of SHPT. When tested in hemodialysis patients with SHPT [73], R-568 improved mineral metabolism but with a remarkable pharmacokinetic variability, which required significantly different doses and time-schedules to get adequate blood concentrations. Accordingly, the drug was excluded from further clinical research.

The second calcimimetic drug developed for clinical uses is AMG-073 (Cinacalcet) (Fig. 31.2) **AMG-073** is the R-enantiomer of a small organic compound with an aromatic ring. After oral administration, its bioavailability is high (>74 %) and the absorbed drug is highly protein bound (more than 95 %). Its metabolism occurs through hepatic and renal cytochromes (CYP1A2 and CYP3A4) with a relative clearance of roughly 30 and 50 %. Increasing oral test dose evidenced a close relationship between administered dose, Cmax and AUC0-24. In front of a wide inter-individual variability of pharmacokinetic parameters, a positive relationship exists between reached C-max and suppressive effect on PTH [74].

By modulating CaSR, Cinacalcet reduces PTH secretion and proliferation in normal ad uremic parathyroid glands [75]. Moreover, it increases the expression of CaSR and VDR on parathyroid cells in both normal and uremic models [76]. These experimental evidences have found clinic confirmation in human parathyroid from uremic patients [77]. Moreover, recent evidence suggests that CaM might increase parathyroid cells apoptosis in humans [78]. On practice, CaM is a powerful suppressor of PTH secretion in HD patients with SHPT [73, 79–81].

Besides PTH mediated effects, CaSR modulators could also exert direct effects on bone cells. CaM had, a direct regulatory role on osteoclast proliferation in experimental conditions and reduced FGF23 serum levels in hemodialysis (HD) patients possibly through a direct effect on bone [82, 83]. Recent data from the BONAFIDE study report improvement of renal osteodystrophy (biopsy parameters of bone turnover), in HD patients treated with cinacalcet [84]. Furthermore, CaM could have a direct effect on vascular calcification in chronic kidney disease (CKD). Cultured vascular smooth muscle cells (VSMCs) exposed to variable concentrations of calcium and phosphate in the medium showed reduced calcification in the presence of CaM [85]. This evidence was confirmed in uremic rats where the use of Cinacalcet reduced the development of vascular calcification [86]. Importantly, experimental in vitro studies suggest that reduced expression of CaSR at the levels of vessel walls is associated with increased calcification. Treatment with CaM, by increasing expression of CaSR, could be relevant for prevention of vascular calcification [87].

Clinical use of Cinacalcet is univocally associated with improved PTH control in HD patients [73, 79–81]. Typically, however some significant side effects occur like nausea, vomiting and diarrhea, which represent a major cause of non-compliance and discontinuation of treatment. These side effects are considered to be related to direct effects of the drug on gastric acid secretion and on activation of CaSR in the central nervous system [88].

31.3.6   AMG-416

Etelcalcetide is the third calcimimetic available for clinical use, whose formulation allows intravenous administration. Its eight amino acids chain is characterized by a disulfide bond (Fig. 31.2). At variance with Cinacalcet, AMG-416 has been shown to exert some direct stimulatory effects on CaSR even in the absence of Ca ions [89].

In phase 1 studies in healthy subjects, administration of i.v. AMG-416 significantly reduced serum PTH levels after only 30 min, with a clear dose dependency [90]. With a half-life of 18–20 h, a clearance of 5–8 L/h and a distribution volume of 112–115 L it is expected to have a longer biological action as compared to Cinacalcet. Half-life increases in mouse models of CRF with evidence of reduced PTH secretion and parathyroid gland hyperplasia. Also, during therapy, CaSR and VDR expression is increased in parathyroid cells. In addition since, serum FGF23 levels are lower in treated animals, a possible role on bone cell is suggested. In patients on HD, half-life of the drug increases up to 3–7 days [91, 92] according to the different doses employed. Eventually, serum PTH levels show a proportional reduction. In the study by Bell [92], which enrolled a limited number of subjects, Etelcalcetide reduced PTH levels by 49.4 % and 33.0 % respectively as compared to basal values, with i.v. boluses of 5 and 10 mg administered thrice weekly at the end of dialysis. Serum levels of Ca dropped, thus resulting in higher doses of vitamin D and/or increased prescription of Ca based phosphate binders. Prevalence of gastrointestinal (GI) side effects is similar to oral formulation, similarly to hypocalcemia, which occurs without evidence of ECG modifications [92]. No study is available to compare prevalence of side effects with oral and i.v. calcimimetic.

31.4   Interactions Between Vitamin D and Ca-Mimetics in CKD

As illustrated in Table 31.3, different types of organs and cells, not necessarily involved with mineral homeostasis, share VDR and CaSR. Further, we know that vitamin D administration can increase the expression of CaSR [34] and that, reciprocally, CaSR activation by Ca or calcimimetics can increase VDR expression [33]. The interaction and the relative homeostatic functions of these two receptors have been explored in different experimental conditions involving transgenic animals with conditional knockouts aiming at deciphering the specific physiologic role at the level of parathyroid, kidney, intestine and bone. Also, functional interactions have been explored in keratinocytes and colon cells, where activation of these two receptors regulates cell proliferation and differentiation, with potential clinical implications. It seems in general that at cellular level VDR and CaSR can have synergistic or antagonistic effects [93].

With these premises, possible therapeutic interactions have been searched for Vitamin D and Calcimimetics in experimental uremia, where the two drugs can be successfully employed to treat SHPT. In uremic rats vitamin D therapy (with calcitriol in particular) not only suppresses PTH but also increases extra-osseous calcifications, progression of renal insufficiency and mortality [94]. Importantly, these undesirable effects can be significantly reduced by co-administration of calcimimetics [95]. These results suggest that administering vitamin D (active natural or analogs) together with calcimimetic can not only improve biochemical control of SHPT, but also improve other hard outcomes like progression of renal failure and mortality. In this context, it is interesting the study by Mary et al. [96] in which

Table 31.3 Tissue expression of VDR and CaSR

Organ/tissue/system		CaSR	VDR
Endocrine	Parathyroid	+	+
	Pancreas	+	+
	Thyroid C-cells	+	+
Renal	Juxtaglomerular cells	+	+
	Tubules	+	+
Bone	Osteoblast	+	+
	Osteoclast	+	+
	Chodrocytes	+	+
Cardiovascular	Heart	+	+
	Smooth muscle cells	+	+
Gastrointestinal	Esophagus	−	+
	Stomach	+	+
	Intestine	+	+
	Colon	+	+
	Liver parenchyma cells	−	+
Reproductive	Testis	−	+
	Ovary	−	+
	Placenta	+	+
	Uterus	−	+
	Endometrium	−	+
Immune	Thymus	−	+
	Bone marrow	+	+
	B cells	−	+
	T cells	−	+
	Monocytes	+	−
	Macrophages	+	−
Epidermis	Skin	+	+
	Breast	+	+
	Hair follicles	−	+
Central nervous system	Brain	+	+

+: expression; −: absent

Abbreviations: VDR vitamin receptor, *CaSR* calcium-sensing receptor

human vascular smooth muscle cells have been exposed to increasing concentrations of calcitriol (0.01–10 nmol/L) in non-calcifying (1.8 mmol/L) or pro-calcifying Ca++ conditions (5.0 mmol/L). A significant increase in CaSR expression was evident after 48 h with calcitriol concentrations within 0.5 and 5 nmol/L, (with maximum effect at 1 nmol/L) and no effect with lower or even higher concentrations. Importantly, in pro-calcifying milieu, vitamin D blocked the Ca-induced decrease in CaSR expression and protected against mineralization. It is thus suggested that nanomolar concentrations of $1,25(OH)_2D_3$ induce a CaSR-dependent protection against vascular calcifications. Indeed, the protective role of increased CaSR expression on vascular calcifications has been evidenced in other studies [87]. There is thus experimental evidence that vitamin D and calcimimetic, by modulating expression of their receptors can improve not only the biochemical control of SHPT, but also other systemic clinical outcomes.

In patients with end stage renal disease active vitamin D compounds and Cinacalcet (currently the only available calcimimetic for clinical uses) are both successfully administered to inhibit PTH hypersecretion. However, while Vitamin D compounds dose dependently increase serum levels of calcium and phosphate, Cinacalcet simultaneously decrease serum levels of these two ions. Whether there are reasons to prefer calcimimetics to active vitamin D derivatives and whether combined administration offers advantages compared with any of the two administered alone is still an open question. Obviously, besides biochemical effects, it is the impact of these therapies alone or in combination on hard outcomes, like cardiovascular events and mortality, that deserves specific attention [97]. Vitamin D has been the only and most effective suppressive therapy of SHPT for years. Availability of Cinacalcet represented a new and possibly alternative suppressive therapy. However, on practical ground, the hypocalcemic effect of Cinacalcet almost invariably claimed for vitamin D administration and, as a consequence, the two drugs have been almost invariably employed together. In the absence of definitive evidence, examining the available studies in CRF patients, in which the two drugs have been described and tentatively compared, can be useful.

In the CONTROL study, 72 adult hemodialysis patients receiving the vitamin D analog paricalcitol (or an equipotent dose of an alternative active vitamin D derivative) at doses >6 mcg/week and who had SHPT controlled by this therapy (biointact PTH [biPTH] 80–160 pg/mL) but at the price of increased $Ca \times P$ product (>55 mg^2/dL^2), were enrolled. At the start of the study the dose of vitamin D derivatives was lowered to 6 ug/week and cinacalcet was introduced. During the study, which lasted 16 weeks, the starting dose of Cinacalcet (30 mg/day) could be titrated up to a maximum of 180 mg/day. At the end of the study the Kidney Disease Outcomes Quality Initiative (KDOQI) targets for biPTH (<150 pg/mL) and for $Ca \times P$ (<55 mg^2/dL^2) were achieved respectively in 85 % and 72 % of the patients, and both targets were achieved in 47 %. Therefore, this study underlines the usefulness of Cinacalcet to improve biochemical control in patients with already controlled SHPT [98].

In the OPTIMA study, at variance with previous study, enrolled patients had poorly controlled SHPT (intact PTH = 300–800 pg/mL). In this multicenter, open-label study, the efficacy of a cinacalcet-based regimen was compared with that of an unrestricted conventional strategy with vitamin D and phosphate binders. Primary end-point was achievement of the KDOQI targets. Patients were randomized to conventional care ($n=184$) or cinacalcet-based regimen ($n=368$). During the study doses of cinacalcet, vitamin D sterols, and phosphate binders were adjusted according to an algorithm allowing contemporary administration of cinacalcet and vitamin D. A higher proportion of patients receiving the cinacalcet-based regimen versus conventional care achieved the targets for PTH (71 % vs 22 %, respectively; $P<0.001$), $Ca \times P$ (77 versus 58 %, respectively; $P<0.001$), calcium (76 % versus 33 %, respectively; $P<0.001$) and phosphorus (63 % versus 50 %, respectively; $P<0.002$). In addition, a higher proportion of patients in the cinacalcet group simultaneously achieved target values of both PTH and Ca×P compared with the conventional care group (59% versus 16%, respectively; $P<0.001$). Most patients (65%) used cinacalcet doses of 60 mg/day or less with only 6% requiring the maximum allowed dose of 180 mg/day. At the end of the study there was an increased proportion of patients treated with vitamin D sterols in both the conventional care group (from 66 to 81%) and in the cinacalcet group (from 68 to 73%). On average, however, the doses of vitamin D employed were lower than baseline. Thus, the addition of cinacalcet to vitamin D therapy improved serum levels of iPTH in patients with poorly controlled SHPT and previous treatment failure with vitamin D alone. Importantly, the decrease in iPTH values obtained with cinacalcet was associated with reductions in calcium, phosphate and Ca × P product, consistent with other studies reporting on the clinical efficacy of Cinacalcet [81]. This study has been the first to directly compare the efficacy of cinacalcet with unrestricted conventional care in patients with poorly controlled SHPT. The clinical efficacy of a cinacalcet-based regimen in achieving the KDOQI targets is underlined also by the fact that these targets were attained with a lower dose of vitamin D sterols [99].

Aim of the ACHIEVE study was to compare two treatment strategies for achieving KDOQI biochemical targets in patients with mild SHPT. Enrolled patients were on hemodialysis, were receiving active vitamin D sterols and had intact PTH values within 150 and 800 pg/mL. Subjects were randomly assigned to either cinacalcet and low-dose vitamin D (Cinacalcet-D group) or flexible vitamin D alone (Flex-D group). After 33 weeks, as compared to the Flex-D group, a greater proportion of patients in the Cinacalcet-D group had a >30% reduction in PTH (68% versus 36%, $P<0.001$) as well as PTH <300 pg/mL (44% versus 23%, $P<0.006$). The advantage of adding cinacalcet to vitamin D for achieving KDOQI targets was again underlined [100].

Another study aiming at comparing vitamin D or Cinacalcet based therapy is the multicenter IMPACT-SHPT study, in which hemodialysis patients were enrolled if they had PTH values within 300 and 800 pg/mL, were not hypercalcemic and had only mild hyperphosphatemia. Treatment strategies were paricalcitol-centered or cinacalcet-centered. In the former, paricalcitol was dose-titrated to achieve biochemical targets and Cinacalcet could be added only in case of hypercalcemia. In the latter, a fixed low-dose of vitamin D was allowed, while cinacalcet was dose titrated. Dose adjustments were based on iPTH, calcium and Ca × P levels. Randomized patients (1:1 to either therapy) received an initial IV paricalcitol dose 0.07 μg/kg or an initial oral paricalcitol dose equal to iPTH/60 in the paricalcitol-centered therapy and a fixed-dose of IV doxercalciferol (1.0 μg three times a week) or of oral alfacalcidol (0.25 μg/day) in the cinacalcet-centered therapy. In this later group the initial oral cinacalcet dose was 30 mg/day. During an observation period of 28 weeks, only four patients (8%) receiving IV paricalcitol developed hypercalcaemia and required supplementary cinacalcet. No episode of hypercalcaemia was recorded in the paricalcitol-centered oral stratum. As a comparison, hypercalcemia in the paricalcitol group (calcium >10.5 mg/dL) was less frequent than hypocalcaemia (calcium <8.4 mg/dL) in the cinacalcet group (57,7% versus 32.7%, p=0.016 in the IV group, and 54.4% versus 43.4% in the oral group, p=0.260). Compared to cinacalcet-centered strategy, target iPTH levels (i.e. 150–300 pg/mL) were reached in a greater proportion of patients in the paricalcitol-centered treatment. Further, in the paricalcitol-centered group serum iPTH levels decreased from baseline and reached KDOQI targets more frequently than in the cinacalcet-centered group. Serum levels of calcium and phosphate remained constant with both treatments [101]. It seems therefore that the less calcemic vitamin D analog, paricalcitol, less frequently needs the help of calcimimetic, at least in patients with mild to moderate SHPT.

Data from this study have been examined in a post-hoc analysis aiming at evaluating more specifically the effects of the two therapies on biomarkers of bone cells activity: Alkaline Phosphatase (AP), Bone Alkaline Phosphatase (BALP) and FGF23 [102]. Interestingly, while both therapies significantly reduced circulating levels of AP and BALP – thus indicating a similar effect of reduction of bone turnover, paricalcitol treated patients showed significantly increased levels of FGF23, at variance with a trend to reduction in the cinacalcet group. Regrettably in this study no histologic nor radiologic evaluation of bone was done. Nonetheless, these contrasting results indicate that the mechanisms of action of the two drugs are different. Cinacalcet, by increasing sensitivity of CaSR to circulating calcium not only inhibits PTH synthesis by parathyroid glands [103] but also FGF23 production by osteocytes [104]. At variance, paricalcitol by activating VDRs in the same tissues, similarly inhibits parathyroid glands but at the same time activates the vitamin D response element located within the FGF23 promoter [105] thus enhancing its synthesis. Since increased levels of both AP [106] and FGF23 [107] are predictive of increased mortality in dialysis patients, we could guess that paricalcitol-centered therapy, by increasing FGF23, could worse prognosis in treated patients as compared to those receiving cinacalcet. However, paricalcitol therapy has been almost invariably associated with improved survival as compared to patients treated with calcitriol or not receiving vitamin D in large observational studies [108, 109]. Accordingly, further research is necessary to unravel the net clinical effect resulting from these therapies.

Recently, the PARADIGM study tried a more direct comparison of cinacalcet and vitamin D analogs as monotherapies to control PTH [110]. In a prospective, multicenter, open-label study 312 adult HD patients with PTH >450 pg/mL were randomized 1:1 to either cinacalcet (n = 155) or vitamin D analogs (n = 157). After 12 months the mean percent reduction of PTH was −12.1 % (−20.0 to −4.1 %) in the cinacalcet arm and −7.0 % (−14.9 to 0.8 %) in the vitamin D analog arm, with no significant difference (p = 0.35). Similarly not different were the percentages of patients reaching PTH values ≤300 pg/ml or the percentages of those experiencing a PTH reduction >30 %. Although there was evidence of local policies effect (greater response to cinacalcet compared with vitamin D analogs in non-United States participants), the conclusion is that the two drugs are similarly effective in controlling SHPT. Thus, the overall impression is that either cinacalcet or vitamin D analogs (paricalcitol in particular) can similarly improve biochemical control of SHPT in end-stage renal disease (ESRD). However, their association may be particularly useful in specific groups of patients (e.g. with more severe disease or challenging levels of divalent ions).

The potential positive effect of cinacalcet on vascular calcification, evidenced by experimental studies, has been evaluated in the ADVANCE study. In this observation the progression of vascular and cardiac valve calcification has been compared in 360 prevalent adult hemodialysis patients with SHPT, treated with either cinacalcet plus low-dose vitamin D sterols or flexible doses of vitamin D sterols alone. Eligible subjects had intact PTH values >300 pg/mL or within the reference range (150–300 pg/ml) but with Ca × P product >50 mg^2/dL^2 while receiving vitamin D. All subjects received calcium-based phosphate binders. Coronary artery and aorta and cardiac valve calcification were measured by multi-detector computed tomography (using Agatston and Volume scores). Only patients with some degree of calcification (Agatston score ≥30) were enrolled and randomized to cinacalcet (30–180 mg/day) plus low-dose calcitriol or vitamin D analog (≤2 μg paricalcitol equivalent/dialysis), or flexible vitamin D therapy. Coronary calcium score increased, without significant differences, in both groups (24 % and 31 % respectively in the cinacalcet and in the flexible vitamin D group). Changes in Volume score were nonetheless more favorable in the cinacalcet group (+22 % versus +30 %; p=0.009). Also calcification scores in the aortic valve increased significantly less in the cinacalcet group. These data suggest but do not demonstrate that cinacalcet therapy can be associated with lower progression of vascular calcification at least in patients clinically similar to those included in this study [111].

Given the hypothesis of possibly different impact on vascular calcification, the further step was a comparison on hard outcomes like overall and CV mortality. This was assessed in the EVOLVE study, which involved 3,883 hemodialysis patients with moderate-to-severe SHPT (median baseline intact PTH: 693 pg/mL, range 363–1,694), randomized to receive either cinacalcet or placebo (intended as conventional therapy including phosphate binders, vitamin D sterols, or both). After 21.2 months of follow-up in the cinacalcet group, and 17.5 months in the placebo group, no difference was evident in the prevalence of hard outcomes (the primary composite end point was reached in 938 of 1,948 patients (48.2 %) in the cinacalcet group and 952 of 1,935 patients (49.2 %) in the placebo group; HR=0.93; 95 % confidence interval, 0.85–1.02; p=0.11) [112]. A lower prevalence of parathyroidectomy was nonetheless evident in the cinacalcet group.

Data of this study have been used for further post-hoc analyses. One of these studies evaluated the role of FGF23, as a surrogate biomarker of CV risk. Besides confirming the association between baseline serum FGF23 levels and CV events and/or mortality, this analysis evidenced a significant lowering effect of cinacalcet therapy on serum FGF23 levels. A reduction of at least 30 % in serum FGF23 levels was recorded in roughly two thirds of patients randomized to cinacalcet. Importantly, these sizable reductions were associated with lower risks of the primary composite end point (heart failure and sudden death) [113]. Another post-hoc analysis of the Evolve study evaluated fracture events and showed a reduced rate of clinical fracture by 16–29 % in the cinacalcet group [114].

The clinical use of cinacalcet, compared with vitamin D, has been attempted in renal patients not on dialysis and has been shown to effectively suppress PTH, however at the price of increasing serum phosphate, which is now regarded as a definitely undesirable effect [115] which precluded further clinical employment. Therefore limited evidence is available on the therapeutic role of contemporary administration of Cinacalcet and vitamin D in conservative chronic kidney disease (CKD). This precludes any speculation on the possible role to slower progression of renal insufficiency, as described in experimental conditions.

31.5 Conclusions

In conclusion, there is experimental evidence that vitamin D (and its analogs) and calcimimetics can consistently interact when used contemporarily. This interaction occurs through reciprocal effects on their receptors. Most of the clinical advantages resulting from combined therapeutic employment are evident for targeting biochemical parameters of SHPT. Other potential positive interactions on hard outcomes are still in need of further research.

References

1. Mazzaferro S, Pasquali M. Vitamin D: a dynamic molecule. How relevant might the dynamism for a vitamin be? Nephrol Dial Transplant. 2016;31:23–30.
2. Parfitt A. The actions of parathyroid hormone on bone: relation to bone remodeling and turnover, calcium homeostasis, and metabolic bone diseases. Metabolism. 1976;25(8):909–55.
3. Brent G, Leboff M, Seely E, Conlin P, Brown E. Relationship between the concentration and rate of change of calcium and serum intact parathyroid hormone levels in normal humans. J Clin Endocrinol Metab. 1988;67(5):944–50.
4. Brown E, Gardner D, Brennan M, Marx S, Spiegel A, Attie M, et al. Calcium-regulated parathyroid hormone release in primary hyperparathyroidism. Am J Med. 1979;66(6):923–31.
5. Brown E, Gamba G, Riccardi D, Lombardi M, Butters R, Kifor O, et al. Cloning and characterization of an extracellular Ca2+-sensing receptor from bovine parathyroid. Nature. 1993;366(6455):575–80.
6. Capuano I, Garrett J, Hammerland L, Hung B, Brown E, Hebert S, et al. Molecular cloning and functional expression of human parathyroid calcium receptor cDNAs. J Biol Chem. 1995;270(21):12919–25.
7. Hubbard P, Canário A. Evidence that olfactory sensitivities to calcium and sodium are mediated by different mechanisms in the goldfish Carassiusauratus. Neurosci Lett. 2007;414(1):90–3.
8. Nearing J, Betka M, Quinn S, Hentschel H, Elger M, Baum M, et al. Polyvalent cation receptor proteins (CaRs) are salinity sensors in fish. Proc Natl Acad Sci U S A. 2002;99(14):9231–6.
9. Kolakowski LF. GCRDb: a G protein coupled receptor database. Recept Channels. 1994;2(1):1–7.
10. Fan G, Ray K, Zhao X, Goldsmith P, Spiegel A. Mutational analysis of the cysteines in the extracellular domain of the human Ca2+ receptor: effects on cell surface expression, dimerization and signal transduction. FEBS Lett. 1998;436(3):353–6.
11. Brown EM, MacLeod RJ. Extracellular calcium sensing and extracellular calcium signaling. Physiol Rev. 2001;81:239–97.

12. Silve C, Petrel C, Leroy C, Bruel H, Mallet E, Rognan D, et al. Delineating a Ca2+ binding pocket within the venus flytrap module of the human calcium-sensing receptor. J Biol Chem. 2005;280(45):37917–23.
13. Hendy G, Canaff L, Cole D. The CASR gene: alternative splicing and transcriptional control, and calcium-sensing receptor (CaSR) protein: structure and ligand binding sites. Best Pract Res Clin Endocrinol Metab. 2013;27(3):285–301.
14. Tfelt-Hansen J, Brown E. The calcium-sensing receptor in normal physiology and pathophysiology: a review. Crit Rev Clin Lab Sci. 2005;42(1):35–70.
15. Hurowitz E, Melnyk J, Chen Y, Kouros-Mehr H, Simon M, Shizuya H. Genomic characterization of the human heterotrimeric G protein nd subunit genes. DNA Res. 2000;7(2):111–20.
16. Ward D. Calcium receptor-mediated intracellular signalling. Cell Calcium. 2004;35(3):217–28.
17. Hofer A, Brown E. Calcium: extracellular calcium sensing and signalling. Nat Rev Mol Cell Biol. 2003;4(7):530–8.
18. Rogers K, Dunn C, Hebert S, Brown E, Nemeth E. Pharmacological comparison of bovine parathyroid, human parathyroid, and rat kidney calcium receptors expressed in HEK 293 cells. J Bone Miner Res. 1995;10(Suppl1):S48.
19. Corbetta S, Lania A, Filopanti M, Vicentini L, Ballaré E, Spada A. Mitogen-activated protein kinase cascade in human normal and tumoral parathyroid cells. J Clin Endocrinol Metab. 2002;87(5):2201–5.
20. Emanuel R, Adler G, Kifor O, Quinn S, Fuller F, Krapcho K, et al. Calcium-sensing receptor expression and regulation by extracellular calcium in the AtT-20 pituitary cell line. Mol Endocrinol. 1996;10(5):555–65.
21. Romoli R, Lania A, Mantovani G, Corbetta S, Persani L, Spada A. Expression of calcium-sensing receptor and characterization of intracellular signaling in human pituitary adenomas 1. J Clin Endocrinol Metab. 1999;84(8):2848–53.
22. Leclercq-Meyer V, Marchand J, Leclercq R, Malaisse W. Calcium deprivation enhances glucagon release in the presence of 2-ketoisocaproate. Endocrinology. 1981;108(6):2093–7.
23. Procino G, Carmosino M, Tamma G, Gouraud S, Laera A, Riccardi D, et al. Extracellular calcium antagonizes forskolin-induced aquaporin 2 trafficking in collecting duct cells. Kidney Int. 2004;66(6):2245–55.
24. Valle C, Rodriguez M, Santamaria R, Almaden Y, Rodriguez M, Canadillas S, et al. Cinacalcet reduces the set point of the PTH-calcium curve. J Am Soc Nephrol. 2008;19(12):2430–6.
25. Nechama M, Ben-Dov I, Silver J, Naveh-Many T. Regulation of PTH mRNA stability by the calcimimetic R568 and the phosphorus binder lanthanum carbonate in CKD. Am J Physiol Ren Physiol. 2009;296(4):F795–800.
26. Marx SJ. Hyperplasia in glands with hormone excess. Endocr Relat Cancer. 2016;23:R1–14.
27. Diaz R, Hurwitz S, Chattopadhyay N, Pines M, Yang Y, Kifor O, Einat MS, Butters R, Hebert SC, Brown EM. Cloning, expression, and tissue localization of the calcium-sensing receptor in chicken (Gallus domesticus). Am J Physiol Regul Integr Comp Physiol. 1997;273:R1008–16.
28. Kifor O, Moore F, Wang P, Goldstein M, Vassilev P, Kifor I, et al. Reduced immunostaining for the extracellular Ca2+-sensing receptor in primary and uremic secondary hyperparathyroidism. J Clin Endocrinol Metab. 1996;81(4):1598–606.
29. Gogusev J, Duchambon P, Hory B, Giovannini M, Goureau Y, Sarfati E, et al. Depressed expression of calcium receptor in parathyroid gland tissue of patients with hyperparathyroidism. Kidney Int. 1997;51(1):328–36.
30. Ritter C, Finch J, Slatopolsky E, Brown A. Parathyroid hyperplasia in uremic rats precedes down-regulation of the calcium receptor. Kidney Int. 2001;60(5):1737–44.
31. Cozzolino M, Lu Y, Finch J, Slatopolsky E, Dusso A. p21WAF1 and TGF-α mediate parathyroid growth arrest by vitamin D and high calcium. Kidney Int. 2001;60(6):2109–17.
32. Yarden N, Lavelin I, Genina O, Hurwitz S, Diaz R, Brown E, et al. Expression of calcium-sensing receptor gene by avian parathyroid gland in vivo: relationship to plasma calcium. Gen Comp Endocrinol. 2000;117(2):173–81.

33. Mendoza F, Lopez I, Canalejo R, Almaden Y, Martin D, Aguilera-Tejero E, et al. Direct upregulation of parathyroid calcium-sensing receptor and vitamin D receptor by calcimimetics in uremic rats. Am J Physiol Ren Physiol. 2008;296(3):F605–13.
34. Carrillo-Lopez N, Alvarez-Hernandez D, Gonzalez-Suarez I, Roman-Garcia P, Valdivielso J, Fernandez-Martin J, et al. Simultaneous changes in the calcium-sensing receptor and the vitamin D receptor under the influence of calcium and calcitriol. Nephrol Dial Transplant. 2008;23(11):3479–84.
35. Boynton AL. Calcium and epithelial cell proliferation. Miner Electrolyte Metab. 1988;14:86–94.
36. Canaff L, Hendy G. Human calcium-sensing receptor gene. Vitamin d response elements in promoters p1 and p2 confer transcriptional responsiveness to 1,25-dihydroxyvitamin d. J Biol Chem. 2002;277(33):30337–50.
37. Aida K, Koishi S, Tawata M, Onaya T. Molecular cloning of a putative Ca2+-sensing receptor cDNA from human kidney. Biochem Biophys Res Comm. 1995;214(2):524–9.
38. Chattopadhyay N, Baum M, Bai M, Riccardi D, Hebert SC, Harris HW, Brown EM. Ontogeny of the extracellular calcium-sensing receptor in rat kidney. Am J Physiol Renal Fluid Electrolyte Physiol. 1996;271:F736–43.
39. Riccardi D, Park J, Lee W, Gamba G, Brown E, Hebert S. Cloning and functional expression of a rat kidney extracellular calcium/polyvalent cation-sensing receptor. Proc Nat Acad Sci. 1995;92(1):131–5.
40. Toka H, Al-Romaih K, Koshy J, DiBartolo S, Kos C, Quinn S, et al. Deficiency of the calcium-sensing receptor in the kidney causes parathyroid hormone-independent hypocalciuria. J Am Soc Nephrol. 2012;23(11):1879–90.
41. Bajwa A, Forster M, Maiti A, Woolbright B, Beckman M. Specific regulation of CYP27B1 and VDR in proximal versus distal renal cells. Arch Biochem Biophys. 2008;477(1):33–42.
42. Maiti A, Hait N, Beckman M. Extracellular calcium-sensing receptor activation induces vitamin D receptor levels in proximal kidney HK-2G cells by a mechanism that requires phosphorylation of p38 MAPK. J Biol Chem. 2007;283(1):175–83.
43. Levi M, Molitoris BA, Burke TJ, Schrier RW, Simon FR. Effects of vitamin D-induced chronic hypercalcemia on rat renal cortical plasma membranes and mitochondria. Am J Physiol Renal Fluid Electrolyte Physiol. 1987;252:F267–75.
44. Wang W, Lu M, Balazy M, Hebert SC. Phospholipase A2 is involved in mediating the effect of extracellular Ca2_ on apical K_ channels in ratTAL. Am J Physiol Renal Physiol. 1997;273:F421–9.
45. Sands JM, Flores FX, Kato A, Baum MA, Brown EM, Ward DT, Hebert SC, Harris HW. Vasopressin-elicited water and urea permeabilities are altered in IMCD in hypercalcemic rats. Am J Physiol Renal Physiol. 1998;274:F978–85.
46. Topala C, Schoeber J, Searchfield L, Riccardi D, Hoenderop J, Bindels R. Activation of the Ca2+-sensing receptor stimulates the activity of the epithelial Ca2+ channel TRPV5. Cell Calcium. 2009;45(4):331–9.
47. Hoenderop J. Modulation of renal Ca2+ transport protein genes by dietary Ca2+ and 1,25-dihydroxyvitamin D3 in 25-hydroxyvitamin D3-1alpha-hydroxylase knockout mice. FASEB J. 2002;16(11):1398–406.
48. Mentaverri R, Yano S, Chattopadhyay N, Petit L, Kifor O, Kamel S, et al. The calcium sensing receptor is directly involved in both osteoclast differentiation and apoptosis. FASEB J. 2006;20(14):2562–4.
49. Kameda T, Mano H, Yamada Y, Takai H, Amizuka N, Kobori M, et al. Calcium-sensing receptor in mature osteoclasts, which are bone resorbing cells. Biochem Biophys Res Comm. 1998;245(2):419–22.
50. Kanatani M, Sugimoto T, Kanzawa M, Yano S, Chihara K. High extracellular calcium inhibits osteoclast-like cell formation by directly acting on the calcium-sensing receptor existing in osteoclast precursor cells. Biochem Biophys Res Comm. 1999;261(1):144–8.
51. Chattopadhyay N, Yano S, Tfelt-Hansen J, Rooney P, Kanuparthi D, Bandyopadhyay S, et al. Mitogenic action of calcium-sensing receptor on rat calvarial osteoblasts. Endocrinology. 2004;145(7):3451–62.

52. Dvorak M, Siddiqua A, Ward D, Carter D, Dallas S, Nemeth E, et al. Physiological changes in extracellular calcium concentration directly control osteoblast function in the absence of calciotropic hormones. Proc Nat Acad Sci. 2004;101(14):5140–5.

53. Chang W, Tu C, Chen T, Bikle D, Shoback D. The extracellular calcium-sensing receptor (CaSR) is a critical modulator of skeletal development. Sci Signal. 2008;1(35):ra1.

54. Carlstedt F, Lind L, Rastad J, Stjernstrom H, Wide L, Ljunghall S. Parathyroid hormone and ionized calcium levels are related to the severity of illness and survival in critically ill patients. Eur J Clin Invest. 1998;28(11):898–903.

55. Nielsen P, Rasmussen Å, Butters R, Feldt-Rasmussen U, Bendtzen K, Diaz R, et al. Inhibition of PTH secretion by interleukin-1β in bovine parathyroid glandsin vitro is associated with an up-regulation of the calcium-sensing receptor mRNA. Biochem Biophys Res Comm. 1997;238(3):880–5.

56. Canaff L, Hendy G. Calcium-sensing receptor gene transcription is up-regulated by the pro-inflammatory cytokine, interleukin-1: role of the nf- b pathway and b elements. J Biol Chem. 2005;280(14):14177–88.

57. Carlstedt E, Ridefelt P, Lind L, Rastad J. Interleukin-6 induced suppression of bovine parathyroid hormone secretion. Biosci Rep. 1999;19:35–42.

58. Brown A, Ritter C, Finch J, Slatopolsky E. Decreased calcium-sensing receptor expression in hyperplastic parathyroid glands of uremic rats: role of dietary phosphate. Kidney Int. 1999;55(4):1284–92.

59. Ritter C, Martin D, Lu Y, Slatopolsky E, Brown A. Reversal of secondary hyperparathyroidism by phosphate restriction restores parathyroid calcium-sensing receptor expression and function. J Bone Miner Res. 2002;17(12):2206–13.

60. Urena P, Frazao J. Calcimimetic agents: review and perspectives. Kidney Int. 2003;63(s85): 91–6.

61. Aida K. Familial hypocalciuric hypercalcemia associated with mutation in the human Ca(2+)-sensing receptor gene. J Clin Endocrinol Metab. 1995;80(9):2594–8.

62. Quitterer U, Hoffmann M, Freichel M, Lohse M. Paradoxical block of parathormone secretion is mediated by increased activity of galpha subunits. J Biol Chem. 2000;276(9):6763–9.

63. Higashijima T, Ferguson KM, Sternweis PC, Smigel MD, Gilman AG. Effects of Mg2+ and the beta gamma-subunit complex on the interactions of guanine nucleotides with G proteins. J Biol Chem. 1987;262(2):762–6.

64. La Piana G, Gorgoglione V, Laraspata D, Marzulli D, Lofrumento N. Effect of magnesium ions on the activity of the cytosolic NADH/cytochrome c electron transport system. FEBS J. 2008;275(24):6168–79.

65. McLarnon S, Holden D, Ward D, Jones M, Elliott A, Riccardi D. Aminoglycoside antibiotics induce pH-sensitive activation of the calcium-sensing receptor. Biochem Biophys Res Comm. 2002;297(1):71–7.

66. Ward D. Aminoglycosides induce acute cell signaling and chronic cell death in renal cells that express the calcium-sensing receptor. J Am Soc Nephrol. 2005;16(5):1236–44.

67. Conigrave A, Mun H, Brennan S. Physiological significance of L-amino acid sensing by extracellular Ca 2+ -sensing receptors. Biochem Soc Trans. 2007;35(5):1195–8.

68. Busque S. L-type amino acids stimulate gastric acid secretion by activation of the calcium-sensing receptor in parietal cells. Am J Physiol Gastrointest Liver Physiol. 2005;289:G1084–90.

69. Dawson-Hughes B, Harris S, Rasmussen H, Dallal G. Comparative effects of oral aromatic and branched-chain amino acids on urine calcium excretion in humans. Osteop Int. 2007;18(7):955–61.

70. Conigrave A, et al. L-Amino acid sensing by the calcium-sensing receptor: a general mechanism for coupling protein and calcium metabolism? Eur J Clin Nutr. 2003;57(7):879.

71. Hira T, Nakajima S, Eto Y, Hara H. Calcium-sensing receptor mediates phenylalanine-induced cholecystokinin secretion in enteroendocrine STC-1 cells. FEBS J. 2008;275(18):4620–6.

72. Nemeth E, Steffey M, Hammerland L, Hung B, Van Wagenen B, DelMar E, et al. Calcimimetics with potent and selective activity on the parathyroid calcium receptor. Proc Nat Acad Sci. 1998;95(7):4040–5.

73. Goodman W, Frazao J, Goodkin D, Turner S, Liu W, Coburn J. A calcimimetic agent lowers plasma parathyroid hormone levels in patients with secondary hyperparathyroidism. Kidney Int. 2000;58(1):436–45.

74. Messa P, Alfieri C, Brezzi B. Cinacalcet: pharmacological and clinical aspects. Expert Opin Drug Metab Toxicol. 2008;4(12):1551–60.

75. Miller G, Davis J, Shatzen E, Colloton M, Martin D, Henley C. Cinacalcet HCl prevents development of parathyroid gland hyperplasia and reverses established parathyroid gland hyperplasia in a rodent model of CKD. Nephrol Dial Transplant. 2011;27(6):2198–205.

76. Rodriguez M, Almaden Y, Canadillas S, Canalejo A, Siendones E, Lopez I, et al. The calcimimetic R-568 increases vitamin D receptor expression in rat parathyroid glands. Am J Physiol Ren Physiol. 2007;292(5):F1390–5.

77. Sumida K, Nakamura M, Ubara Y, Marui Y, Tanaka K, Takaichi K, et al. Cinacalcet upregulates calcium-sensing receptors of parathyroid glands in hemodialysis patients. Am J Nephrol. 2013;37(5):405–12.

78. Tatsumi R, Komaba H, Kanai G, Miyakogawa T, Sawada K, Kakuta T, et al. Cinacalcet induces apoptosis in parathyroid cells in patients with secondary hyperparathyroidism: histological and cytological analyses. Nephron Clin Pract. 2013;124(3–4):224–31.

79. Quarles L. The calcimimetic AMG 073 as a potential treatment for secondary hyperparathyroidism of end-stage renal disease. J Am Soc Nephrol. 2003;14(3):575–83.

80. Lindberg J, Moe S, Goodman W, Coburn J, Sprague S, Liu W, et al. The calcimimetic AMG 073 reduces parathyroid hormone and calcium x phosphorus in secondary hyperparathyroidism. Kidney Int. 2003;63(1):248–54.

81. Block GA, Martin KJ, de Francisco AL, Turner SA, Avram MM, Suranyi MG, et al. Cinacalcet for secondary hyperparathyroidism in patients receiving hemodialysis. N Engl J Med. 2004;350(15):1516–25.

82. Komaba H, Koizumi M, Tanaka H, Takahashi H, Sawada K, Kakuta T, et al. Effects of cinacalcet treatment on serum soluble Klotho levels in haemodialysis patients with secondary hyperparathyroidism. Nephrol Dial Transplant. 2011;27(5):1967–9.

83. Shalhoub V, Grisanti M, Padagas J, Scully E, Rattan A, Qi M, et al. In vitro studies with the calcimimetic, cinacalcet HCl, on normal human adult osteoblastic and osteoclastic cells. Crit Rev Eukaryot Gene Expr. 2003;13(2–4):107–8.

84. Behets G, Spasovski G, Sterling L, Goodman W, Spiegel D, De Broe M, et al. Bone histomorphometry before and after long-term treatment with cinacalcet in dialysis patients with secondary hyperparathyroidism. Kidney Int. 2014;87(4):846–56.

85. Mendoza F, Martinez-Moreno J, Almaden Y, Rodriguez-Ortiz M, Lopez I, Estepa J, et al. Effect of calcium and the calcimimetic AMG 641 on matrix-Gla protein in vascular smooth muscle cells. Calcif Tissue Int. 2010;88(3):169–78.

86. Jung S, Querfeld U, Müller D, Rudolph B, Peters H, Krämer S. Submaximal suppression of parathyroid hormone ameliorates calcitriol-induced aortic calcification and remodeling and myocardial fibrosis in uremic rats. J Hypertens. 2012;30(11):2182–91.

87. Alam M, Kirton J, Wilkinson F, Towers E, Sinha S, Rouhi M, et al. Calcification is associated with loss of functional calcium-sensing receptor in vascular smooth muscle cells. Cardiovasc Res. 2008;81(2):260–8.

88. Zizzo M, Mulè F, Amato A, Maiorana F, Mudò G, Belluardo N, et al. Guanosine negatively modulates the gastric motor function in mouse. Purinergic Signal. 2013;9(4):655–61.

89. Walter S, Baruch A, Dong J, Tomlinson J, Alexander S, Janes J, et al. Pharmacology of AMG 416 (velcalcetide), a novel peptide agonist of the calcium-sensing receptor, for the treatment of secondary hyperparathyroidism in hemodialysis patients. J Pharmacol Exp Ther. 2013;346(2):229–40.

90. Martin K, Bell G, Pickthorn K, Huang S, Vick A, Hodsman P, et al. Velcalcetide (AMG 416), a novel peptide agonist of the calcium-sensing receptor, reduces serum parathyroid hormone and FGF23 levels in healthy male subjects. Nephrol Dial Transplant. 2013;29(2):385–92.

91. Martin K, Pickthorn K, Huang S, Block G, Vick A, Mount P, et al. AMG 416 (velcalcetide) is a novel peptide for the treatment of secondary hyperparathyroidism in a single-dose study in hemodialysis patients. Kidney Int. 2013;85(1):191–7.

92. Bell G, Huang S, Martin K, Block G. A randomized, double-blind, phase 2 study evaluating the safety and efficacy of AMG 416 for the treatment of secondary hyperparathyroidism in hemodialysis patients. Curr Med Res Opin. 2015;31(5):943–52.
93. Brown EM. Vitamin D and the calcium sensing receptor. In: Feldman D, Pike JW, Adams JS, editors. Vitamin D. 3rd ed. Oxford, UK: Elsevier; 2011. p. 425–56.
94. Rodriguez M, Aguilera-Tejero E, Mendoza FJ, Guerrero F, López I. Effects of calcimimetics on extraskeletal calcifications in chronic kidney disease. Kidney Int Suppl. 2008;111:S50–4.
95. Lopez I, Aguilera-Tejero E, Mendoza FJ, Almaden Y, Perez J, Martin D, Rodriguez M. Calcimimetic R-568 decreases extraosseous calcifications in uremic rats treated with calcitriol. J Am Soc Nephrol. 2006;17(3):795–804.
96. Mary A, Hénaut L, Boudot C, et al. Calcitriol prevents in vitro vascular smooth muscle cell mineralization by regulating calcium-sensing receptor expression. Endocrinology. 2015;156(6):1965–74.
97. Drüeke TB, Ritz E. Treatment of secondary hyperparathyroidism in CKD patients with cinacalcet and/or vitamin D derivatives. Clin J Am Soc Nephrol. 2009;4(1):234–41.
98. Chertow GM, Blumenthal S, Turner S, Roppolo M, Stern L, Chi EM, Reed J, CONTROL Investigators. Cinacalcet hydrochloride (Sensipar) in hemodialysis patients on active vitamin D derivatives with controlled PTH and elevated calcium x phosphate. Clin J Am Soc Nephrol. 2006;1(2):305–12.
99. Messa P, Macário F, Yaqoob M, et al. The OPTIMA study: assessing a new cinacalcet (Sensipar/Mimpara) treatment algorithm for secondary hyperparathyroidism. Clin J Am Soc Nephrol. 2008;3(1):36–45.
100. Fishbane S, Shapiro WB, Corry DB, et al. CinacalcetHCl and concurrent low-dose vitamin D improves treatment of secondary hyperparathyroidism in dialysis patients compared with vitamin D alone: the ACHIEVE study results. Clin J Am Soc Nephrol. 2008;3(6):1718–25.
101. Ketteler M, Martin KJ, Wolf M, et al. Paricalcitol versus cinacalcet plus low-dose vitamin D therapy for the treatment of secondary hyperparathyroidism in patients receiving haemodialysis: results of the IMPACT SHPT study. Nephrol Dial Transplant. 2012;27(8):3270–8.
102. Cozzolino M, Ketteler M, Martin KJ, Sharma A, Goldsmith D, Khan S. Paricalcitol- or cinacalcet-centred therapy affects markers of bone mineral disease in patients with secondary hyperparathyroidism receiving haemodialysis: results of the IMPACT-SHPT study. Nephrol Dial Transplant. 2014;29(4):899–905.
103. Lewis R. Mineral and bone disorders in chronic kidney disease: new insights into mechanism and management. Ann Clin Biochem. 2012;49(5):432–40.
104. Koizumi M, Komaba H, Nakanishi S, et al. Cinacalcet treatment and serum FGF23 levels in haemodialysis patients with secondary hyperparathyroidism. Nephrol Dial Transplant. 2012;27(2):784–90.
105. Liu S, Tang W, Zhou J, et al. Fibroblast growth factor 23 is a counter-regulatory phosphaturic hormone for vitamin D. J Am Soc Nephrol. 2006;17(5):1305–15.
106. Drechsler C, Verduijn M, Pilz S, et al. Bone alkaline phosphatase and mortality in dialysis patients. Clin J Am Soc Nephrol. 2011;6:1752–9.
107. Gutiérrez OM, Mannstadt M, Isakova T, et al. Fibroblast growth factor 23 and mortality among patients undergoing hemodialysis. N Engl J Med. 2008;359(6):584–92.
108. Lee GH, Benner D, Regidor DL, et al. Impact of kidney bone disease and its management on survival of patients on dialysis. J Ren Nutr. 2007;17(1):38–44.
109. Tentori F, Hunt WC, Stidley CA, for the Medical Directors of Dialysis Clinic Inc, et al. Mortality risk among hemodialysis patients receiving different vitamin D analogs. Kidney Int. 2006;70(10):1858–65.
110. Wetmore JB, Gurevich K, Sprague S, et al. A randomized trial of cinacalcet versus vitamin D analogs as monotherapy in secondary hyperparathyroidism (PARADIGM). Clin J Am Soc Nephrol. 2015;10(6):1031–40.
111. Raggi P, Chertow GM, Urena Torres P, on behalf of the ADVANCE Study Group, et al. The ADVANCE study: a randomized study to evaluate the effects of cinacalcet plus low-dose vitamin D on vascular calcification in patients on hemodialysis. Nephrol Dial Transplant. 2011;26(4):1327–39.

112. Chertow GM, Block GA, Correa-Rotter R, et al. Effect of cinacalcet on cardiovascular disease in patients undergoing dialysis. EVOLVE Trial Investigators. N Engl J Med. 2012;367(26):2482–94.
113. Moe SM, Chertow GM, Parfrey PS, Evaluation of CinacalcetHCl Therapy to Lower Cardiovascular Events (EVOLVE) Trial Investigators*, et al. Cinacalcet, fibroblast growth factor-23, and cardiovascular disease in hemodialysis: the Evaluation of CinacalcetHCl Therapy to Lower Cardiovascular Events (EVOLVE) Trial. Circulation. 2015;132(1):27–39.
114. Moe SM, Abdalla S, Chertow GM, et al. Effects of cinacalcet on fracture events in patients receiving hemodialysis: the EVOLVE Trial. J Am Soc Nephrol. 2015;26(6):1466–75.
115. Montenegro J, Cornago I, Gallardo I, et al. Efficacy and safety of cinacalcet for the treatment of secondary hyperparathyroidism in patients with advanced chronic kidney disease before initiation of regular dialysis. Nephrol (Carlton). 2012;17(1):26–31.

Index

A

Active vitamin D, in CKD patients
  mineral and skeletal outcomes, 501–502
  oral calcitriol and survival, 503–504
  survival and cardiovascular outcomes
    oral active vitamin D analogues, 505
    parenteral active vitamin D analogues,
      505–506
Acute cellular rejection, 445, 449
Adynamic bone disease (ABD), 219
  aflacalcidol, 517
  in pediatrics, 234–235
  sclerostin, 209
Adynamic osteopathy, 170, 173, 221
Alfacalcidol
  comparison studies of, 519–520
  doxercalciferol, 520–522
  kidney transplant recipients, 518–519
  non-dialysis CKD, 517–518
Allosteric CaSR activators
  AMG 416, 549–550
  aromatic L-amino acids, 548
  pharmacological modulation, 548
  R-568, 548–549
  vitamin D and CaMim, CKD
    ACHIEVE study, 553
    ADVANCE study, 555
    bone cells biomarkers, 554
    cinacalcet, 552
    CONTROL study, 552
    EVOLVE study, 555

FGF23, 554, 555
KDOQI targets, 553
OPTIMA study, 552
PARADIGM study, 554
SHPT, 550
vascular calcifications, 551
VDR expression, 550, 551
Anemia
  causes, in CKD patients, 392–393
  definition, 391–392
  iron deficiency, 393–394
  prevalence, 391–392
  symptoms, 392
  treatment of, 401–402
  vitamin D and
    association of, 393
    erythropoiesis and, 395–397
    erythropoietin deficiency, 395
    HIF metabolism, 397–398
    and inflammation, 398–399
    and PTH, 399
    resistance, 393–395
    role of, 393–395
    vitamin D receptor, 399–400
Angiogenesis, 346, 347, 480
Australian Diabetes Obesity and Lifestyle
      Study (AusDiab), 27, 37
Autosomal dominant hypoparathyroidism
      (ADH), 150
Autosomal dominant hypophosphatemic
      rickets (ADHR), 180

© Springer International Publishing Switzerland 2016
P.A. Urena Torres et al. (eds.), *Vitamin D in Chronic Kidney Disease*,
DOI 10.1007/978-3-319-32507-1

B
Bone alkaline phosphatase (BALP), 331,
    518, 554
Bone health
    renal transplantation
        efficacy, vitamin D supplementation,
            430–431
        epidemiology of, 428
        low BMD and fractures, 430
        risk factors and pathophysiology of,
            428–430
        safety, vitamin D supplementation,
            431–432
    sclerostin, 210, 214
Bone morphogenetic protein 2 (BMP2), 368
Bovine parathyroid calcium receptor
    (BoPCaR), 538

C
Calcific uremic arteriolopathy (CUA). *See*
    Calciphylaxis
Calcimimetics (CaM)
    allosteric CaSR activators (*see* Allosteric
        CaSR activators)
    aminoglycoside antibiotics, 546–547
    CaSR (*see* Calcium sensing receptor
        (CaSR))
    magnesium, 546
    orthosteric CaSR activators, 546
    in pediatric CKD, 239–240
Calcineurin inhibitor (CNI), 426
Calciphylaxis
    calcitol, 104
    chronic hemodialysis, 379
    clinical picture of, 381–382
    CUA treatment, 386–387
    EVOLVE study, 384
    German calciphylaxis registry, 380
    historical perspective, 380–381
    international registry initiatives, 388
    risk factors, 382–383
    sodium thiosulfate, 387–388
    vitamin D, 383–384
    vitamin K, 385
Calcitriol, 406, 446
    anti-atherosclerotic actions, 268
    anti-hypertrophic and fibrotic
        properties, 268
    anti-inflammatory properties, 268
    anti-oxidative effects, 268
    diabetes mellitus, 268, 272
    FGF23 (*see* Fibroblast growth factor 23
        (FGF23))

natural vitamin D, 468–469
oral active vitamin D, 503–504
parathyroid pre-pro-PTH mRNA levels,
    reduction of, 149
parathyroid VDR expression, regulation of,
    152–154
serum PTH level reduction, in dialysis
    patients, 149
SHPT, 149, 154–156
vascular calcification, 268
Calcium sensing receptor (CaSR)
    allosteric CaSR activators (*see* Allosteric
        CaSR activators)
    identification of, 538–539
    mineral metabolism
        bone, 544–545
        CaSR expression, 545
        and kidney, 544
        parathyroid glands, 542–544
    orthosteric CaSR activators, 546
    parathyroid hormone
        secretion control, 149–151
        VDR, in SHPT, 155–158
    structure of, 539–541
CaM. *See* Calcimimetics (CaM)
Cancer
    mortality risk, 413–414
    natural vitamin D, 480
    renal transplant recipients, 434
Cardiovascular calcification
    CKD–MBD, 362
    uraemic toxins, 361
    vascular calcification
        direct effects of, 365–369
        systemic and indirect effects of,
            369–371
    VDRAs, 363
    vitamin D, CKD
        animal models, 365
        ESRD, 363–364
        supplementation, 364
Cardiovascular disease (CVD), 344
    heart structure and function
        25-hydroxyvitamin D, 325–326
        vitamin D genetics, 326
    mortality risk, 408
Cardiovascular magnetic resonance (CMR), 525
Cardiovascular (CV) risk, nutritional vitamin D
    in CKD patients, 499–501
    in general population, 498–499
CaSR. *See* Calcium sensing receptor (CaSR)
C3-epimer of 25(OH)D, 15
Childhood chronic kidney disease. *See*
    Pediatrics

Cholecalciferol
    analytical characteristics of, 120, 121
    natural vitamin D
        biochemical and pharmacological
            properties, 469–471
        DBP and VDR, 472
        recommended intake and dosage,
            472–473
        structure, 469, 470
        synthetic compounds, 468
    structure of, 5
    synthesis of, 4–5
Chronic kidney disease-mineral and bone
        disorder (CKD-MBD)
    extra-skeletal complications, 218
    fractures
        and BMD, 222
        bone quantity and quality,
            reduction of, 222
        cortical bone, 222
        femoral fractures, risk of, 221–222
        high bone remodeling, 223
        hip fracture, risk of, 221, 223
        peripheral fractures, incidence of, 222
        PTH levels, 222, 223
        treatment of, 223–225
    KDIGO guidelines, 118
    klotho-FGF23 axis, role of
        bone metabolism, 184
        ESRD patients, 182–183
        hypertension, 182
        left ventricular hypertrophy, 182
        parathyroid gland, 183–184
        secondary hyperparathyroidism, 182
        urinary phosphate excretion, 181–182
        vascular calcification, 184
        volume expansion, 182
    metabolic abnormalities, 218
    renal osteodystrophy, forms of, 219–221
    sclerostin, 210, 214
    soluble klotho, role of, 189–190
    vitamin D insufficiency and deficiency,
        impact of, 223
    vitamin D metabolism, 218–220, 467
Chronic kidney disease (CKD), vitamin D
    abnormal bone remodeling, 52
    active vitamin D
        mineral and skeletal outcomes,
            501–502
        oral calcitriol and survival, 503–504
        survival and cardiovascular outcomes,
            505–506
    anemia (see Anemia)
    anti-hypertensive effects

        cardiovascular events, risk of, 254
        paricalcitol, 254
        RAAS, 252–253
        secondary hyperparathyroidism, 254
    anti-proteinuric effect, 251–252
    bioactivation, abnormalities in, 52–54
    cardiovascular calcification (see
            Cardiovascular calcification)
    in children (see Pediatrics)
    defective mineralization, 52
    endothelial dysfunction
        diabetes, 350
        dyslipidemia, 351–352
        hypertension, 350–351
        inflammation, 352–353
        klotho-fibroblast growth factor-23,
            353–354
        SHPT, 353
    glomerular filtration rate, 260–261
    hyperphosphatemia, FGF23/klotho
            complex, 64–66, 68
    hypertension, 52
    inflammation, 257–258
        anti-inflammatory effects of, VDRA,
            311–313
        low-grade inflammation, 306
        systemic inflammation, 307
    innate immune responses, 257–258
    insulin resistance, 256
    lipid metabolism, 257
    mortality risk
        cardiac morphology, 410
        hypertension, 409
        management in, 416
        physiological role for, 407, 415
        progression, 411
    multiple organ damage, 52
    natural vitamin D
        calcidiol–DBP complex, 474–475
        calcidiol deficiency, 474
        calcitriol–VDR-RXR complex, 475
        fracture and vitamin D status, 475
        mineral bone density, 475
        randomized clinical trials, 476–477
        supplementation, 476
    non RAAS-mediated effects,
            cardiovascular system, 255–256
    nutritional vitamin D
        cardiovascular risk, 499–501
        infection reduction, 501
    nutrition and dietary (see Nutrition and
            dietary vitamin D, in CKD)
    obesity, 257
    parathyroid hyperplasia, 59–61

Chronic kidney disease (CKD), vitamin D (*cont.*)
   phosphate retention, 250
   pro-aging features, 52
   PTH synthesis, suppression of, 58–61
   randomized clinical trials, 261
   renal fibrosis and nephropathy, 258–260
   renal klotho, 52
      ADAM17/TGFα signals, 66–67
      anti-aging actions, induction of, 67
   sclerostin (*see* Sclerostin)
   skeletal development and mineralization,
      61–64
   skeletal muscle, vitamin D
      supplementation
      contractile function, 289–290
      insulin resistance, 290–291
      muscle mass and function, 286–287
      pathophysiology, 287
   systemic inflammation, 52
   vitamin D receptor
      calcium concentration, 99–100
      CaSR expression, 100
      complex inter-relationships, 101
      $1,25(OH)_2D_3$ resistance, 95–96
      genomic calcitriol, abnormalities in,
         54–56
      1α-hydroxylase, 101
      klotho-FGFR1 complex, 100
      lower density and binding capacity,
         98–99
      non-genomic calcitriol, abnormalities
         in, 57
      renal failure, 96
      secondary hyperparathyroidism in, 82
      selective VDR activators, 101–105
      uremic toxins, effect of, 96–98
      vitamin D3 treatment, 250
Chronic Renal Insufficiency Cohort (CRIC)
      study, 27, 37
Ciclosporine A (CsA), 448
CKD-MBD. *See* Chronic kidney
      disease-mineral and bone disorder
      (CKD-MBD)
Coronary calcification (CAC), 409
C-reactive protein (CRP), 275, 298, 307, 309, 369
CVD. *See* Cardiovascular disease (CVD)
Cyclic adenosine monophosphate (cAMP), 350
Cyclooxygenase 1 (COX1), 345
Cytomegalovirus (CMV), 434

D
Diabetes mellitus (DM)
   CKD, vitamin D, 272–273
      biochemistry, 269

calcitriol, 268, 272
   mechanism of action, 271
   oxidative stress, 270
   palmitate, 271
   pancreatic function, 270
   patients with, 276, 280
   proteinuria, 280
   renal disease, progression of, 281
   ROS, 271
   treatment, 275–279
   type-1 diabetes, 273–274
   type-2 diabetes, 274–275
   vitamin D supplementation, 281–282
   endothelial dysfunction, 350
   epidemiology of, 272
   natural vitamin D, 480
   racial and ethnic differences, 138
Diabetic nephropathy (DN), 280
24,25-Dihydroxyvitamin D ($24,25(OH)_2D$),
      13–14
Dyslipidemia, 351–352

E
Endocrine nuclear receptors, 76
Endothelial dysfunction (ED)
   diabetes, 350
   dyslipidemia, 351–352
   hypertension, 350–351
   inflammation, 352–353
   klotho-fibroblast growth factor-23, 353–354
   SHPT, 353
Endothelial nitric oxide synthase 3 (eNOS), 345
Endothelium
   dysfunction (*see* Endothelial
      dysfunction (ED))
   functions, 344–345
   smooth muscle cell proliferation, 345
   VEGF, 345
   vitamin D and
      in CKD, 347–349
      general population and experimental
         studies, 345–347
Endothelium-derived contracting factors
      (EDCF), 351
End-stage renal disease (ESRD), 296, 347,
      363, 380, 495, 554
   klotho-FGF23 axis, 182–183
   serum PTH level reduction, $1,25(OH)_2D_3$
      administration, 149
   VDRA, 516
Ergocalciferol
   biochemical and pharmacological
      properties, 470–472
   DBP and VDR, 472

recommended intake and dosage, 472–473
structure, 5, 470, 471
synthetic compounds, 468
Erythropoiesis, 393, 395–397
Erythropoietin stimulating agents (ESA), 395
Etelcalcetide, 549, 550

F
Familial hypocalciuric hypocalcemia
    (FHH), 150
Fibroblast growth factor 23 (FGF23),
    181, 268, 353–354
  anti-FGF23 antibodies, 203
  calcitriol
    CYP24A1 and CYP27B1
        expression, 198
    deleterious cardiac effects, in CKD
        patients, 202
    FGFR, stimulation of, 198
    glomerular filtration rate, 201–202
    hypophosphatemia, 198
    plasma intact FGF23 concentration,
        increase in, 199
    production, 200
    treatment, 202–203
    VDR, 199–200
  cleavage and inactivation, 196–197
  FGF23 mRNA, 196
  and klotho
    ADHR and TIO, 180
    CKD-MBD, 181–184
    1,25(OH)₂D suppression, 180
    FGFR1c, 180–181
    in vivo studies, 181
    αklotho expression, 197
    liver cirrhosis, 196
    osteocytes and osteoblast, 196
    plasma phosphate concentration,
        197–199
    renal insufficiency, 196
    renal sodium-phosphate
        co-transporters, inhibition of, 203
    soluble klotho, 188
    urinary phosphate excretion, 180
    vitamin D, in pediatric CKD patients,
        235–237
Flow mediated dilatation (FMD), 346
Fractures
  and BMD, 222
  bone quantity and quality,
      reduction of, 222
  cortical bone, 222
  femoral fractures, risk of, 221–222
  high bone remodeling, 223

hip fracture, risk of, 221, 223
in pediatrics, 234
peripheral fractures, incidence of, 222
PTH levels, 222, 223
treatment of, 223–225
vitamin D deficiency,
    impact of, 223
Framingham Offspring Study, 498
Free fatty acids (FFA), 270, 271

G
German calciphylaxis registry, 380
Glomerular filtration rate (GFR), 344, 495
    FGF23 concentration and
        SHPT, 201–202
    vitamin D receptor activation, 260–261
Glucocorticoids, 428–429
Guanosine diphosphate (GDP), 540
Guanosine triphosphate (GTP), 540

H
Health Professionals Follow-up Study
    (HPFS), 498
Heart structure and function
  active vitamin D treatment
    observational and uncontrolled studies,
        328–329
    RCTs, 329–331
  cardiovascular disease, 326
  natural vitamin D treatment
    observational and uncontrolled studies,
        326–327
    RCTs, 327–328
  VDR activation
    aggravated fibrosis, 324
    and cardiovascular risk factors, 325
    interstitial fibrosis, 324
    myocardium, 323
    vessels, 324–325
High-density lipoprotein (HDL), 351
Homeostasis model assessment of insulin
    resistance (HOMA-IR), 291
Hypertension, 182
  endothelial dysfunction, 350–351
  klotho-FGF23 axis, role of, 182
  mortality risk, 409

I
Immunity, vitamin D
  adaptive immunity, 298
  and inflammation, 298–299
  and innate immunity, 297–298

Inflammation
    CKD patients
        anti-inflammatory effects of, VDRA,
            311–313
        low-grade inflammation, 306
        systemic inflammation, 307
    endothelial dysfunction, 352–353
    vitamin D
        anemia, 398–399
        cardiovascular disease, 307–308
        mechanisms, 308–311
    vitamin D deficiency, 296–297
Intercellular adhesion molecule 1 (ICAM-1),
    325, 348
Iron deficiency, 393–394

J
Jansen's disease, 170

K
Kaplan-Meier analysis, 505
Kidney Disease Improving Global Outcome
        (KDIGO) guidelines, 118, 391, 516
Kidney Disease Outcomes Quality Initiative
        (KDOQI) guidelines, 529, 552
Kidney transplantation, vitamin D
    CANDLE-KIT study, 449
    health, 424
    kidney graft rejection
        acute kidney allograft rejection,
            445–446
        chronic renal allograft rejection,
            446–447
        renoprotective effects of, 446–447
    optimal dosage scheme, 445
    renal transplant recipients
        bone health in (see Bone health)
        1,25(OH)₂D levels, 426
        25(OH)D levels, 425–426
        non-MBD effects, 433–434
        non-renal outcomes, 427
        vascular calcification, 432–433
    risk reduction, fracture, 434, 435
    VITA-D study, 449
    VITALE study, 448
    vitamin D insufficiency, 444
Klotho, 190–191
    and FGF23
        ADHR and TIO, 180
        CKD-MBD, 181–184
        1,25(OH)₂D suppression, 180
        FGFR1c, 180–181

in vivo studies, 181
        urinary phosphate excretion, 180
    function of, 180
    physiological roles, 180
    premature-aging phenotype, 181
    soluble klotho
        calcium reabsorption, 187
        characteristics of, 184–186
        CKD-MBD, 189–190
        as endocrine factor, 187
        FGF23 production and secretion,
            regulation of, 188
        metabolism of, 186
        NaPi-2a inhibition, 188
        phosphate transport inhibition, 188
        renoprotective action of, 188–189
        secretion and clearance of, 186–187
        source of production, 186
        urinary phosphate excretion, 187–188
    transmembrane forms
        characteristics of, 184–186
        function of, 187, 188
Korean National Health and Nutrition
        Examination Survey (KNAHES
        IV), 27, 37

L
Left ventricular hypertrophy (LVH),
        182, 525
Left ventricular mass index (LVMI), 410,
        525, 526
Ligand-binding domain (LBD), 82–86
Liquid chromatographs coupled with two mass
        spectrometers in tandem
        (LC-MS/MS) method
    1,25(OH)₂D, 123
    24,25(OH)₂D, 123
    25(OH)D, 121–122
    VDBP, 125

M
Matrix extracellular phosphoglycoprotein
        (MEPE), 209
Matrix-Gla protein (MGP), 385
Mediator-D complex, 92–93
Metabolites, vitamin D
    analytical characteristics of, 121
    23- and 26-hydroxylated metabolites, 15
    C3-epimer of 25(OH)D, 15
    cholecalciferol, 120
    circulating DBP concentration, 5–6
    1,25(OH)₂D, 122–123

calcium and phosphorus homeostasis,
    regulation of, 8–10
and 25(OH)D, 16
extra-renal production, 10
in kidney, 6–8
VDR, 12–13
vitamin D-dependent rickets type I, 10
24,25(OH)$_2$D, 13–14, 123–124
25(OH)D, 121–122
24(OH)D$_2$ and 1,24(OH)$_2$D$_2$, 15
pre-pro-PTH levels, inhibition of, 149
1,24,25-trihydroxyvitamin D, 13–14
VDBP, 124–126
Mitogen activated protein kinases
    (MAPKs), 540–541
Mortality risk
biological plausibility, 406–407
cancer, 413–414
cardiovascular disease, 408
cardiovascular events, 411–413
CKD
    cardiac morphology, 410
    hypertension, 409
    management in, 416
    progression, 411
endothelial dysfunction, 408–409
historical issues, 406
infections, 413
native vitamin D/active VDRA
    compound, 414
vascular calcification, 408–409
vascular stiffness, 408–409
vitamin D
    deficiency and CKD, 408
    physiological role for, 407, 415
Mycobacterium tuberculosis, 257, 297, 298

N
National Health and Nutrition Examination
    Survey (NHANES III), 27, 36
Natural vitamin D
adverse effects of, 480–481
bone tissue mineralization, defects in, 466
calcitriol, VDR, 468–469
cancer protecting effect, 480
cholecalciferol
    biochemical and pharmacological
        properties, 469–471
    DBP and VDR, 472
    recommended intake and dosage,
        472–473
    structure, 469, 470
    synthetic compounds, 468

in CKD patients
    calcidiol–DBP complex, 474–475
    calcidiol deficiency, 474
    calcitriol–VDR-RXR complex, 475
    fracture and vitamin D status, 475
    mineral bone density, 475
    randomized clinical
        trials, 476–477
    supplementation, 476
diabetes, 480
ergocalciferol
    biochemical and pharmacological
        properties, 470–472
    DBP and VDR, 472
    recommended intake and dosage,
        472–473
    structure, 470, 471
    synthetic compounds, 468
    25(OH)D$_3$, 473–474
rickets, treatment of, 468
skeletal and survival outcomes, RCTs,
    481–485
supplements, effects of, 466
    cardiovascular system, 479
    immune system, 479–480
    kidney and nephroprotection, 478
    mineral and bone disorders, 466
    muscles, 477–478
vitamin D$_4$, 474
Neonatal severe hyperparathyroidism
    (NSHPT), 150
Nicotinamide, 203
Nutritional vitamin D
bone and mineral metabolism, deficiency
    effects, 496–497
cardiovascular risk
    in CKD patients, 499–501
    in general population, 498–499
optimal levels, 506–507
required supplementation dose, 506–507
supplementation effects
    bone and mineral metabolism, 497
    infection reduction, in CKD
        patients, 501
    non-classical actions of, 500
toxicity, 506–507
Nutrition and dietary vitamin D, in CKD
1,25(OH)$_2$D, 455
25(OH)D, 456–457
food-fortification, 457–458
hydroxylation, 454
optimal vitamin D status, 458–460
simplified representation of, 454
vitamin D$_2$ and vitamin D$_3$, 455–456

O
Osteoporosis, 168

P
Parathyroid hormone (PTH), 268, 410, 411,
        495, 538
    calcitriol
        parathyroid function, regulation of,
            148–149
        SHPT, pathophysiology of, 154–156
        VDR expression, regulation of,
            152–154
    calcium/phosphate homeostasis,
        regulator of, 164
    calcium-sensing receptor
        mineral metabolism, 542–544
        secretion control, 149–151
        and VDR, in SHPT, 155–158
    cardiovascular risk factors, VDR
        activation, 325
    definition, 164
    FGF23, 197–198, 200
    mineral metabolism, 148
    physiological functions, 164
    PTH1R (see Parathyroid hormone type 1
        receptor (PTH1R))
    PTH2R (see Parathyroid hormone type 2
        receptor (PTH2R))
    suppression of, 58–61
Parathyroid hormone-related peptide (PTHrP),
        165, 171–172
Parathyroid hormone type 1 receptor (PTH1R)
    adynamic osteopathy, 170
    autosomal recessive chondrodysplasia, 170
    characteristics of, 168
    chronic kidney disease, 169
    endochondral bone, development of, 170
    intracellular signaling pathways, 166–167
    Jansen's disease, 170
    mineral ion homeostasis, regulation of, 164
    molecular structure, 167
    mutations, 170
    PTH1R gene polymorphism, 168
    PTHrP, 171–172
    renal and bone PTH1R, 1,25(OH)$_2$D$_3$, 171
    SHPT, development of, 165, 169–170
Parathyroid hormone type 2 receptor (PTH2R)
    features of, 167, 168
    TIP39, 165, 166
Parathyroid hormone type 3 receptor
        (PTH3R), 168
Paricalcitol
    albuminuria reduction, 523–525

    cardiac structure and function, 525–527
    SHPT treatment, 529–532
Paricalcitol Capsule Benefits in Renal
        Failure-induced cardiac Morbidity
        (PRIMO) trial, 330
Pediatrics
    bone metabolism
        bone formation, 231
        longitudinal growth, 230–231
        vitamins D, role of, 231–232
    CKD patients, vitamin D metabolism in
        active vitamin D sterols, 238–239
        adynamic bone disease, 234–235
        calcimimetics, 239–240
        CKD-MBD management, 237
        complications, 230
        25-D deficiency, 230, 232
        FGF23, 235–237
        fracture, 234
        longitudinal growth, 232–233
        renal osteodystrophy, 234
        renal transplantation, 241
        skeletal mineralization, defects in, 234
Peritoneal dialysis (PD), 37–42
Persistent hyperparathyroidism, 429
Phospholipase C (PLC), 166, 540
Plasma renin concentration (PRC), 525
Polyomavirus associated nephropathy
        (PVAN), 434
Pregnane X receptor (PXR), 76
Premature aging syndrome, 181
Prolyl hydroxylases (PHDs), 397
Protein kinase A (PKA), 167
Proximal convoluted tubule (PCT), 544
PTH. See Parathyroid hormone (PTH)
PTH1R. See Parathyroid hormone type 1
        receptor (PTH1R)
PTHrP. See Parathyroid hormone-related
        peptide (PTHrP)
Pulse wave velocity (PWV), 327, 346, 410

R
Racial and ethnic differences, in CKD
    25(OH)D
        activated vitamin D analogs, treatment
            with, 133
        bone structure and function, 136–137
        cardiovascular health, 138, 139
        chronic disease, 138
        DBP concentrations, 134–135,
            138–139
        deficiency, prevalence of, 132, 134
        diabetes, 138

lower calcium intake, 132, 135
  muscle health, 132
  osteoporosis, lower rates of, 132, 135
  rickets, prevalence of, 135
  skeletal fractures, lower rates of, 132
vitamin D deficiency
  ESRD outcomes, 133, 135
  prevalence rates of, 134
Regulated and normal T-cell expressed and
  secreted (RANTES), 311
Renal anemia. *See* Anemia
Renal osteodystrophy (ROD)
  forms of, 219–221
  in pediatrics, 234
Renal transplant recipients
  bone health in (*see* Bone health)
  1,25(OH)$_2$D levels, 426
  25(OH)D levels, 425–426
  vitamin D
    and cancer, 434
    infections, 433–434
    and mortality, 427
    and vascular calcification, 432–433
Renin-angiotensin-aldosterone system
  (RAAS), 252–253, 280, 323, 344,
  447, 524
Renin-angiotensin system (RAS), 408
Retinoid X receptor (RXR), VDR, 494
  coactivators, 85, 88–94
  corepressors, 85, 88, 94–95
  heterodimerization, 83–84, 89
  nuclear receptor-binding sites, 89
  PTH1R expression, 171
  uremic toxins, effect of, 97–98

S
Sclerosteosis, 208
Sclerostin
  in CKD patients
    bone health, 210, 214
    hemodialysis, 209
    mortality, 210–213
    in peritoneal dialysis patients, 209
    renal osteodystrophy, 209
    in renal transplanted patients, 209
    vascular calcifications, 210, 211
  osteoporosis, 208, 214
  sclerosteosis, 208
  SOST gene, 208
  Van Buchem disease, 208
  vitamin D, 213–214
  Wnt/B-catenin signaling pathway,
    208, 214

Secondary hyperparathyroidism (SHPT), 353,
  363, 495, 515, 543
  endothelial dysfunction, 353
  FGF23 and calcitriol
    GFR values, 201–202
    treatment of, 202–203
  parathyroid hormone
    1,25(OH)$_2$D$_3$, 149, 154–156
    VDR and CaR, 155–158
    PTH1R, 164–165, 169–170
  treatment
    dialysis patients, 527–529
    non-dialysis CKD patients, 522–523
    paricalcitol- and cinacalcet-based
      regimen, 529–532
Selye's theory, 380
Shitake mushroom, 456
Skeletal muscle, vitamin D supplementation
  in CKD patients
    contractile function, 289–290
    insulin resistance, 290–291
    muscle mass and function, 286–287
    pathophysiology, 287
  mode of action, 288
  muscle function, 288–289
Sodium-dependent hydrogen exchanger
  regulatory factor-1 (NHERF-1), 166
Sodium-thiosulfate (STS), 387–388
Steroid receptor coactivator-1 (SRC-1), 88, 92
Steroid receptor coactivators (SRCs), 88, 92

T
Tartrate resistant acid phosphatase
  (TRAP), 221
Transcriptional regulation, 53, 55, 76, 345
Transforming growth factor β-1 (TGFβ1),
  252, 258
Transient receptor potential vanilloid member
  5 (TRPV5), 544
1,24,25-Trihydroxyvitamin D, 13–14
Tuberculosis, 257–258
Tuberoinfundibular peptide 39 (TIP39), 165, 166
Tumor-induced osteomalacia (TIO), 180
Tumor necrosis-α-converting enzyme (TACE),
  79, 309, 310, 352
Tumour necrosis factor-alpha (TNF-α), 325,
  369, 370, 395–396

U
Uremic toxins, 287
Urinary albumin-to-creatinine ratio (UACR),
  252, 524

V
Van Buchem disease, 208
Vascular calcifications (VCs)
    klotho
        and FGF23, 184
        transmembrane klotho, 188
    mortality risk, 408–409
    and sclerostin, in CKD patients, 210, 211
    vitamin D
        direct effects of, 365–369
        systemic and indirect effects of,
            369–371
Vasorelaxation impairment. *See* Endothelial
    dysfunction (ED)
VDBP. *See* Vitamin D binding protein
    (VDBP)
VDR. *See* Vitamin D receptor (VDR)
VDRAs. *See* Vitamin D receptor activators
    (VDRAs)
VDREs. *See* Vitamin D responsive elements
    (VDREs)
Venus flytrap (VFT), 539
Very-low-density lipoproteins
    (VLDLs), 351
Vitamin D
    active vitamin D (*see* Active vitamin D,
        in CKD patients)
    anemia (*see* Anemia)
    calcium homeostasis, 131
    cholecalciferol
        structure of, 5
        synthesis of, 4–5
    classical and non-classical actions of, 496
    ergocalciferol, structure of, 5
    FGF23 (*see* Fibroblast growth factor 23
        (FGF23))
    kidney transplantation (*see* Kidney
        transplantation, vitamin D)
    klotho (*see* Klotho)
    metabolites, measurement of (*see*
        (Metabolites, vitamin D))
    natural vitamin D (*see* Natural vitamin D)
    nutritional vitamin D (*see* Nutritional
        vitamin D)
    pediatrics (*see* Pediatrics)
    physiological systems, regulation of, 131
    physiopathology of, 118–120
    posttransplant CKD-MBD, 429
    prohormone, 4
    sclerostin (*see* Sclerostin)
    sources, 4
    sterols, 494

Vitamin D and Acute Respiratory Infection
    Study (VIDARIS), 500
Vitamin D binding protein (VDBP), 274, 447
    analytical characteristics of, 121
    biological functions, 124
    free and bioavailable 25(OH)D, 125–126
    Gc1F- and Gc1S-allele frequencies, 125
    molar excess, 124–125
    molecular weight of, 124
Vitamin D deficiency, in CKD, 118
    bone metabolism, impact on, 223
    circulating 25(OH)D levels
        age, sex, and region, 23–25
        vitamin D status, definitions of, 21–23
    CVD events, 132
    eGFR/albuminuria levels, in general
        population, 27–31
    end-stage CKD, epidemiology in
        hemodialysis/peritoneal dialysis
            patients, 37–42
        kidney transplant patients, 42–44
    infection
        immune dysfunction (*see* Immunity,
            vitamin D)
        immune impairment, 296–297
        inflammation, 296–297
        intervention trials, 301
        low vitamin D, immune impairment,
            299–300
        observational studies, 300–301
    in non-end-stage CKD, epidemiology in
        AusDiab, 27, 37
        CRIC study, 27, 37
        1,25(OH)$_2$D$_3$ deficiency, prevalence of,
            25–26
        1,25(OH)D$_3$ deficiency, prevalence of,
            25–26
        eGFR/albuminuria levels, clinic-based
            studies, 27, 32–35
        French NephroTest study, 36–37
        Japanese Osaka study, 27
        KNAHES IV, 27, 37
        NHANES III, 27, 36
        Rancho Bernardo study, 27
        reduced kidney function, 25
    in northern countries, incidence in, 4
    prevalence, 467
    risk factors, 20, 24–26, 37, 42
Vitamin D receptor (VDR), 407
    anemia, 399–400
    calcitriol-induced FGF23 synthesis,
        199–200

and CaR, in SHPT, 155–158
CKD
  calcium concentration, 99–100
  CaSR expression, 100
  complex inter-relationships, 101
  1,25(OH)$_2$D$_3$ resistance, 95–96
  genomic calcitriol, abnormalities in,
    54–56
  1α-hydroxylase, 101
  klotho-FGFR1 complex, 100
  lower density and binding capacity,
    98–99
  non-genomic calcitriol, abnormalities
    in, 57
  PTH suppression and parathyroid
    hyperplasia, 58–61
  renal failure, 96
  secondary hyperparathyroidism in, 82
  selective VDR activators, 101–105
  uremic toxins, effect of, 96–98
1,25(OH)$_2$D, 12–13
1,25(OH)$_2$D$_3$
  adaptive immune system, control of, 79
  antiproliferative effects, 78
  bone remodeling, impacts on, 77
  calcium and phosphate homeostasis, 77
  cathelicidin expression, regulator of, 79
  cellular proliferation, regulator of, 78
  CYP24A1, 77–78
  DNA repair enzymes, 78
  fatty acid β-oxidation, 79
  FGF23, 78
  gene expression, control of, 77
  hair growth, regulators of, 79
  health and longevity, benefits in, 78
  innate immune system, 79
  insulin resistance, 79
  klotho, up-regulation of, 78
  lipid and amino acid metabolism, role
    in, 79
  local generation of, 79, 81
  megalin, 77
  in mineralization, 77
  osteoblast apoptosis, prevention of, 77
  osteoblastogenesis, 77
  osteoid matrix, formation of, 77
  parathyroid function, inhibition of,
    152–154
  premature aging, prevention of, 78
  renin-angiotensin system,
    inhibition of, 79
  RXR heterodimerization, 83–84, 89

secondary bile acids, 79
specific and high-affinity binding, 81
TACE inhibition, 79
TGF-α-ADAM17-EGFR pathway,
  79–80
therapeutic roles, 78–79
vascular calcification, inhibition of, 77
Wnt/β-catenin signaling pathway, 80
xenobiotic detoxification, 79
degradation and transcriptional
  regulation, 53
discovery of, 151
DNA-binding domain, 82–84
functional domains, 151
gene expression, regulation of, 81
gene transcription, inhibition of, 151–152
heart structure and function
  aggravated fibrosis, 324
  and cardiovascular risk factors, 325
  interstitial fibrosis, 324
  myocardium, 323
  vessels, 324–325
high-volume and fracture-resistant bone,
  formation of, 77
ligand-binding domain, 82–86
mutations in, 80
nutritional lipids, 81
polymorphisms, 82
PXR, 76
in target tissues and cell lines, 81
unliganded function, 81
and vitamin D response elements
  chromatin unit, structure of, 86–87
  corepressors, 85, 88, 94–95
  CYP27B1 gene, down-regulation of,
    87–88
  gene repression, 87
  remote and multiple VDREs, 86–87
  retinoid X receptor and coregulators,
    85, 88–94
Vitamin D receptor activators (VDRAs), 362
  alfacalcidol
    comparison studies of, 519–520
    doxercalciferol, 520–522
    kidney transplant recipients, 518–519
    non-dialysis CKD, 517–518
  ESRD, 516
  paricalcitol
    albuminuria reduction, 523–525
    cardiac structure and function, 525–527
    SHPT treatment, 529–532
  vitamin D sterols, 516

Vitamin D responsive elements (VDREs), 12
   parathyroid CaR expression, 150
   vitamin D receptor
      chromatin unit, structure of, 86–87
      corepressors, 85, 88, 94–95
      CYP27B1 gene, down-regulation of,
         87–88
      gene repression, 87
      heterodimerization, 83–84, 89
      remote and multiple VDREs, 86–87

   renal failure, 96
   retinoid X receptor and coregulators,
      85, 88–94
   uremic toxins, RXR, 97–98
Vitamin K antagonist (VKA), 385

W
Walker carcinoma tumor, 171

Printed by Printforce, the Netherlands